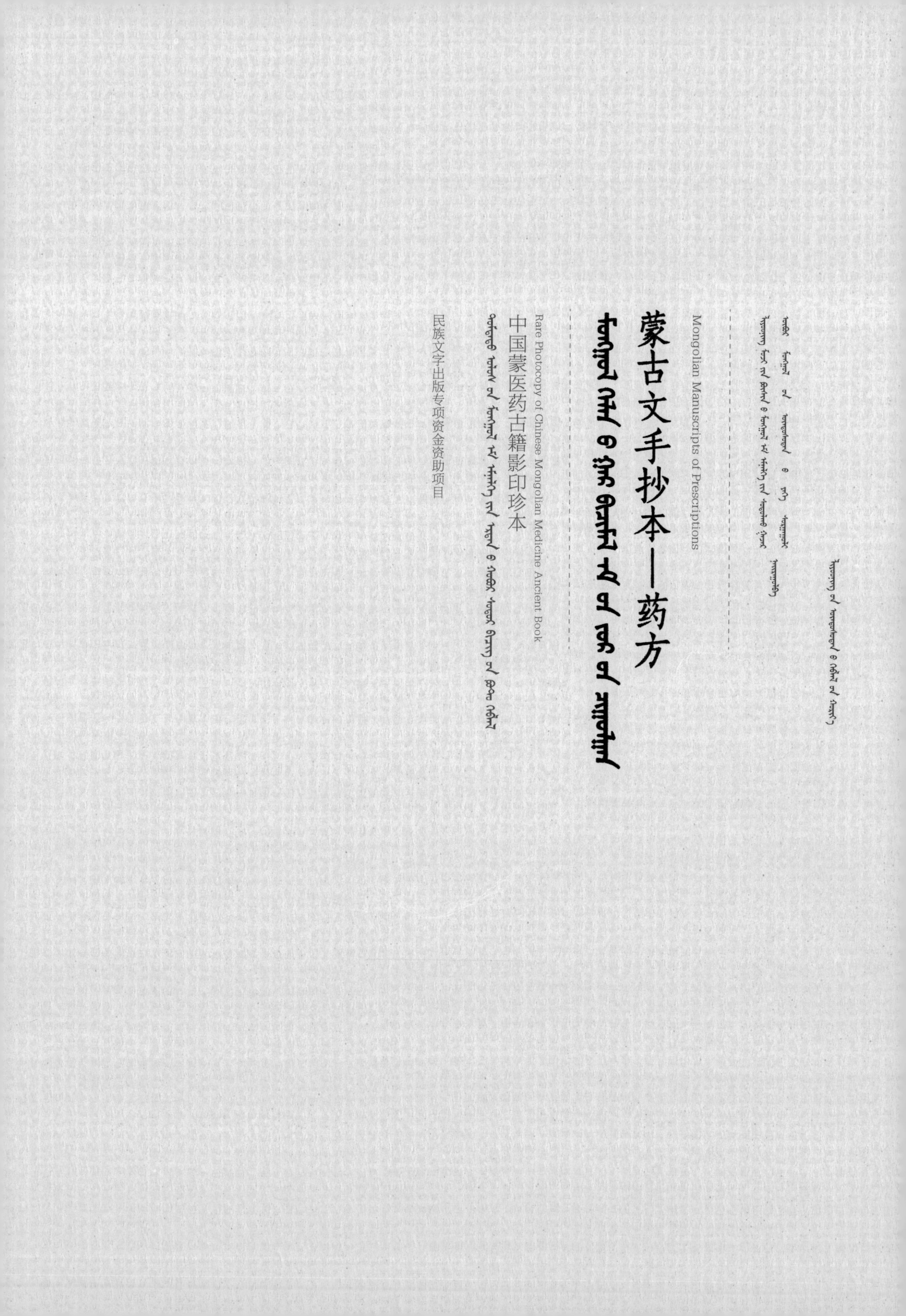

蒙古文手抄本——药方

Mongolian Manuscripts of Prescriptions

中国蒙医药古籍影印珍本

Rare Photocopy of Chinese Mongolian Medicine Ancient Book

民族文字出版专项资金资助项目

图书在版编目（CIP）数据

蒙古文手抄本—药方：蒙古文 / 辽宁省阜新蒙医药研究所，内蒙古民族大学编．—沈阳：辽宁民族出版社，2018.7

（中国蒙医药古籍影印珍本）

ISBN 978-7-5497-1859-7

Ⅰ．①蒙… Ⅱ．①辽… ②内… Ⅲ．①蒙医—药方—汇编—蒙古语（中国少数民族语言） Ⅳ．①R291.2

中国版本图书馆CIP数据核字（2018）第166855号

蒙古文手抄本—药方

MENGGUWENSHOUCHAOBEN-YAOFANG

出版发行者：辽宁民族出版社

地　　址：沈阳市和平区十一纬路25号　邮编：110003

印 刷 者：辽宁奥美雅印刷有限公司

幅面尺寸：210mm×285mm

印　　张：37

字　　数：720千字

印　　数：1-400

出版时间：2018年7月第1版

印刷时间：2018年7月第1次印刷

责任编辑：白兰英

封面设计：杜　江

责任印制：杨　雪

责任校对：代智敏

标准书号：ISBN 978-7-5497-1859-7

定　　价：480.00元

网　　址：www.lnmzcbs.com　　邮购热线：024-23284335

淘宝网店：http://lnmz2013.taobao.com

如有印装质量问题，请与出版社联系调换　联系电话：024-23284340

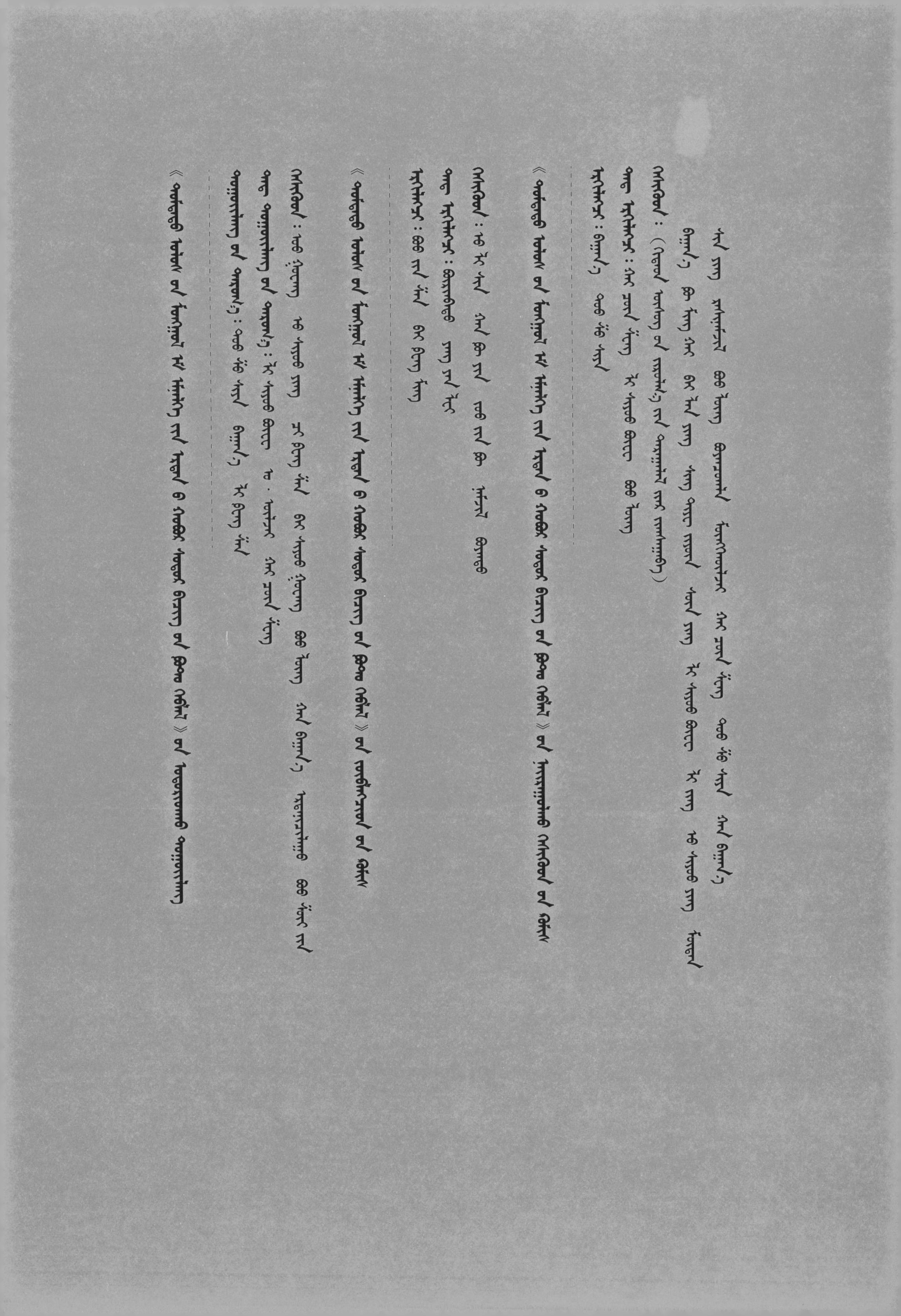

《中国蒙医药古籍影印珍本》领导小组

《中国蒙医药古籍影印珍本》顾问委员会

《中国蒙医药古籍影印珍本》编辑委员会

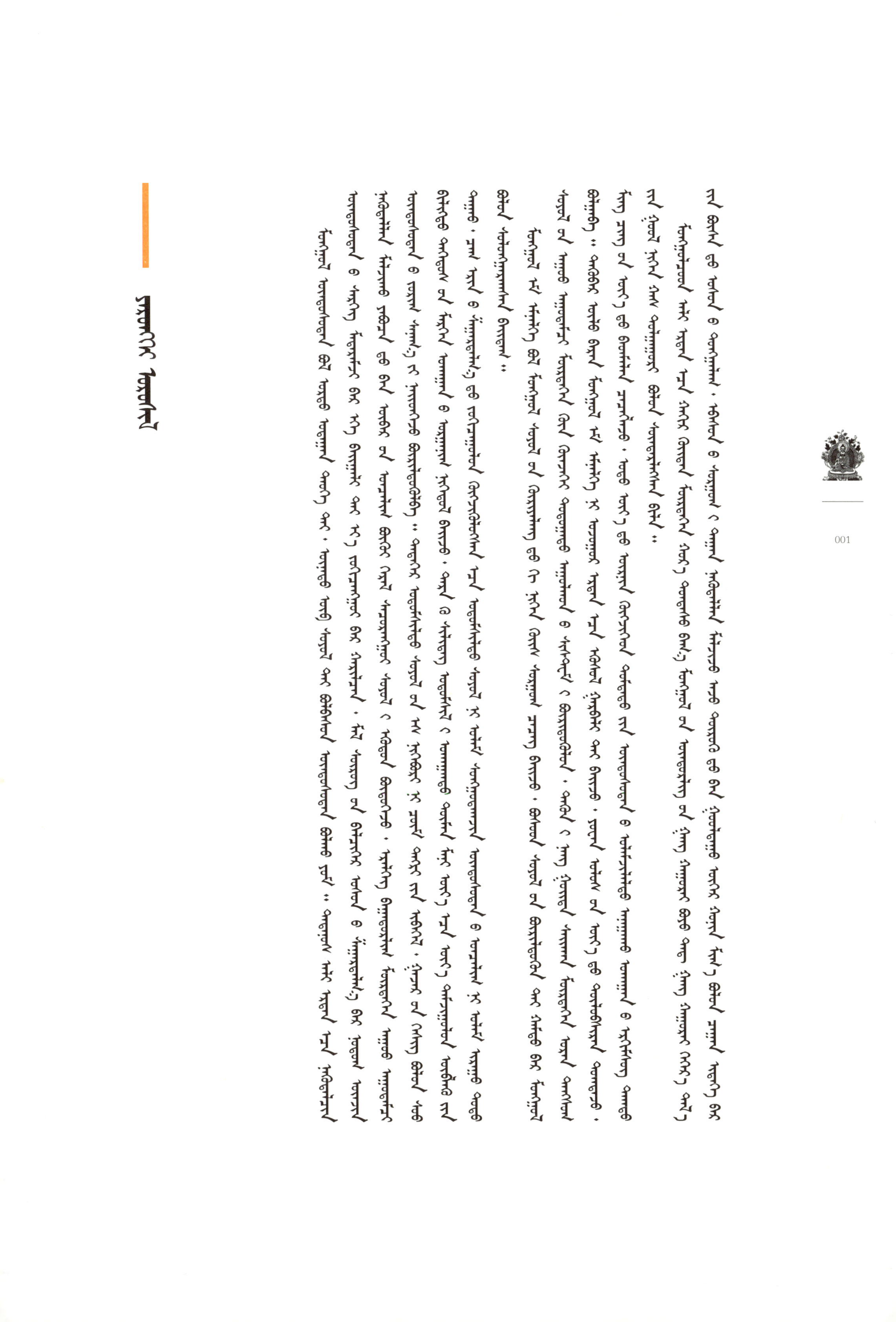

ᠮᠠᠨ ᠤ 16 ᠳᠤᠭᠠᠷ ᠵᠠᠭᠤᠨ ᠡᠴᠡ ᠡᠬᠢᠯᠡᠨ ᠮᠣᠩᠭᠣᠯ ᠤᠨ ᠪᠢᠴᠢᠭ ᠦᠨ ᠬᠡᠪᠯᠡᠯ ᠦᠨ ᠦᠢᠯᠡᠳᠪᠦᠷᠢ ᠪᠣᠢ ᠪᠣᠯᠤᠭᠰᠠᠨ ᠪᠠᠢᠨ᠎ᠠ ᠃ ᠃ ᠪᠢᠳᠡ ᠪᠠᠢᠭ᠎ᠠ ᠮᠣᠩᠭᠣᠯ ᠤᠨ ᠡᠷᠲᠡᠨ ᠦ ᠨᠣᠮ ᠤᠨ ᠰᠤᠷᠭᠠᠭᠤᠯᠢ ᠳᠤ ᠰᠤᠷᠭᠠᠭᠰᠠᠨ ᠪᠢᠴᠢᠭ ᠦᠨ ᠰᠤᠷᠭᠠᠭᠤᠯᠢ ᠶᠢᠨ ᠪᠣᠯᠪᠠᠰᠤᠷᠠᠯ ᠢ ᠬᠥᠭᠵᠢᠭᠦᠯᠦᠨ ᠲᠡᠯᠭᠡᠷᠡᠭᠦᠯᠦᠭᠰᠡᠨ ᠃ ᠃ ᠬᠡᠪᠯᠡᠯ ᠦᠨ ᠪᠦᠲᠦᠭᠡᠯ ᠤᠨ ᠪᠠᠷᠢᠮᠲᠠ ᠶᠢᠨ ᠬᠣᠶᠠᠷ ᠳᠤᠭᠠᠷ ᠪᠠᠢᠳᠠᠯ ᠪᠣᠯᠪᠠᠰᠤ ᠪᠠᠢᠨ᠎ᠠ ᠃ ᠃ ᠬᠢᠳ ᠦᠨ ᠪᠢᠴᠢᠭ ᠦᠨ ᠪᠦᠲᠦᠭᠡᠯ ᠢ ᠮᠣᠩᠭᠣᠯ ᠤᠨ ᠣᠷᠣᠨ ᠳᠤ ᠰᠢᠨ᠎ᠡ ᠪᠢᠴᠢᠭ ᠦᠨ ᠰᠤᠷᠭᠠᠭᠤᠯᠢ ᠶᠢᠨ 《 ᠬᠡᠪᠯᠡᠯ ᠦᠨ ᠬᠡᠷᠡᠭ ᠦᠨ ᠲᠠᠯ᠎ᠠ ᠪᠢᠴᠢᠭ 》 ᠬᠡᠮᠡᠬᠦ ᠮᠣᠩᠭᠣᠯ ᠪᠢᠴᠢᠭ ᠦᠨ ᠰᠤᠷᠬᠠᠢ ᠪᠢᠴᠢᠭ ᠦᠨ ᠬᠡᠪᠯᠡᠯ ᠦᠨ ᠦᠢᠯᠡᠳᠪᠦᠷᠢ ᠶᠢᠨ ᠮᠣᠩᠭᠣᠯ ᠪᠢᠴᠢᠭ ᠦᠨ ᠲᠦᠷᠦᠯ ᠢ ᠪᠠᠢᠭᠤᠯᠤᠭᠰᠠᠨ ᠲᠣᠭ᠎ᠠ ᠶᠢᠨ ᠪᠦᠲᠦᠭᠡᠯ ᠦᠳ ᠢ ᠪᠠᠢᠭᠤᠯᠤᠭᠰᠠᠨ ᠪᠠᠢᠨ᠎ᠠ ᠃ ᠃ ᠬᠣᠶᠠᠷ ᠳᠤᠭᠠᠷ ᠳᠤ ᠂ ᠪᠢᠴᠢᠭ ᠦᠨ ᠪᠠᠢᠯᠭ᠎ᠠ ᠶᠢᠨ ᠬᠡᠪᠯᠡᠯ ᠦᠨ ᠬᠡᠷᠡᠭ ᠂ ᠬᠡᠪᠯᠡᠯ ᠦᠨ ᠬᠡᠷᠡᠭ ᠂ ᠮᠣᠩᠭᠣᠯ ᠬᠡᠪᠯᠡᠯ ᠦᠨ ᠬᠡᠷᠡᠭ ᠲᠦ ᠰᠢᠨᠡᠳᠬᠡᠯ ᠮᠣᠩᠭᠣᠯ ᠬᠡᠯᠡ ᠶᠢ ᠬᠡᠪᠯᠡᠯ ᠦᠨ 《 ᠮᠣᠩᠭᠣᠯ ᠪᠢᠴᠢᠭ ᠦᠨ ᠪᠦᠲᠦᠭᠡᠯ ᠦᠨ ᠰᠣᠨᠢᠨ ᠪᠢᠴᠢᠭ 》 ᠬᠢᠭᠡᠳ 《 ᠰᠢᠨᠡ ᠮᠣᠩᠭᠣᠯ ᠪᠢᠴᠢᠭ 》 ᠵᠡᠷᠭᠡ ᠪᠦᠲᠦᠭᠡᠯ ᠦᠳ ᠦᠨ ᠬᠡᠪᠯᠡᠯ ᠦᠨ ᠪᠠᠢᠭᠤᠯᠤᠯᠲᠠ ᠶᠢ ᠰᠢᠨᠡᠳᠬᠡᠯ ᠦᠨ ᠬᠡᠷᠡᠭ ᠲᠦ ᠣᠷᠣᠭᠤᠯᠤᠭᠰᠠᠨ ᠪᠠᠢᠨ᠎ᠠ ᠂ ᠮᠣᠩᠭᠣᠯ ᠪᠢᠴᠢᠭ ᠦᠨ ᠬᠡᠪᠯᠡᠯ ᠦᠨ ᠬᠥᠭᠵᠢᠯ ᠂ ᠬᠥᠭᠵᠢᠯ ᠦᠨ ᠪᠠᠢᠳᠠᠯ ᠢ ᠬᠠᠷᠢᠴᠠᠭᠤᠯᠪᠠᠯ ᠬᠡᠪᠯᠡᠯ ᠦᠨ ᠦᠢᠯᠡᠳᠪᠦᠷᠢ ᠶᠢᠨ ᠦᠢᠯᠡ ᠬᠡᠷᠡᠭ ᠲᠦ ᠶᠡᠬᠡ ᠬᠥᠭᠵᠢᠯ ᠭᠠᠷᠭᠠᠭᠰᠠᠨ ᠪᠠᠢᠨ᠎ᠠ ᠃ ᠃ ᠬᠡᠪᠯᠡᠯ ᠦᠨ ᠬᠡᠷᠡᠭ ᠲᠦ ᠮᠣᠩᠭᠣᠯ ᠪᠢᠴᠢᠭ ᠦᠨ ᠬᠡᠪᠯᠡᠯ ᠦᠨ ᠲᠤᠰᠬᠠᠢ ᠪᠦᠲᠦᠭᠡᠯ ᠦᠳ ᠢ ᠬᠡᠪᠯᠡᠨ ᠭᠠᠷᠭᠠᠭᠰᠠᠨ ᠪᠠᠢᠨ᠎ᠠ ᠃ ᠃

ᠰᠣᠨᠢᠨ ᠬᠡᠪᠯᠡᠯ ᠦᠨ ᠬᠡᠷᠡᠭ ᠲᠦ ᠮᠣᠩᠭᠣᠯ ᠪᠢᠴᠢᠭ ᠦᠨ ᠬᠡᠪᠯᠡᠯ ᠦᠨ ᠬᠡᠷᠡᠭᠯᠡᠭᠡᠨ ᠦ ᠪᠠᠢᠳᠠᠯ ᠢ ᠬᠠᠷᠢᠴᠠᠭᠤᠯᠪᠠᠯ ᠂ ᠮᠣᠩᠭᠣᠯ ᠪᠢᠴᠢᠭ ᠦᠨ ᠬᠡᠪᠯᠡᠯ ᠦᠨ ᠪᠦᠲᠦᠭᠡᠯ ᠦᠳ ᠦᠨ ᠲᠣᠭ᠎ᠠ ᠨᠢ ᠤᠯᠠᠮ ᠨᠡᠮᠡᠭ᠍ᠳᠡᠵᠦ ᠂ ᠬᠡᠪᠯᠡᠯ ᠦᠨ ᠠᠷᠭ᠎ᠠ ᠪᠠᠷ ᠪᠦᠲᠦᠭᠡᠭᠰᠡᠨ ᠪᠢᠴᠢᠭ ᠦᠨ ᠬᠡᠪᠯᠡᠯ ᠦᠨ ᠲᠥᠷᠦᠯ ᠵᠦᠢᠯ ᠂ ᠬᠡᠪᠯᠡᠯ ᠦᠨ ᠴᠢᠨᠠᠷ ᠂ ᠬᠡᠪᠯᠡᠯ ᠦᠨ ᠠᠷᠭ᠎ᠠ ᠂ ᠬᠡᠪᠯᠡᠯ ᠦᠨ ᠬᠡᠷᠡᠭᠰᠡᠯ ᠵᠡᠷᠭᠡ ᠪᠦᠬᠦ ᠲᠠᠯ᠎ᠠ ᠪᠠᠷ ᠬᠥᠭᠵᠢᠭᠰᠡᠨ ᠪᠠᠢᠨ᠎ᠠ ᠃ ᠃

ᠮᠣᠩᠭᠣᠯ ᠪᠢᠴᠢᠭ ᠦᠨ ᠬᠡᠪᠯᠡᠯ ᠦᠨ ᠦᠢᠯᠡᠳᠪᠦᠷᠢ ᠨᠢ ᠡᠷᠲᠡ ᠡᠴᠡ ᠡᠬᠢᠯᠡᠨ ᠮᠣᠩᠭᠣᠯ ᠦᠨᠳᠦᠰᠦᠲᠡᠨ ᠦ ᠰᠣᠶᠣᠯ ᠤᠨ ᠬᠥᠭᠵᠢᠯ ᠳᠦ ᠴᠢᠬᠤᠯᠠ ᠨᠥᠯᠦᠭᠡ ᠦᠵᠡᠭᠦᠯᠦᠭᠰᠡᠨ ᠪᠦᠭᠡᠳ ᠂ ᠮᠣᠩᠭᠣᠯ ᠪᠢᠴᠢᠭ ᠦᠨ ᠬᠡᠪᠯᠡᠯ ᠦᠨ ᠲᠡᠦᠬᠡ ᠶᠢ ᠰᠤᠳᠤᠯᠬᠤ ᠨᠢ ᠮᠣᠩᠭᠣᠯ ᠰᠣᠶᠣᠯ ᠤᠨ ᠲᠡᠦᠬᠡ ᠶᠢ ᠰᠤᠳᠤᠯᠬᠤ ᠳᠤ ᠴᠢᠬᠤᠯᠠ ᠠᠴᠠ ᠬᠤᠯᠢᠭ ᠢ ᠦᠵᠡᠭᠦᠯᠬᠦ ᠪᠣᠯᠤᠨ᠎ᠠ ᠃ ᠃

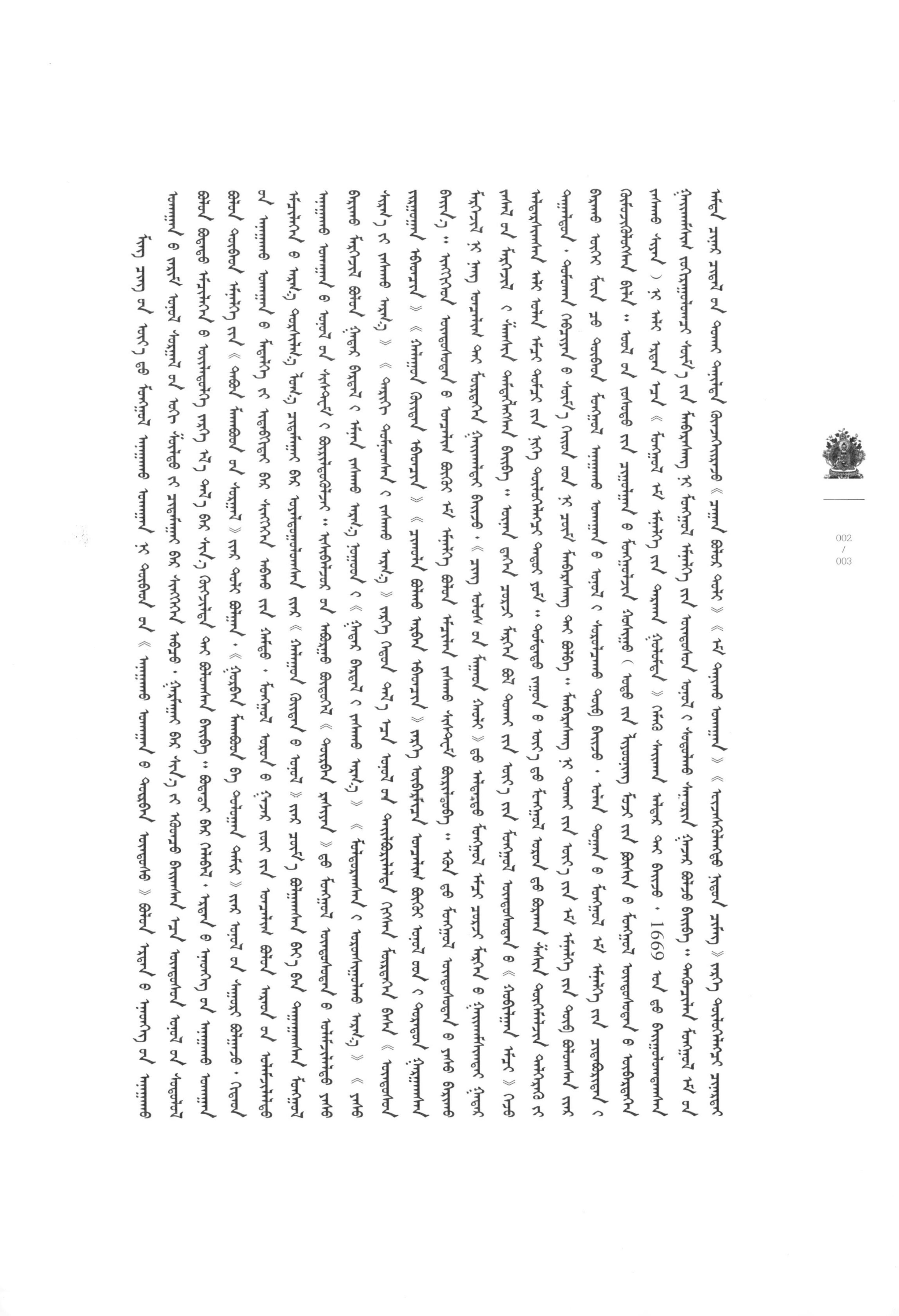

[illegible] 1669 [illegible]

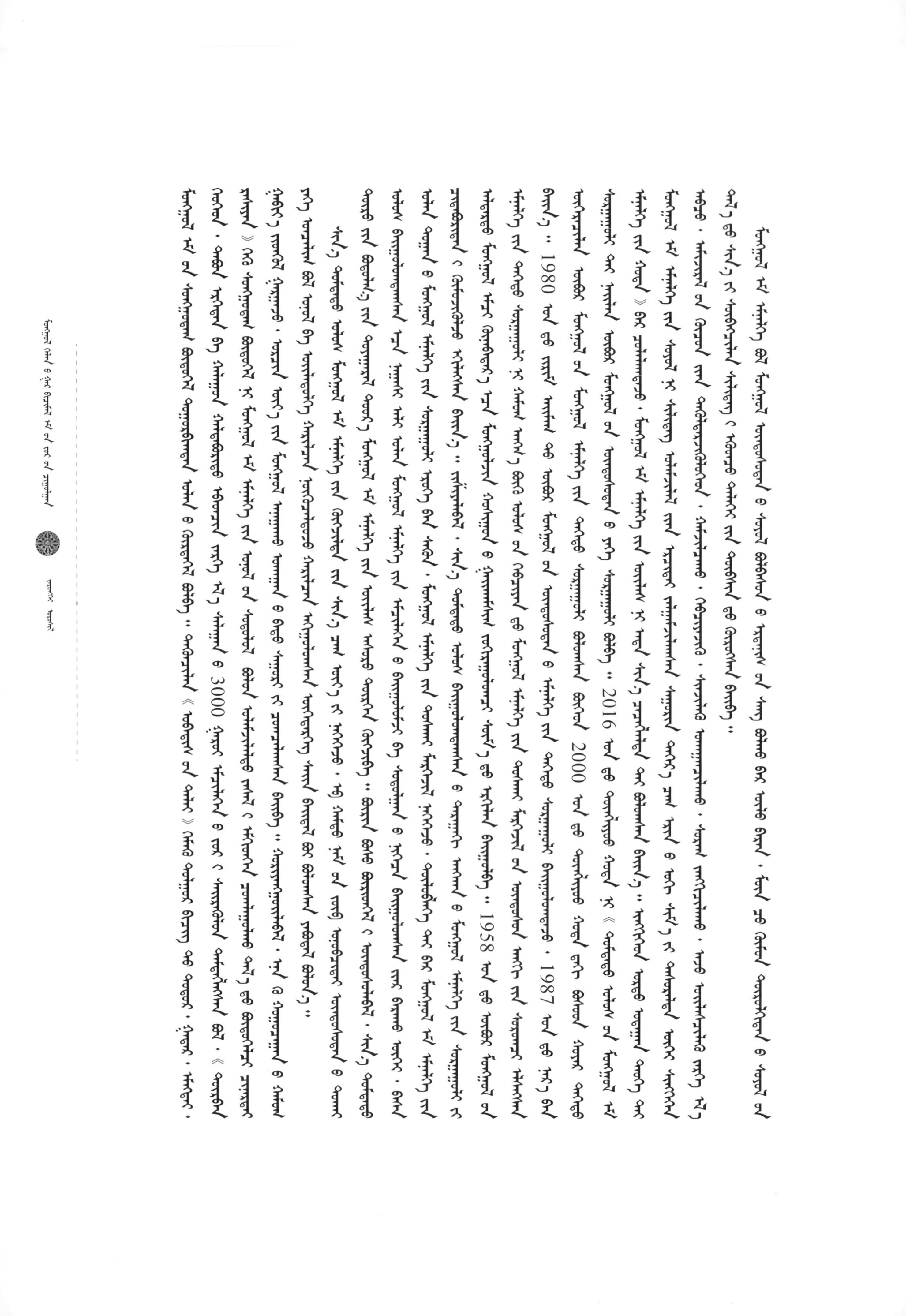

… 2016 … 2000 … 1980 … 1987 … 1958 … 3000 …

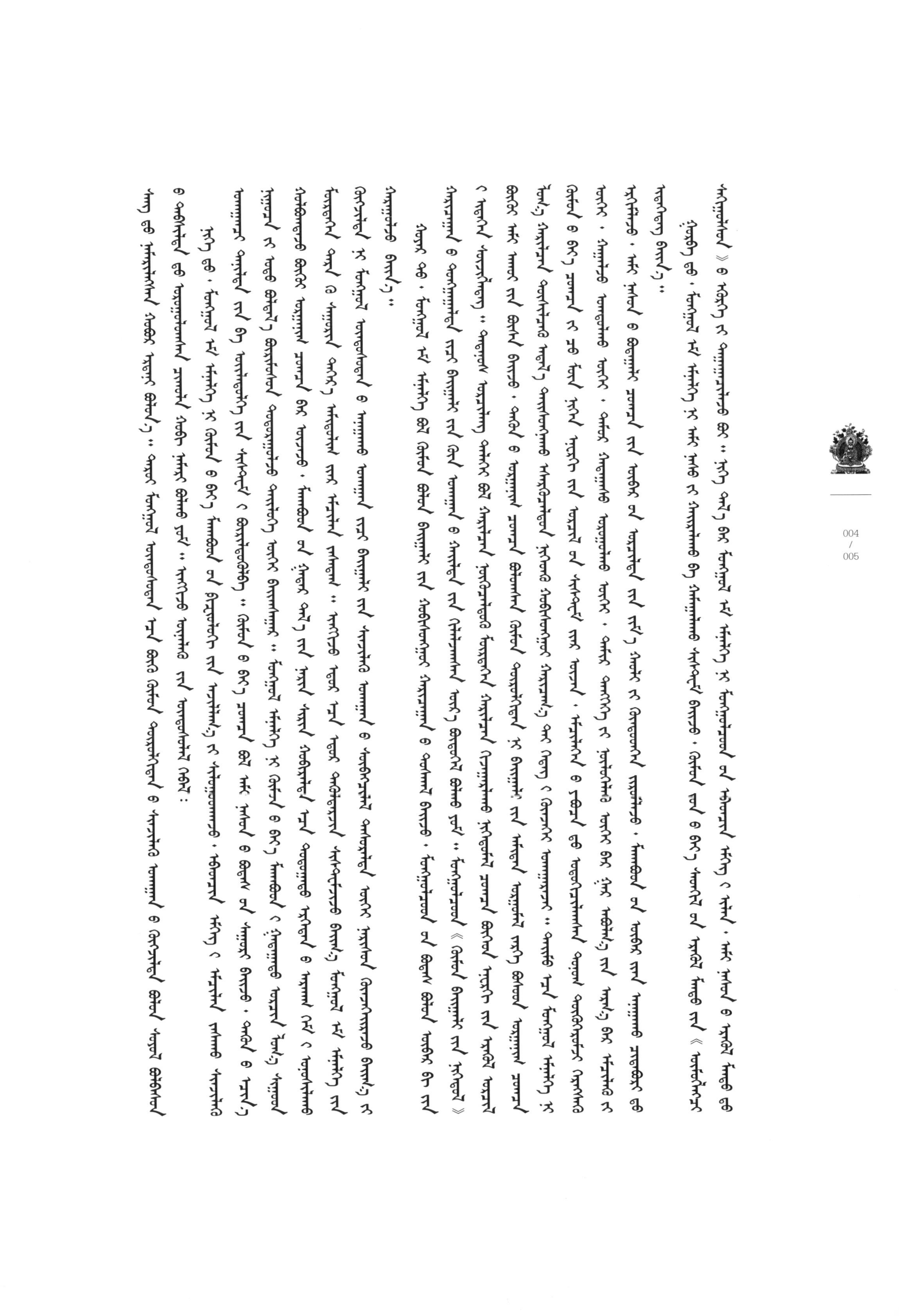

ᠬᠦᠮᠦᠨ ᠢ ᠬᠥᠮᠦᠵᠢᠭᠦᠯᠬᠦ ᠶᠢᠨ ᠰᠤᠷᠭᠠᠯ᠂ ᠮᠣᠩᠭᠣᠯ ᠬᠡᠯᠡ ᠪᠢᠴᠢᠭ ᠦᠨ ᠰᠤᠷᠭᠠᠯᠲᠠ ᠶᠢᠨ ᠰᠤᠳᠤᠯᠭᠠ ᠶᠢ ᠪᠣᠯᠪᠠᠰᠤᠷᠠᠭᠤᠯᠬᠤ ᠳᠤ ᠴᠢᠬᠤᠯᠠ ᠠᠴᠢ ᠬᠣᠯᠪᠣᠭᠳᠠᠯ ᠲᠠᠢ ᠪᠣᠯᠤᠨ᠎ᠠ ᠃ ᠮᠣᠩᠭᠣᠯ ᠬᠡᠯᠡ ᠪᠢᠴᠢᠭ ᠦᠨ ᠰᠤᠷᠭᠠᠯᠲᠠ ᠶᠢᠨ ᠰᠤᠳᠤᠯᠭᠠ ᠶᠢ ᠬᠥᠭᠵᠢᠭᠦᠯᠬᠦ ᠳᠤ ᠴᠢᠬᠤᠯᠠ ᠠᠴᠢ ᠬᠣᠯᠪᠣᠭᠳᠠᠯ ᠲᠠᠢ ᠪᠣᠯᠤᠨ᠎ᠠ ᠃

ᠮᠣᠩᠭᠣᠯ ᠬᠡᠯᠡ ᠪᠢᠴᠢᠭ ᠦᠨ ᠰᠤᠷᠭᠠᠯᠲᠠ ᠶᠢᠨ ᠰᠤᠳᠤᠯᠭᠠ ᠶᠢᠨ ᠣᠨᠣᠯ ᠤᠨ ᠰᠠᠭᠤᠷᠢ ᠪᠣᠯᠤᠨ᠎ᠠ ᠃

ᠮᠣᠩᠭᠣᠯ ᠬᠡᠯᠡ ᠪᠢᠴᠢᠭ ᠦᠨ ᠰᠤᠷᠭᠠᠯᠲᠠ ᠶᠢᠨ ᠰᠤᠳᠤᠯᠭᠠ 《ᠮᠣᠩᠭᠣᠯ ᠬᠡᠯᠡ ᠪᠢᠴᠢᠭ》 《ᠮᠣᠩᠭᠣᠯ ᠬᠡᠯᠡ ᠵᠦᠢ》 (ᠨᠢᠭᠡ) ᠂ 《 ᠮᠣᠩᠭᠣᠯ ᠬᠡᠯᠡ ᠵᠦᠢ 》 (ᠬᠣᠶᠠᠷ) ᠂ 《 ᠮᠣᠩᠭᠣᠯ ᠬᠡᠯᠡ ᠵᠦᠢ Ⅱ 》 《 ᠮᠣᠩᠭᠣᠯ ᠬᠡᠯᠡ ᠵᠦᠢ — 》 ᠵᠡᠷᠭᠡ ᠰᠤᠷᠭᠠᠯᠲᠠ ᠶᠢᠨ ᠪᠢᠴᠢᠭ ᠦᠳ ᠢ ᠰᠤᠳᠤᠯᠤᠨ᠎ᠠ ᠃

ᠮᠣᠩᠭᠣᠯ ᠬᠡᠯᠡ ᠪᠢᠴᠢᠭ ᠦᠨ ᠰᠤᠷᠭᠠᠯᠲᠠ ᠶᠢᠨ ᠰᠤᠳᠤᠯᠭᠠ ᠶᠢᠨ ᠠᠷᠭ᠎ᠠ ᠪᠠᠷᠢᠯ ᠢ ᠰᠤᠳᠤᠯᠵᠤ ᠂ ᠮᠣᠩᠭᠣᠯ ᠬᠡᠯᠡ ᠪᠢᠴᠢᠭ ᠦᠨ ᠰᠤᠷᠭᠠᠯᠲᠠ ᠶᠢᠨ ᠣᠨᠣᠯ ᠢ ᠪᠠᠶᠠᠵᠢᠭᠤᠯᠬᠤ ᠳᠤ ᠴᠢᠬᠤᠯᠠ ᠠᠴᠢ ᠬᠣᠯᠪᠣᠭᠳᠠᠯ ᠲᠠᠢ ᠪᠣᠯᠤᠨ᠎ᠠ ᠃

ᠮᠣᠩᠭᠣᠯ ᠬᠡᠯᠡ ᠪᠢᠴᠢᠭ ᠦᠨ ᠰᠤᠷᠭᠠᠯᠲᠠ ᠶᠢᠨ ᠰᠤᠳᠤᠯᠭᠠ ᠶᠢᠨ ᠠᠷᠭ᠎ᠠ ᠪᠠᠷᠢᠯ ᠪᠣᠯᠤᠨ 《ᠮᠣᠩᠭᠣᠯ ᠬᠡᠯᠡ ᠪᠢᠴᠢᠭ ᠦᠨ ᠰᠤᠷᠭᠠᠯᠲᠠ ᠶᠢᠨ ᠰᠤᠳᠤᠯᠭᠠ》 ᠪᠣᠯᠤᠨ᠎ᠠ ᠃

ᠰᠤᠷᠭᠠᠭᠤᠯᠢ ᠶᠢᠨ ᠰᠤᠷᠭᠠᠯᠲᠠ ᠶᠢᠨ ᠠᠵᠢᠯ ᠳᠤ ᠮᠣᠩᠭᠣᠯ ᠬᠡᠯᠡ ᠪᠢᠴᠢᠭ ᠦᠨ ᠰᠤᠷᠭᠠᠯᠲᠠ ᠶᠢᠨ ᠣᠨᠣᠯ ᠢ ᠬᠡᠷᠡᠭᠯᠡᠵᠦ ᠪᠠᠶᠢᠨ᠎ᠠ ᠃ ᠲᠡᠭᠦᠨ ᠡᠴᠡ ᠭᠠᠳᠠᠨ᠎ᠠ ᠮᠣᠩᠭᠣᠯ ᠬᠡᠯᠡ ᠪᠢᠴᠢᠭ ᠦᠨ ᠰᠤᠷᠭᠠᠯᠲᠠ ᠶᠢᠨ

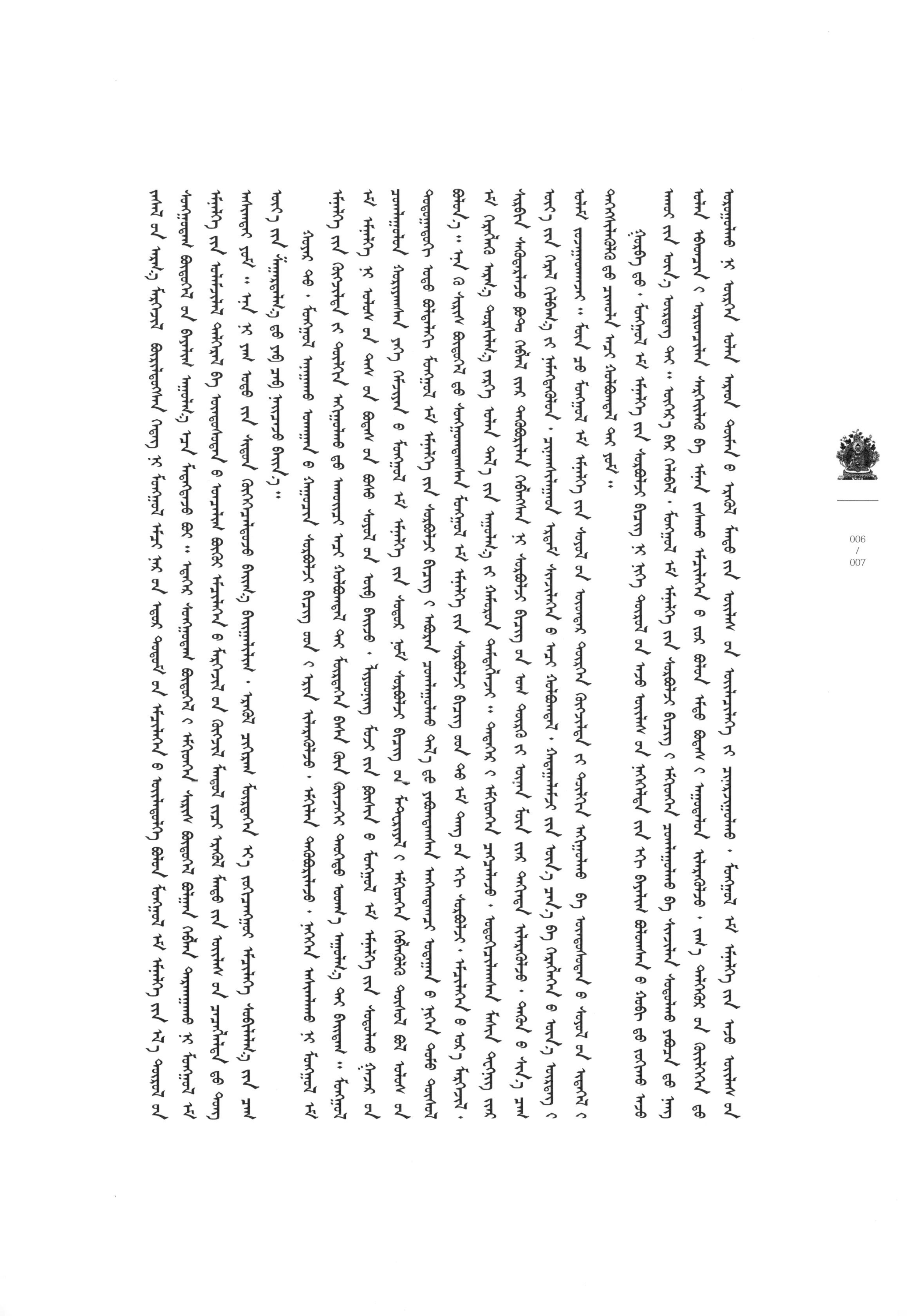

[illegible]

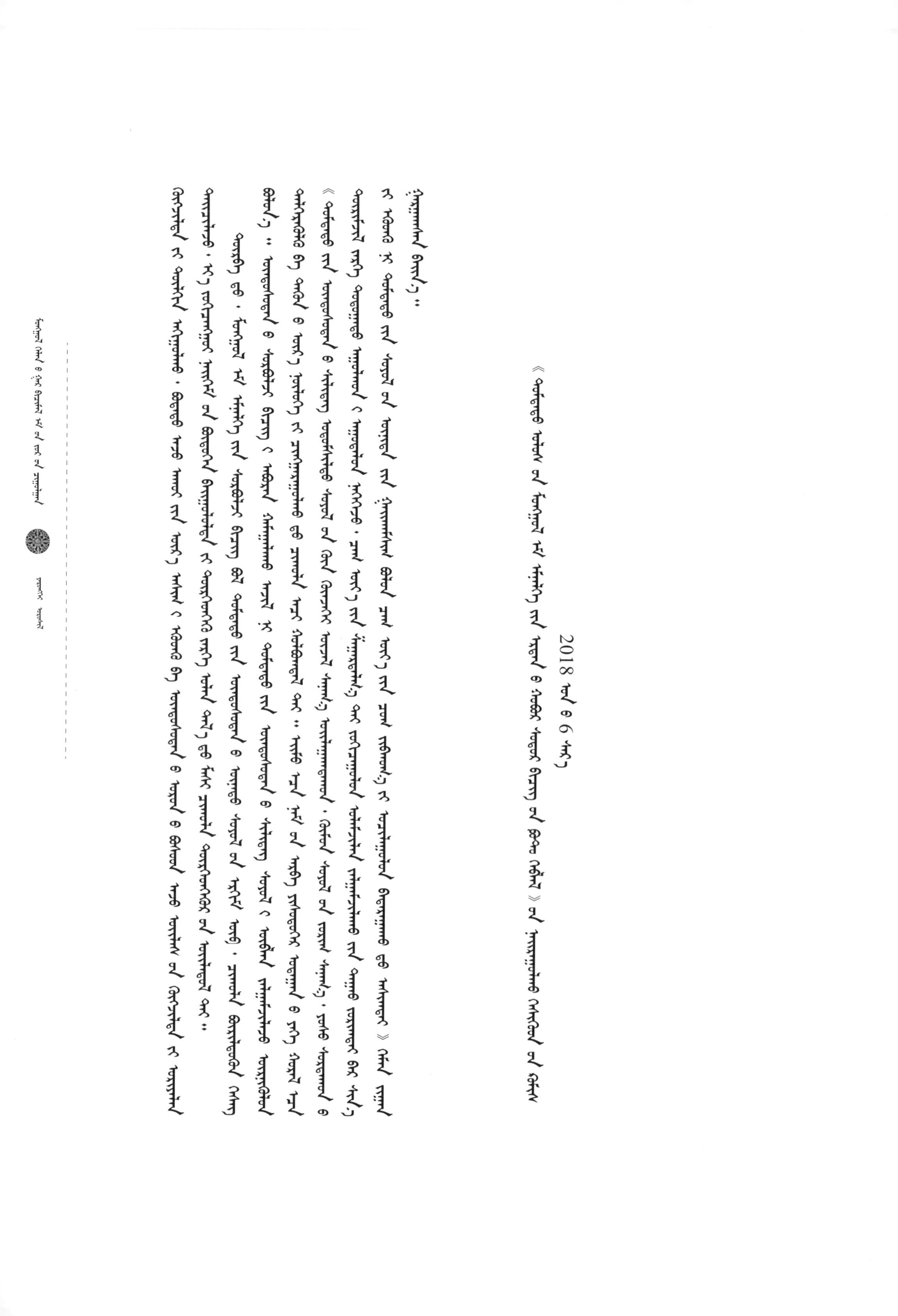

[illegible]

[illegible]

2018 ᠣᠨ ᠤ 6 ᠰᠠᠷ᠎ᠠ

[illegible]

总序

蒙古族是一个历史悠久而又富于传奇色彩的民族。蒙古民族在漫长的历史进程中，形成了博大精深、绚丽多彩的民族文化样态，在居住、饮食、服饰、语言、文字、歌舞、艺术、医药、卫生等多个方面，积累下了丰富的成果，形成了自己的传统。这些传统文化的每一部分，都是凝结天地精气、承传祖先遗训的美丽造物，更是不断吐故纳新、汇聚历史风云的精华结晶。

蒙医药是蒙古民族文化百花园中的绚丽的一枝，它与蒙古族文化的其他部分一起构成了蒙古族文化博大精深的内涵体系，共同把蒙古族文化的百花园装扮得分外美丽。蒙医药源于上古，成于元代，兴于明清，盛于当代，是中华民族传统医学中的瑰宝，在中国杏林中独树一帜。

蒙古族自古以游牧为生，生活在寒冷又干旱、半干旱的草原，主要以牛羊肉和乳制品为食，平日里的骑马放牧、转场迁徙和战时纵马驰骋，极易造成摔伤、骨折、战伤等外伤。这样的气候条件、地理条件、饮食条件和生活情形，促使蒙古族的先民不断体察与大自然中动物、植物的关系，对动植物的营养、毒性等性能和防病治疗等作用，形成了初步的认识和掌握；把在长期狩猎、游牧、农耕生产和迁徙、征战中积累起来的与疾病伤害做斗争的感受和经验，加以分析和总结，从而发明了极具地域特点和民族特色的诊治技术，如灸疗术、整骨术、震脑术以及策格（酸马奶）疗法等。这是蒙医药学的萌芽和雏形阶段。

到了元代，蒙医药学获得了长足发展。这一方面是由于中原内地医学与蒙医药的相互滋养和促进，另一方面，元代蒙医药学获得体制性政策保障，在承袭唐宋时期医疗制度的基础上，国都设立太医院，各地设立惠民局，大力扶持和推广蒙医蒙药，从而为蒙医药的全方位发展提供了良好条件。在原有基础上，骨伤科等蒙古族传统医疗技术获得了新的发展和提高。与此同时，通过博采众长，集思广纳，深入研究，蒙古族先民早已归纳出来的“疾病的本质为寒、热两种”的认识，即“寒热学说”，以及人体解剖知识、药物知识、急救知识和传染病预防知识等传统蒙医药的理论认识得到了进一步丰富和充实。元太医忽思慧撰写的《饮膳正要》是记录蒙医学饮食疗法内容的第一部典籍。这些都为16世纪后蒙医蒙药走向成熟奠定了坚实基础。

明清时期，随着藏医学的《四部医典》和古代印度医学的部分理论陆续传入蒙古地区，蒙医药学得以合理吸收藏医学和印度医学的精华，基础理论研究和临床治疗实践都上升到了新的高度。蒙古族的先民以藏医学及古代印度医学的“五元学说”为借鉴和出发点，以“三根和七素”作为理论基础，兼而吸收中医药知识，并结合蒙古地区的特点和民间疗法，创建了以传统的“寒热学说”为核心主导的独立的蒙医学理论体系。伊喜巴拉珠尔在他的《甘露四部》中，把传统的蒙古骨伤整治术和创伤医疗术，从“创伤医疗术”“脱臼复位术”“骨伤疗法”“震脑疗法”等几个具体的角度，进行了详细的理论阐述和操作说明，内容甚为丰满，提出了“六基症”“寒症”“十大要症”等独特理论。与此同时，在临床治疗经验日渐丰富的基础上，形成了具有民族特点的独特的医疗诊治体系。蒙古族的骨伤整治技术更是独到而神奇，著名蒙医绰尔济莫尔根以其精湛的外科诊治技术享誉漠南，被载入《清史稿》。而他仅仅是众多蒙古族“神医”中的典型代表而已。随着黄教在蒙古的兴盛，规模较大的寺庙都设有曼巴扎仓，这不仅是当地的医疗中心，也是学习和研究藏医、蒙医理论的基地，培养了大批蒙医蒙药人才。地处东部的蒙古勒津（今辽宁阜新），素有“蒙医药发祥地”之称，早在1669年瑞应寺兴建之初，寺内就设有曼巴扎仓。蒙医药理论研究方兴未艾，对蒙药的性味功能也有了更深刻的认识，《认药白晶鉴》《识药学》《蒙药正典》三大蒙药学代表性著作应运而生。《秘诀方海》收载有内、外、妇、儿、五官及热病、传染病等临床各科的3000余种药方，尤其是《甘露四部》在蒙医药学的基础理论探究和传统疗法的整理方面做出了创造性的贡献，奠定了近代蒙医药学理法方药的基础。总之，理论和实践相互印证、相互促进的良好局面的形成，是这一时期蒙医药学发展的一大特征。

新中国成立，迎来了蒙医蒙药发展的新纪元。在党和国家民族政策的光辉照耀下，蒙医蒙药获得了大踏步的发展。据不完全统计，新中国成立以来，不仅建立了许多新的蒙医医疗机构和研究机构，而且也成立了许多蒙医学校，设置蒙医药专业，有计划、有步骤地培养蒙医药人才。如新中国成立后第一所蒙医学校就是著名蒙医古拿巴达拉在辽宁蒙古勒津（阜新）瑞应寺主持建立的。1958年内蒙古医学院在全国西医药院校中第一个设立了蒙医专业本科。1980年在通辽成立了内蒙古民族医学院，1987年更名为内蒙古蒙医学院，2000年与通辽地区其他两所高校合并组建了内蒙古民族大学。2016年通辽市被命名为“中国蒙医药之都”，蒙医药的发展，形成了新的格局，新的境界。在继承传统的基础上，古老的蒙医药体系不断吸收新的时代精华，活力频注，生机勃发，在与国际水平和现代科技接轨方面，在协同化、规模化、科学化、信息化、产业化发展等方面，不断探索和迈进。

纵观蒙医蒙药发展历程，深深感到她是蒙古民族文化宝库，乃至人类文化宝库里的珍宝，散发着璀璨夺目的光芒。蒙医蒙药是蒙古族人民对人类科学进步、文明发展进程做出的极大贡献。

第一，蒙医蒙药是对人体生理机制及疾病治疗的科学认识体系和实践体系。人体是生命的物质基础，一个蕴藏着无数奥秘的神奇所在。蒙医把人体看作是与外界直接联系的有机整体，通过身体表面的细微变化诊察体内的疾病，并在此基础上辨证施治。自成体系、日渐成熟的蒙医蒙药反映着蒙古民族在医学领域的探究深度。

第二，蒙医蒙药是人与大自然辩证关系的折射，是蒙古人在物我关系、自然哲学探究高度的表征。蒙古人信仰“天人一脉”，相信宇宙是个相互联系、彼此制约的系统，是一个能量循环共生的生态圈，人是这个生态圈里的有机部分，与动物、植物等其他部分都有着相生相抵又相依相宜的关系。蒙医把人体本身也看作是一个自我能量循环系统，蒙医的很多治疗手段（比如骨伤术），不使用仪器，不开刀破肤，不打钢钉，不伤元气，全靠手法技术医治的前提，是对个体生命自我循环规律的尊重、顺应和对自愈能力的信任。

第三，蒙医蒙药是生命的珍爱与呵护系统，承担着民众身心健康的“保护神”的使命。一方面，蒙医蒙药反映着蒙古人战胜疾病侵袭、维护生命健康的爱心和仁怀，另一方面，蒙医蒙药反映着蒙古人既诚于顺应自然，又勇于利用自然，并在与自然的关系中，发展出为我所用的实际效能、实际价值的能力。蒙医蒙药是蒙古人源远流长的创新意识和创新能力的实证和“活化石”。

蒙医药学在其发展的各个历史时期形成的文献典籍，不仅是蒙古民族的优秀文化遗产，也是蒙医药学丰富内容的主要载体。为展示蒙医药学博大精深的内容，更好地保护、传承和利用民族优秀文化遗产，辽宁民族出版社组织辽宁省阜新蒙医药研究所和内蒙古民族大学蒙医药专家学者，将辽宁省阜新蒙医药研究所馆藏部分古籍文献进行整理，并影印出版《中国蒙医药古籍影印珍本》。

《中国蒙医药古籍影印珍本》（丛书），共7卷本，包括《兰塔布》《甘露精要八支秘诀续. Ⅰ》《甘露精要八支秘诀续. Ⅱ》《痘症精言》（蒙古文版）、《格体全录》《蒙古文手抄普济杂方》《蒙古文手抄本一药方》，内容涵盖了蒙医药基础理论、临床经验、药物药理、药物方剂、自然疗法等多个层面。

《中国蒙医药古籍影印珍本》的出版，意义重大。

第一，有利于弘扬民族医术，造福人类健康。蒙医药在治病救人、保健益生方面，具有一套科学和谐的理念和独到神奇的技术方法，而这些既体现在蒙医医生的日常医疗活动中，也积淀于各种蒙医药典籍中。将这些典籍集中整理出版，有利于蒙医药学的传播，有利于民族医术的弘扬，更有益于人类健康。这与当下人们追求自然、健康、和谐的医疗保健效果的时代需求，是相契合的。

第二，有利于蒙医药古籍文献的发掘整理利用，以促进蒙医药的振兴和发展，具有强劲的现实意义和深远的历史意义。蒙医药是国家级非物质文化遗产，将辽宁省阜新蒙医药研究所馆藏的大量蒙医药古籍文献资料整理出版，是目前为止国内首个关于蒙医药古籍抢救类大型出版项目。本丛书收录的蒙医药古籍文献中记录了大量医药资源、诊疗技术、用药经验，对其进行整理、梳理，利用现代科学仪器来扫描影印出版，能真实展现古籍原貌，从而让古老典籍焕发时代光彩，极具学术价值、收藏价值和应用价值，有利于促进蒙医药文化的长足发展，提升文化自信。

第三，蒙医药古籍文献作为一种产业开发的资源，具有一定的经济价值。从蒙医药古籍文献整理和研究中挖掘更多的有效预防和治疗疾病的方剂和药物，并将其投入市场，不仅可以为人民群众的健康提供服务，还能带动蒙医药的产业化发展，创造出可观的经济效益，并进而带动民族地区其他行业的发展，加速和谐社会建设进程。

第四，蒙医药古籍文献是中华民族宝贵的文化遗产，是中华文化的重要组成部分，抢救和保护民族古籍，对于传承和弘扬中华优秀传统文化，扩大中华优秀传统文化影响，具有重要意义。党的十九大报告指出：“深入挖掘中华优秀传统文化蕴含的思想观念、人文精神、道德规范，结合时代要求继承创新，让中华文化展现出永久魅力和时代风采。”

《中国蒙医药古籍影印珍本》编辑委员会

2018年6月

General Preface

The Mongolian nationality is a legendary ethnic group with a long history. In the long history process, Mongolians have developed broad, profound and gorgeous cultural patterns in many aspects, such as living, diet, clothing, language, writing, dance, art, medicine and health, which has accumulated tremendous achievements and formed its unique tradition. Each part of this traditional culture is the beautiful creation that condenses the world essence and the ancestral teachings; it is also the cream and crystallization that encourage constant innovations and gather the experience of big historical events.

Mongolian Medicine, is the gorgeous one in the Mongolian cultural garden. With other flowers in this cultural garden, it develops a broad and full Mongolian connotation system, making the garden extraordinarily beautiful. Mongolian Medicine, which originated in ancient times, formed in the Yuan Dynasty, developed in the Ming and Qing dynasties, and flourished in the contemporary era, is the treasure of traditional Chinese Medicine and the unique one in the Chinese medical field.

Mongolians have lived a nomadic life since ancient times. They lived in the cold, arid or semi-arid grassland, and fed on beef, mutton, and dairy products. Riding, grazing, migrating and fast gallop during the war made them easy to suffer from various injuries like bruises, fractures, and war wound. Under such climatic, geographical, dietary and living conditions, Mongolian ancestors insistently observed the relationship between animals and plants in nature, and initially mastered the nutrition, toxicity of animals and plants and their functions to prevent and cure of diseases. Through analyzing and summarizing the experience that has been accumulated to fight against diseases during the long period of hunting, nomadism, agricultural production, migration, and fighting, the Mongolian people invented a series of treatments inclusive of regional and ethnic characteristics. For example, fire therapy to resist cold and dampness, osteopathy featured by bone setting and skull setting, as well as dietotherapy like kumiss therapy based on the nutrition of the dairy product. This period is the bud and embryonic stage of Mongolian medical science.

In the Yuan Dynasty, Mongolian Medicine had made great progress for two reasons. First, the mainland Medicine and Mongolian Medicine nourished and promoted each other mutually. Second, Mongolian Medicine received institutional political security in the Yuan Dynasty. Followed the medical system in the Tang and Song dynasties, the government of the Yuan Dynasty set up The Imperial Hospital and The Medical Institute of Benevolence to support and promote Mongolian Medicine, thus providing a suitable condition for the all-round development of Mongolian Medicine. On the original basis, the traditional Mongolian medical technologies such as orthopedics and traumatology had gained new progress. At the same time, by absorbing, drawing upon all useful opinions and in-depth research, the Mongolian ancestors had already summed up the understanding that "the origins of disease are no more than cold and fever", thus inventing and enriching "Theory of Cold and Fever" and other traditional Mongolian medical theory, such as human anatomy knowledge, medicine knowledge, first-aid knowledge and infectious disease prevention knowledge. Yuan Imperial doctor Husihui's *Yinshan Zhengyao* is the first book of Mongolian medical dietotherapy, which laid the foundation for the maturity of Mongolian Medicine after the 16th century.

In the Ming and Qing dynasties, with the introduction of Tibetan *Rgyud bzhi* and some ancient Indian medical theories, Mongolian Medicine reasonably absorbed the essence of Tibetan Medicine and Indian Medicine. Therefore, its basic theoretical research and clinical treatment practice had reached a new level. Taking Tibetan Medicine and ancient Indian Medicine's "Wuyuan Xueshuo" as references and starting points, on the theoretical basis of "Three Roots and Seven Elements", absorbing the knowledge of traditional Chinese Medicine, and combining the characteristics of Mongolian region and folk therapy, the Mongolian people created an independent Mongolian medical theory system, in which "Theory of Cold and Fever" plays the core leading role. In Ixibalazhuer's book *Ganlu Tetralogy*, he theoretically and practically elaborated the traditional Mongolian Bone Injury Treatment from many specific perspectives, such as "Trauma Surgery", "Dislocation Reduction", "Bone Injury Therapy", "Shaking Brain Therapy",etc. The contents were very substantial, in which the special theories of "Six Basic Diseases", "Cold Diseases", "Top Ten Major Symptoms" were proposed. At the same time, on the basis of the increasingly rich experience of clinical treatment, a unique medical treatment system with ethnic characteristics came into being. Mongolian Bone Injury Treatment is extremely unique and magical. Mongolian medical expert Chuerjimorgen was famous for the exquisite precision of his treatment in surgery. Thus, he was written into *Draft History of the Qing Dynasty.* He is but a typical representative of the large number of Mongolian "Miracle Doctors". With the prosperity of Yellow Sect in the Mongolian region, temples in large-scale all equipped with Mamba Raseng. Mamba Raseng is not only the medical center, but also the base for studying and researching the theories of Mongolian and Tibetan Medicine. It has cultivated a great number of talents in this field. Mongoliajin located in the Eastern part (now Liaoning Fuxin), is known as "The Birthplace of Mongolian Medicine". As early as 1669, Ruiying Temple was built and equipped with Mamba Raseng. Research on Mongolian Medicine theories was just unfolding. Mongolian doctors also achieved more profound understanding of the nature and flavor of Mongolian drugs. Under such situation, three typical masterpieces of Mongolian Medicine appeared. They are *Baijing Drug Recognition and Discrimination*, *Recognition of Drugs*, *Mongolian Medicine Canon.* Another famous book *Magic Code and Recipe* selected more than 3000 prescriptions for internal, external, women, children, facial features, fever and infectious diseases. Especially *Ganlu Tetralogy* which made a creative contribution to exploring the basic theories and sorting the traditional therapies laid a solid foundation for the modern Mongolian Medicine. In a word, the situation that theory and practice mutually confirm and promote each other was a major characteristic of the Mongolian Medicine development in this period.

The founding of New China ushered in a new era of Mongolian Medicine progress. Under the brilliant care of our Party and State, Mongolian Medicine dramatically developed. Preliminary statistics show that, many new Mongolian medical institutions, research centers as well as Mongolian Medicine schools were established to cultivate Mongolian talents purposefully and designedly. For example, the first Mongolian Medicine school was built in Mongoliajin (Fuxin) Ruiying Temple in Liaoning Province by a famous Mongolian doctor Badara. In 1958, Inner Mongolia Medical College, which is famous as a West Medicine college, firstly set up Mongolian Medicine department. In 1980, Inner Mongolian National Medical College was established in Tongliao and renamed Mongolian Medical College of Inner Mongolia in 1987, and expanded as Inner Mongolia University for Nationalities after merging other two colleges in 2000. In 2016, Tongliao was entitled "Mongolian Medicine Capital of China". A new pattern and a new state for the development of Mongolian Medicine came into being. On the basis of inheriting its tradition, ancient Mongolian Medicine absorbs the essence of the contemporary era, brimming over with vigor and vitality. It insistently explores and progresses in many aspects such as the connection with global society and modern science and technology, as well as its collaboratization, scientization, scale expansion, informatization and industrialization.

From an overview of the development history of Mongolian Medicine, it can be drawn that she is a priceless treasure of Mongolian culture, and even the treasure of human culture, exuding dazzling light. It is Mongolians' great contribution to the development of human science and the development of civilization.

First, Mongolian Medicine is a scientific understanding system and practical system of human physiological mechanism and disease treatment. Human body is the material basis of life, a place containing countless mysteries. Mongolian Medicine takes the human body as an organic whole that is directly related to the outside world. Disease can be correctly diagnosed and dialectically treated through the subtle changes in the body. The Mongolian Medicine, coming from ancient times, establishing her own system, becoming mature and perfect, reflects the depth of the exploration Mongolian people have done in the field of medical science.

Second, Mongolian Medicine is the reflection of the dialectical relationship between man and nature, and it is the symbol of Mongolians' exploration level in the relationship between man and nature, and natural philosophy. The Mongolians believe in the theory that man is a part of nature. They believe that the universe is an interrelated and restricted system, and it is a symbiotic ecological circle of balanced energy. Human being is an organic part of this ecological circle, keeping a contrarious and dependent relationship with animals and plants. Mongolian Medicine takes the human body as a self-energy circulatory system. There are numerous treatments in Mongolian Medicine (such as Bone Injury Therapy), free from instruments, operations, steel nails and avoiding devitalizing patients. All these treatments are based on manipulative therapy, reflecting Mongolian Medicine's respect for human beings' self-circulation law and confidence for their self-cure ability.

Third, Mongolian Medicine is the precious and caring system of life, bearing the mission of protecting people's physical and mental health. On one hand, Mongolian Medicine reflects the Mongolians' love of conquering the disease and safeguarding the health of life. On the other hand, Mongolian Medicine reflects that Mongolians sincerely obey the rules of nature and bravely make use of nature. In the relationship between man and nature, they develop their abilities of taking every advantage of nature to maximize the actual effects and practical value. Mongolian Medicine is the robust evidence and the "living fossil" of the Mongolian people's long history of innovation and creation.

Ancient and classical works appeared in different period in the process of the Mongolian Medicine development are not only the precious heritage of Mongolian culture, but also the great carrier of the rich content of Mongolian Medicine. In order to show the broad and profound Mongolian Medicine, to better protect, inherit and make use of this precious heritage, Liaoning Nationality Publishing House photocopied and published *Rare Photocopy of Chinese Mongolian Medicine Ancient Book* by organizing the scholars of Liaoning Fuxin Mongolian Medicine Research Institute and Inner Mongolia University for Nationalities to sort the ancient and classical works kept in Liaoning Fuxin Mongolian Medicine Research Institute.

Rare Photocopy of Chinese Mongolian Medicine Ancient Book (series) consists of seven volumes, including *Man Ngag Lhan Thabs*, *The Secret Tantra of Nectar Essence Eight Branches (i.e. Rgyud bzhi) I*, *The Secret Tantra of Nectar Essence Eight Branches (i.e. Rgyud bzhi) II*, *The Fine Words of Smallpox*, *Completely Record of Body*, *Mongolian Manuscripts of Cure-all Prescriptions* and *Mongolian Manuscripts of Prescriptions*. It covers the basic theories of medicine, clinical experience, pharmacology, prescriptions, natural therapies and many other aspects.

It is of profound significance to publish the *Rare Photocopy of Chinese Mongolian Medicine Ancient Book*.

First, it helps to carry forward National Medicine to benefit human health. Mongolian Medicine saves lives and cures of diseases with a set of scientific and harmonious ideas and unique and magical technical methods. These are not only embodied in the daily therapeutic activities of Mongolian Medicine doctors, but also accumulated in various Mongolian Medicine classics. Centralization and publication of these classics are conducive to the spread of Mongolian Medicine, to the promotion of National Medicine and human health. This is in harmony with the demand of the contemporary time that people pursue the pure, healthy and harmonious health care.

Second, it is beneficial to the exploitation and utilization of ancient literature of Mongolian Medicine in order to promote Mongolian Medicine's rejuvenation and development, which has strong practical significance and far-reaching historical significance. Mongolian Medicine is a state-level intangible cultural heritage. Editing and publishing a large number of Mongolian Medicine ancient literature from Liaoning

Fuxin Mongolian Medicine Research Institute is the first large-scale project on the rescue of Mongolian Medicine ancient classics in our country. This book contains a mass of medical resources, diagnosis and treatment technologies and medication experience. Sorting and photocopying this great work with modern scientific instruments can truly display these ancient classics and let them glow splendid brilliance, which is of great academic value, collection value and application value. It is also contributes to the rapid development and increasing self-confidence of Mongolian Medicine culture.

Third, as a kind of cultural resource, the ancient literature of Mongolian Medicine has certain economic value. During the process of sorting and researching these ancient classics, some prescriptions and medicine that can effectively cure of and prevent diseases were discovered. Putting them into the market, not only can provide service for people's health keeping, but also can drive the development of Mongolian Medicine industrialization, creating considerable economic benefits, promoting the development of other industries in ethnic areas and accelerating the process of building a harmonious society.

Fourth, the ancient literature of Mongolian Medicine is the precious cultural heritage of China, and is an important part of Chinese culture. Rescuing and protecting national ancient books is of great significance for inheriting and carrying forward Chinese excellent traditional culture and expanding the influence of Chinese excellent traditional culture. The 19th National Congress of the Communist Party of China pointed out: "Dig into the ideas, spirit and moral norms of Chinese elite traditional culture. Inherit and innovate Chinese elite traditional culture to meet the requirements of the contemporary era. Let Chinese culture show its permanent charm and time features."

Rare Photocopy of Chinese Mongolian Medicine Ancient Book

Editorial Committee

June, 2018

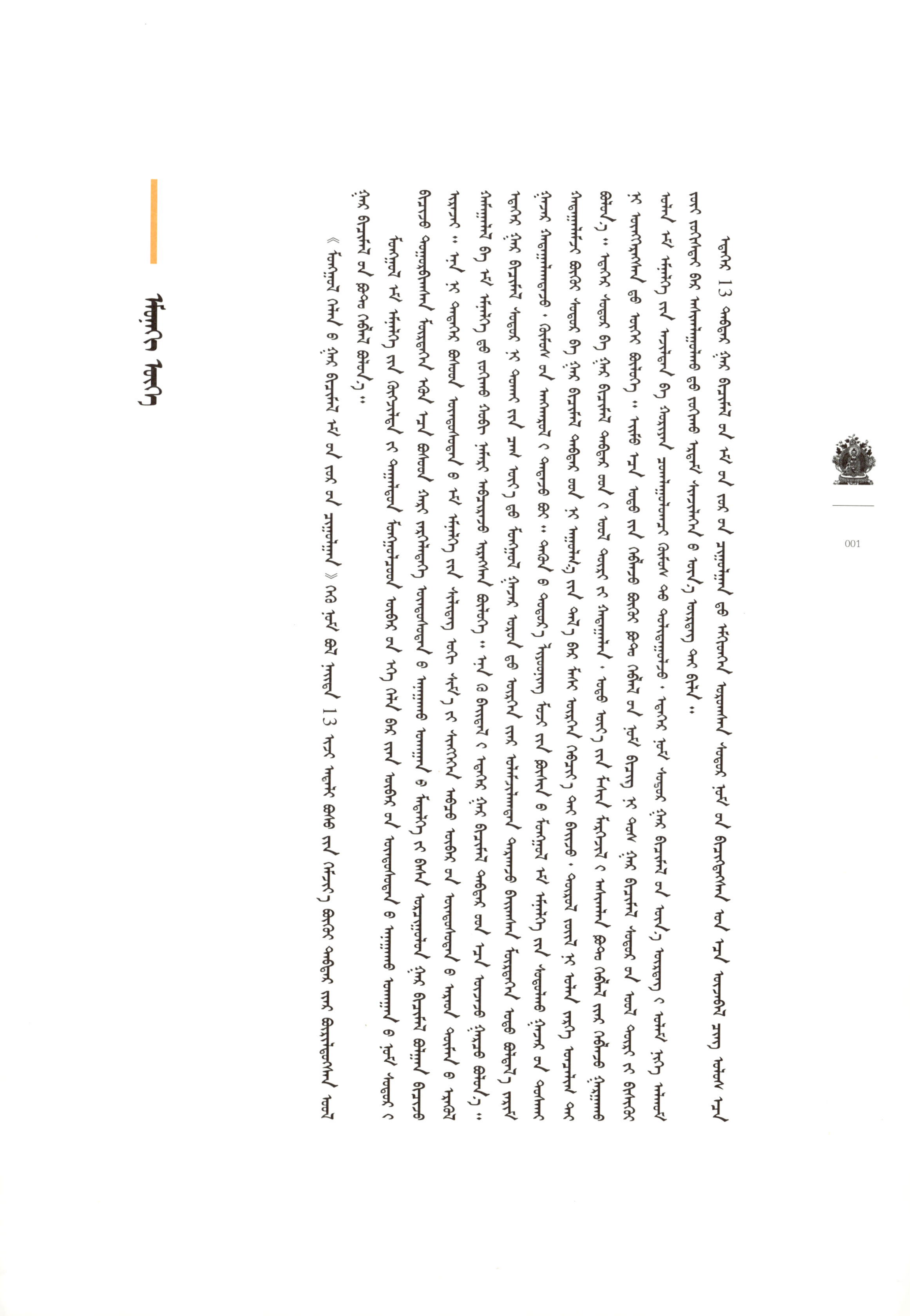

ᠡᠮᠦᠨᠡᠬᠢ ᠦᠭᠡ

ᠰᠠᠶᠢᠬᠠᠨ ᠮᠠᠰᠢ ᠵᠢᠨ᠎ᠠ ᠄ ᠬᠡᠯᠡᠯᠴᠡ ᠮᠠᠨᠠᠢ ᠬᠡᠯᠡᠭᠰᠡᠨ ᠬᠡᠷᠡᠭ ᠶᠢᠨ ᠰᠠᠨᠠᠭ᠎ᠠ ᠰᠣᠶᠣᠯᠭᠠᠪᠠ ᠬᠡᠮᠡᠨ ᠪᠣᠯᠪᠠ ᠳᠠᠭᠠᠭᠠᠳ ᠤ ᠪᠣᠯᠤᠨ᠎ᠠ —᠂

ᠲᠡᠷᠡ ᠪᠣᠯ ᠬᠦᠮᠦᠨ ᠦ ᠰᠠᠨᠠᠭᠠᠯᠲᠠ ᠶᠢᠨ ᠡᠬᠢ ᠳᠦ ᠶᠠᠪᠤ ᠶᠠᠪᠤᠭᠠ ᠶᠢᠨ ᠠᠷᠭ᠎ᠠ ᠪᠣᠯᠤᠨ ᠬᠡᠷᠡᠭ ᠳᠡᠭᠡᠷᠡ ᠳᠤ ᠬᠡᠷᠡᠭᠯᠡᠬᠦ ᠶᠠᠭᠤᠮ ᠶᠢᠨ ᠪᠣᠳᠤᠭ ᠮᠣᠩᠭᠣᠯ ᠪᠠᠢᠢᠳᠠᠯ ᠲᠠᠯ᠎ᠠ ᠪᠠᠢᠢᠭ᠎ᠠ ᠶᠢ

ᠬᠦᠮᠦᠨᠵᠢᠷᠡᠯ ᠳᠤ ᠮᠡᠳᠡᠭᠳᠡᠬᠦᠨ ᠦ ᠡᠬᠢᠨ ᠳᠤ ᠰᠣᠨᠢᠨ ᠶᠠᠭᠤ ᠮᠠᠨᠢ ᠪᠠᠶᠢᠳᠠᠯ ᠳᠤ ᠪᠣᠯᠤᠨ ᠪᠠᠨ ᠲᠡᠷᠡ ᠡᠬᠢᠨ ᠪᠣᠯᠭᠠᠭᠰᠠᠨ ᠵᠢᠨ᠎ᠠ ᠄

ᠪᠡᠷ ᠲᠡᠷᠡ ᠮᠠᠨᠢ ᠲᠡᠷᠡ ᠶᠢᠨ ᠡᠷᠬᠢᠮ ᠲᠡᠷᠡ ᠲᠡᠷᠡᠭᠦᠨ ᠮᠡᠳᠡᠭᠰᠡᠨ ᠪᠡᠷ ᠮᠠᠨᠠᠢ ᠳᠤ ᠡᠷᠬᠢ ᠶᠢᠨ ᠰᠠᠨᠠᠭ᠎ᠠ ᠶᠢᠨ ᠪᠣᠯᠭᠠᠨ ᠠ ᠪᠠᠶᠢᠭᠰᠠᠨ ᠮᠠᠨᠢ ᠲᠡᠷᠡ ᠲᠡᠷᠡᠭᠦᠳ

ᠲᠡᠷᠡ ᠮᠡᠳᠡᠭᠰᠡᠨ ᠦ ᠡᠬᠢᠨ ᠨᠢ ᠮᠠᠨᠢ ᠶᠠᠭᠤᠨ ᠤ ᠶᠠᠪᠤᠭᠰᠠᠭᠠᠷ ᠠ ᠪᠣᠯᠤᠭᠰᠠᠨ ᠪᠡᠷ ᠮᠣᠩᠭᠣᠯ ᠪᠠᠨ ᠳᠤ ᠮᠠᠨ ᠲᠡᠷᠡᠭᠡ ᠠ ᠪᠠᠶᠢᠭ᠎ᠠ ᠪᠠᠶᠢᠳᠠᠯ ᠮᠠᠨᠠᠢᠰᠠᠭᠠᠷ ᠂ ᠪᠠᠶᠢᠭᠠᠯᠭᠠᠭᠰᠠᠨ ᠶᠠᠪᠤᠭᠰᠠᠭᠠᠷ

ᠲᠡᠭᠦᠨ ᠦ ᠬᠡᠯᠡᠭᠰᠡᠨ ᠪᠡᠷ ᠰᠣᠶᠣᠯᠤᠨ ᠪᠣᠯᠭᠠᠭᠰᠠᠨ ᠤ ᠲᠡᠮᠳᠡᠭᠯᠡᠭᠰᠡᠨ ᠮᠡᠳᠡᠭᠰᠡᠭᠰᠡᠨ ᠪᠣᠯᠤᠨ᠎ᠠ ᠄

ᠮᠡᠳᠡᠭᠰᠡᠨ ᠦ ᠮᠣᠩᠭᠣᠯᠴᠤᠳ ᠤᠨ ᠰᠣᠶᠣᠯᠬᠠᠨᠲᠠᠨ ᠲᠡᠷᠡ ᠪᠠᠶᠢᠭ᠎ᠠ ᠮᠠᠨᠢ ᠮᠠᠨᠢ ᠪᠣᠯᠤᠨ ᠬᠡᠮᠡᠬᠦ ᠲᠡᠷᠡ ᠮᠣᠩᠭᠣᠯᠴᠤᠳ ᠪᠡᠷ ᠲᠡᠷᠡ ᠶᠠᠭᠤ ᠮᠠᠨᠠᠢ ᠲᠡᠮᠳᠡᠭ ᠦ ᠬᠡᠷ ᠮᠡᠳᠡᠭᠰᠡᠨ ᠲᠡᠷᠡ ᠲᠡᠷᠡᠭᠦᠨ ᠰᠣᠶᠣᠯᠬᠠᠯ

ᠮᠠᠨᠢ ᠨᠢᠭᠡ ᠪᠣᠯᠭᠠᠨ ᠶᠠᠪᠤᠭᠰᠠᠨ ᠲᠡᠷᠡ ᠶᠠᠭᠤ ᠮᠠᠨᠠᠭᠤ ᠳᠦ ᠂ ᠲᠡᠷᠡᠭᠦᠨ ᠲᠡᠷᠡ ᠮᠣᠩᠭᠣᠯ ᠲᠡᠷᠡ ᠬᠡᠷ ᠮᠣᠩᠭᠣᠯᠴᠤᠳ ᠲᠡᠷᠡ ᠮᠠᠨᠢ ᠬᠡᠯᠡᠭᠰᠡᠭᠰᠡᠨ ᠪᠣᠯᠤᠨ᠎ᠠ ᠮᠠᠨᠢᠨ ᠲᠤ ᠲᠠᠭᠠᠯᠠᠨ ᠮᠣᠩᠭᠣᠯᠴᠤᠳ ᠮᠡᠳᠡᠭᠰᠡᠨ

ᠰᠣᠶᠣᠯᠬᠠᠨ ᠮᠡᠳᠡᠭᠰᠡᠨ ᠦ ᠮᠠᠨᠢᠬᠦᠪᠦᠭᠦᠨ ᠰᠠᠨᠠᠭᠠᠯᠲᠠᠨ ᠮᠠᠨᠠᠢ ᠲᠡᠷᠡ ᠶᠠᠭᠤ ᠨᠢᠭᠤᠴᠠ ᠪᠠᠢᠢᠭ᠎ᠠ ᠰᠠᠨᠠᠭᠠᠨ ᠮᠣᠩᠭᠣᠯᠴᠤᠳ ᠲᠡᠷᠡ ᠲᠡᠷᠡ ᠰᠣᠶᠣᠯᠬᠠᠨ ᠪᠣᠯᠤᠭᠰᠠᠨ ᠄

ᠰᠠᠨᠠᠭ᠎ᠠ ᠮᠣᠩᠭᠣᠯᠴᠤᠳ ᠤᠨ ᠰᠢᠨᠵᠢᠯᠡᠯᠲᠡ ᠲᠡᠮᠳᠡᠭ ᠮᠠᠨᠢᠨ ᠪᠡᠷ ᠮᠣᠩᠭᠣᠯᠴᠤᠳ ᠤᠨ ᠮᠡᠳᠡᠭᠰᠡᠭᠰᠡᠨ ᠨᠢᠭᠤᠴᠠ ᠪᠣᠯᠭᠠᠨ ᠪᠣᠯᠤᠨ ᠲᠡᠮᠳᠡᠭᠯᠡᠭᠰᠡᠨ ᠪᠣᠯ ᠄ ᠮᠣᠩᠭᠣᠯ ᠳᠦ ᠪᠣᠯᠤᠨ᠎ᠠ ᠲᠡᠷᠡ ᠶᠢᠨ ᠪᠣᠯᠤᠭᠰᠠᠨ ᠢ ᠲᠡᠮᠳᠡᠭᠯᠡᠨ ᠮᠡᠳᠡᠭᠰᠡᠨ

ᠮᠠᠨᠢ ᠳᠦ ᠮᠣᠩᠭᠣᠯ ᠬᠡᠷ ᠪᠡᠷ ᠮᠣᠩᠭᠣᠯ ᠲᠡᠷᠡ ᠮᠡᠳᠡᠭᠰᠡᠨ ᠦ ᠰᠠᠨᠠᠭᠰᠠᠨ ᠪᠣᠯᠤᠨ ᠨᠢᠭᠤᠴᠠ ᠮᠣᠩᠭᠣᠯᠴᠤᠳ ᠲᠡᠷᠡ ᠪᠣᠯᠭᠠᠨ ᠰᠣᠶᠣᠯᠬᠠᠨᠲᠠᠨ ᠪᠠᠶᠢᠭᠰᠠᠨ ᠢ ᠮᠣᠩᠭᠣᠯᠴᠤᠳ ᠄ ᠮᠣᠩᠭᠣᠯ ᠲᠡᠷᠡ ᠨᠢᠭᠤᠴᠠ ᠂ ᠮᠠᠨᠠᠢ ᠰᠢᠨᠵᠢᠯᠡᠭᠰᠡᠨ

ᠬᠦᠮᠦᠨᠢᠢᠨ ᠪᠣᠯᠭᠠᠭᠰᠠᠨ ᠰᠠᠨᠠᠭᠠᠨ ᠪᠠᠶᠢᠭᠰᠠᠨ ᠲᠡᠷᠡ ᠪᠣᠯᠤᠭᠰᠠᠨ ᠂ ᠮᠣᠩᠭᠣᠯᠴᠤᠳ ᠢ ᠮᠣᠩᠭᠣᠯᠴᠤᠳ ᠳᠦ ᠮᠠᠨᠢᠬᠦᠪᠦᠭᠦᠨ ᠰᠠᠨᠠᠭᠠᠯᠲᠠᠨ ᠮᠣᠩᠭᠣᠯ ᠤᠨ ᠲᠡᠷᠡ ᠪᠡᠷ ᠮᠠᠨᠢ ᠤᠨ ᠮᠡᠳᠡᠭᠰᠡᠨ ᠨᠢᠭᠤᠴᠠ ᠪᠣᠯᠤᠭᠰᠠᠨ ᠂ ᠲᠡᠷᠡ ᠲᠡᠷᠡ

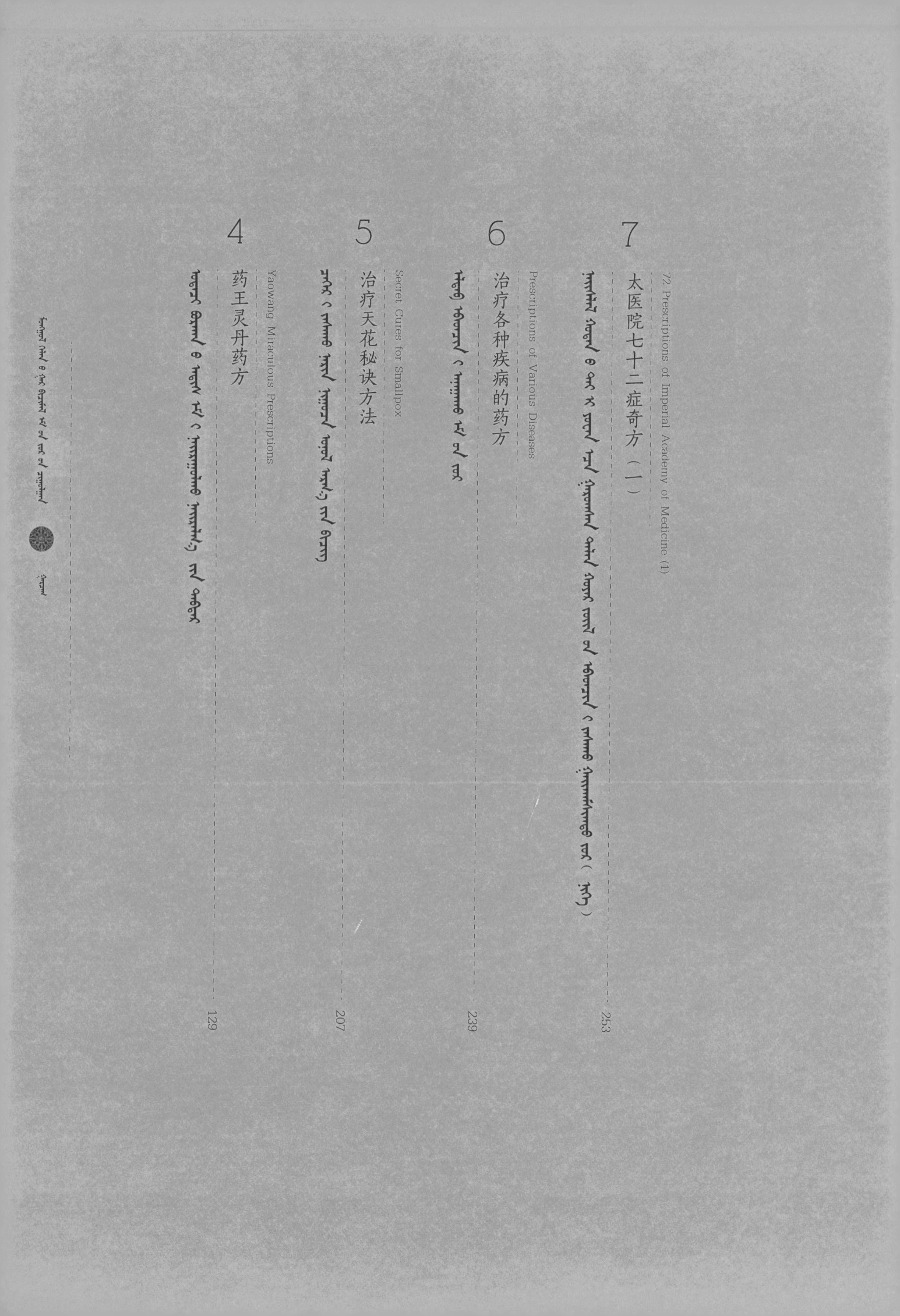

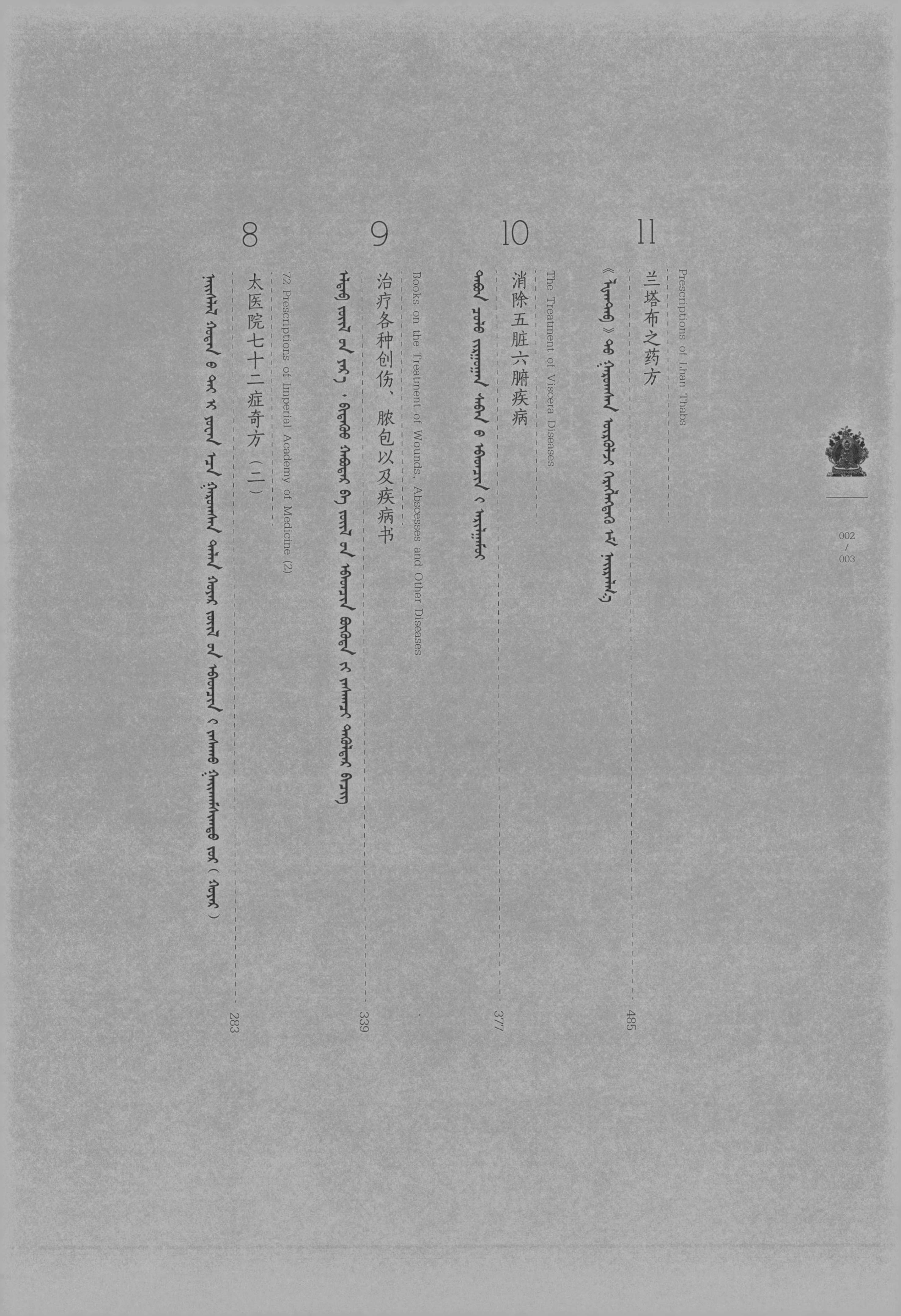

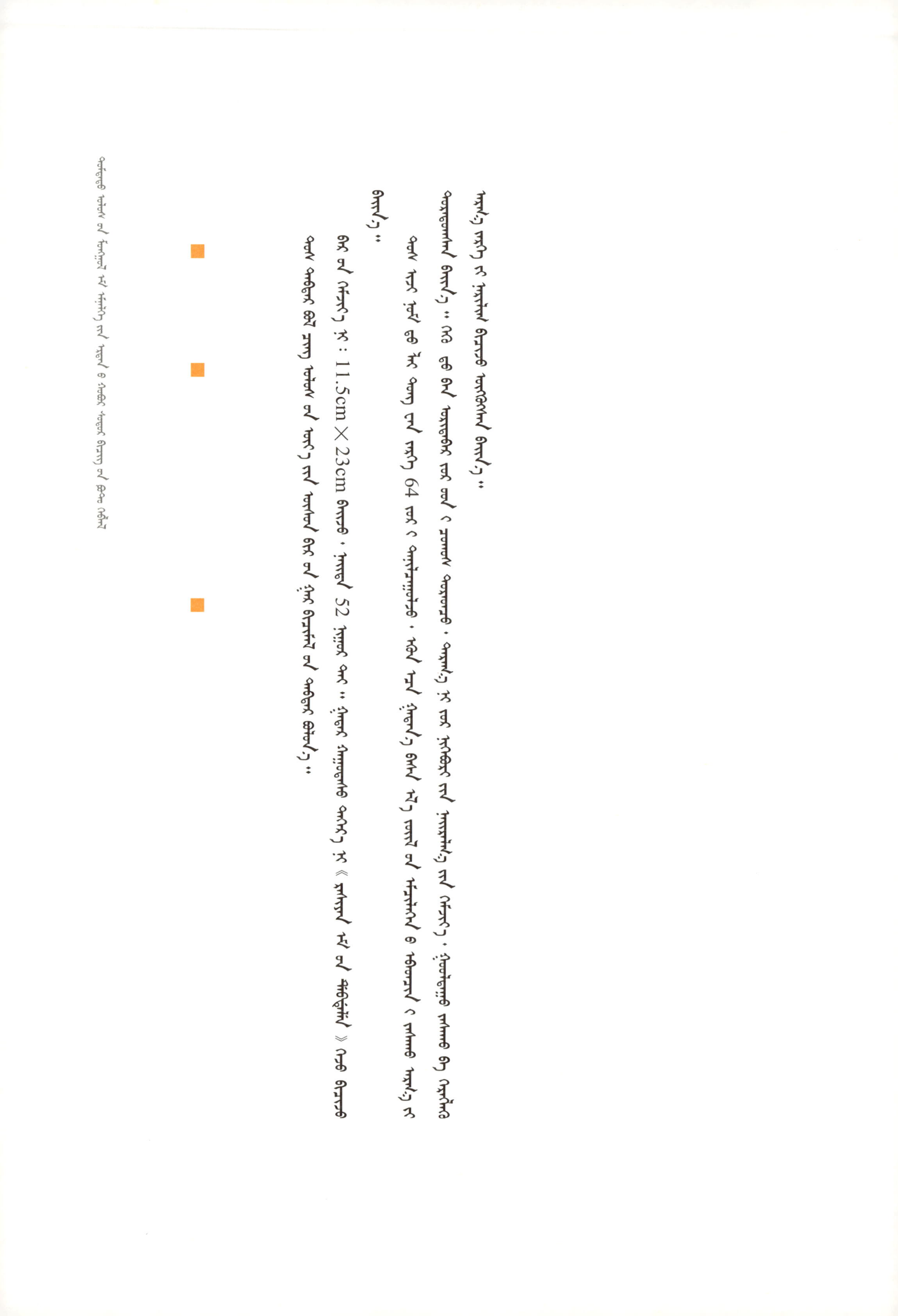

ᠡᠨᠡ ᠨᠢ ᠬᠡᠮᠵᠢᠶ᠎ᠡ ᠨᠢ: 11.5cm × 23cm ᠪᠣᠯᠤᠨ᠎ᠠ᠂ ᠨᠢᠭᠤᠷ 52 ᠬᠤᠪᠢ ᠲᠠᠢ᠃ ᠬᠠᠪᠲᠠᠰᠤ ᠰᠢᠷᠬᠡᠭᠰᠡᠨ ᠲᠡᠷᠢᠭᠦᠨ ᠳᠦ《ᠰᠠᠩᠰᠤᠷ ᠤᠨ ᠨᠢ ᠮᠠᠨᠳᠠᠯ》ᠭᠡᠵᠦ ᠪᠢᠴᠢᠵᠦ

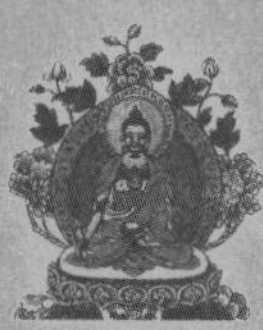

Prescriptions

药方

1

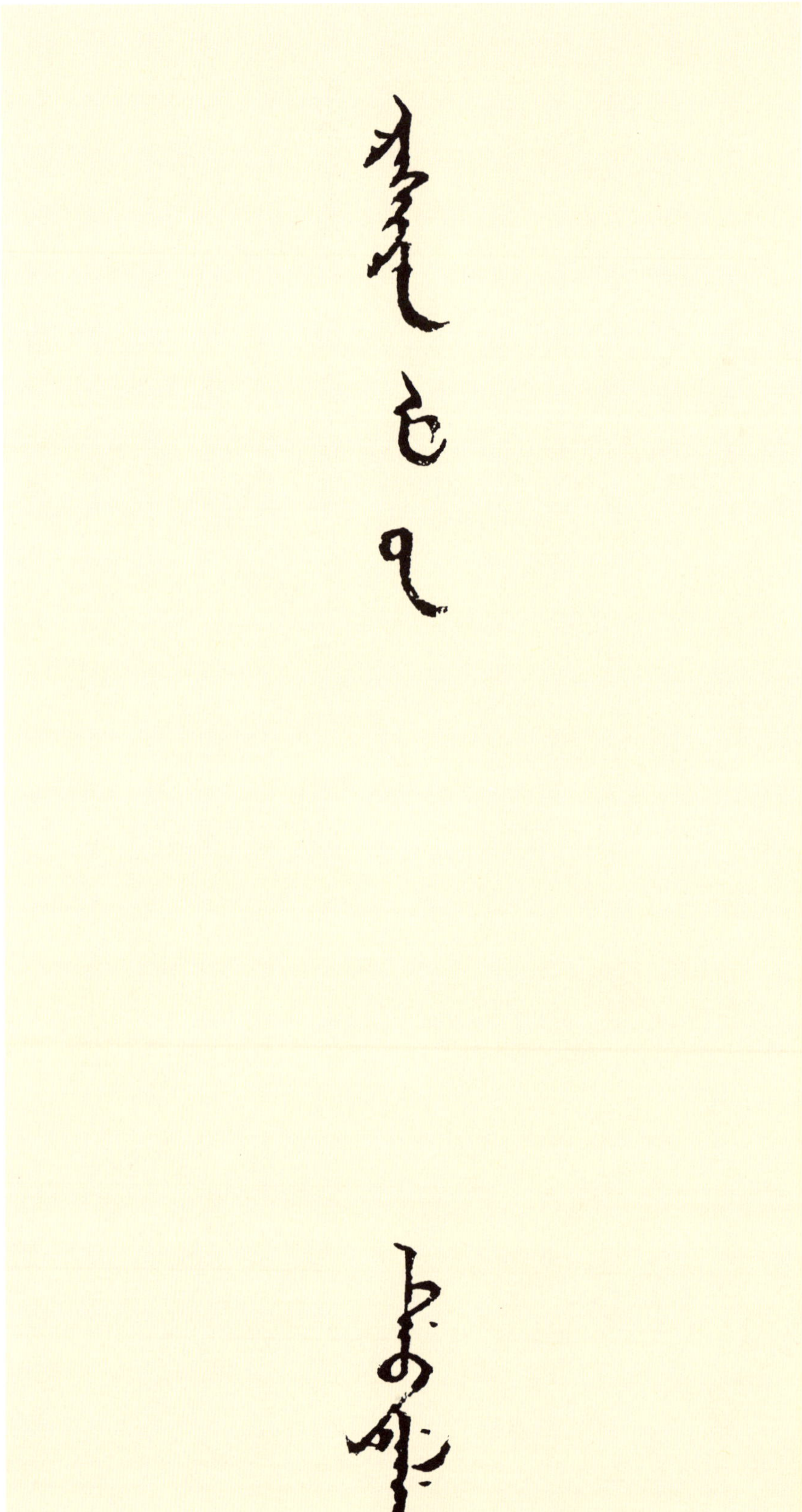

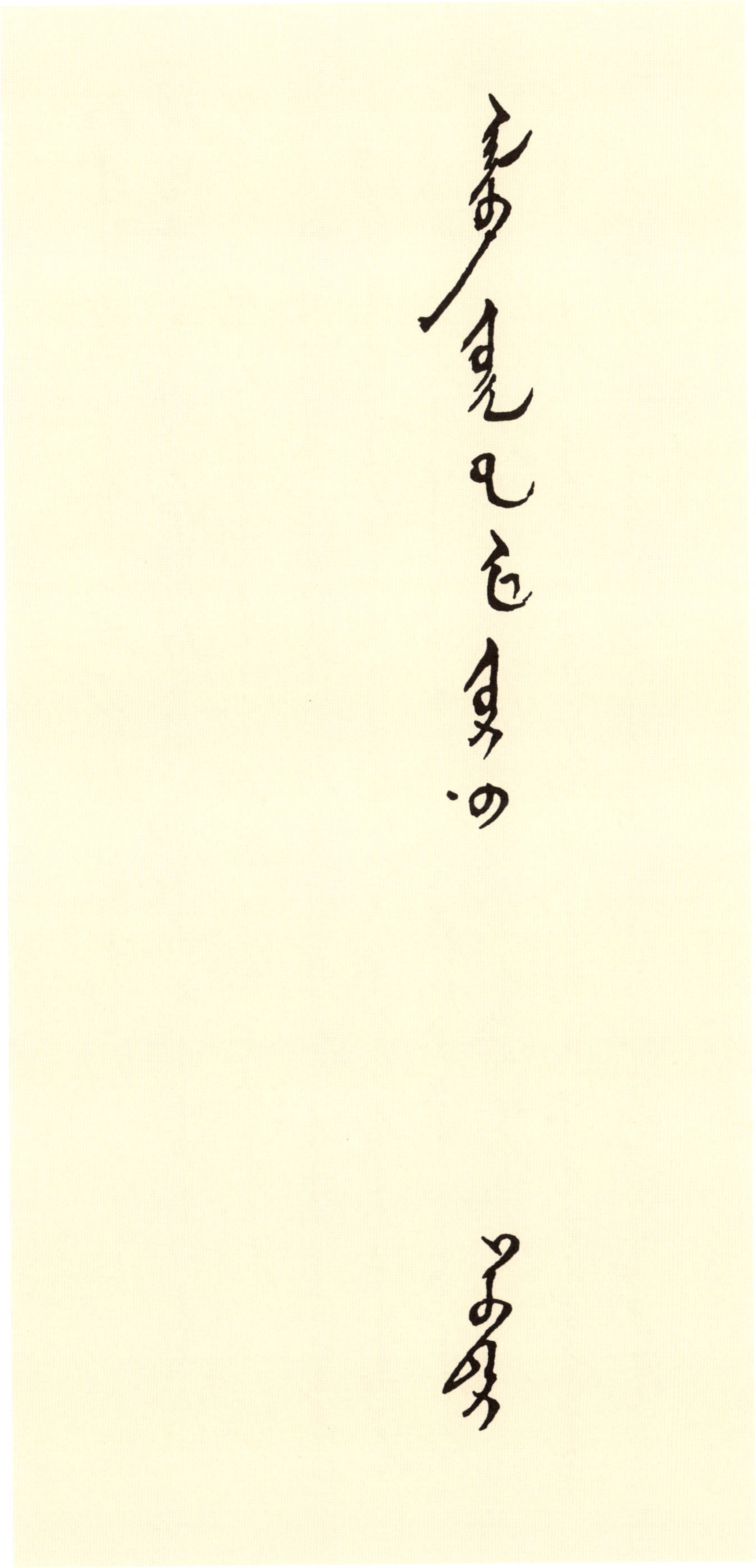

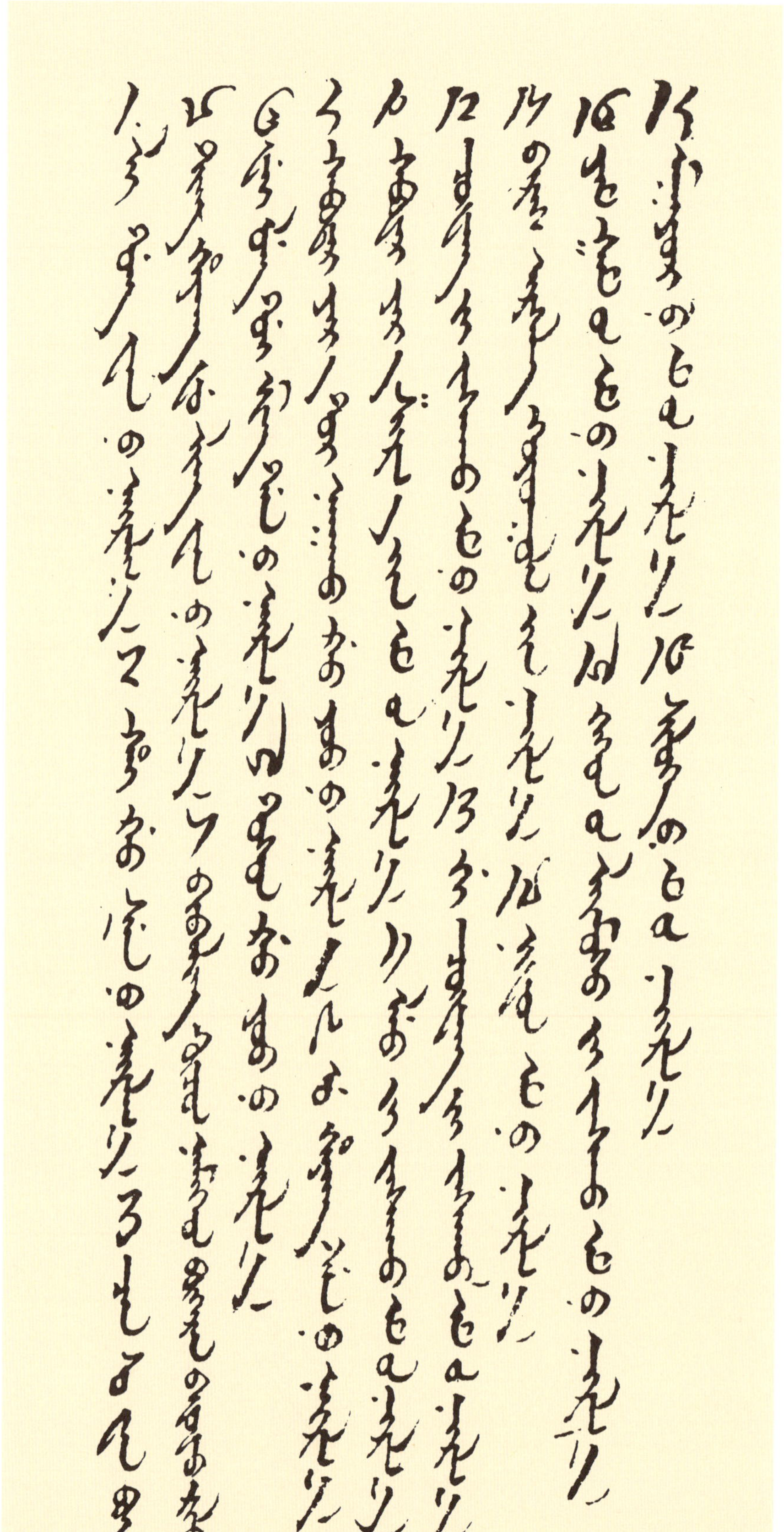

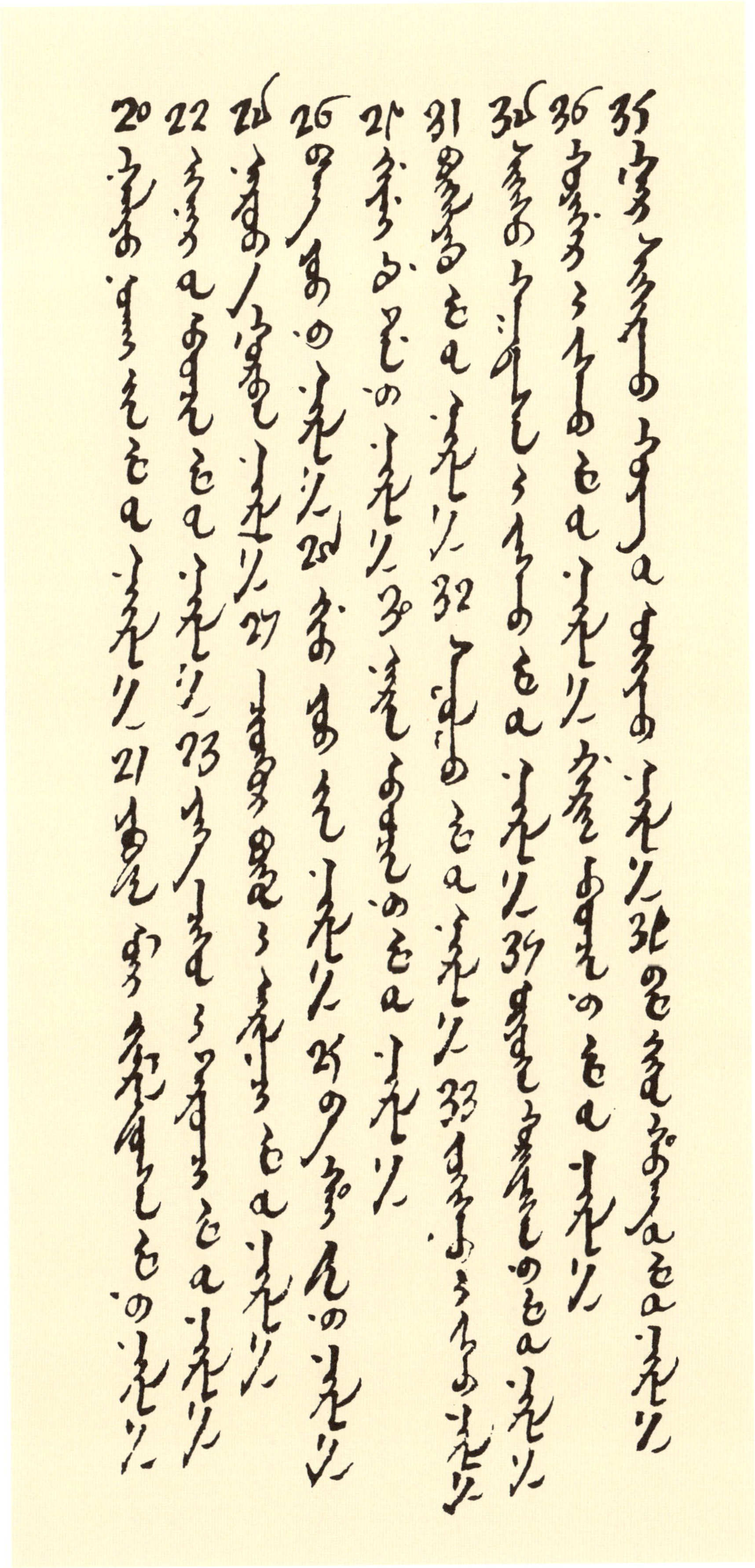

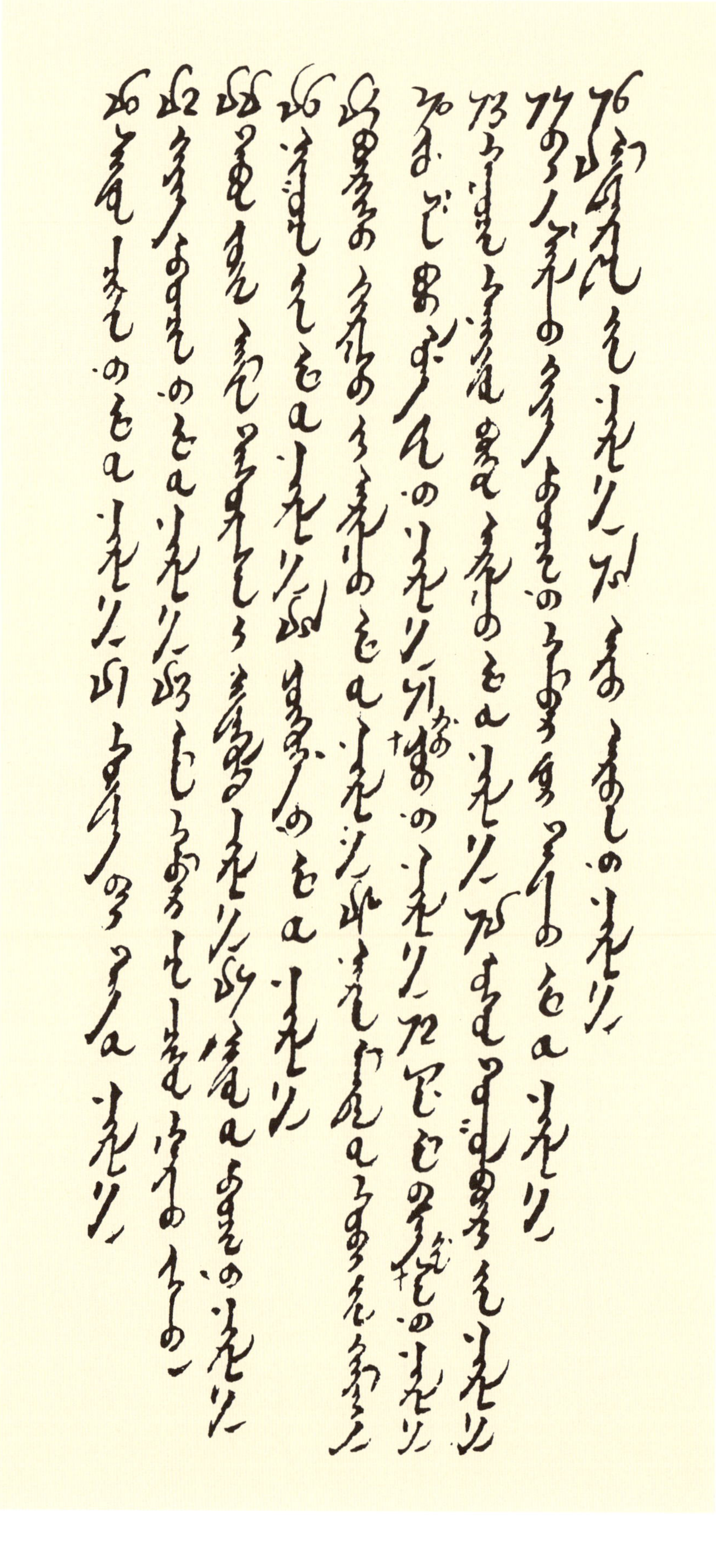

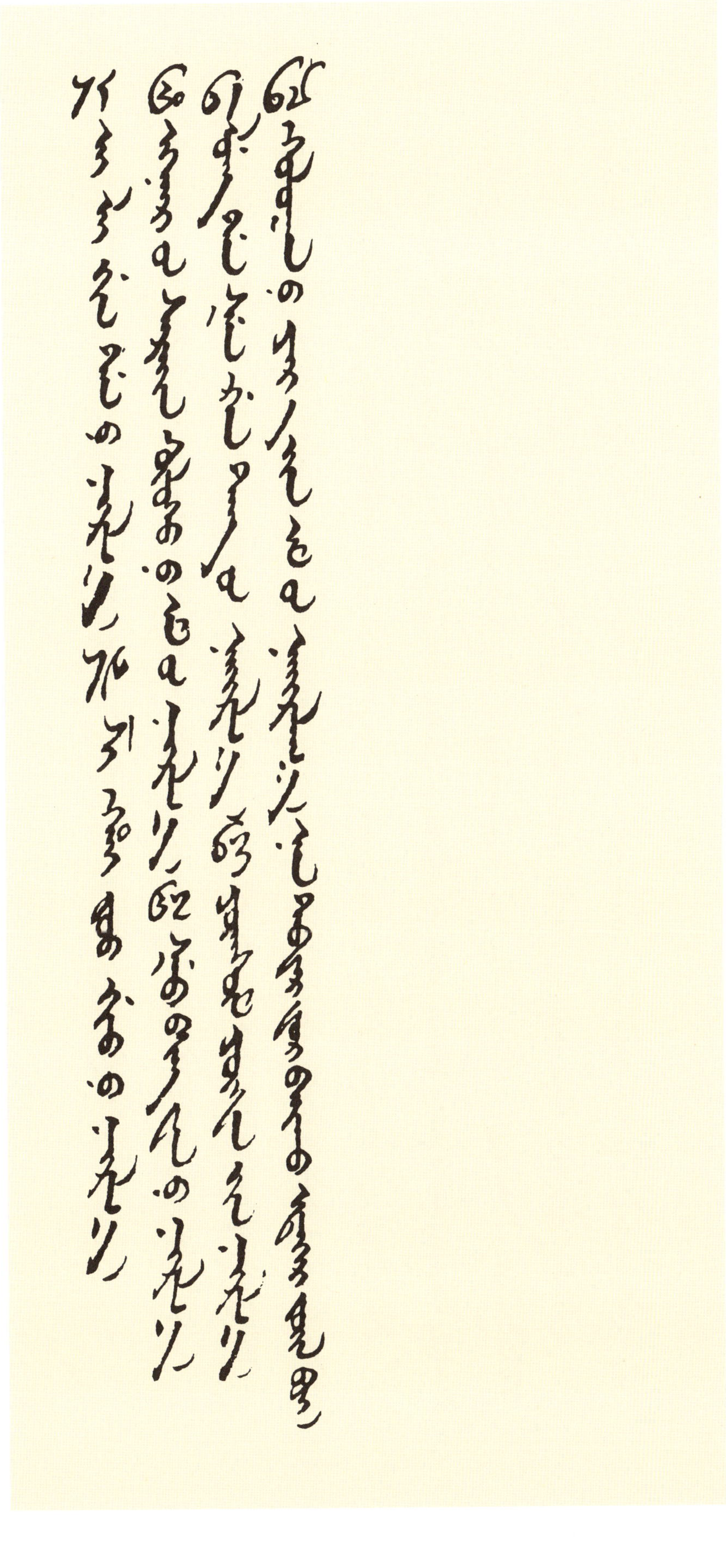

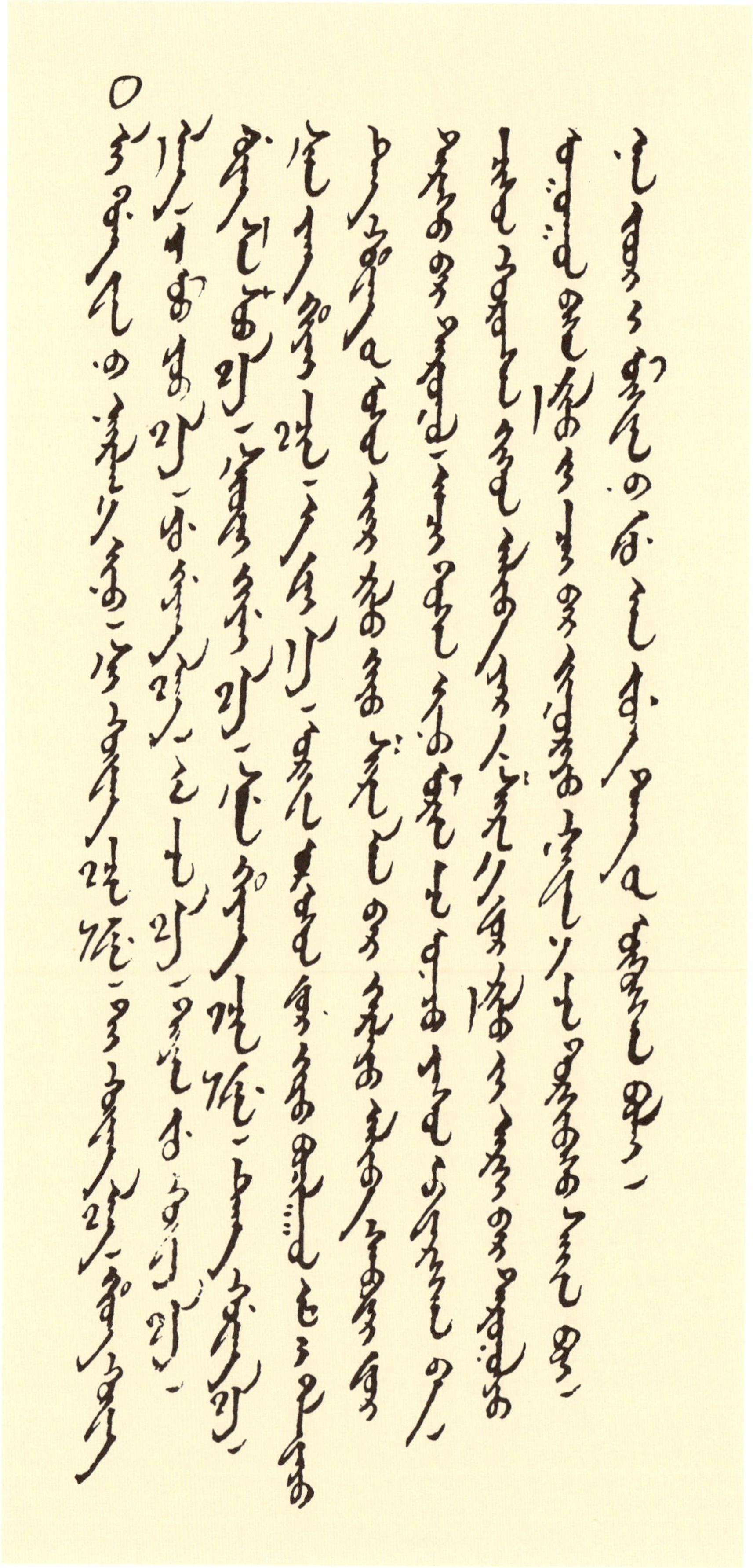

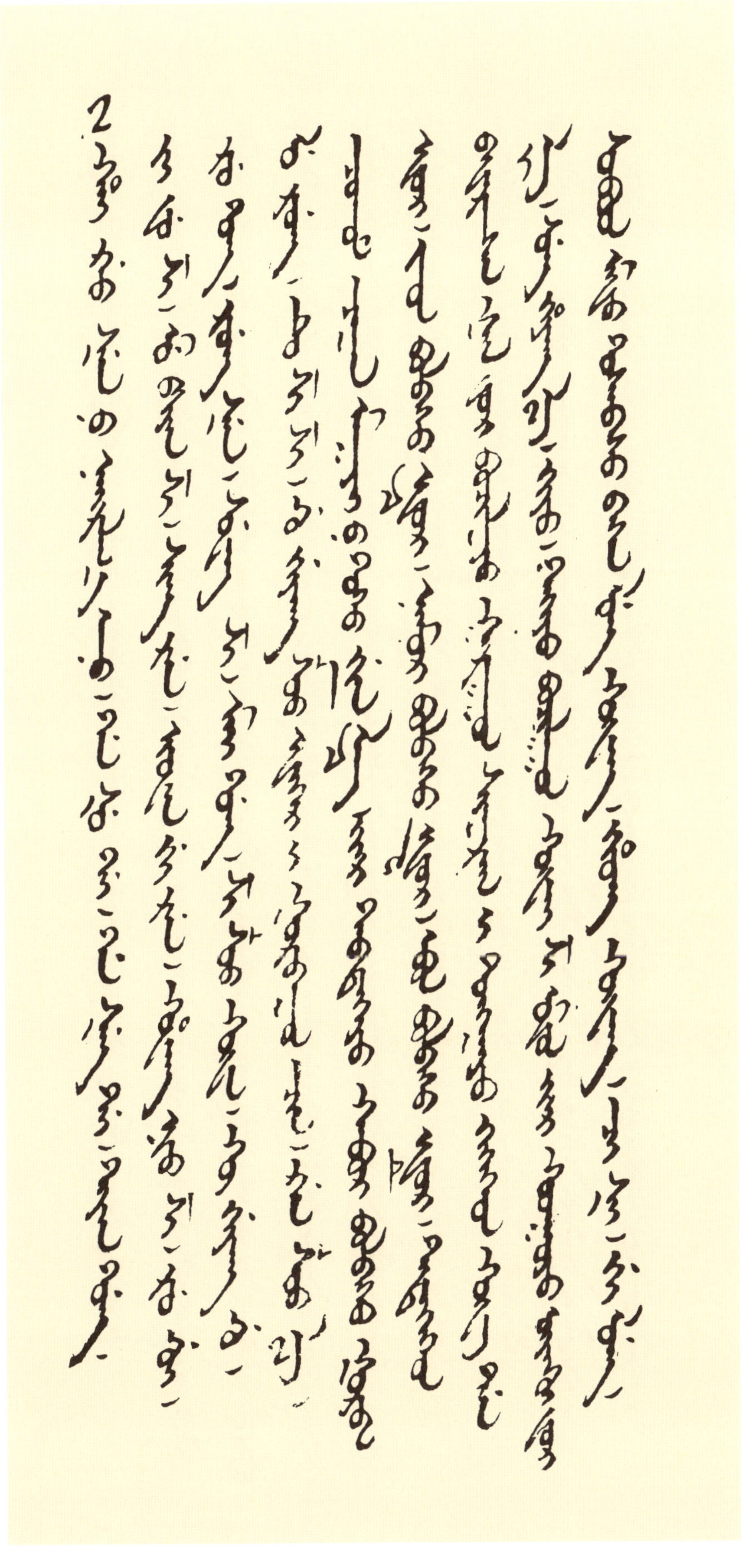

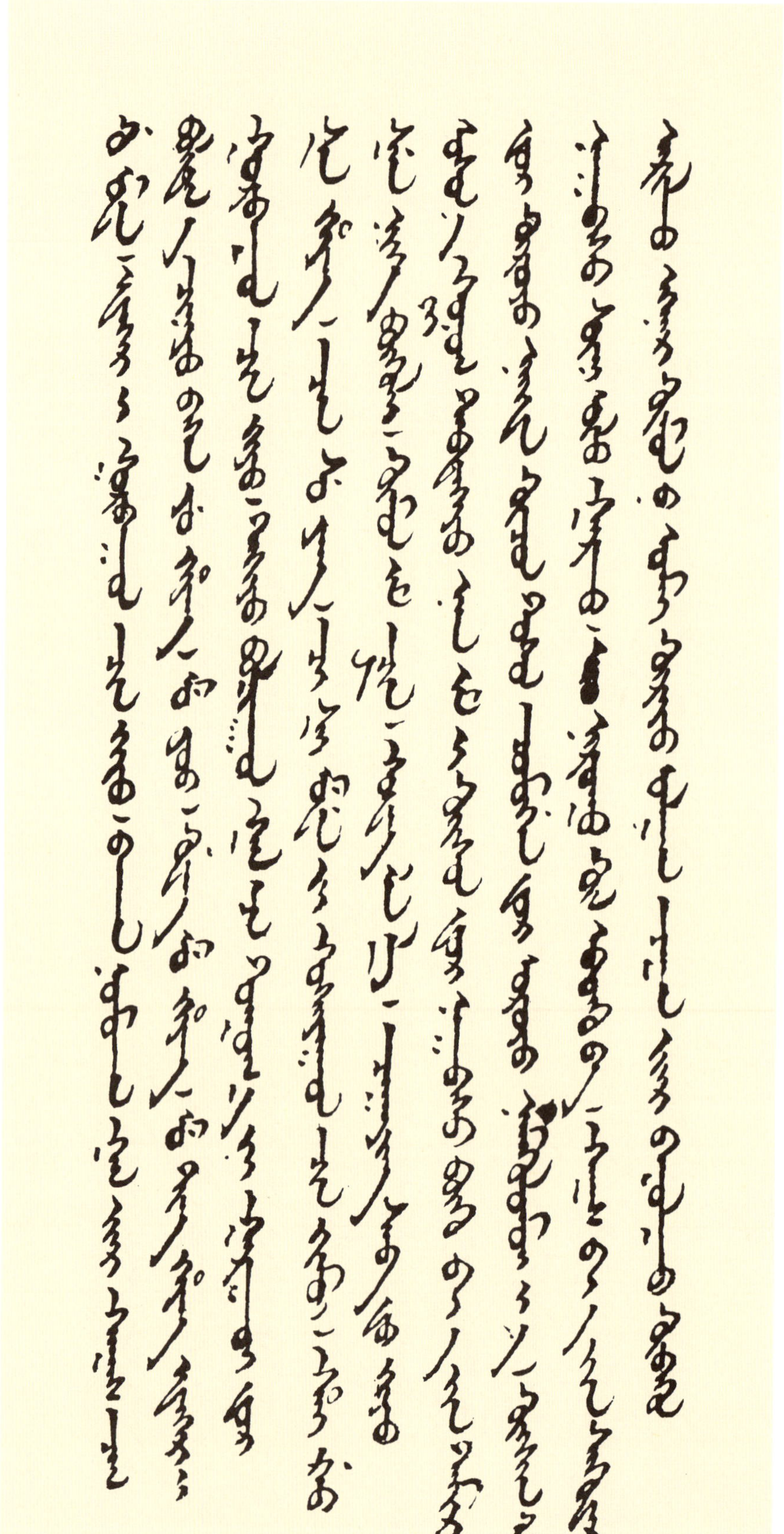

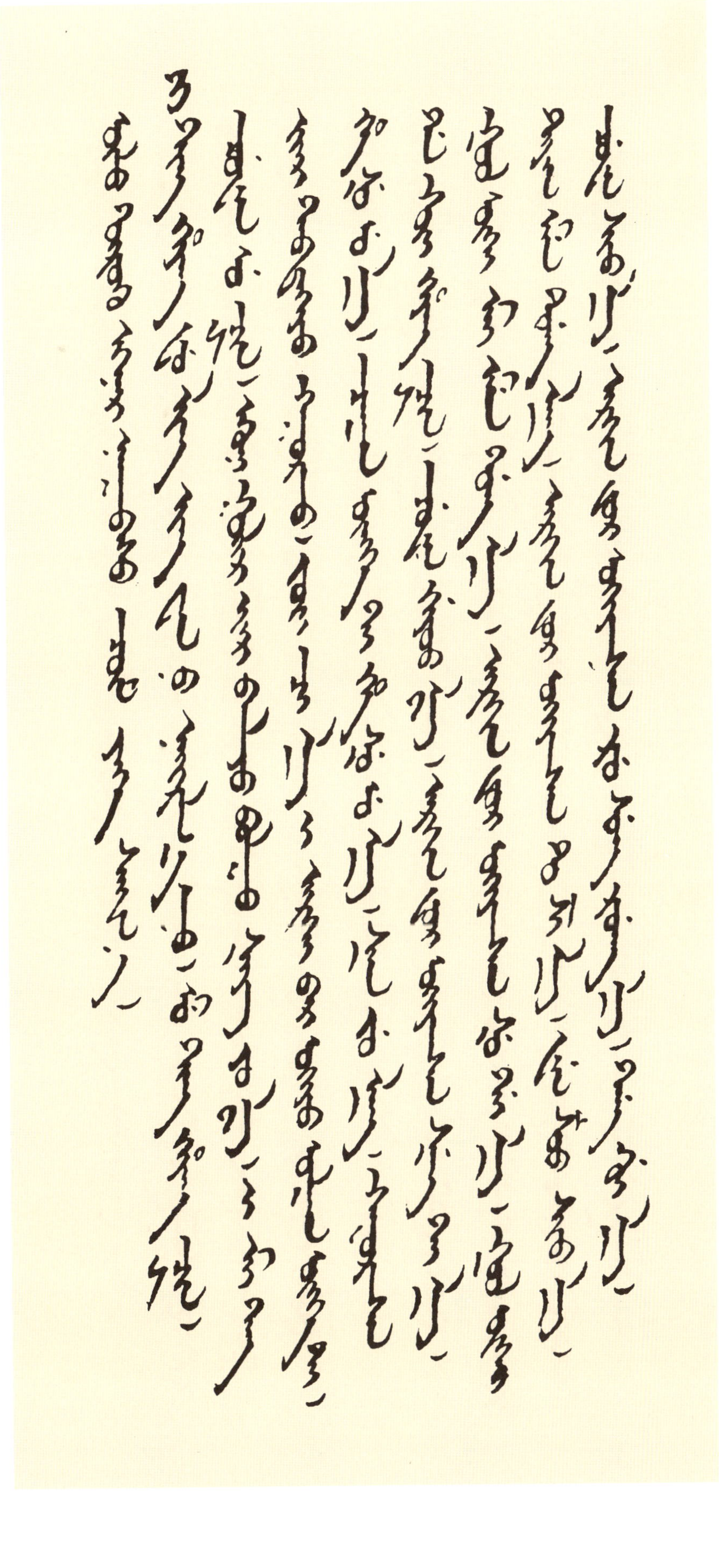

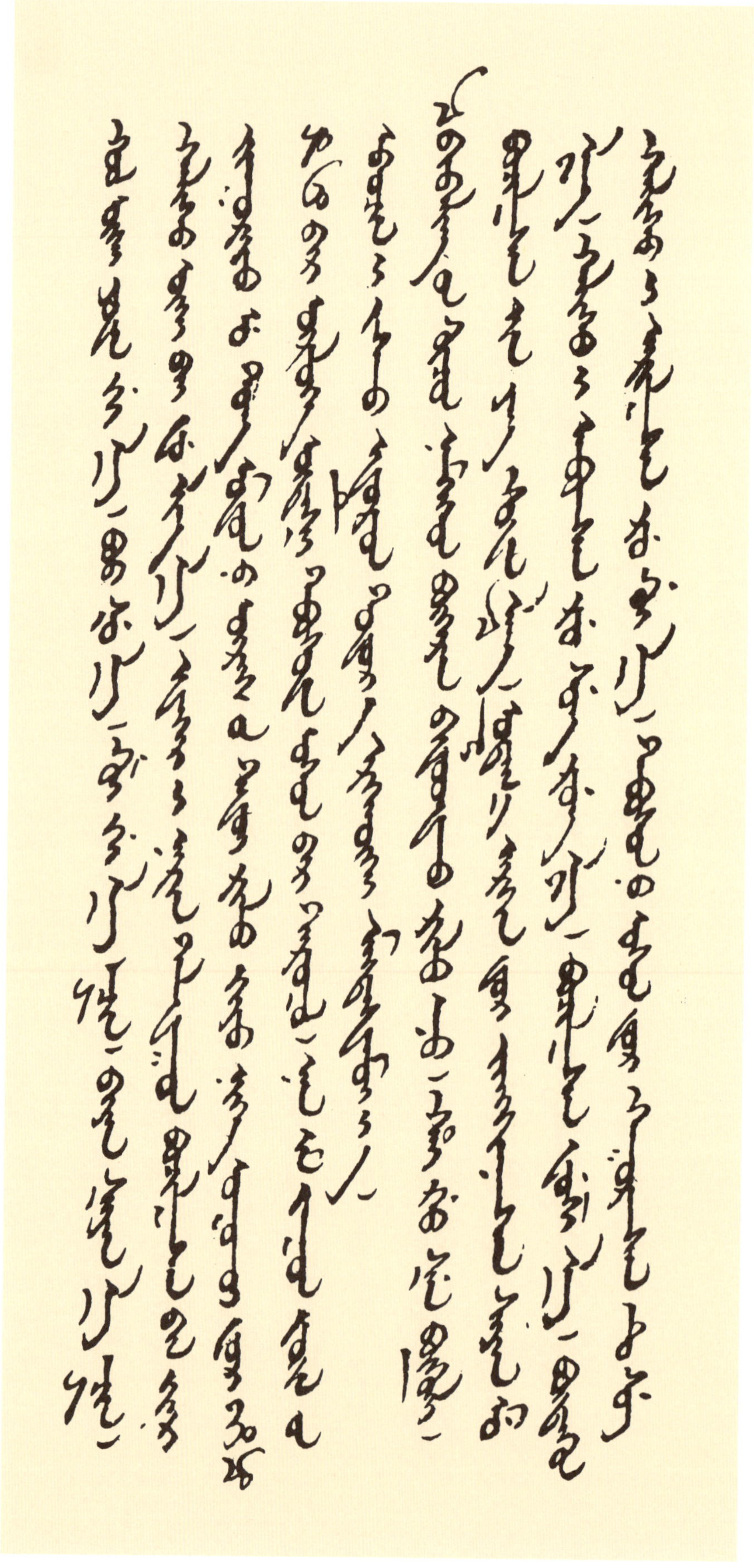

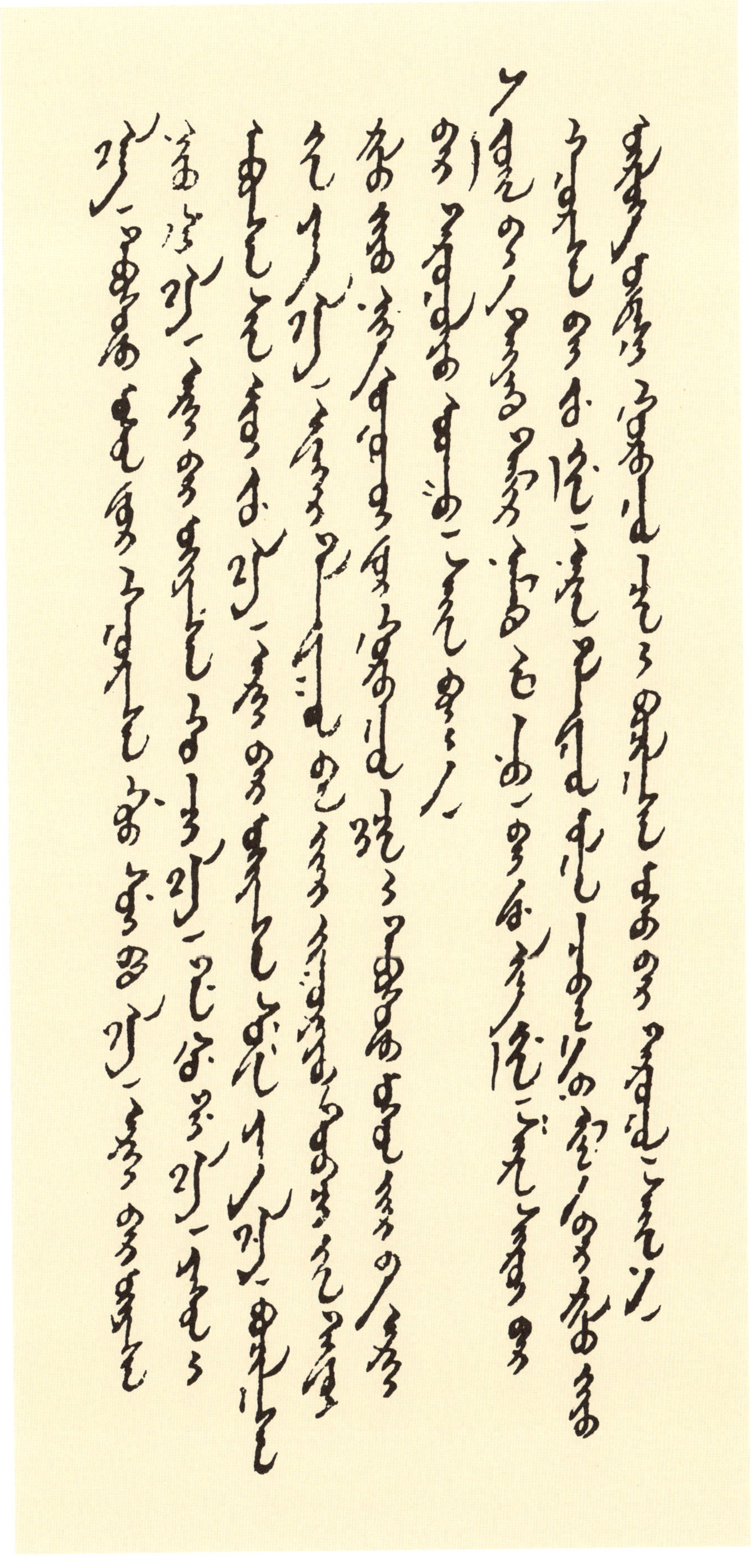

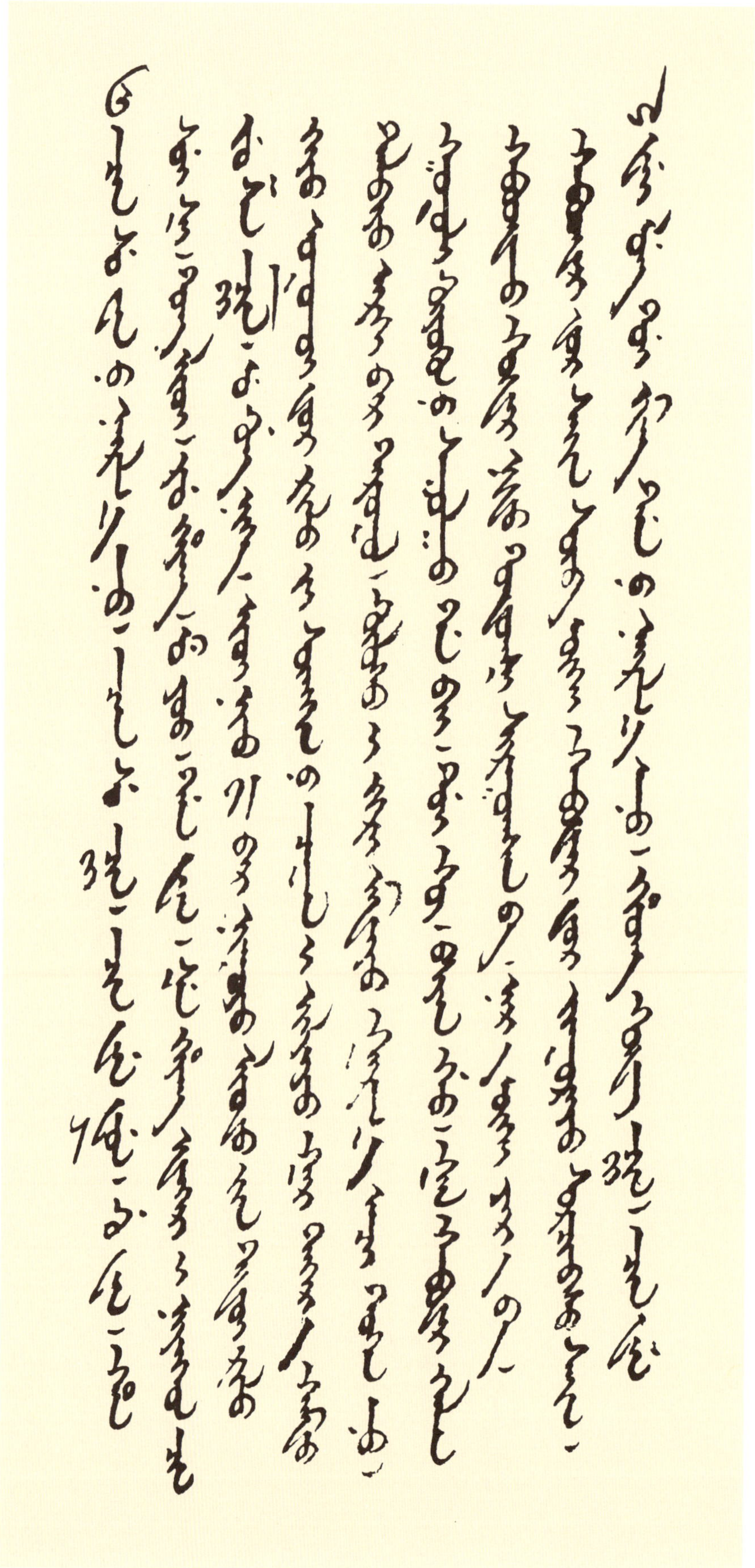

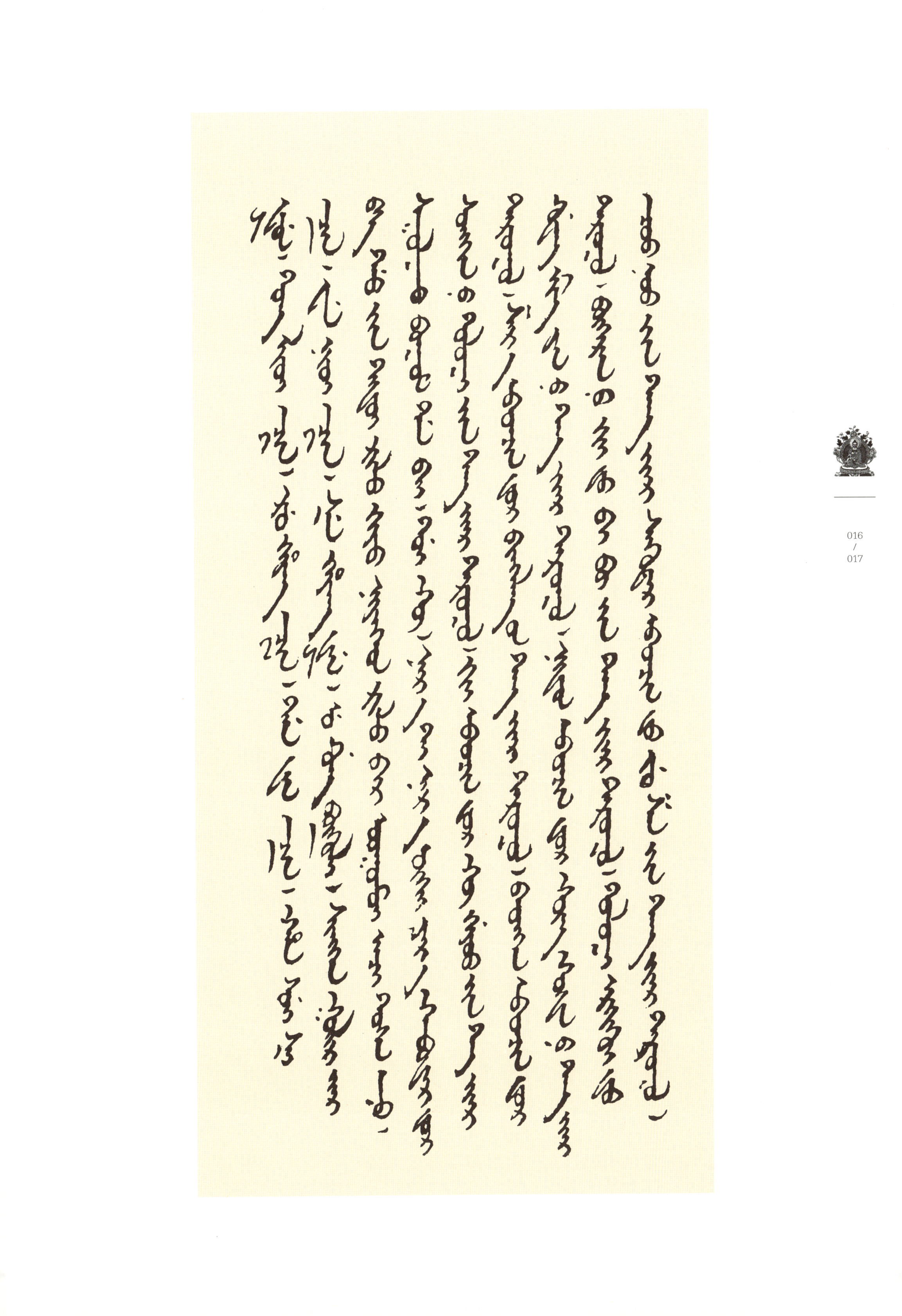

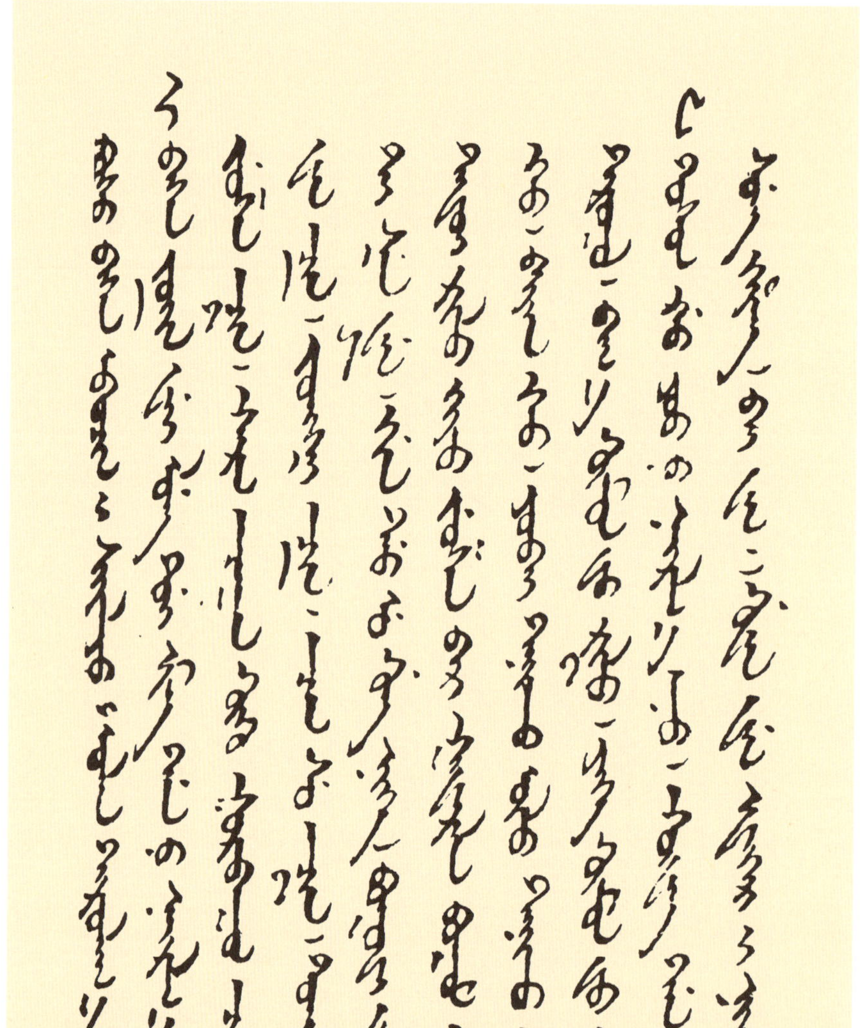

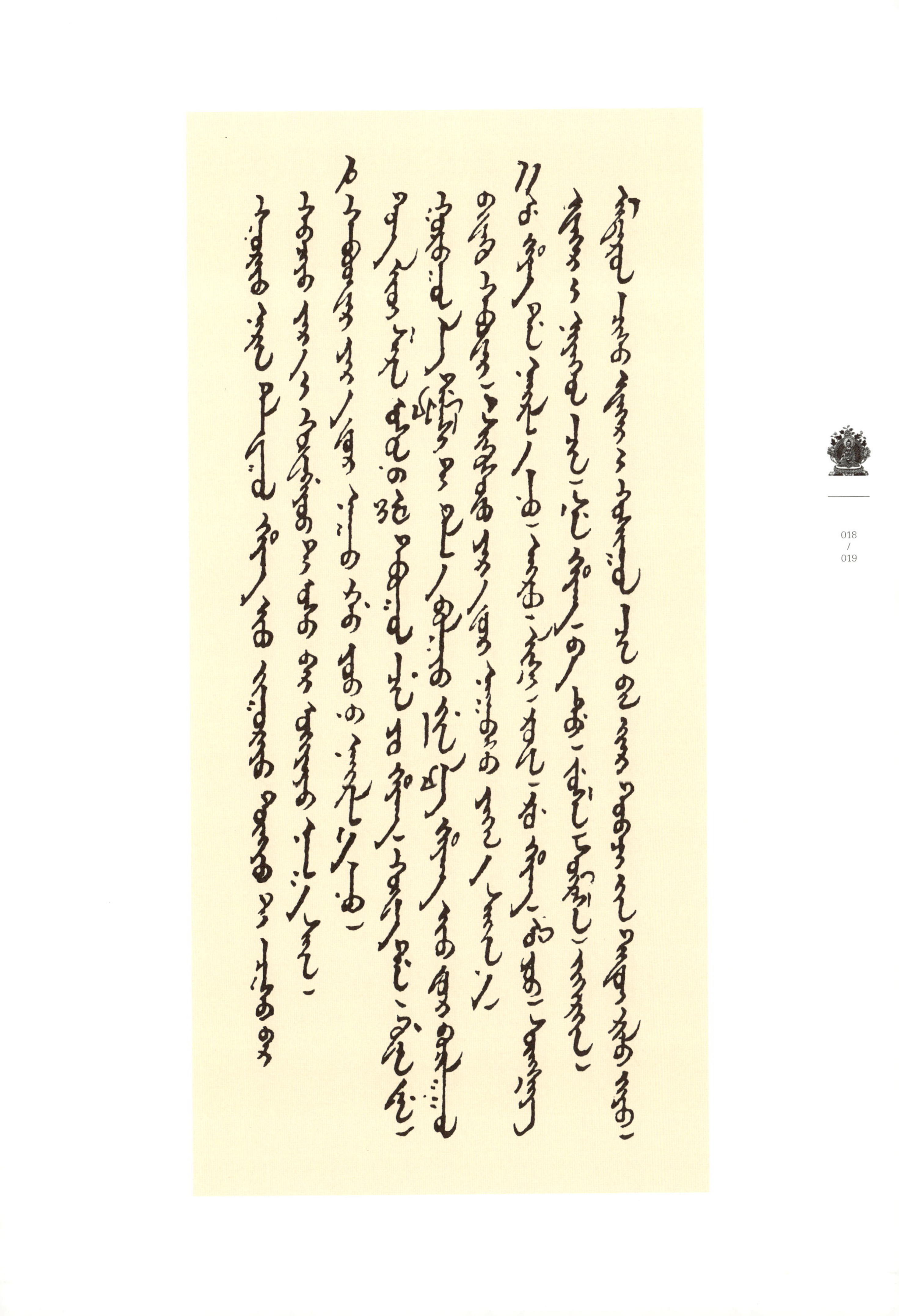

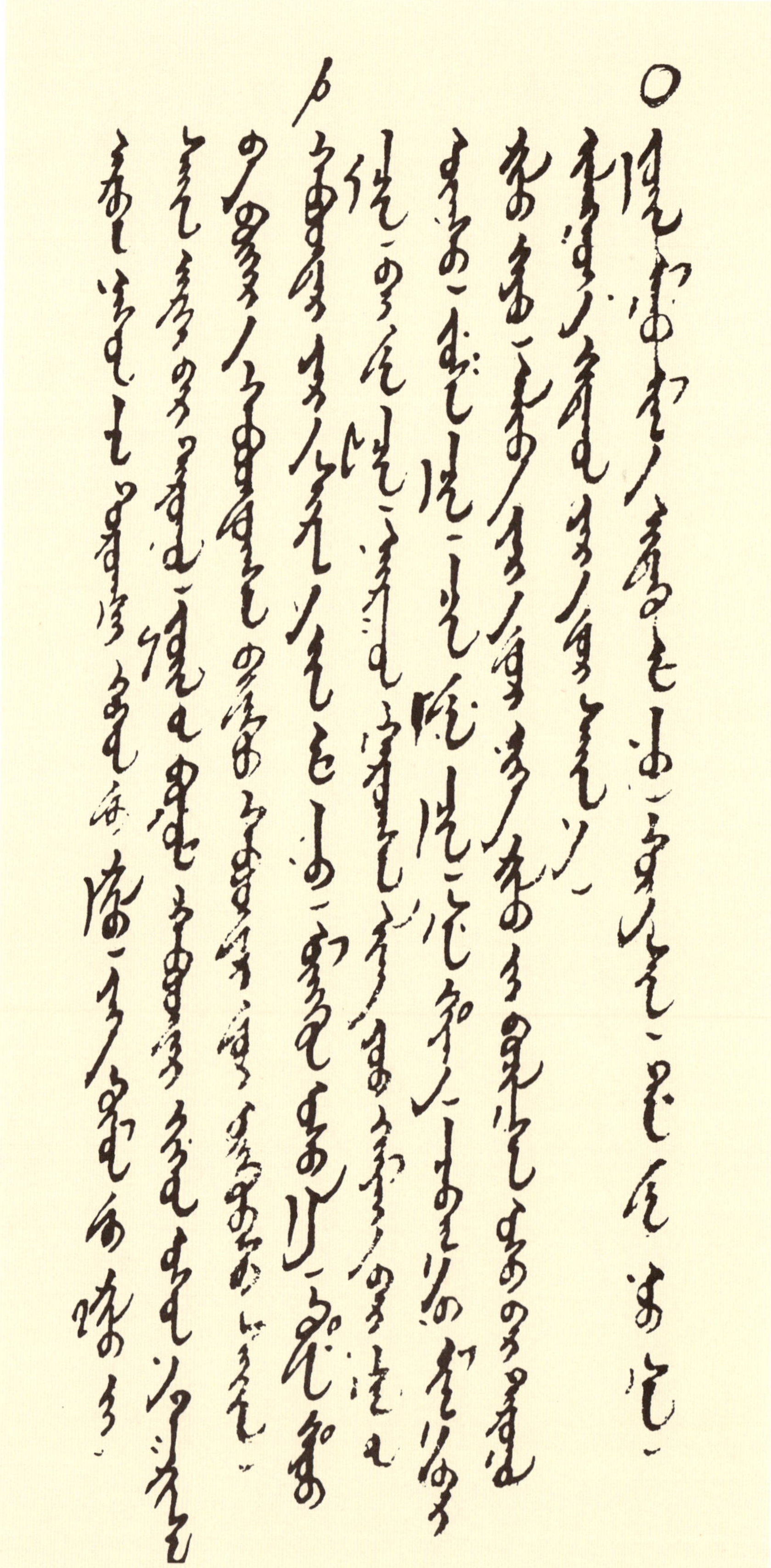

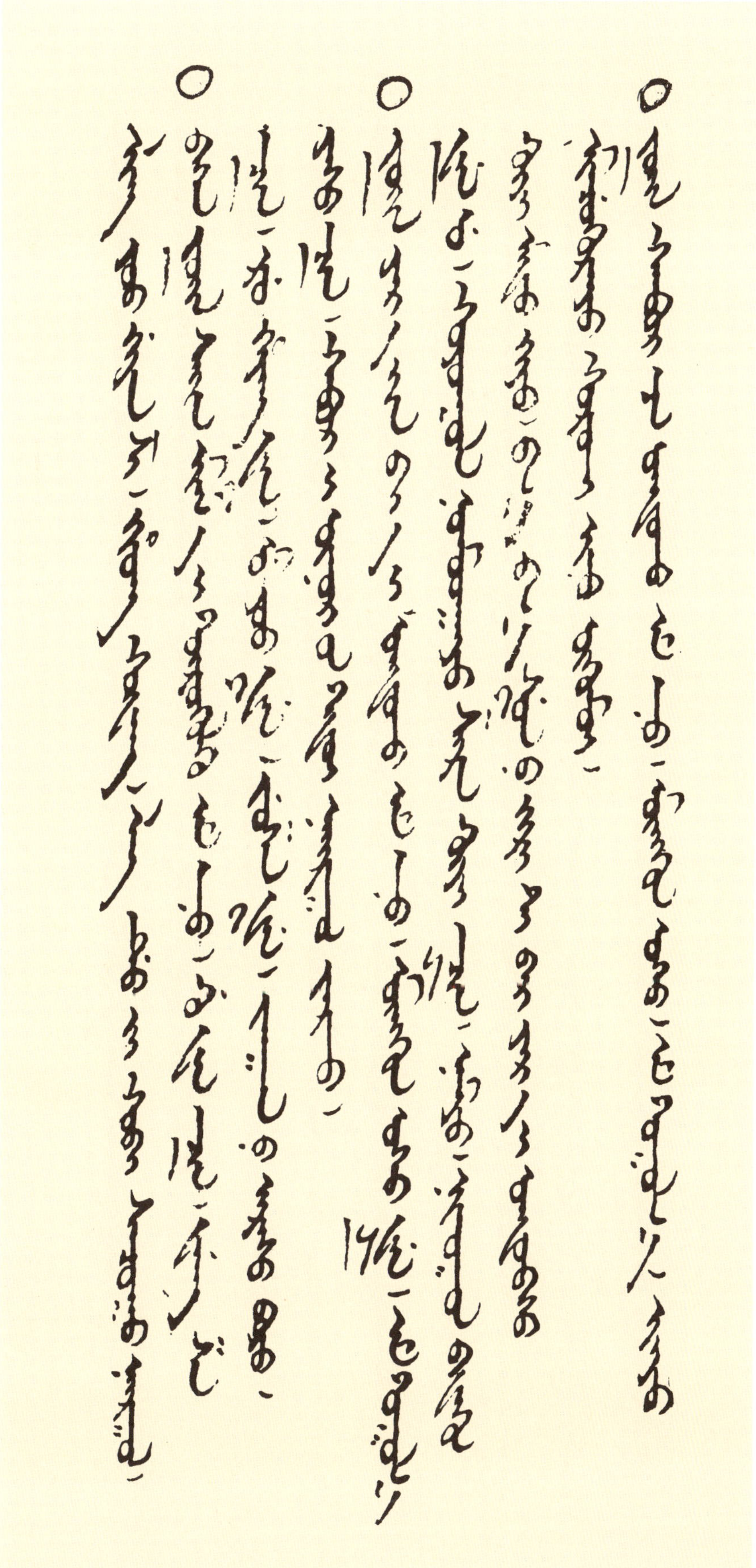

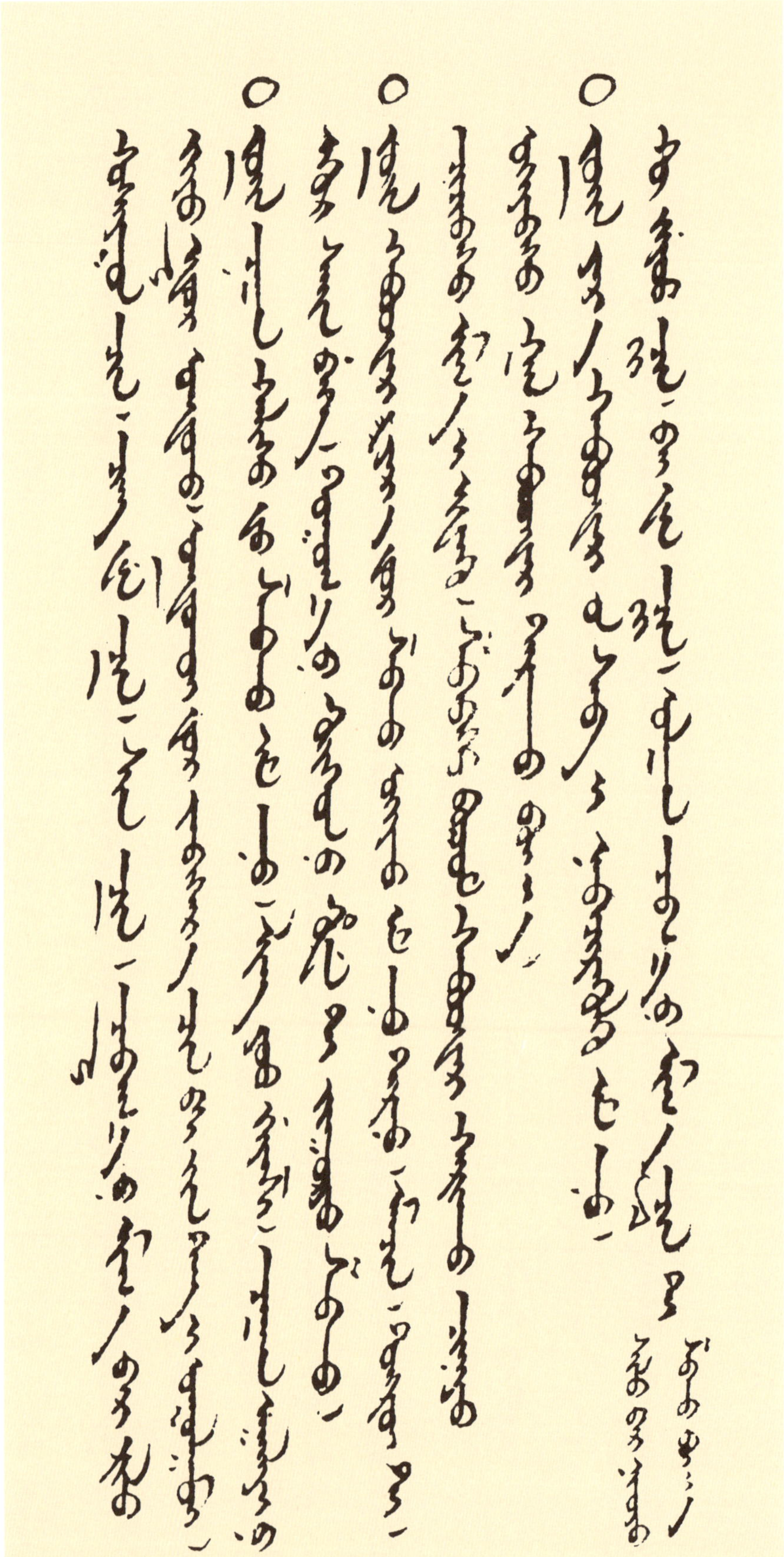

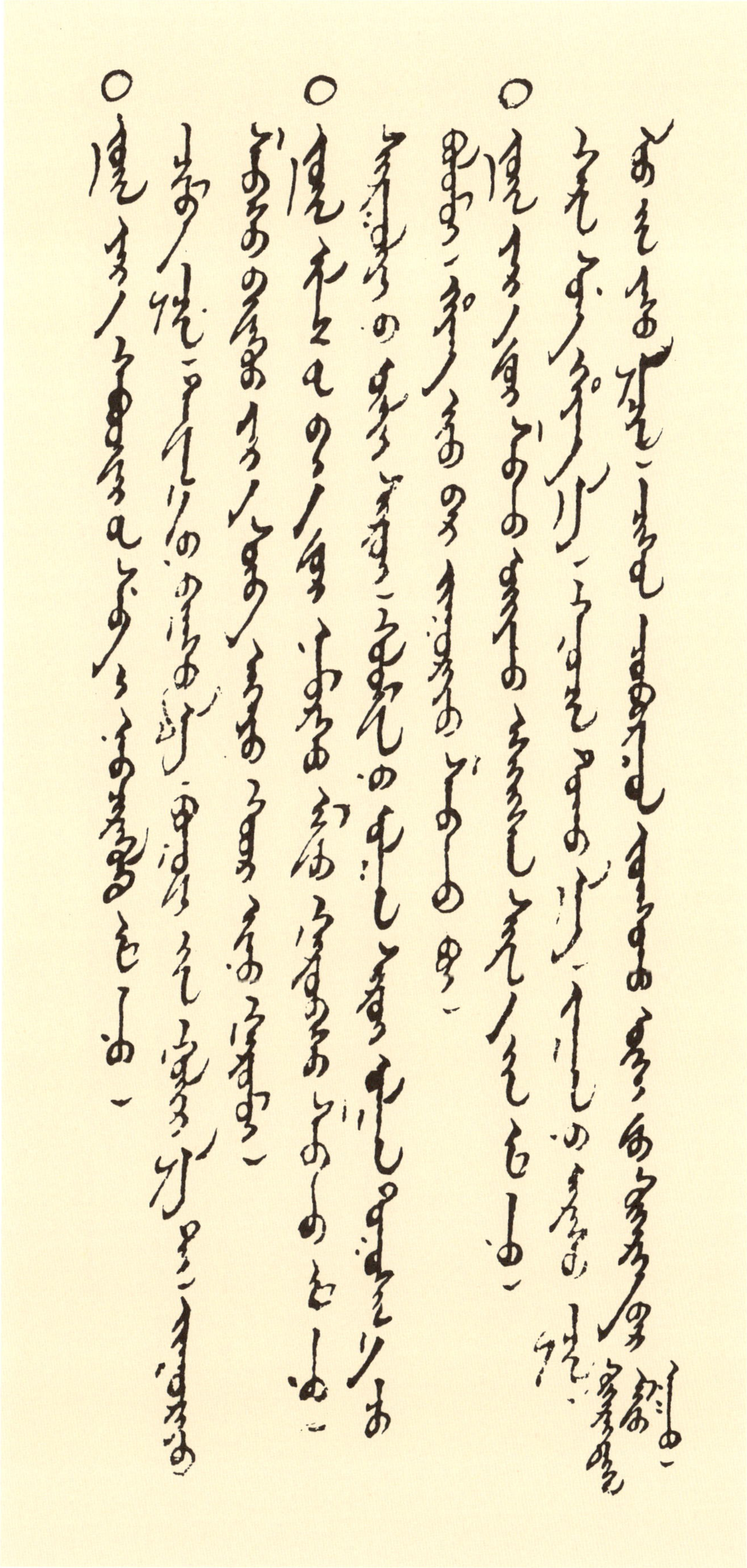

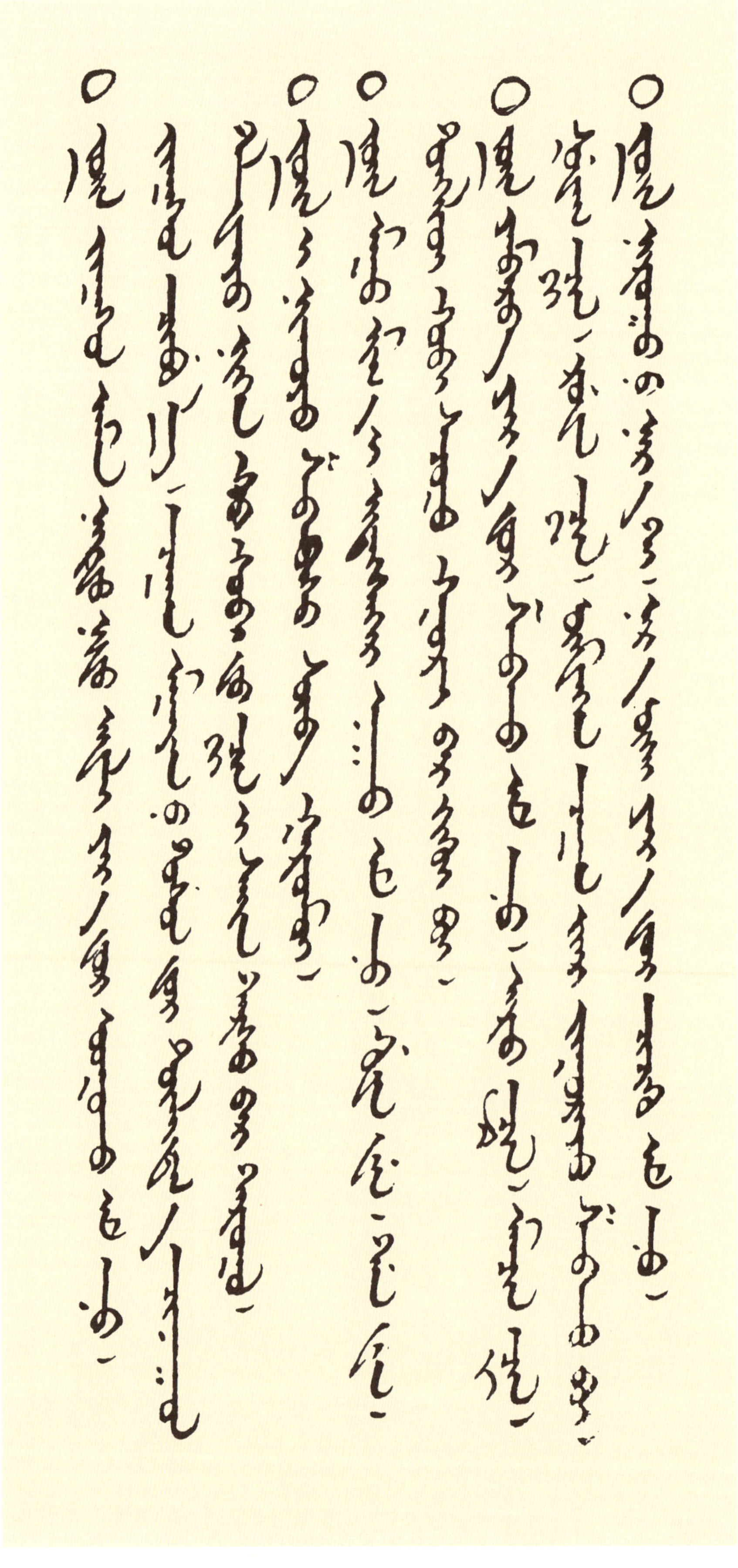

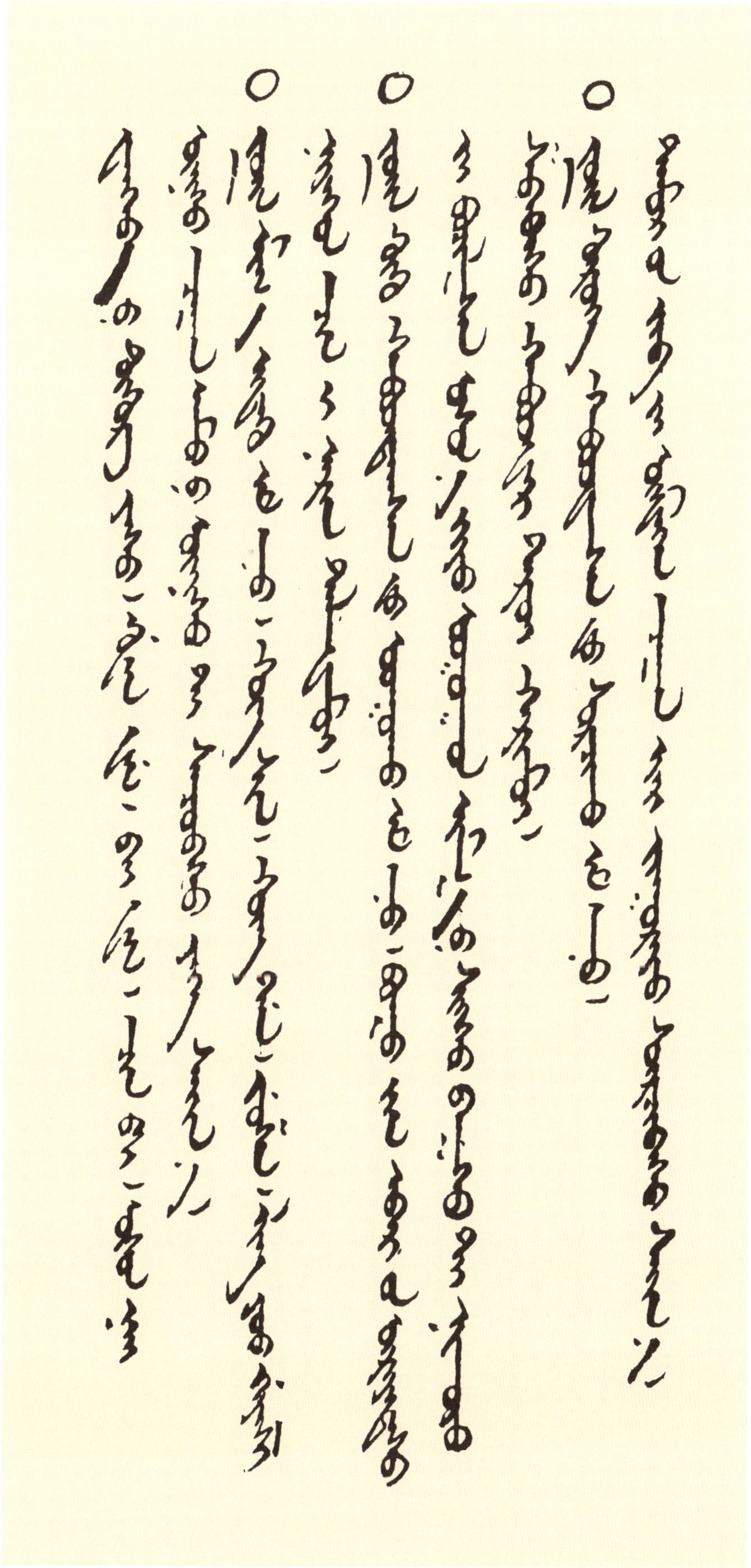

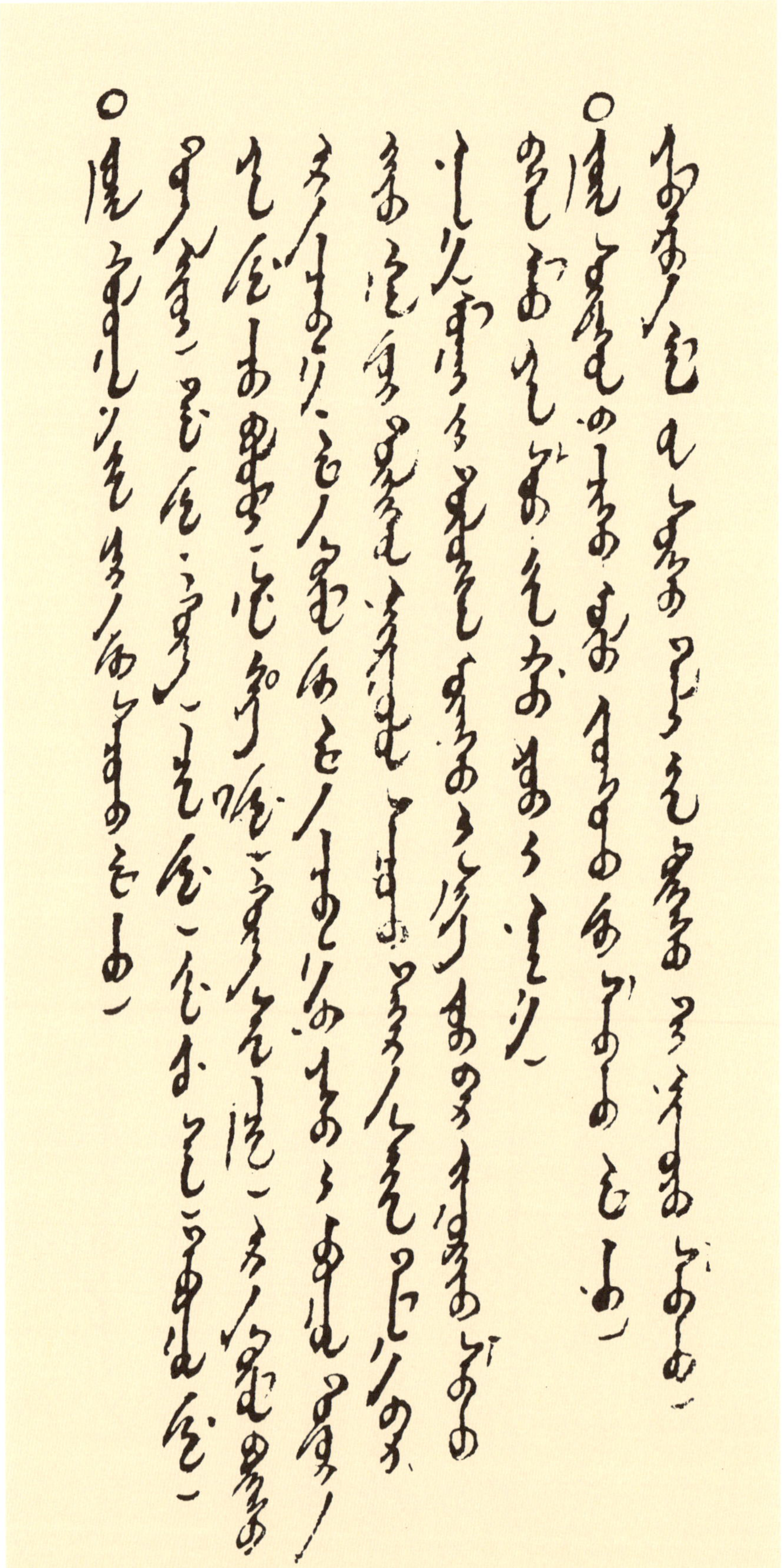

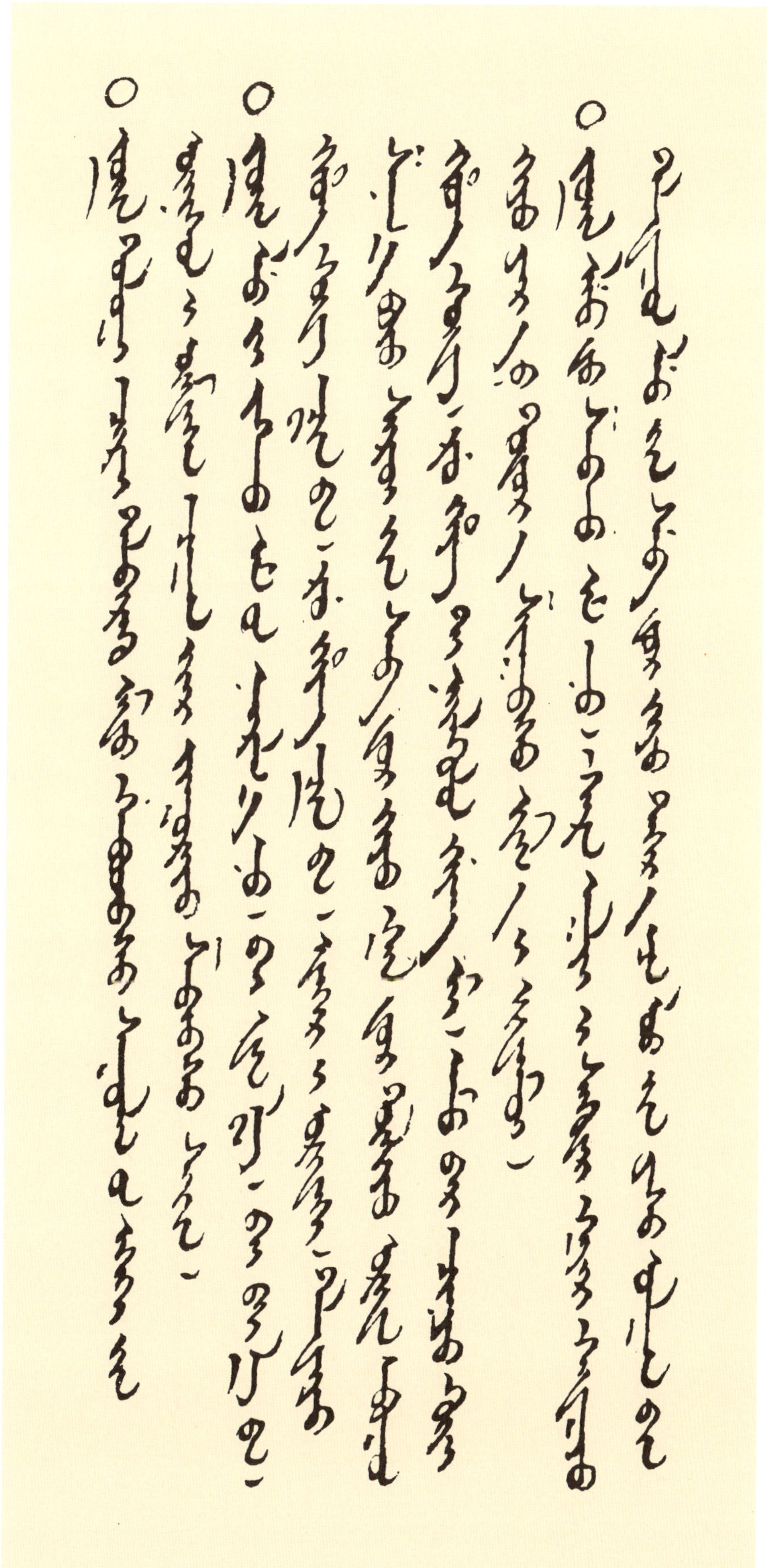

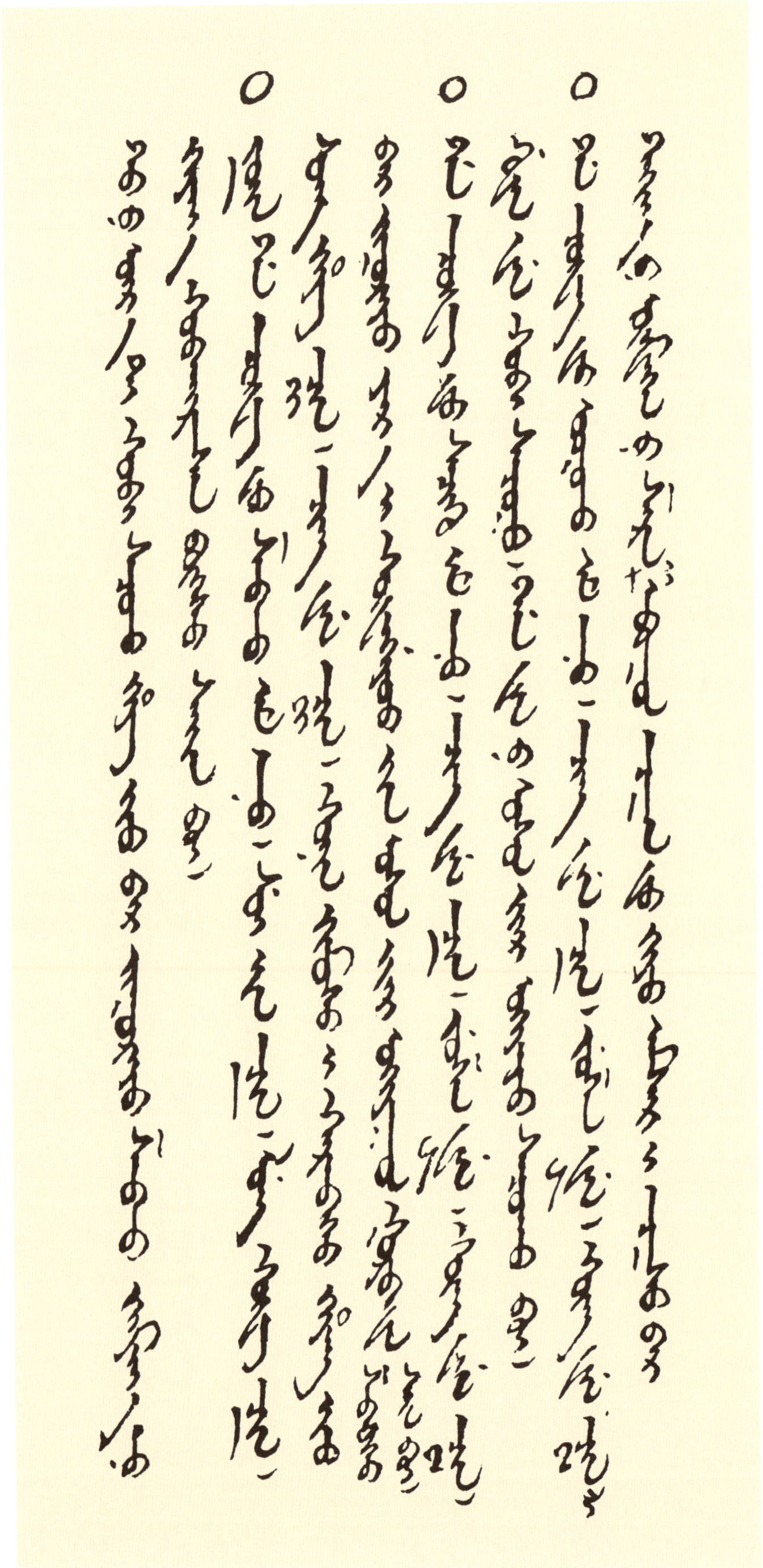

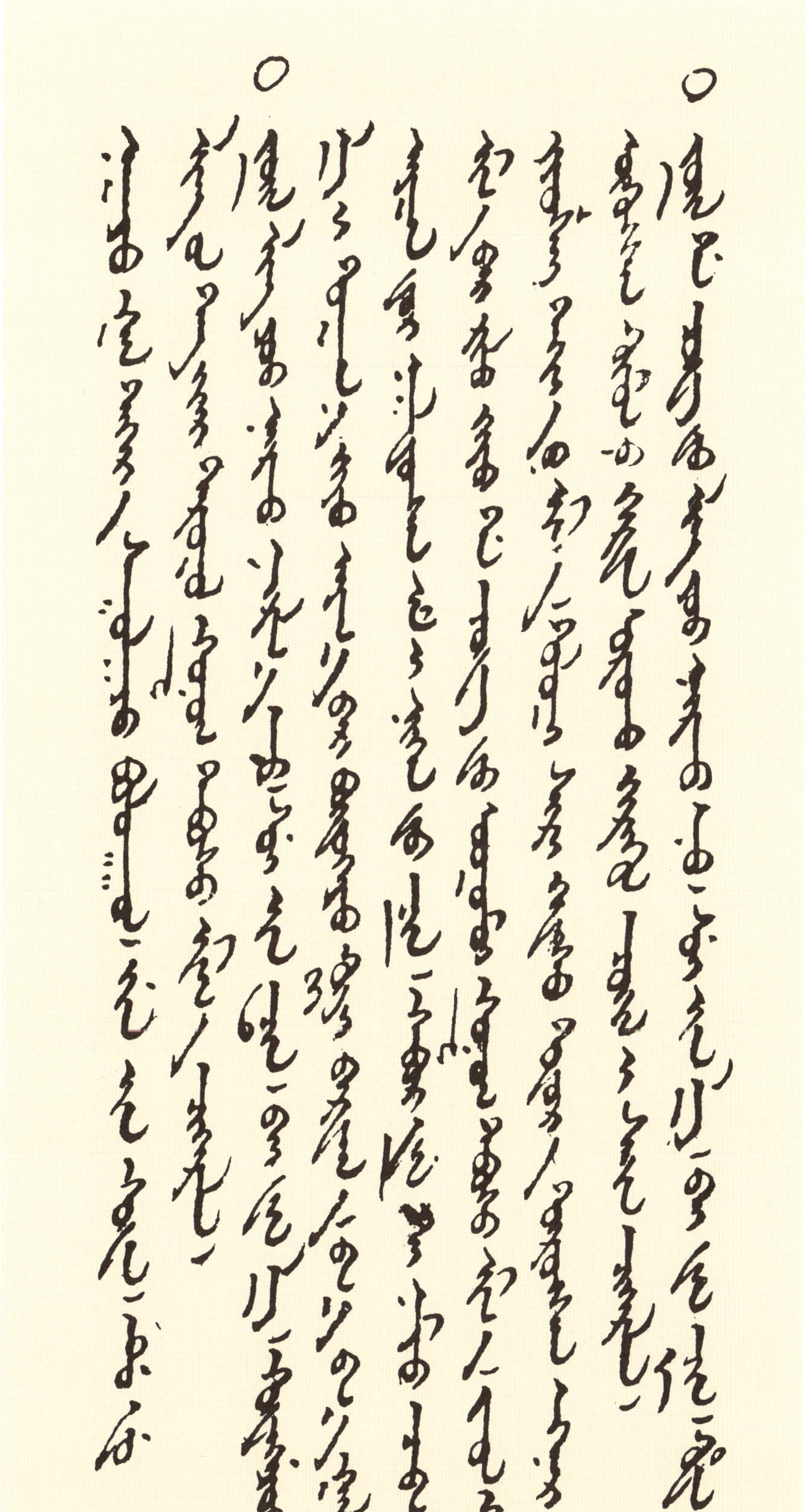

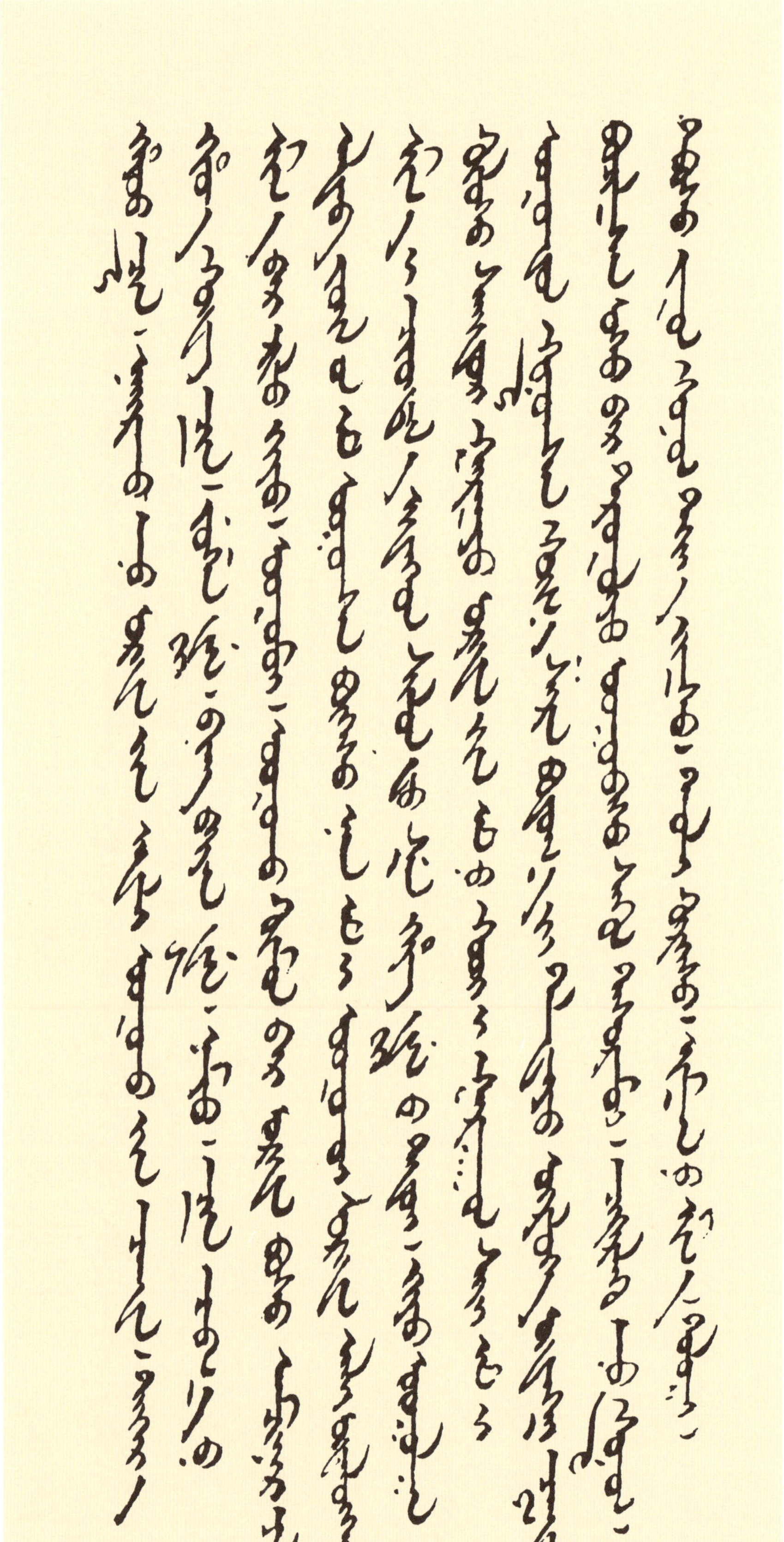

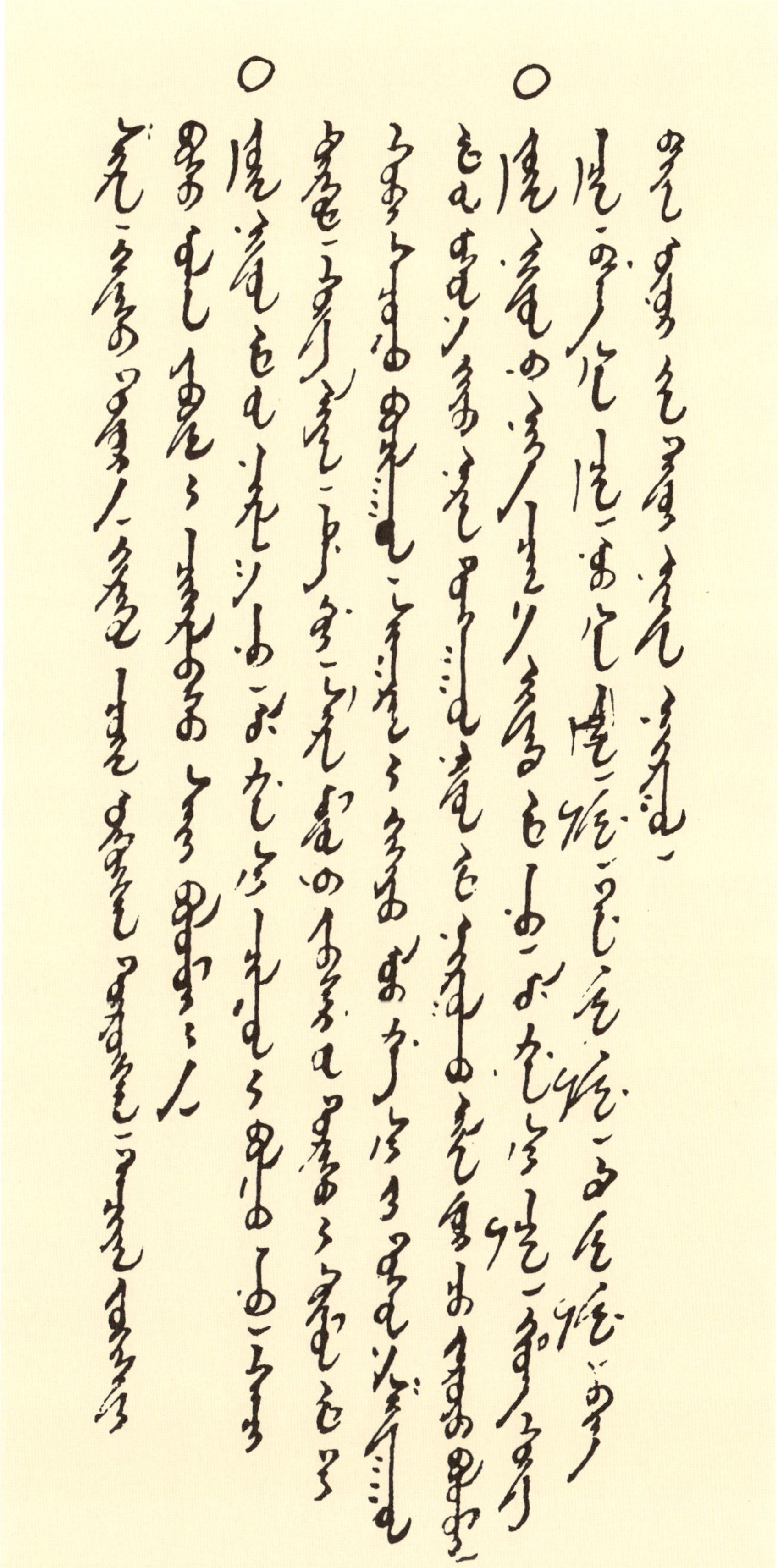

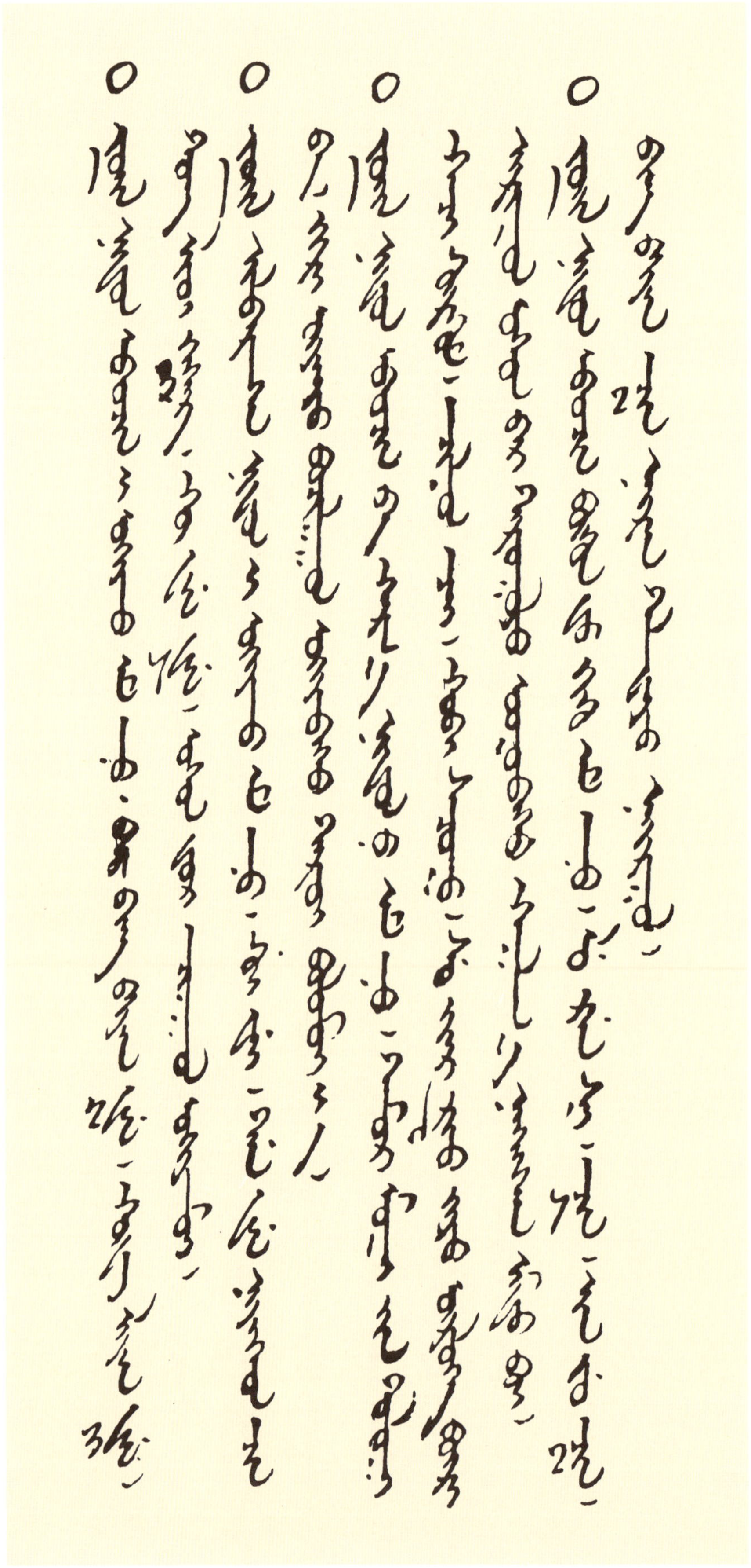

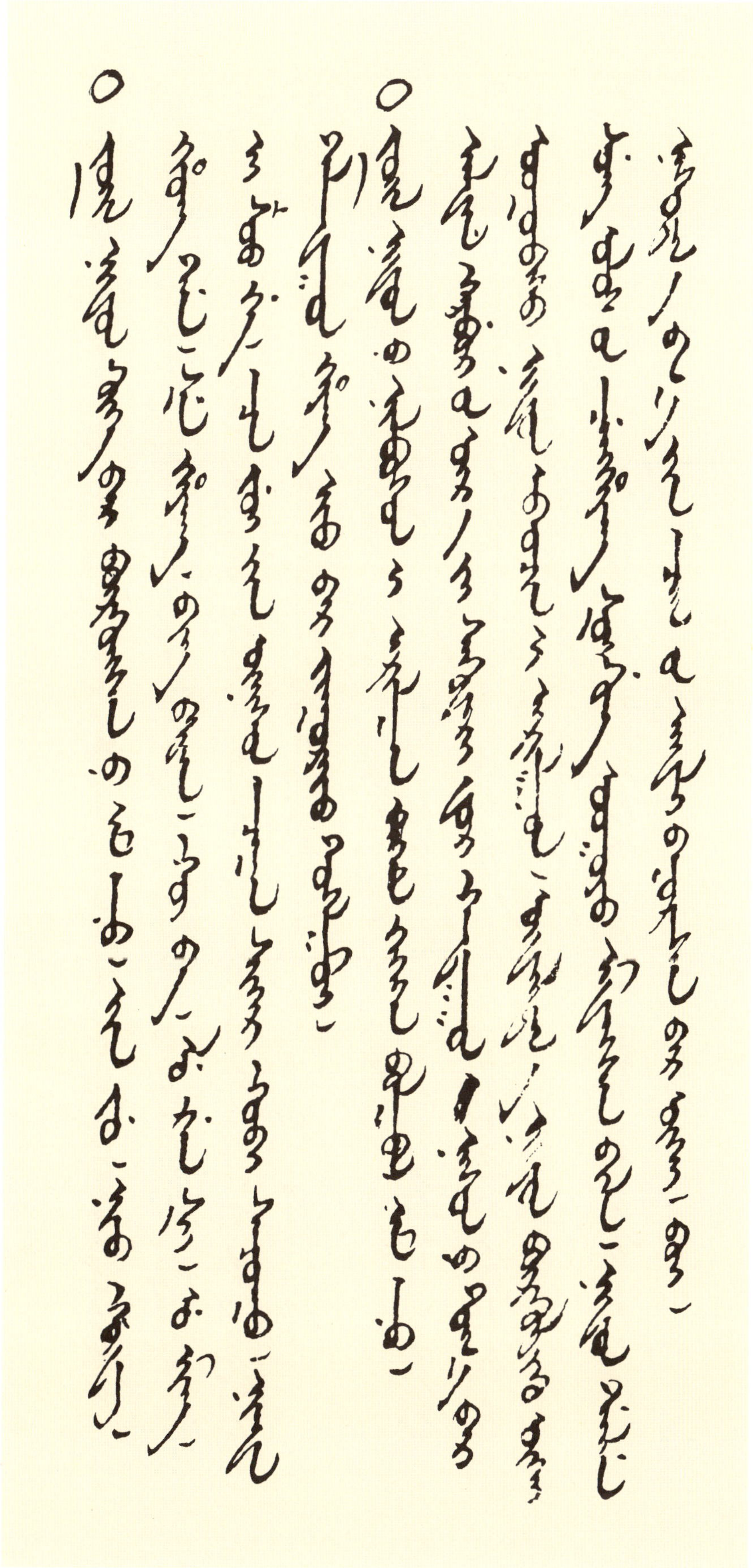

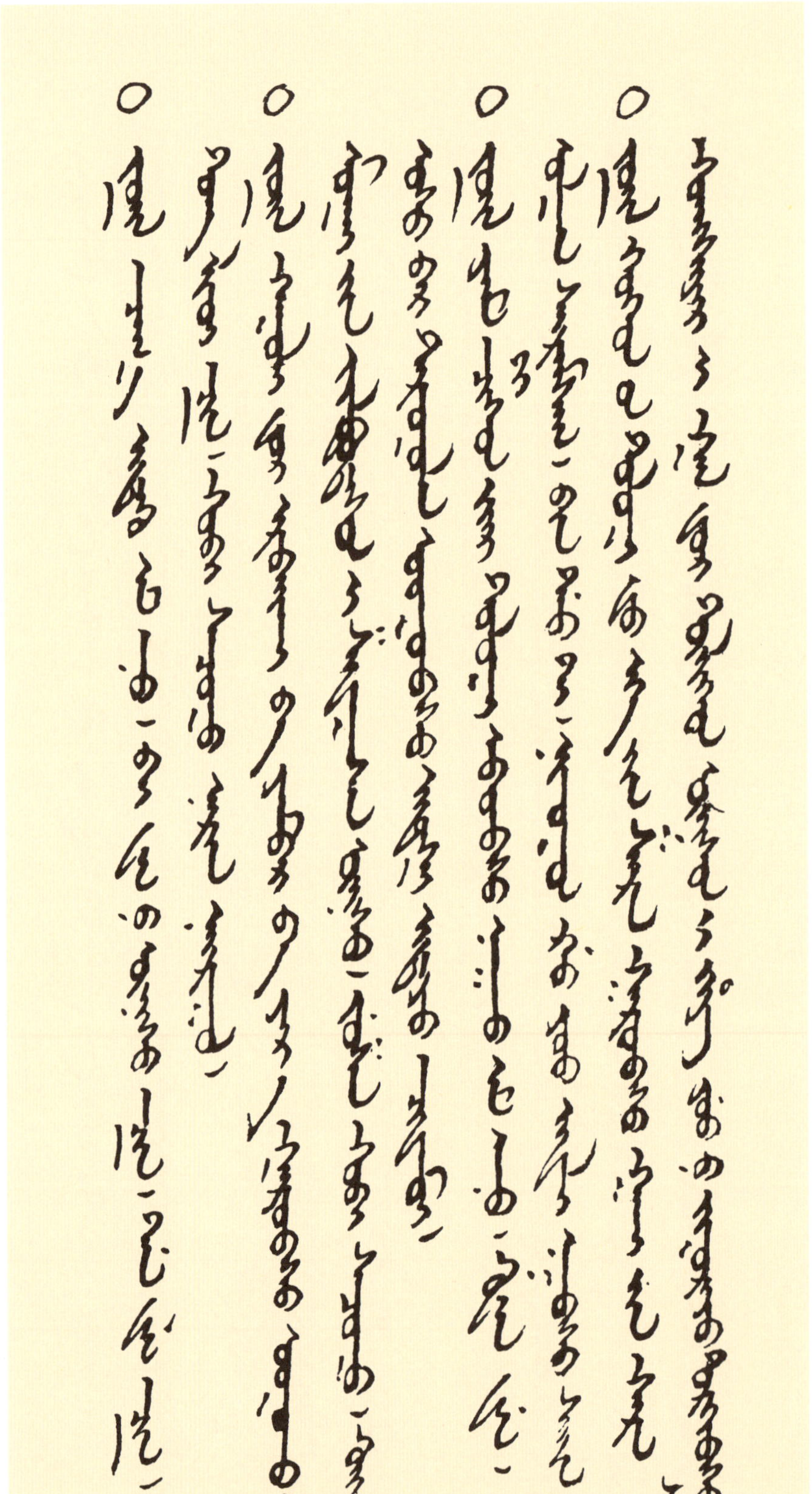

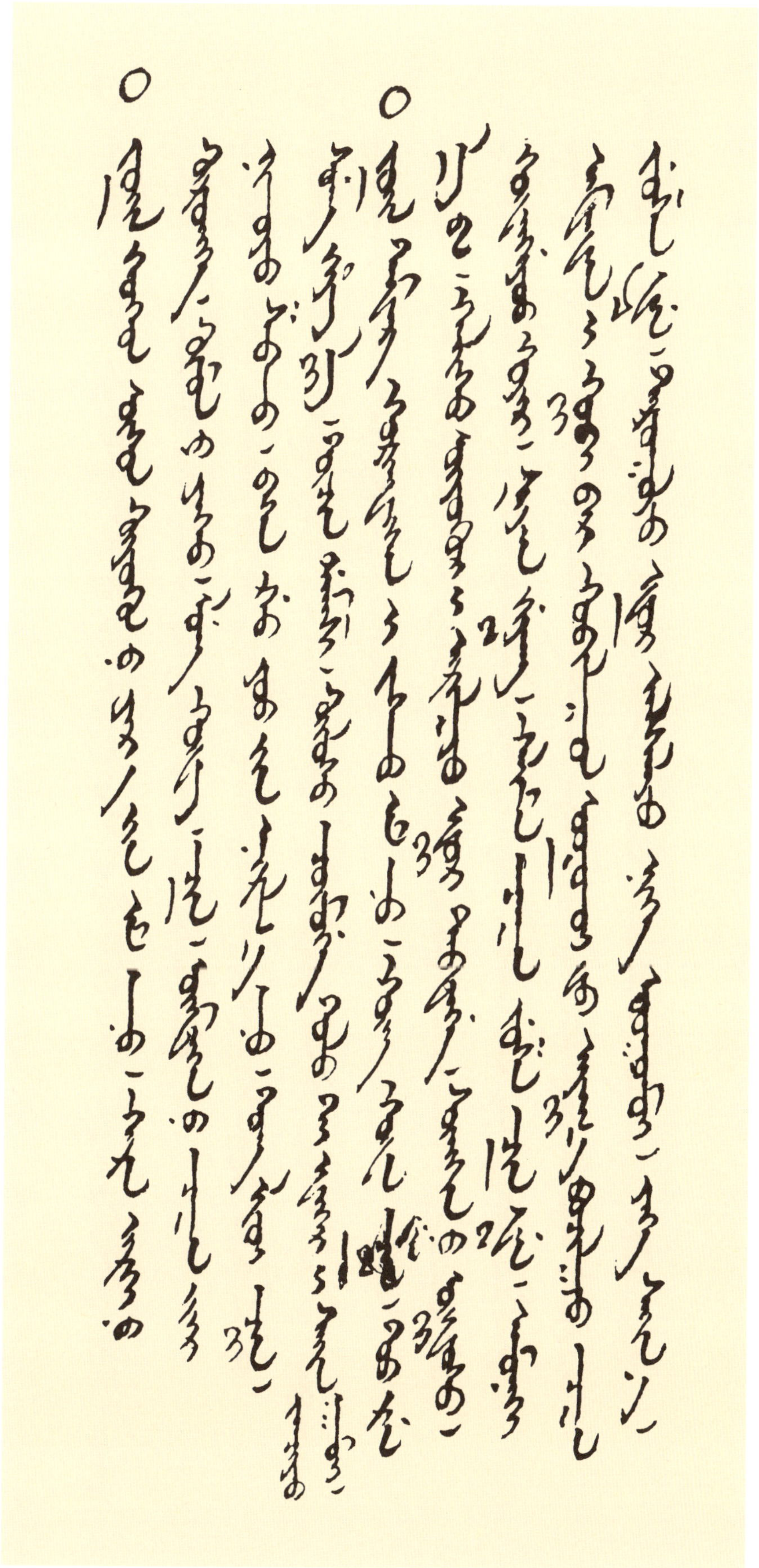

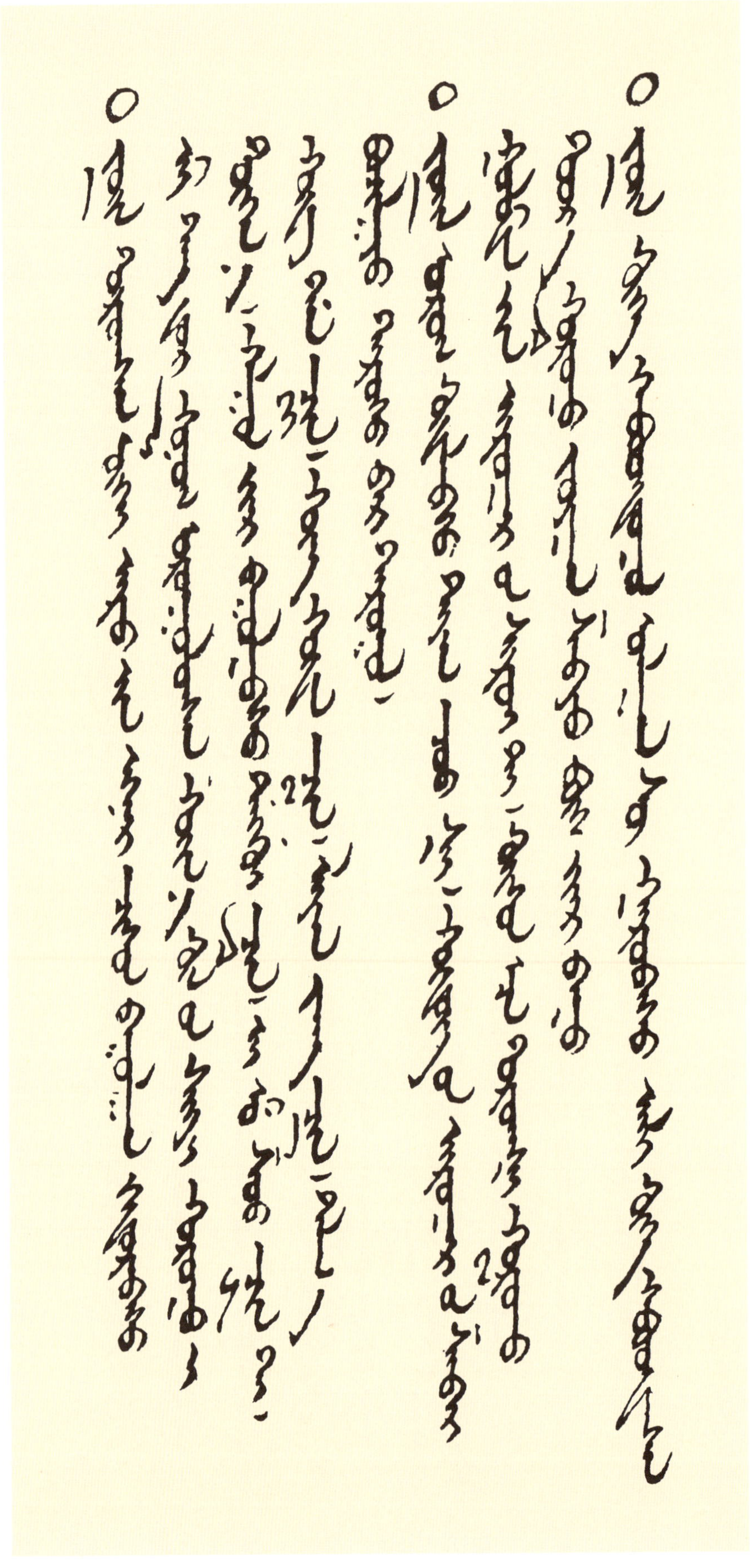

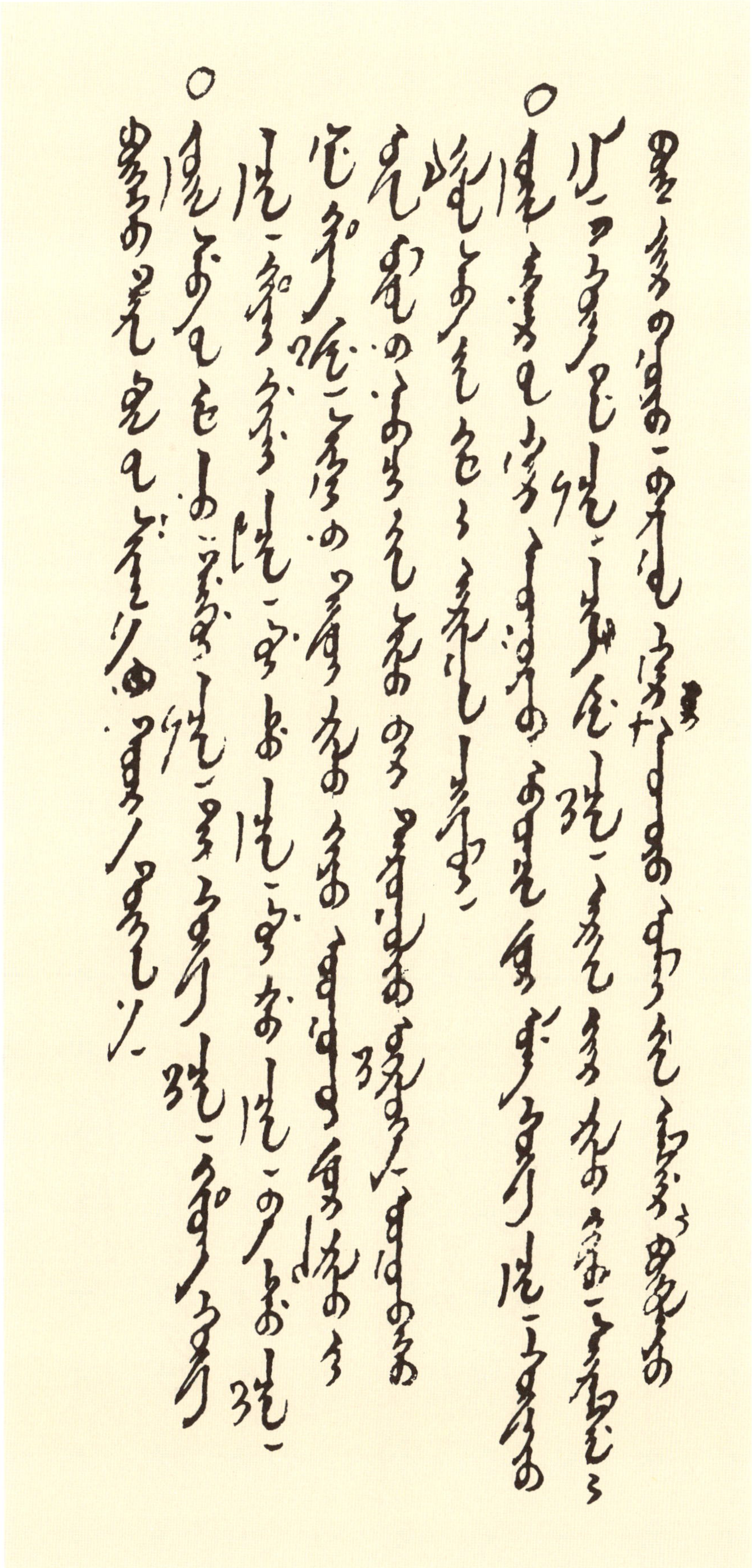

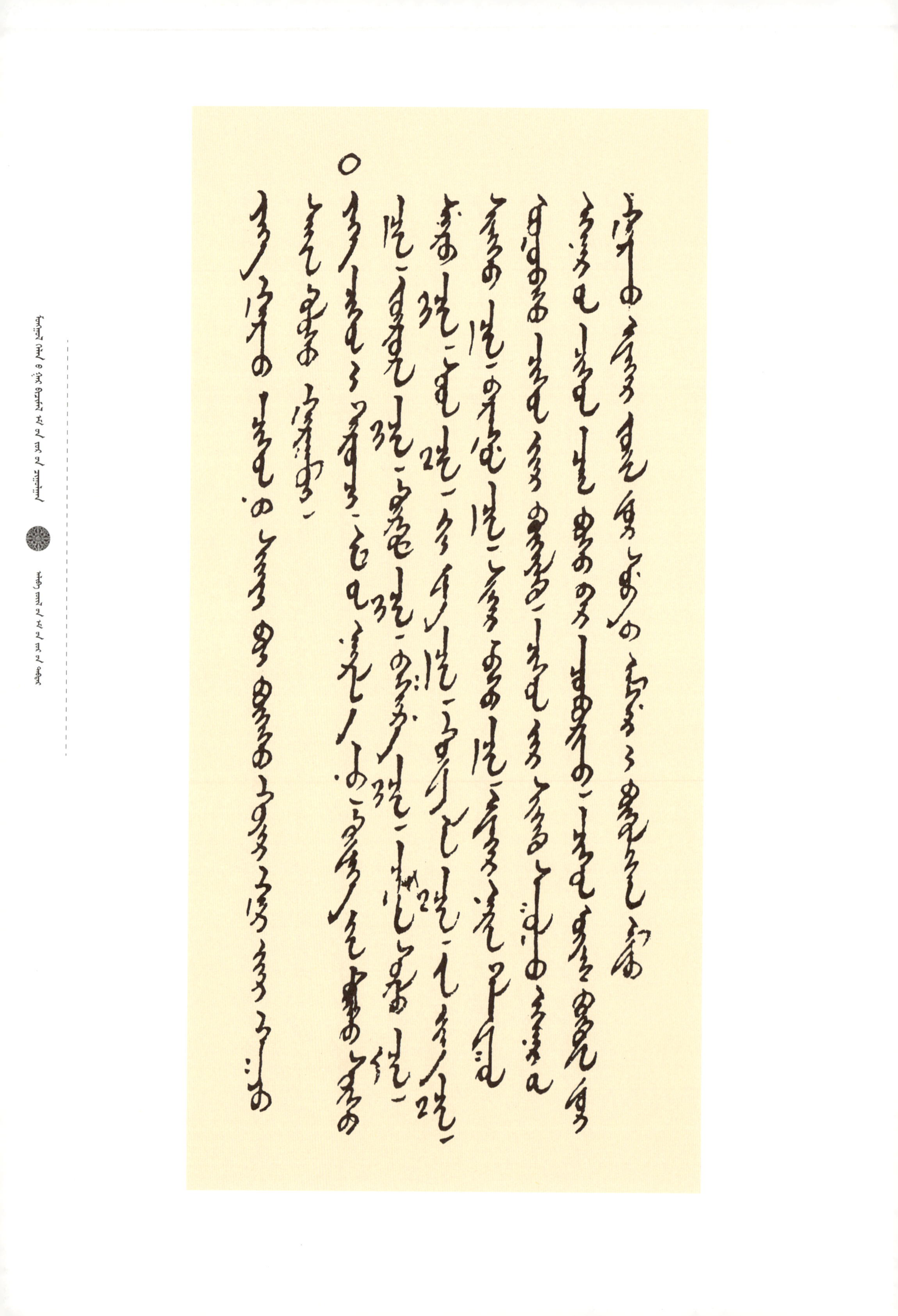

[illegible]

[illegible]

[illegible]

[illegible]

[illegible]

[illegible]

[illegible]

[illegible]

[illegible]

○

[illegible]

[illegible]

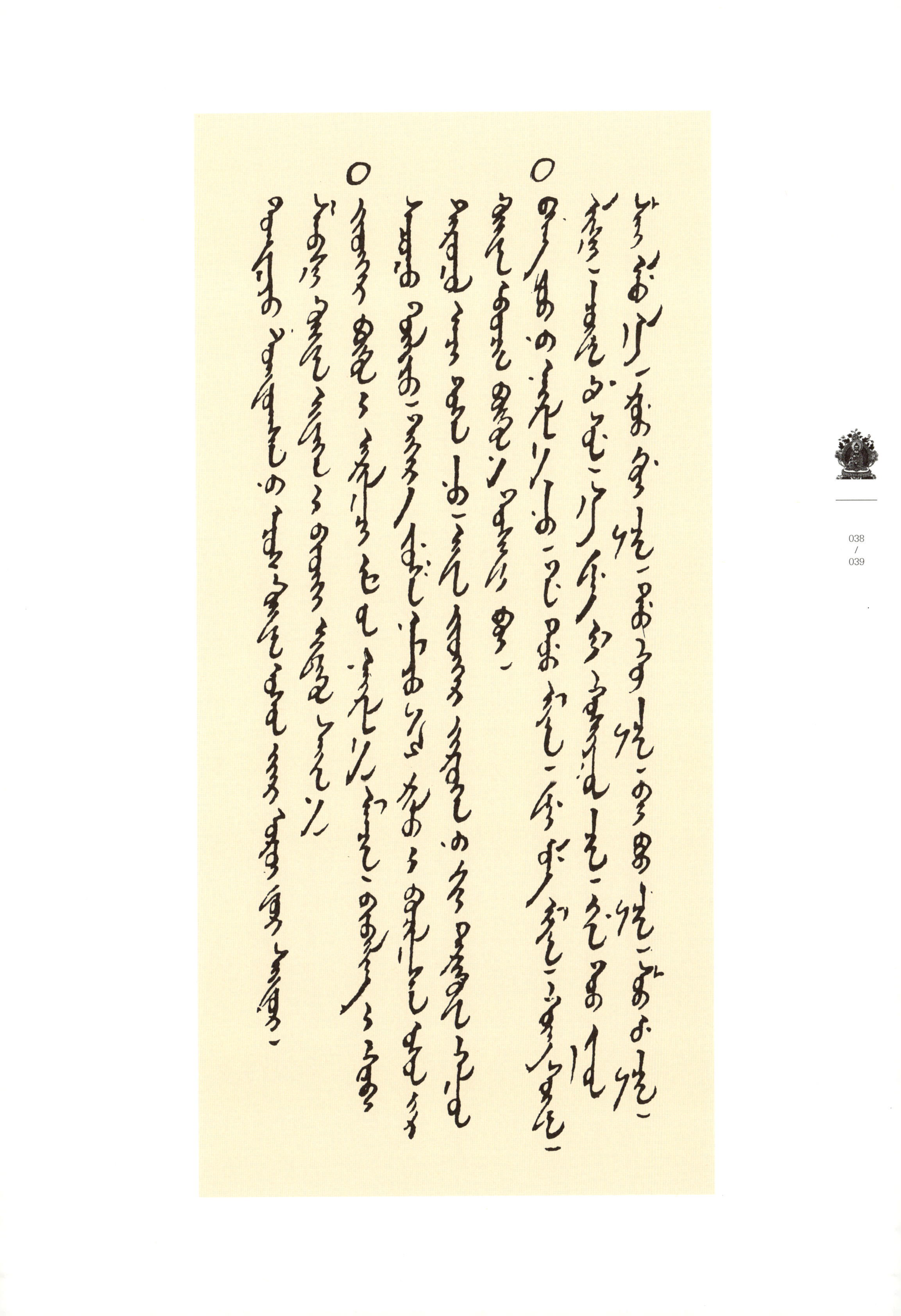

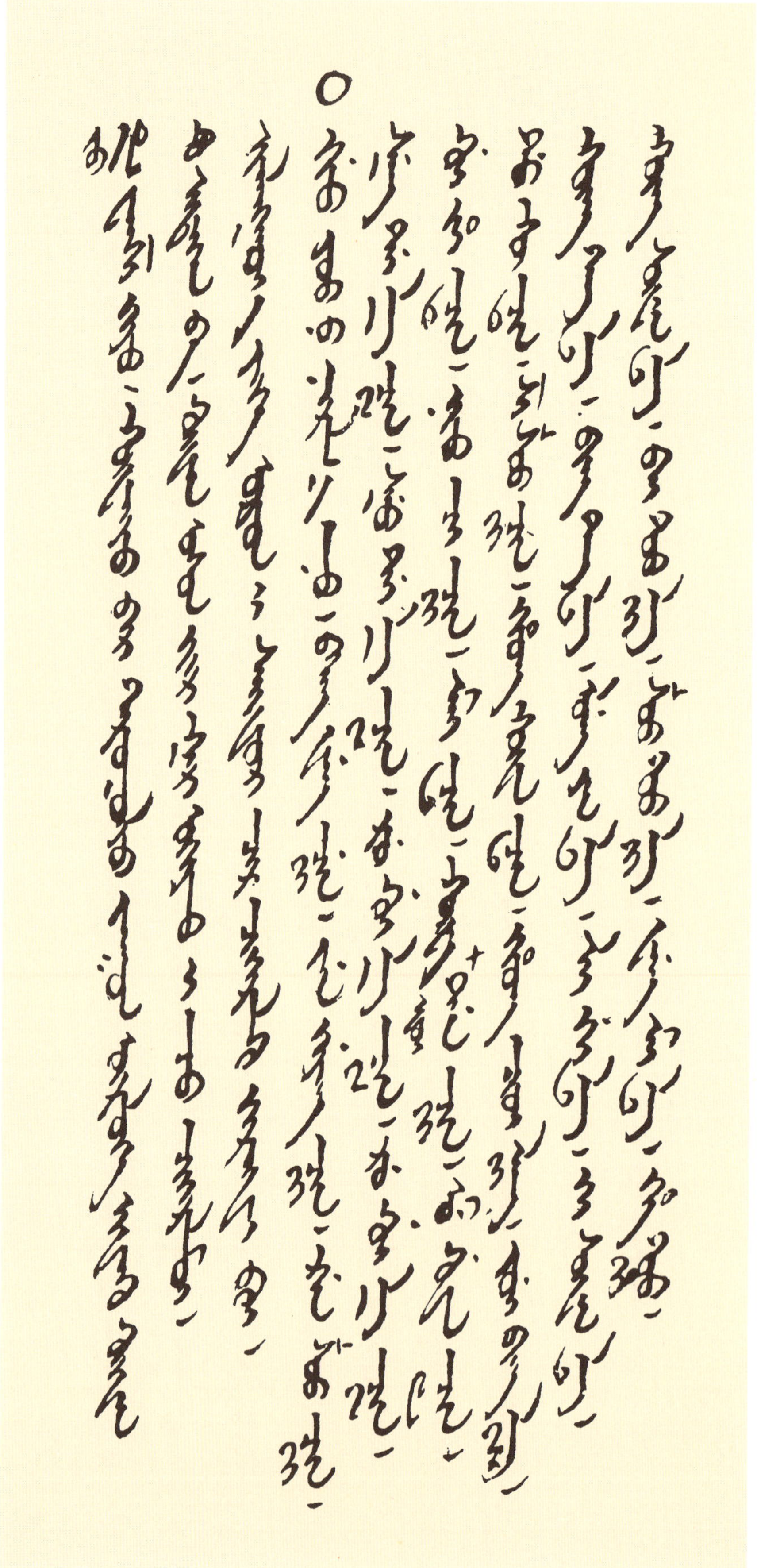

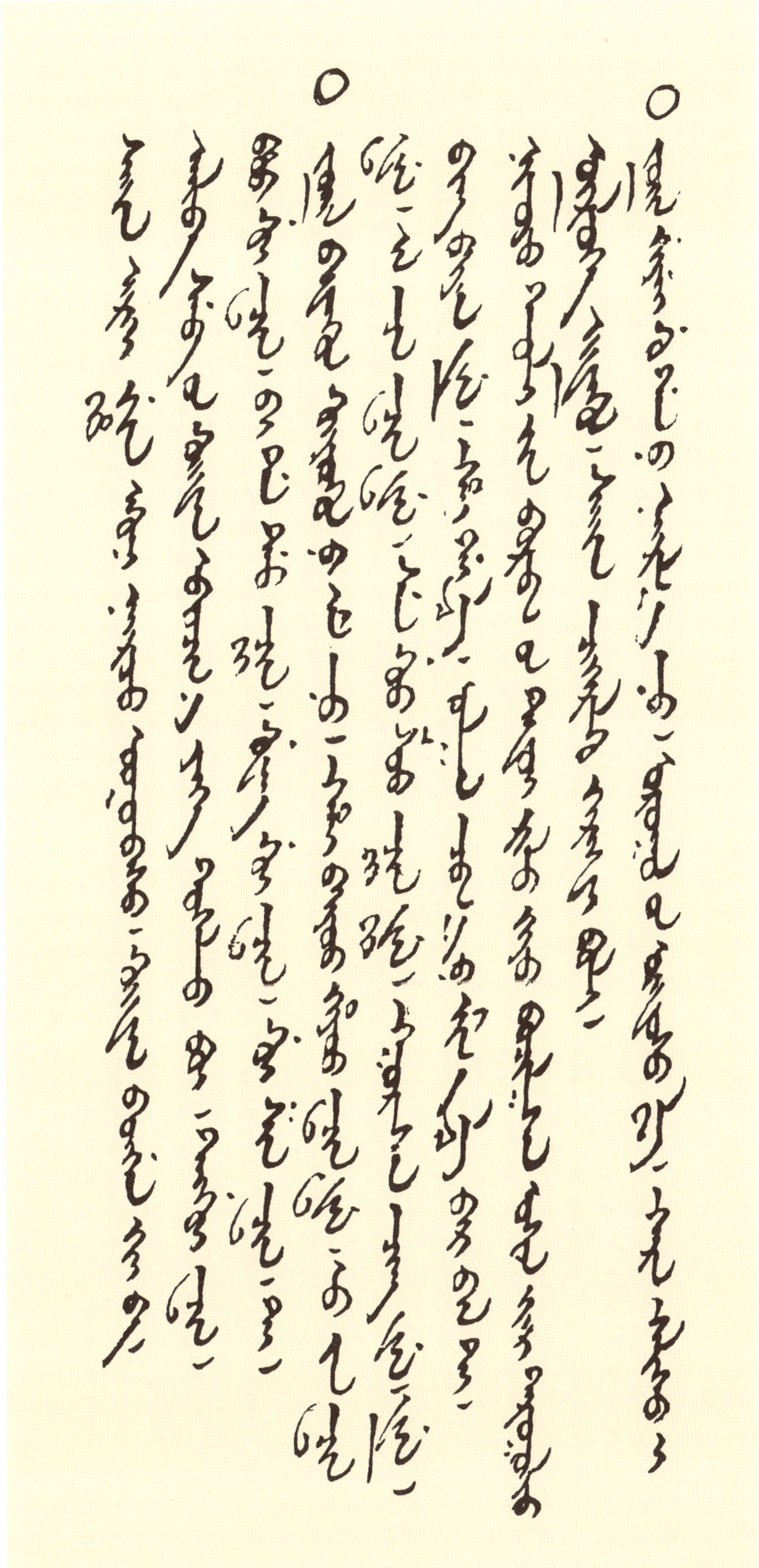

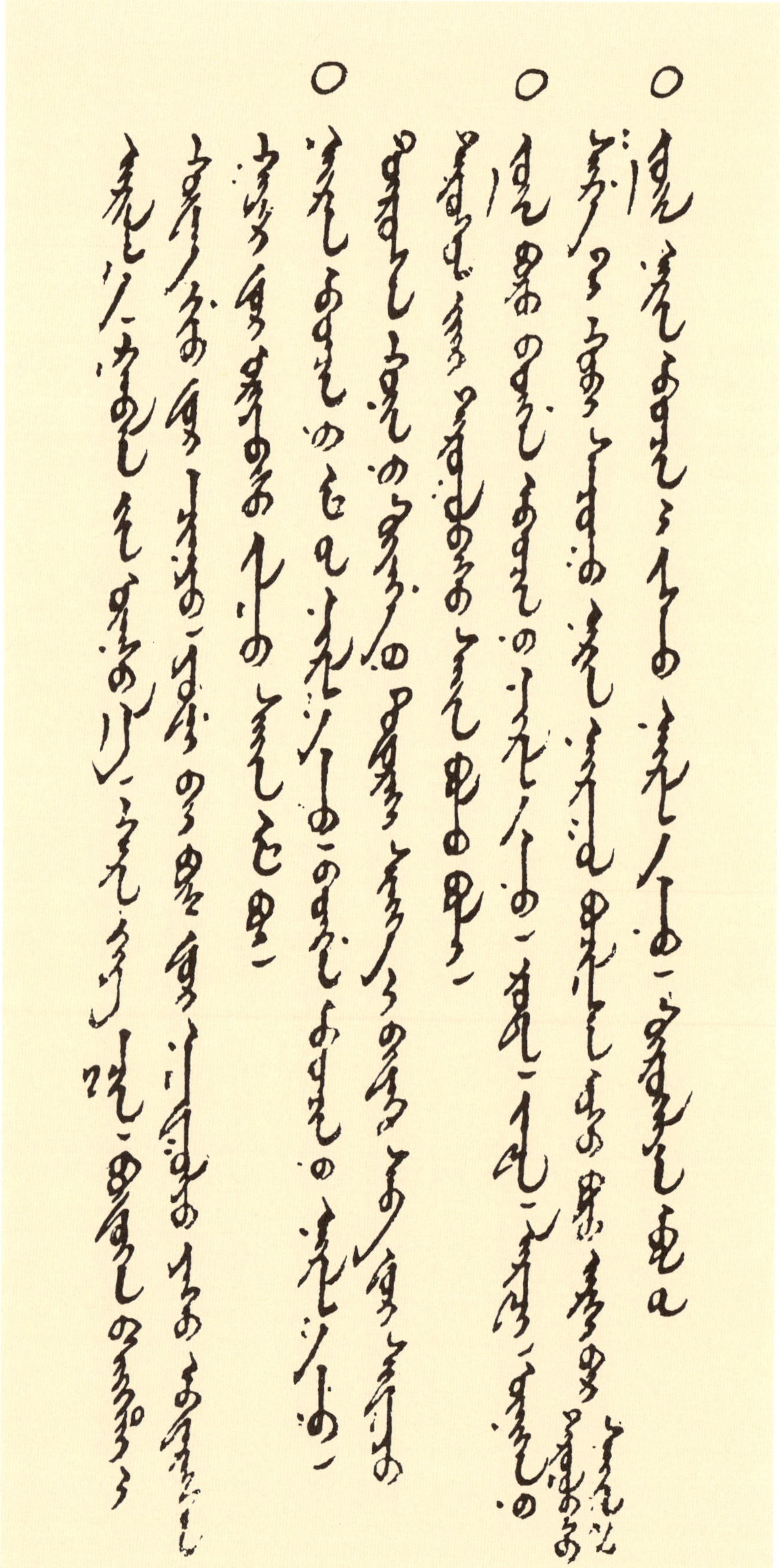

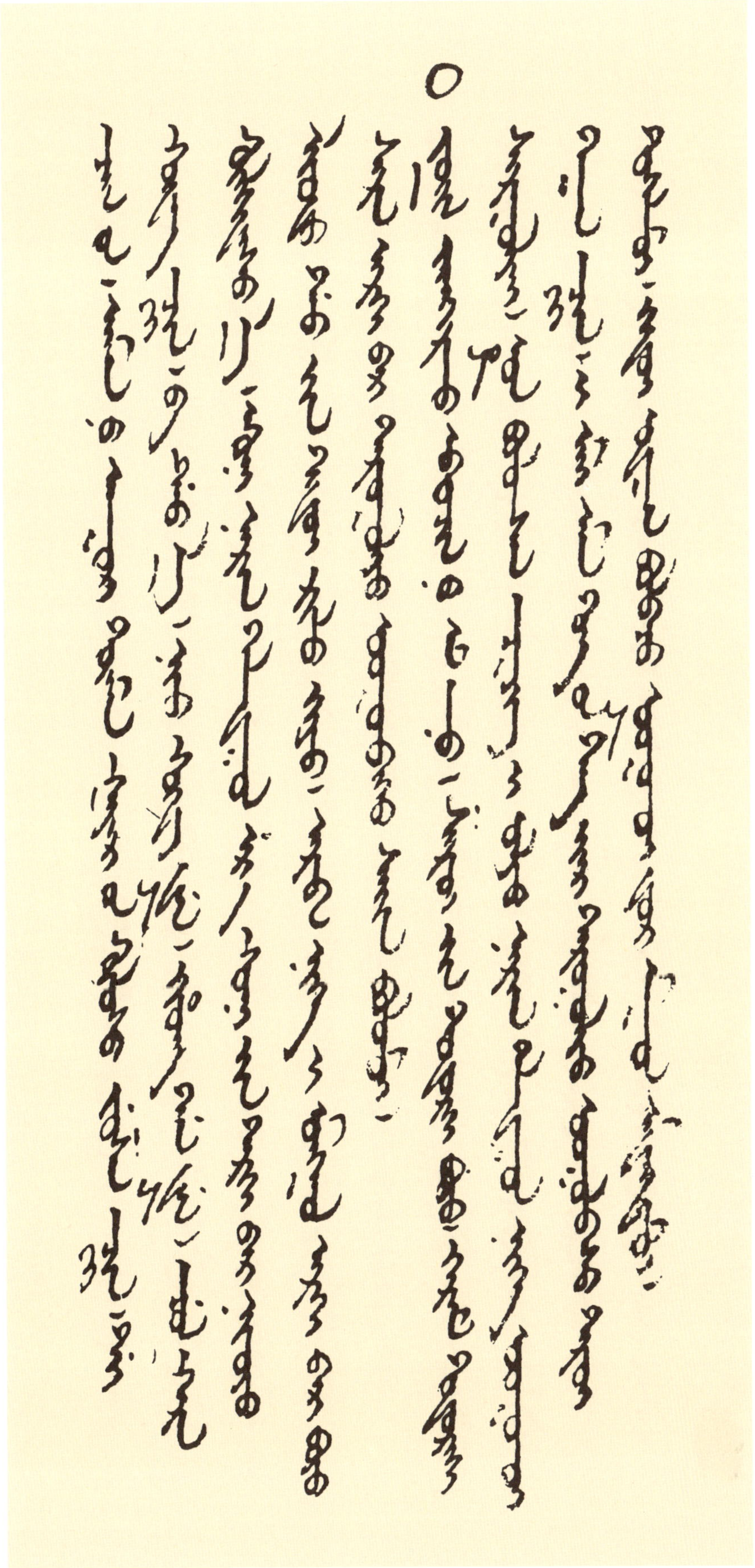

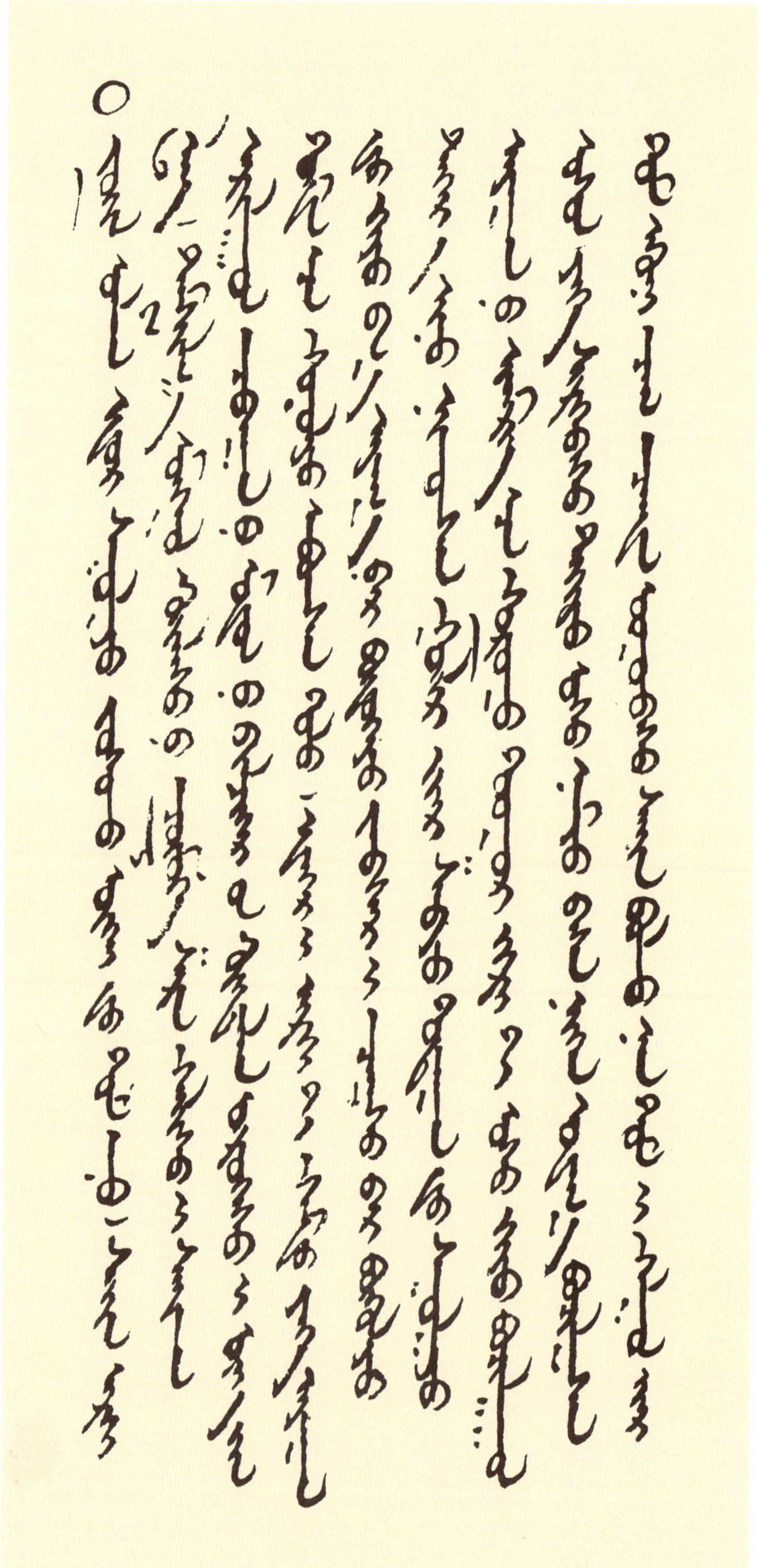

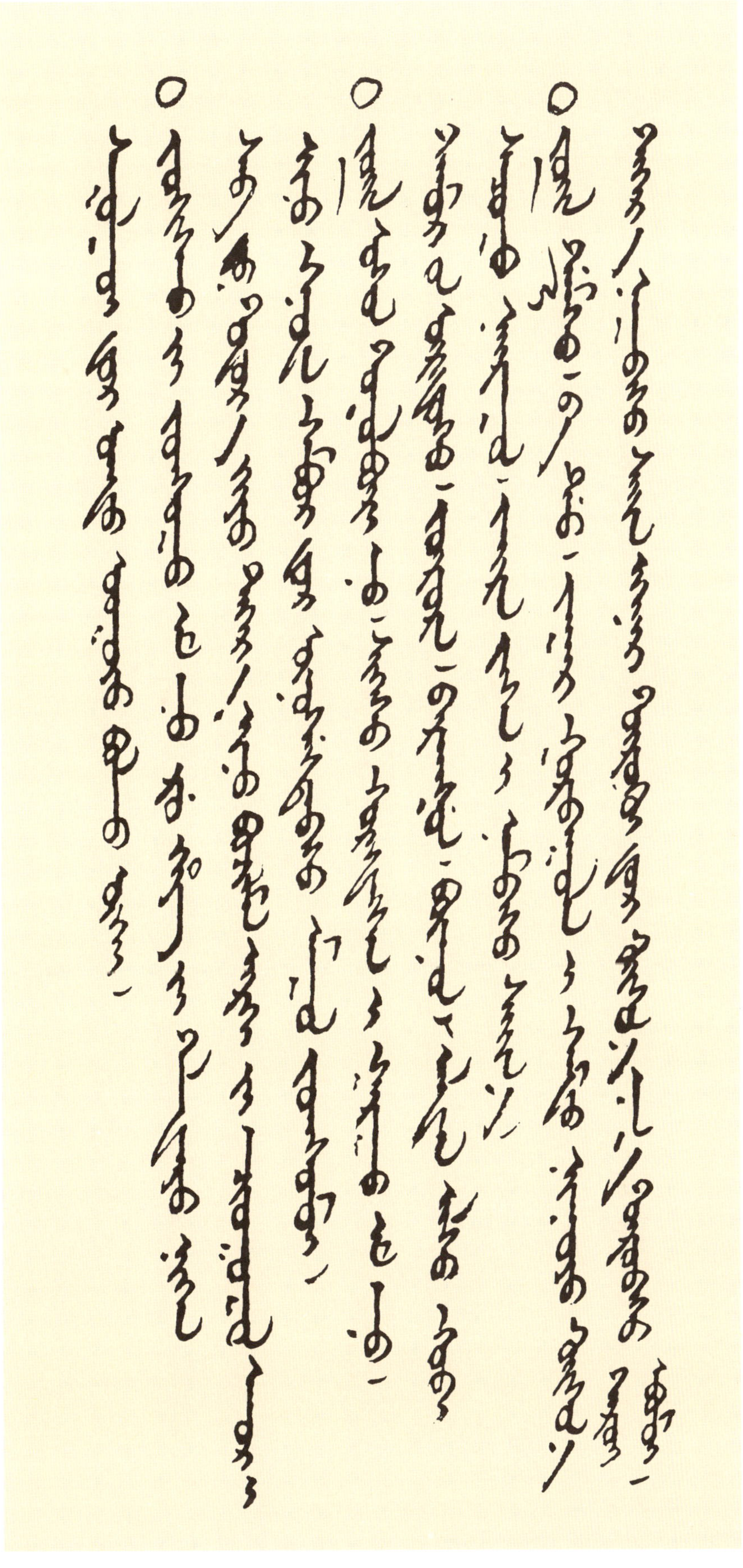

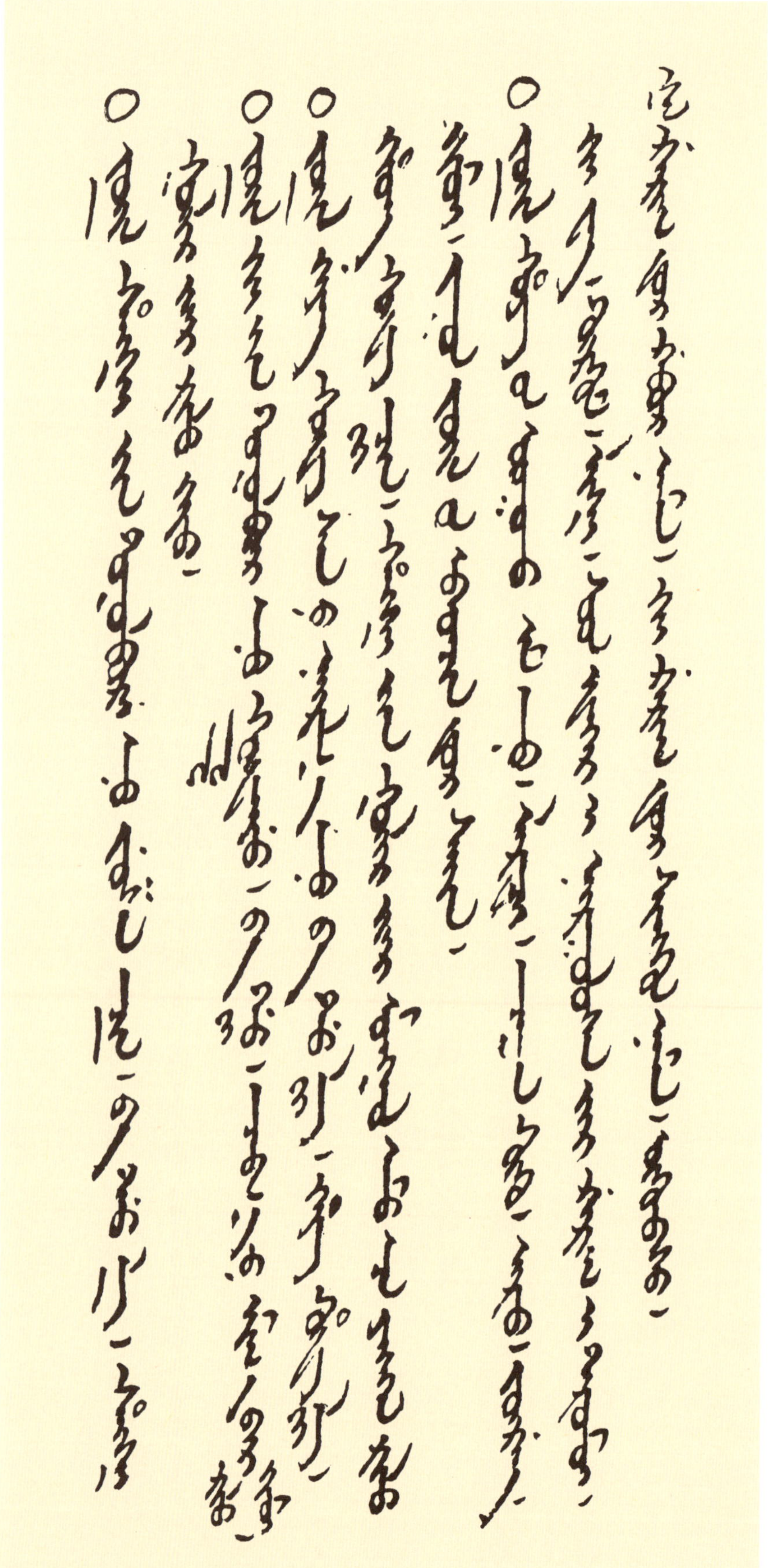

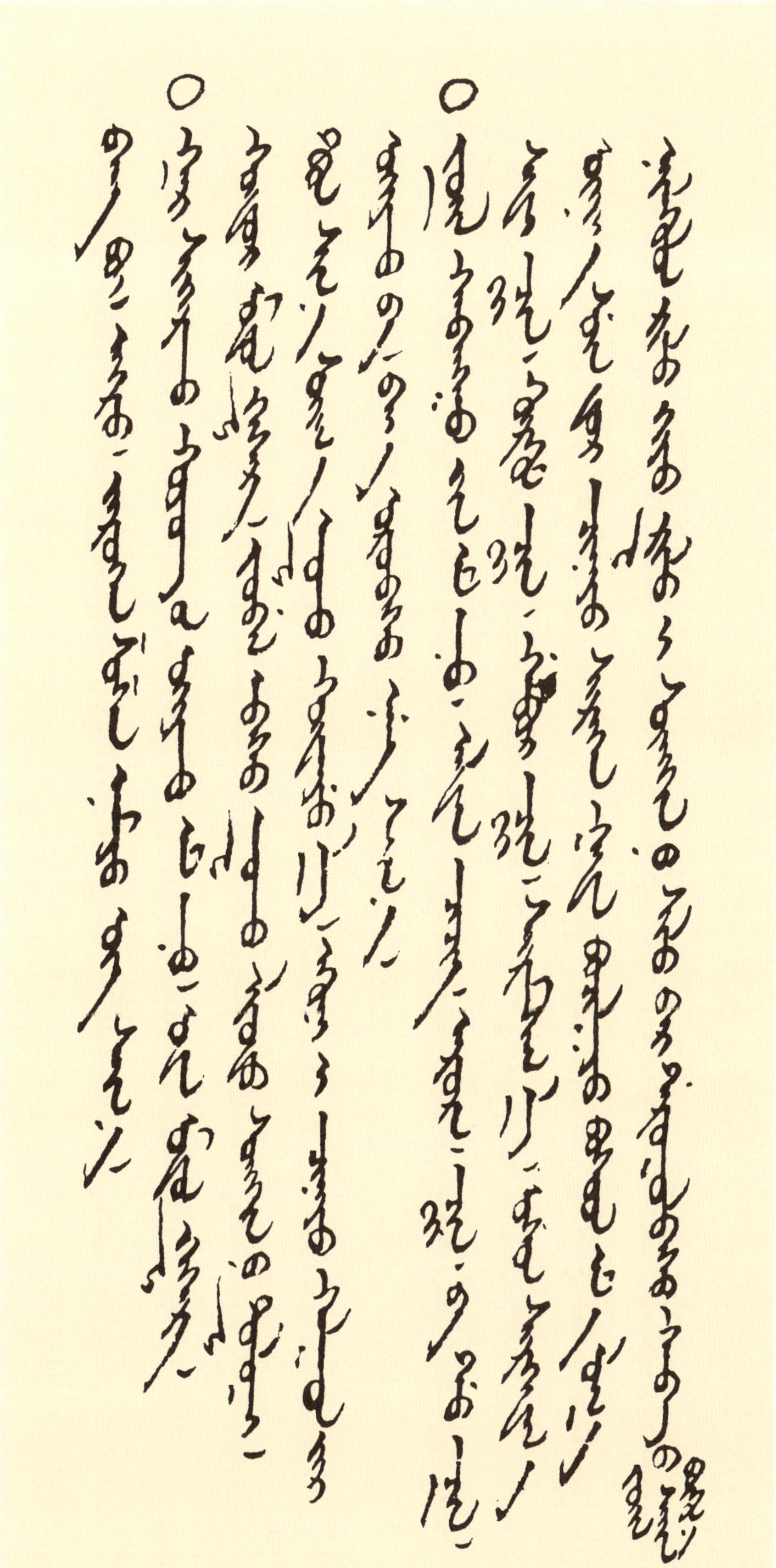

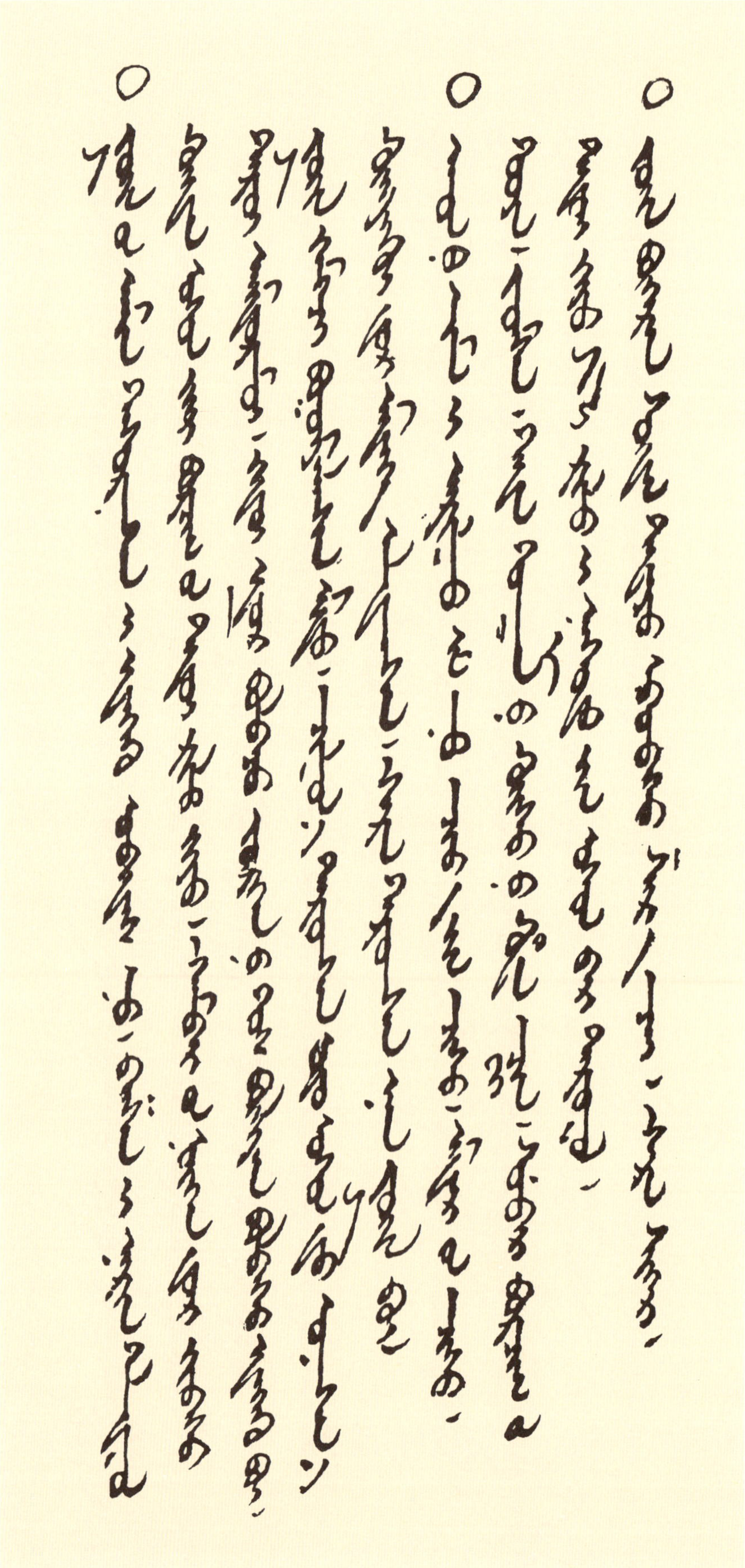

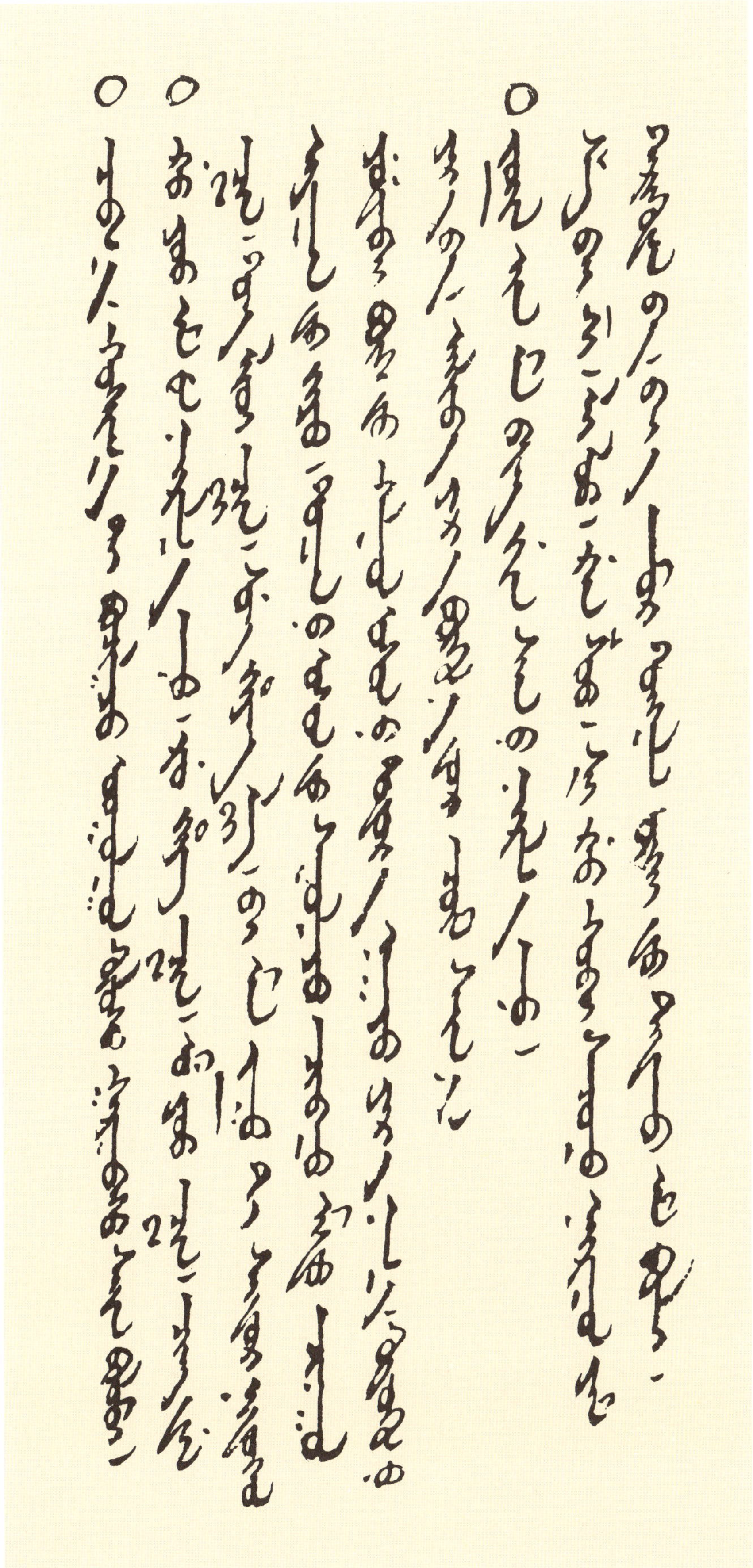

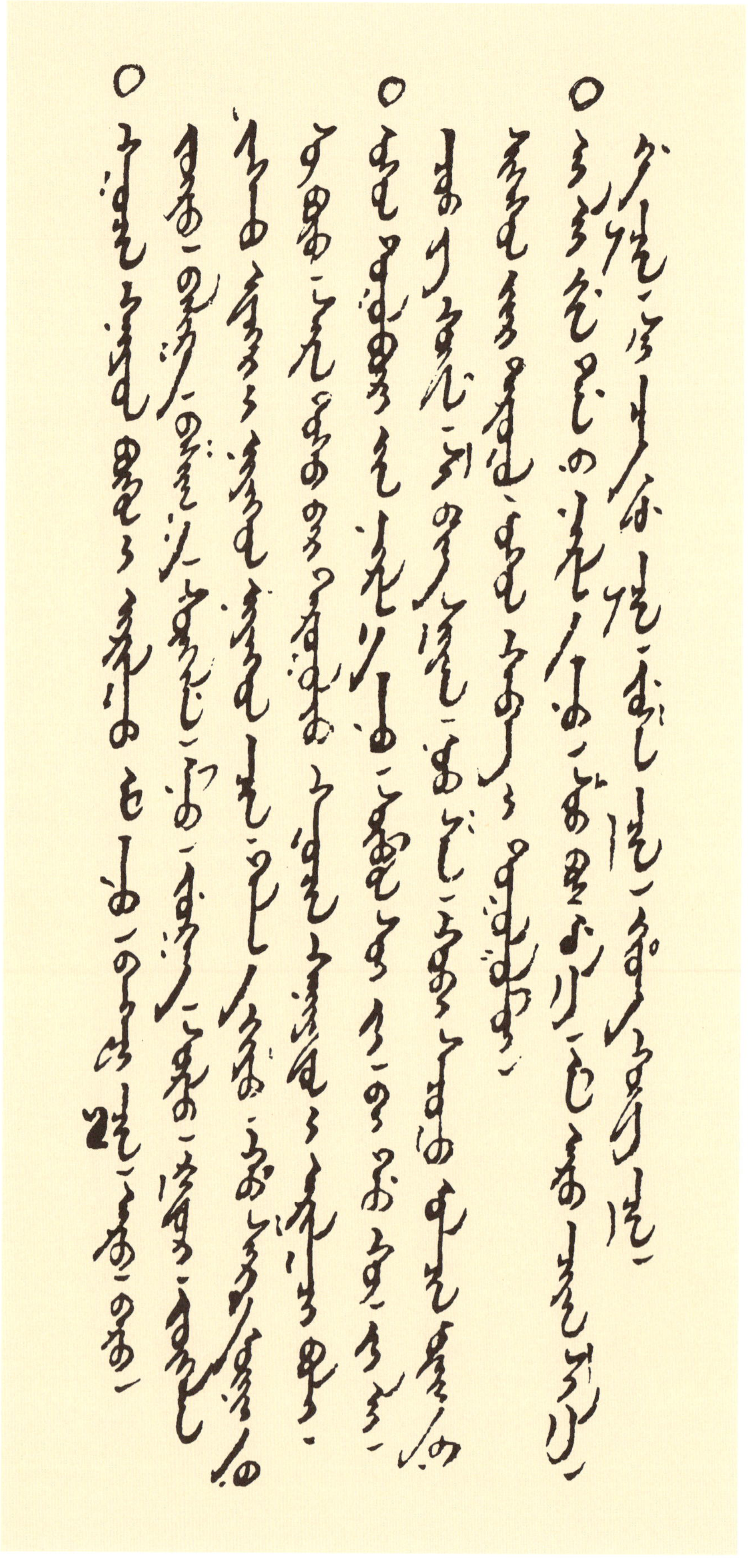

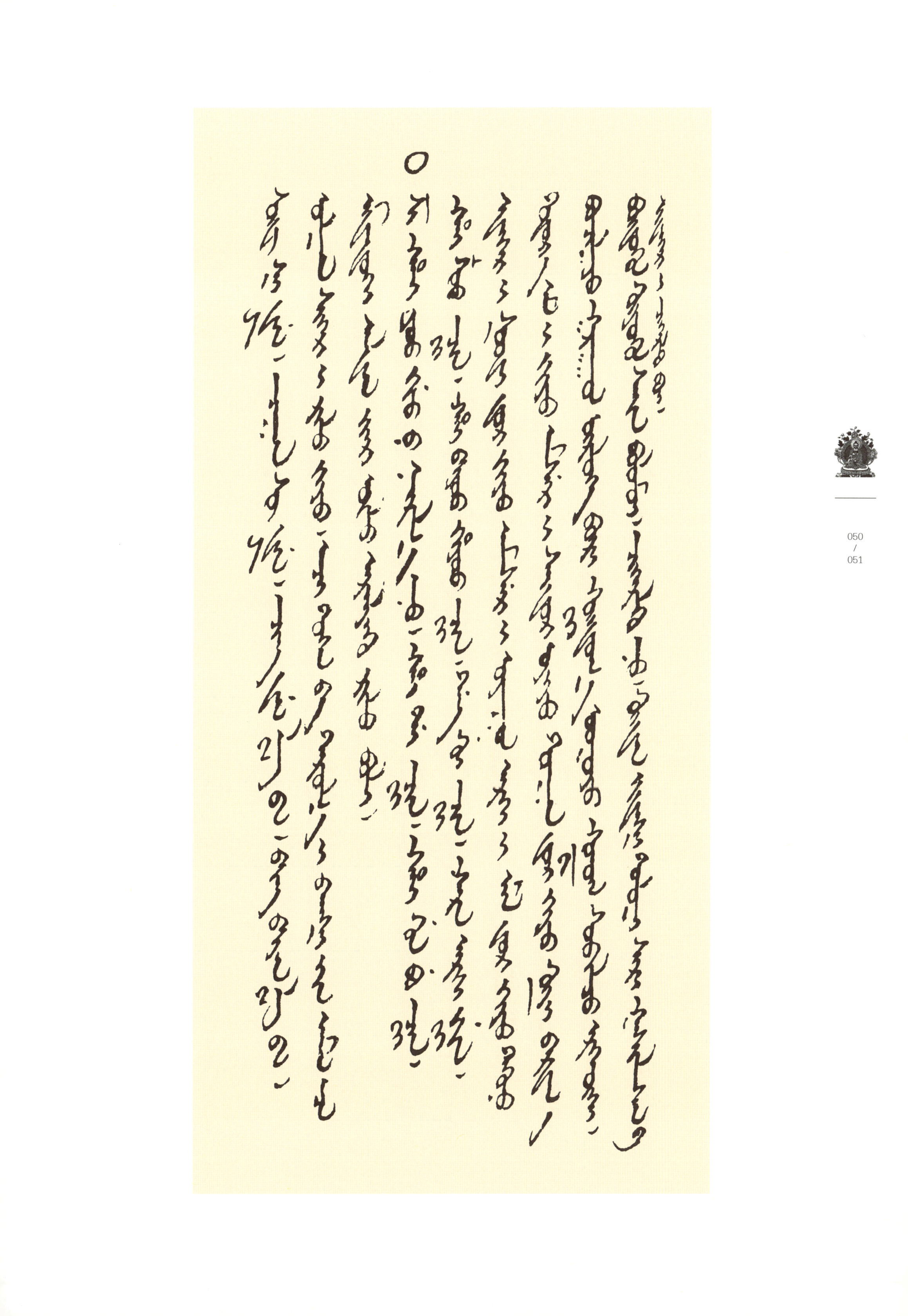

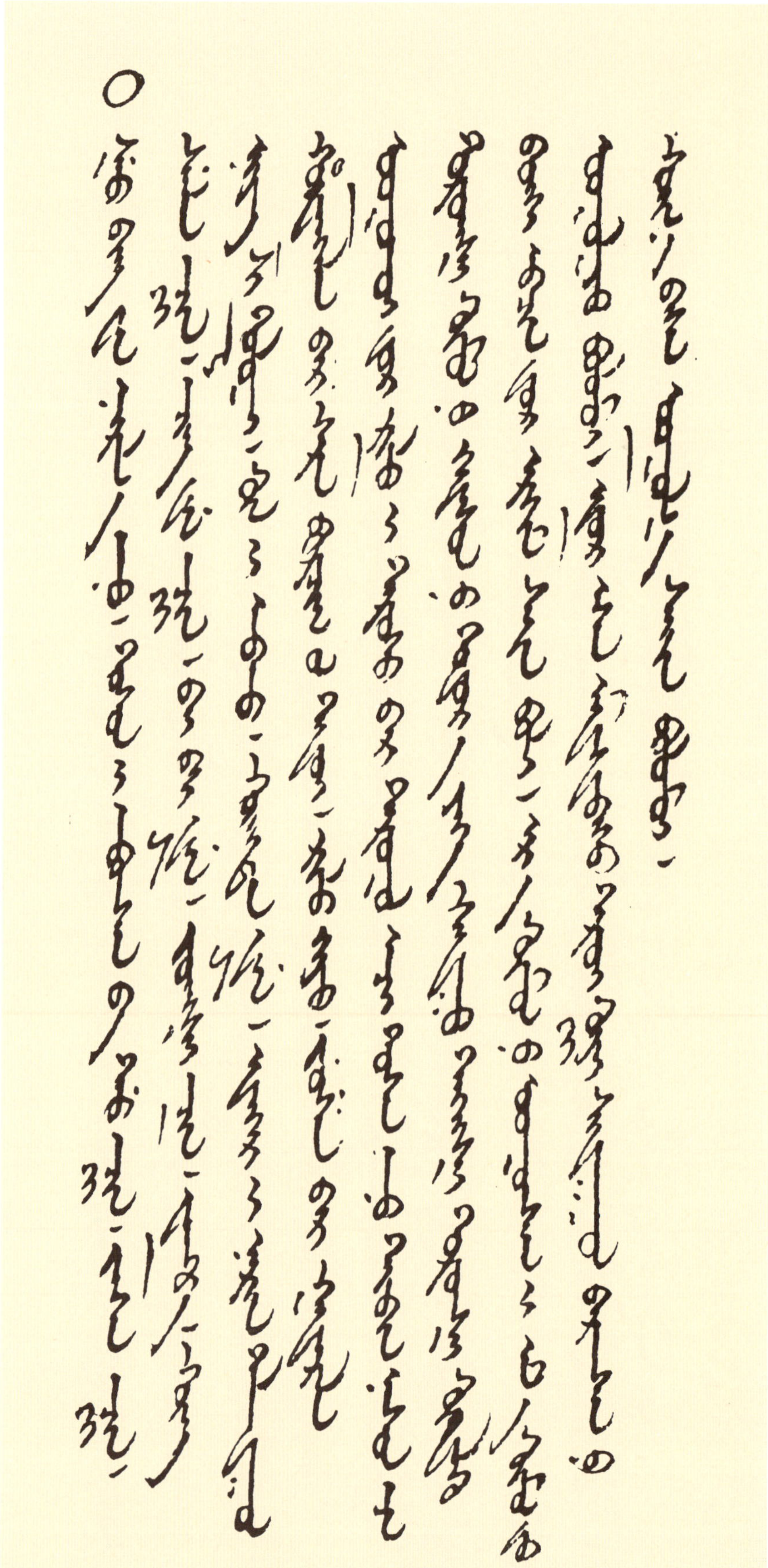

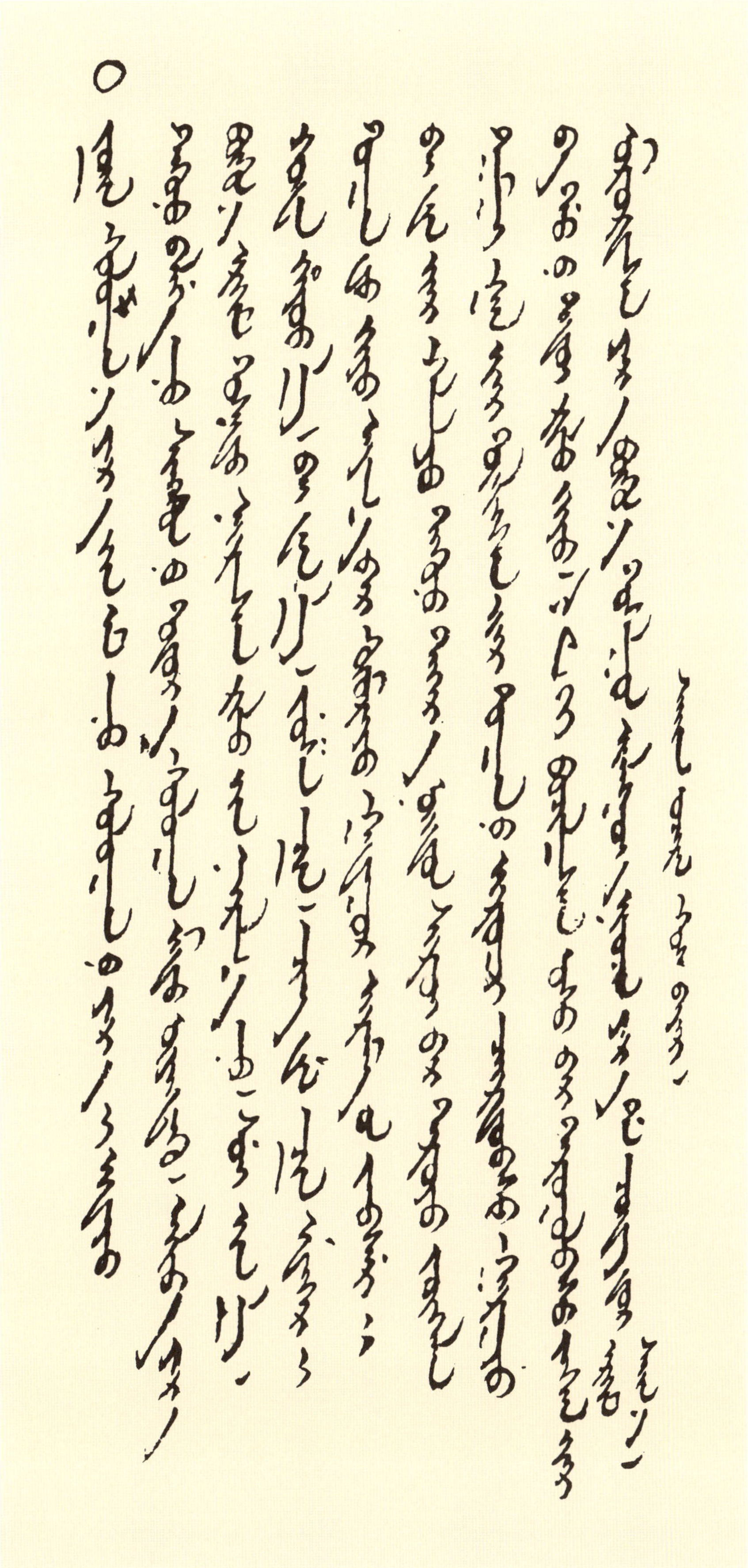

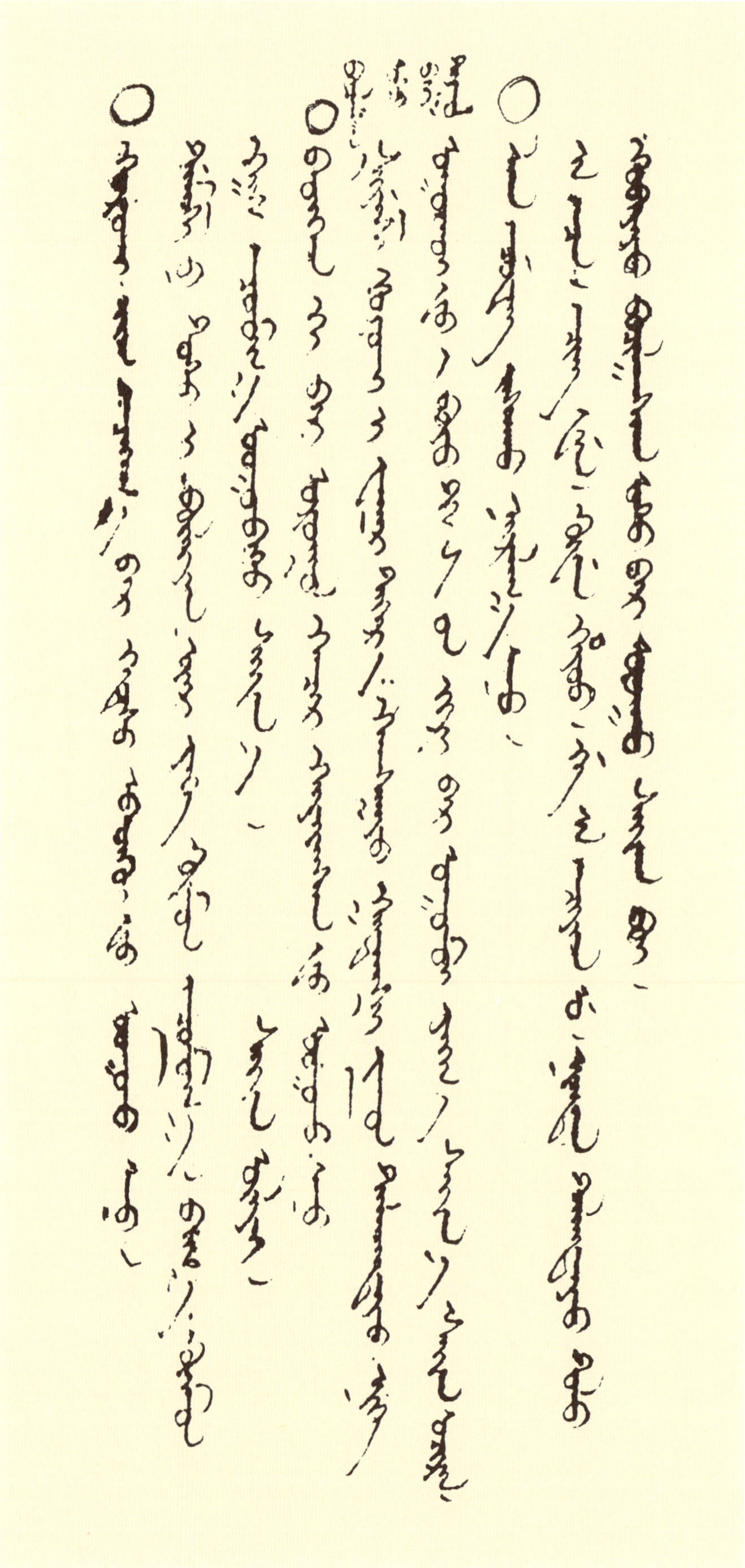

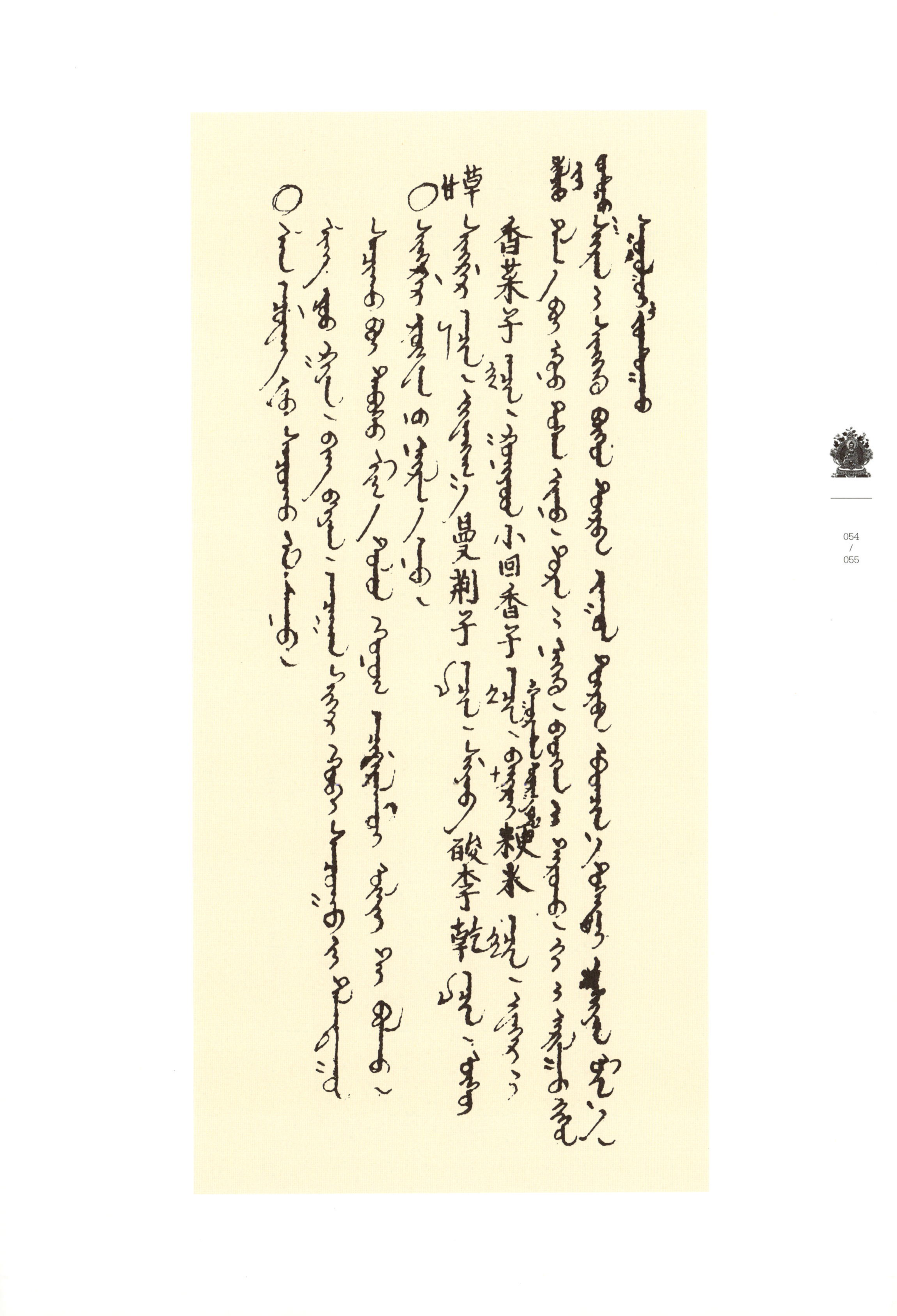

○ [illegible]

[illegible]

[illegible]

○ [illegible]

甘草 [illegible] 蔓荆子 [illegible] 酸李乾 [illegible]

香菜子 [illegible] 小回香子 [illegible] 粳米 [illegible]

[illegible]

[illegible]

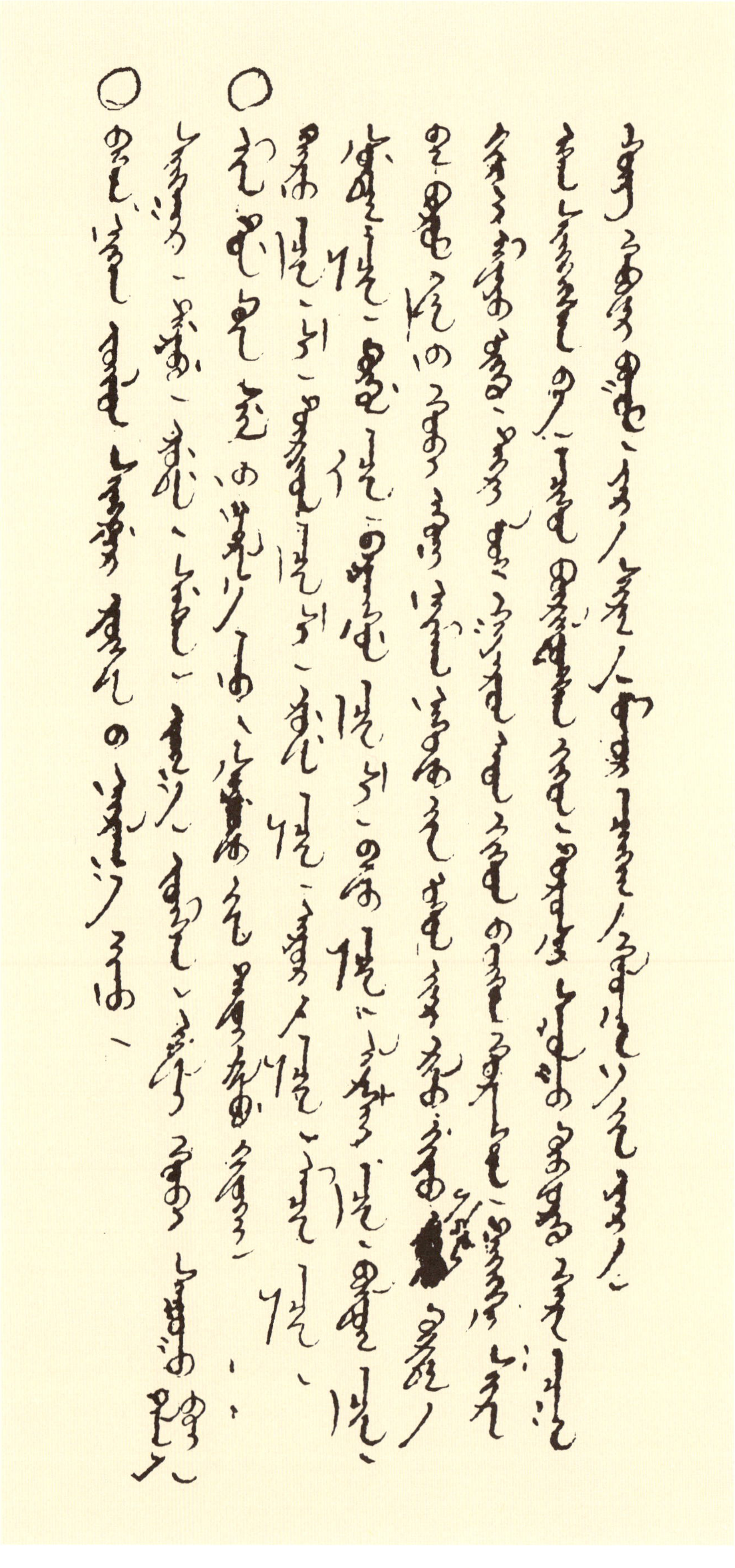

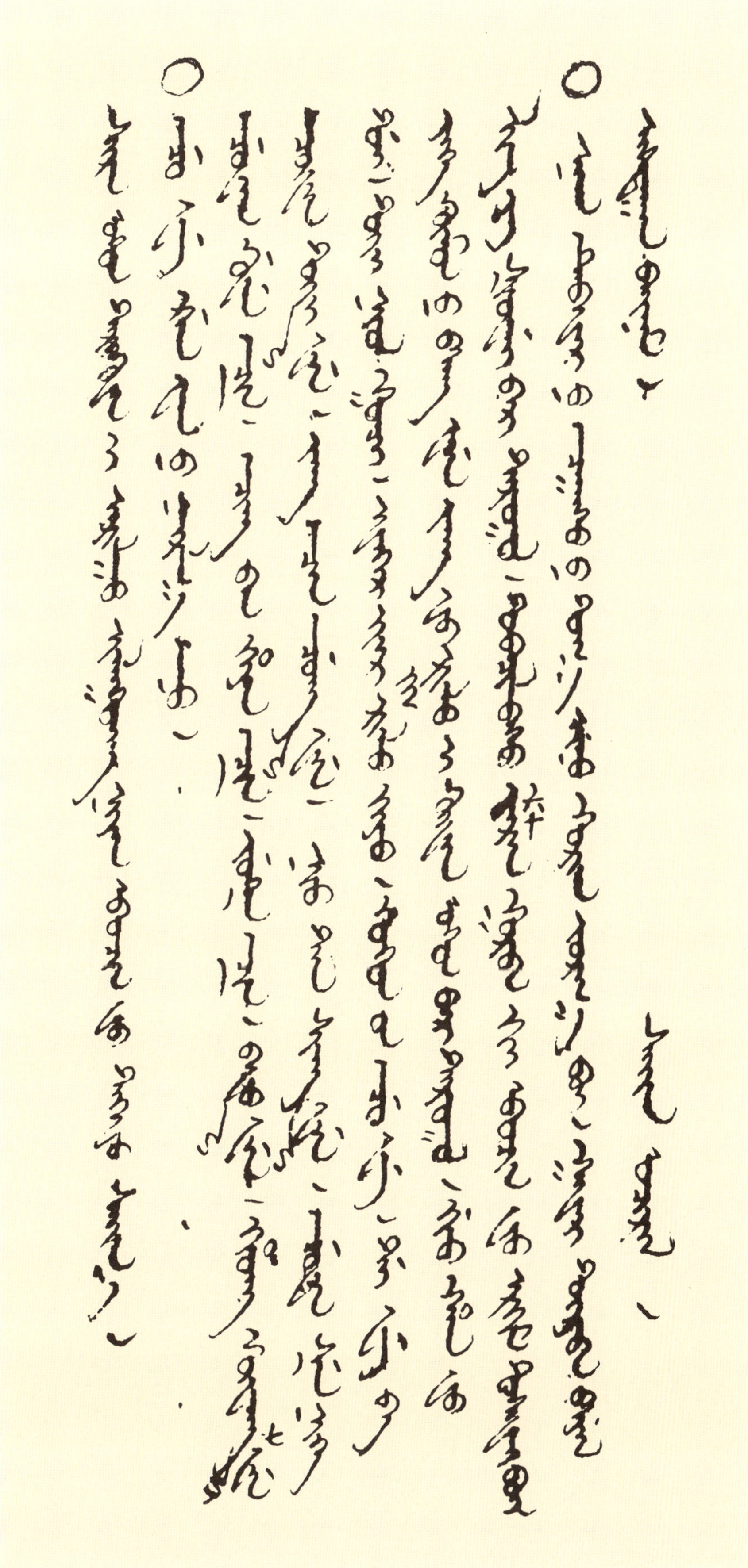

ᠪᠢᠴᠢᠭ ᠦᠨ ᠬᠡᠮᠵᠢᠶ᠎ᠡ ᠨᠢ : 12cm × 23.3cm ᠪᠣᠯᠤᠨ᠎ᠠ · ᠨᠡᠢᠲᠡ 34 ᠨᠢᠭᠤᠷ ᠲᠠᠢ :: ᠳᠣᠲᠣᠷ᠎ᠠ ᠰᠤᠳᠤᠯᠤᠭᠰᠠᠨ ᠭᠠᠷᠴᠠᠭ ᠨᠢ 《 ᠬᠡᠪᠯᠡᠯ ᠬᠡᠪᠯᠡᠭᠰᠡᠨ ᠦ ᠪᠢᠴᠢᠭᠯᠡᠯ 》ᠭᠡᠳᠡᠭ ᠪᠢᠴᠢᠭ

甘露精要八支秘诀续——根本续

The Secret Tantra of Nectar Essence Eight Branches (i.e. Rgyud bzhi) –Rtsa Rgyud

2

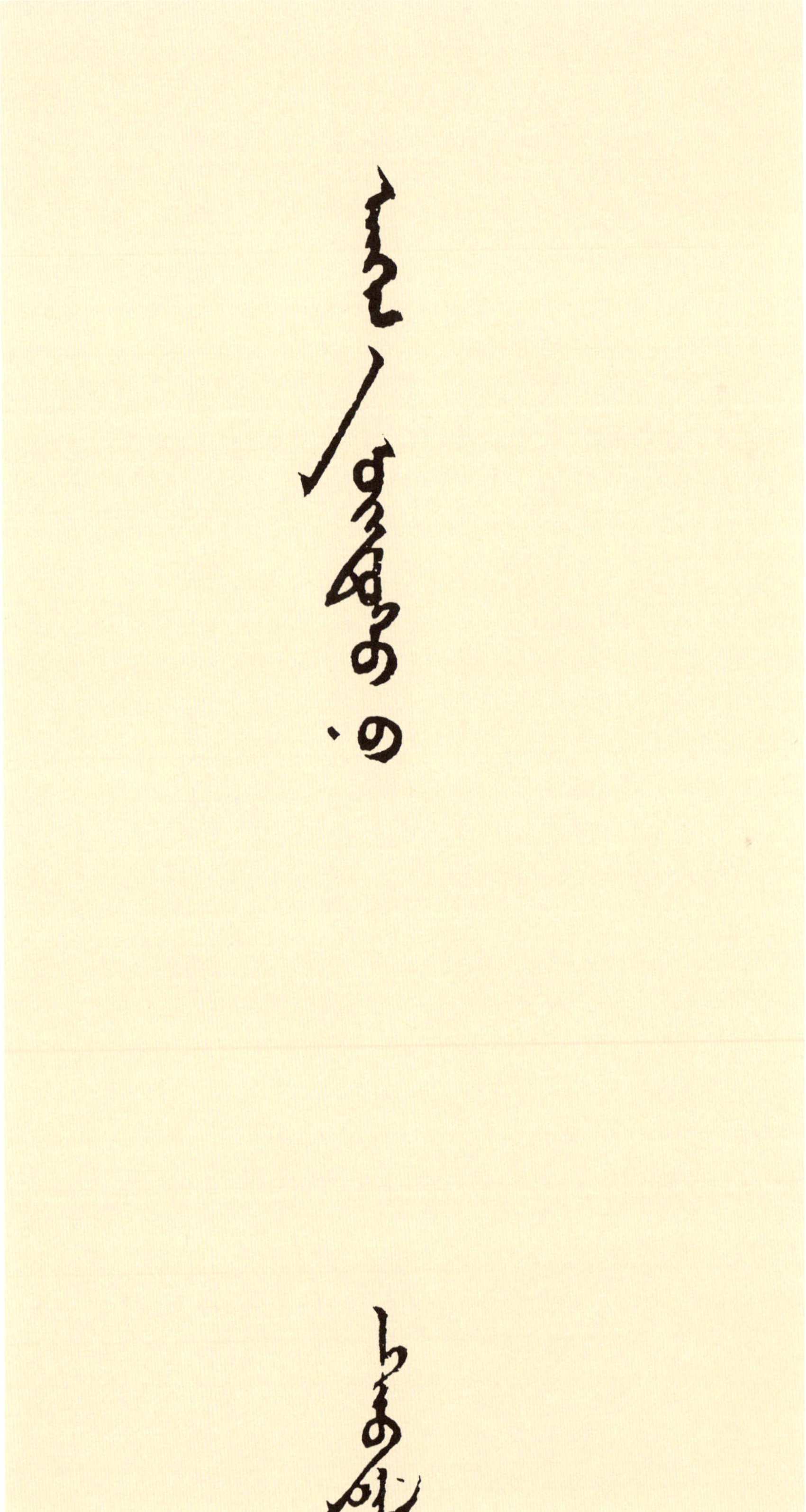

ᠮᠥᠩᠬᠡ ᠮᠥᠩᠭᠡᠯᠢ ᠤ ᠪᠥᠬᠡ ᠰᠦᠷᠯᠢ ᠮᠥᠩᠭᠦ ᠮᠥᠩᠬᠡᠷᠡᠨ ::

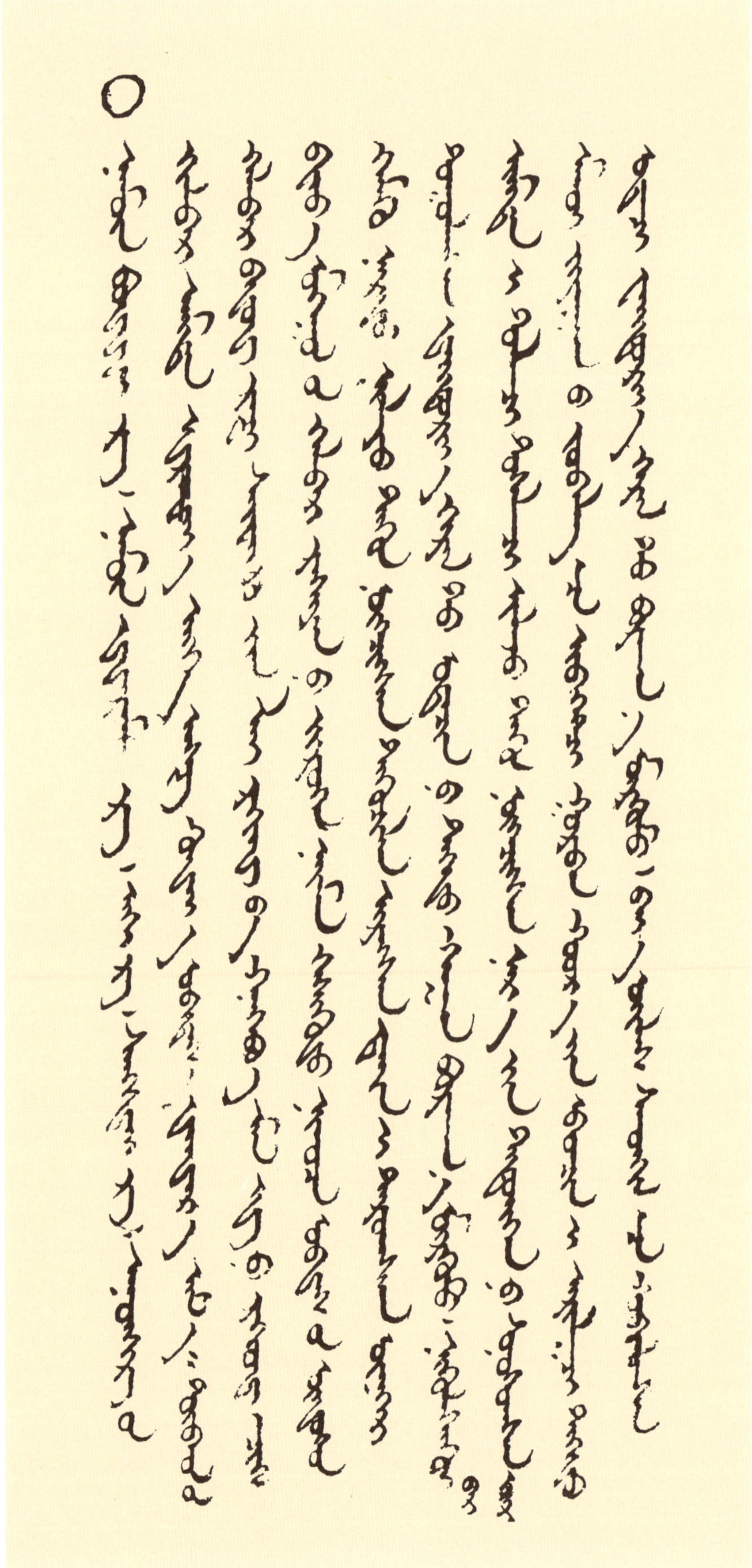

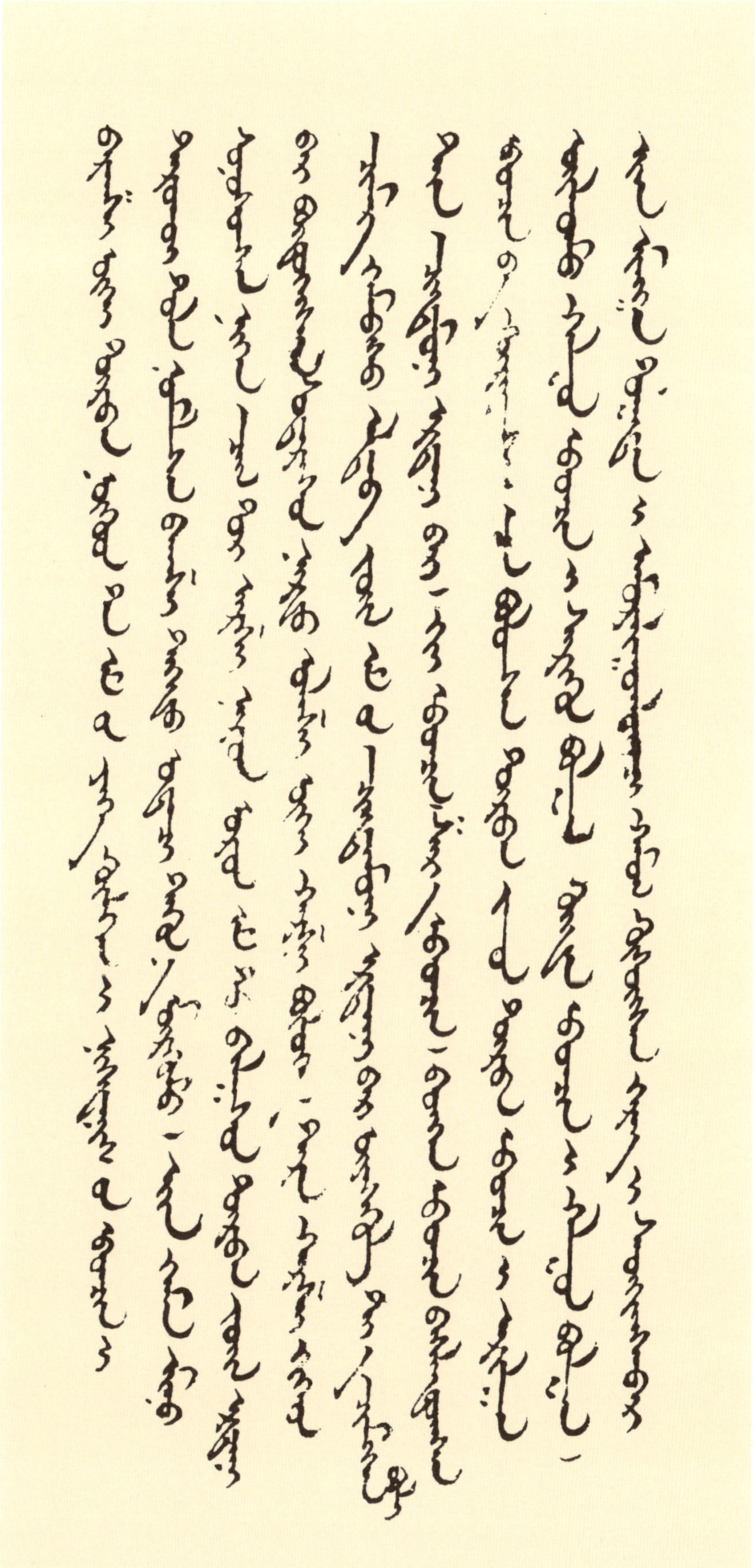

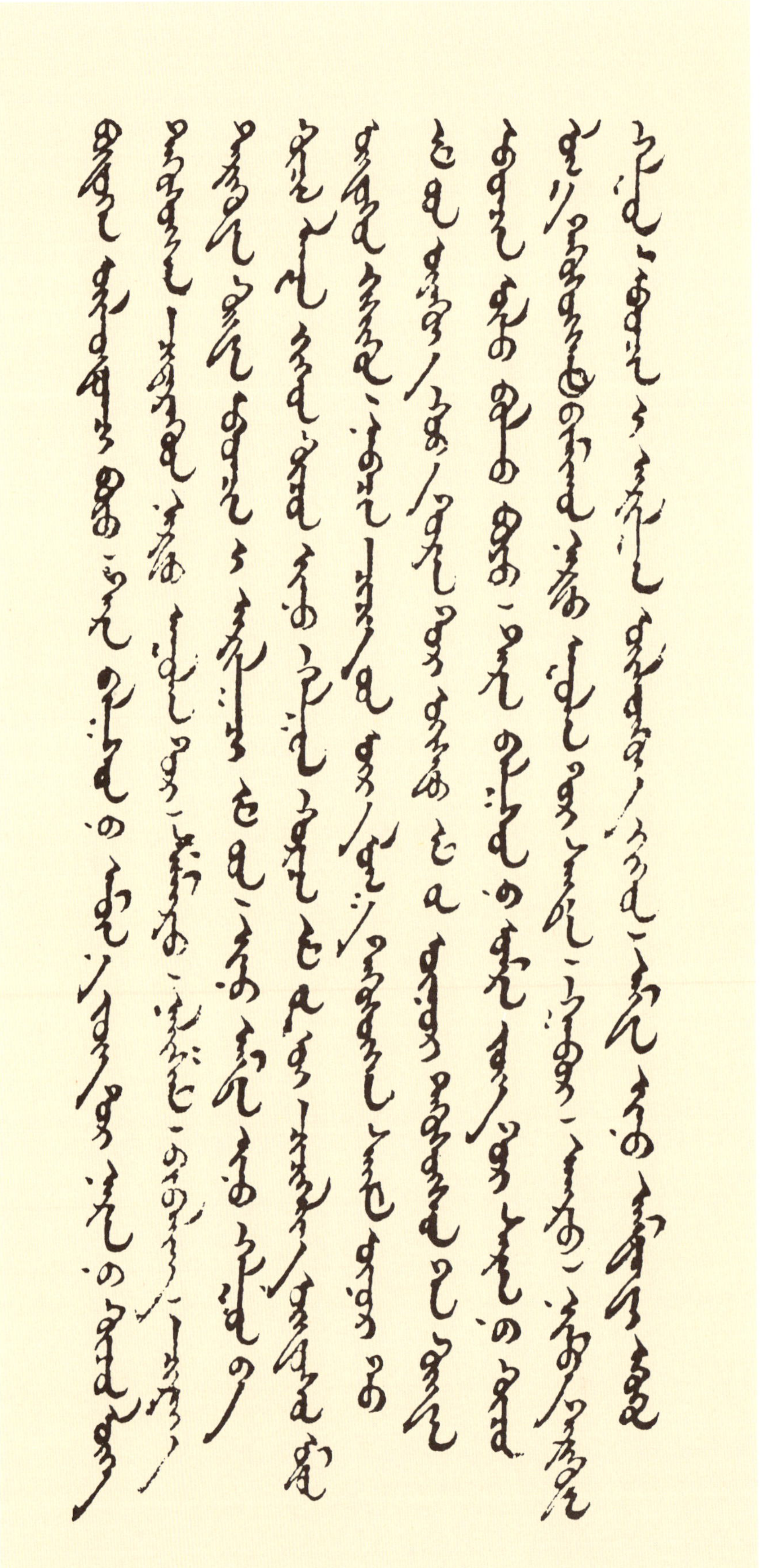

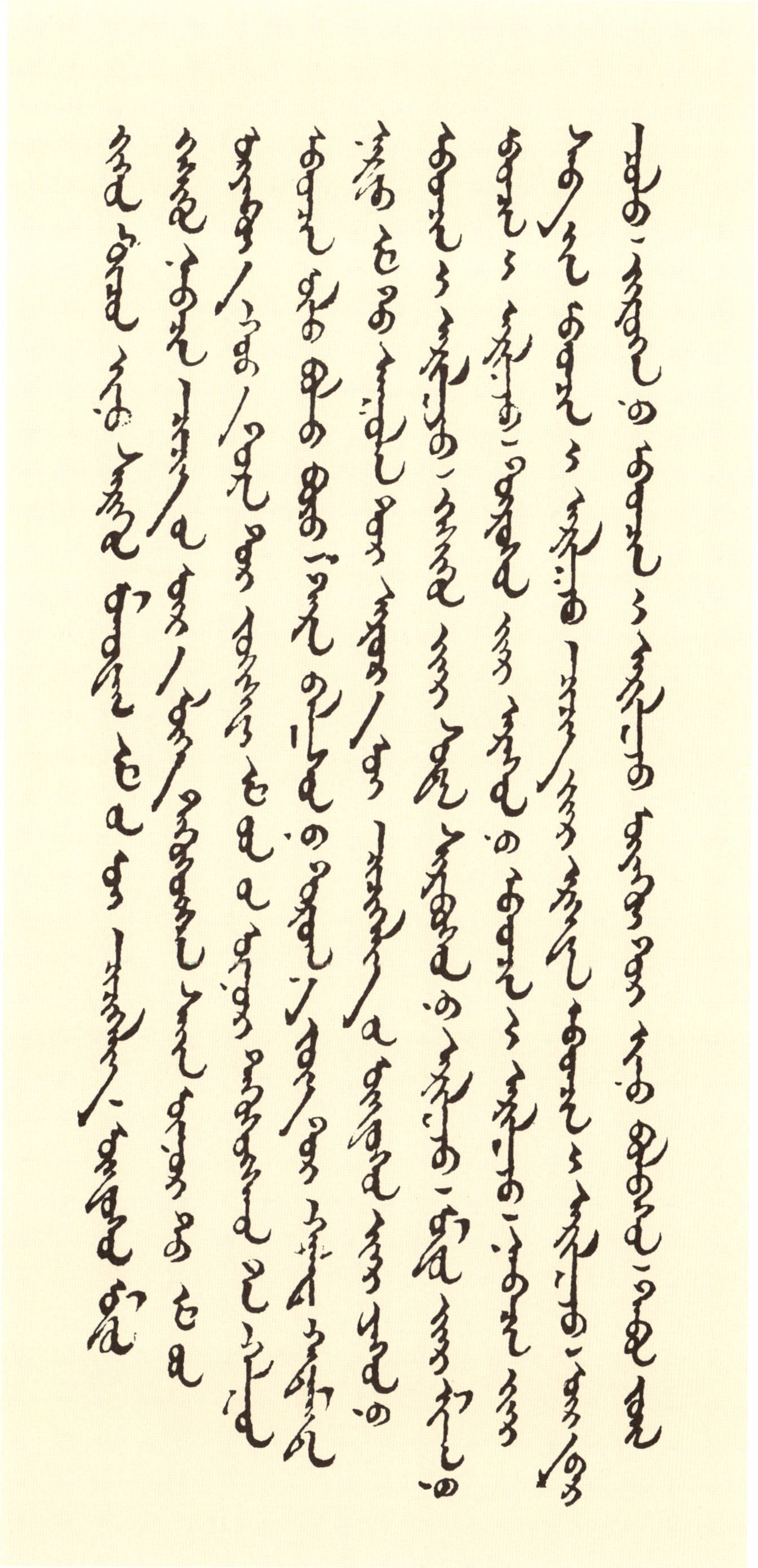

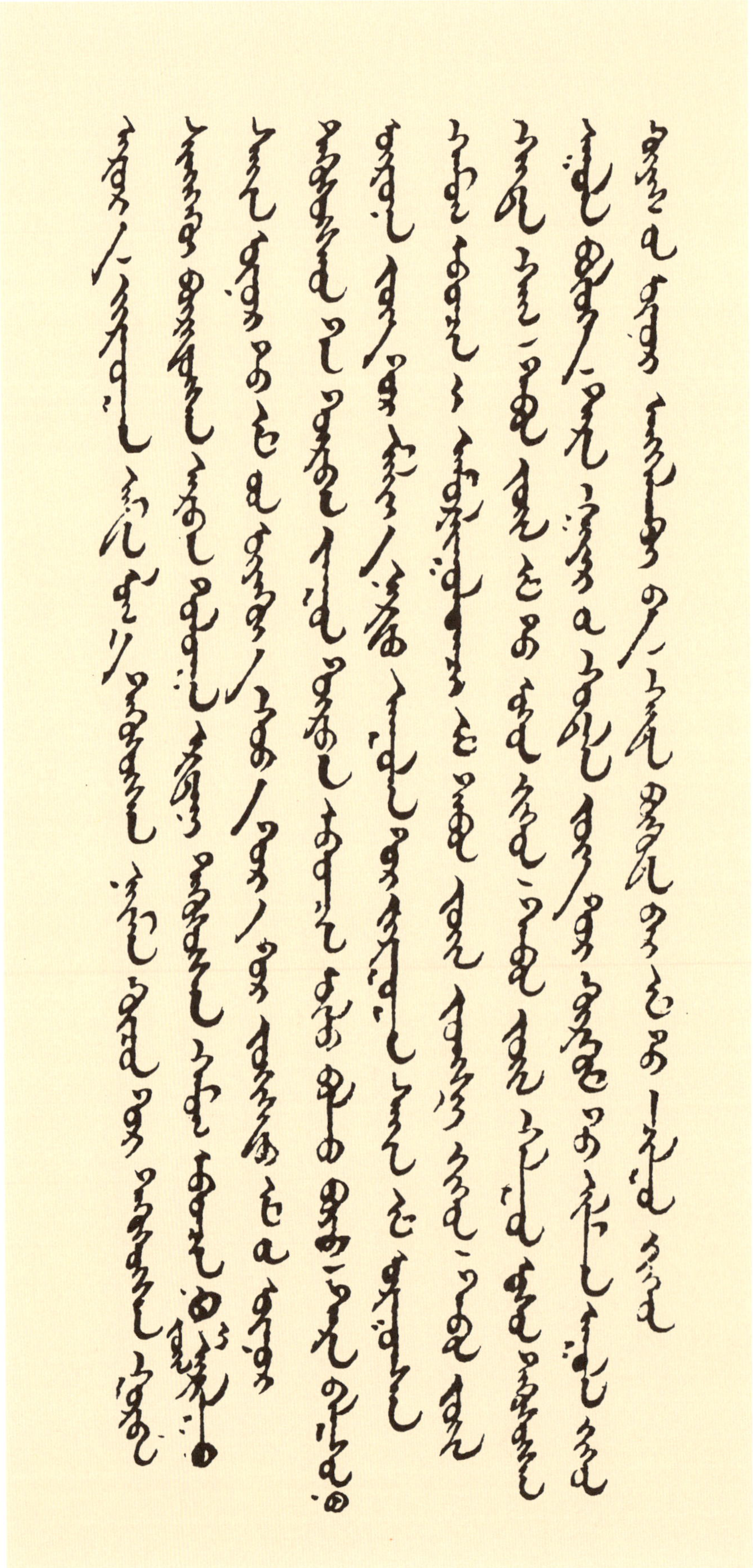

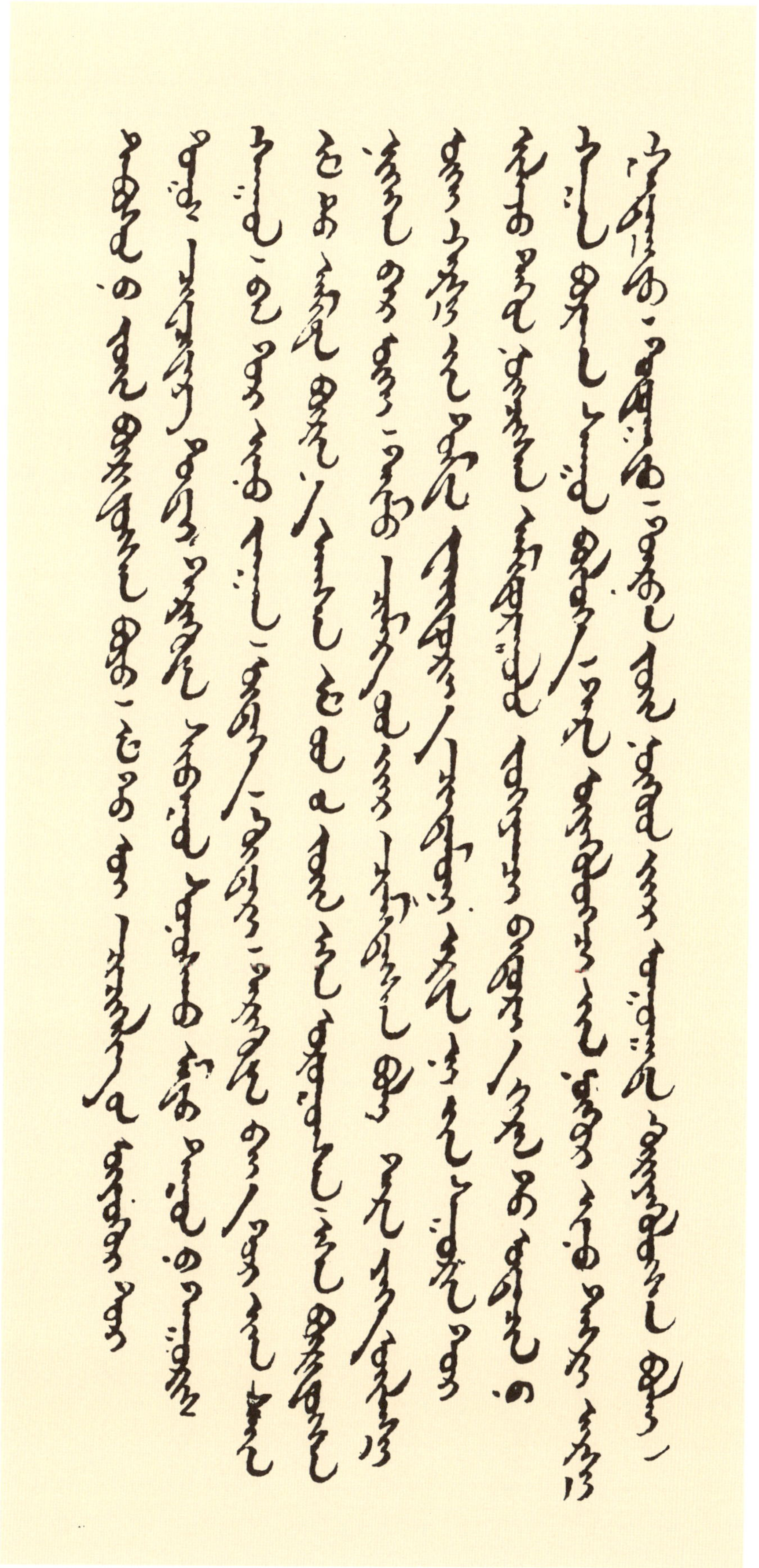

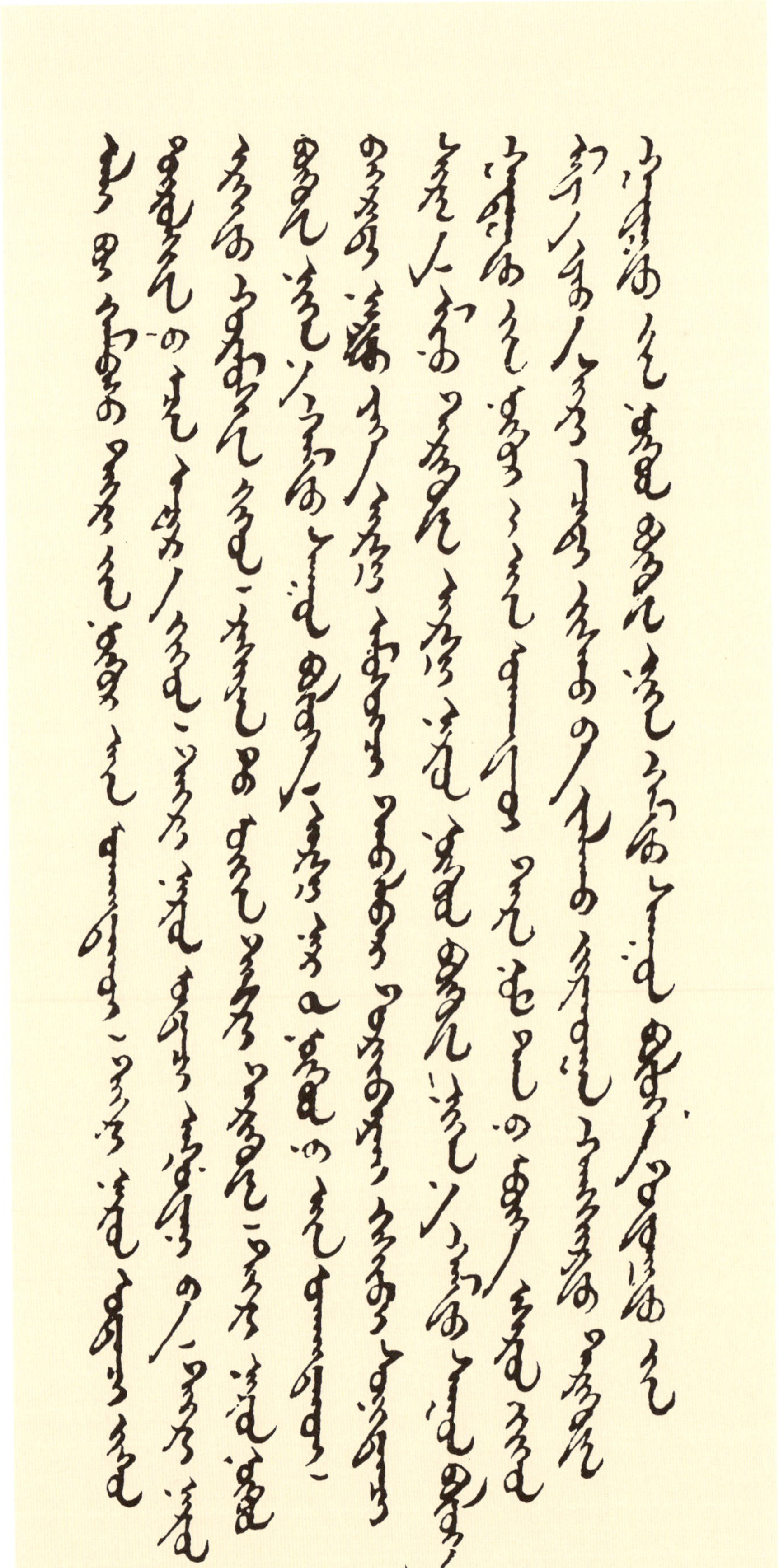

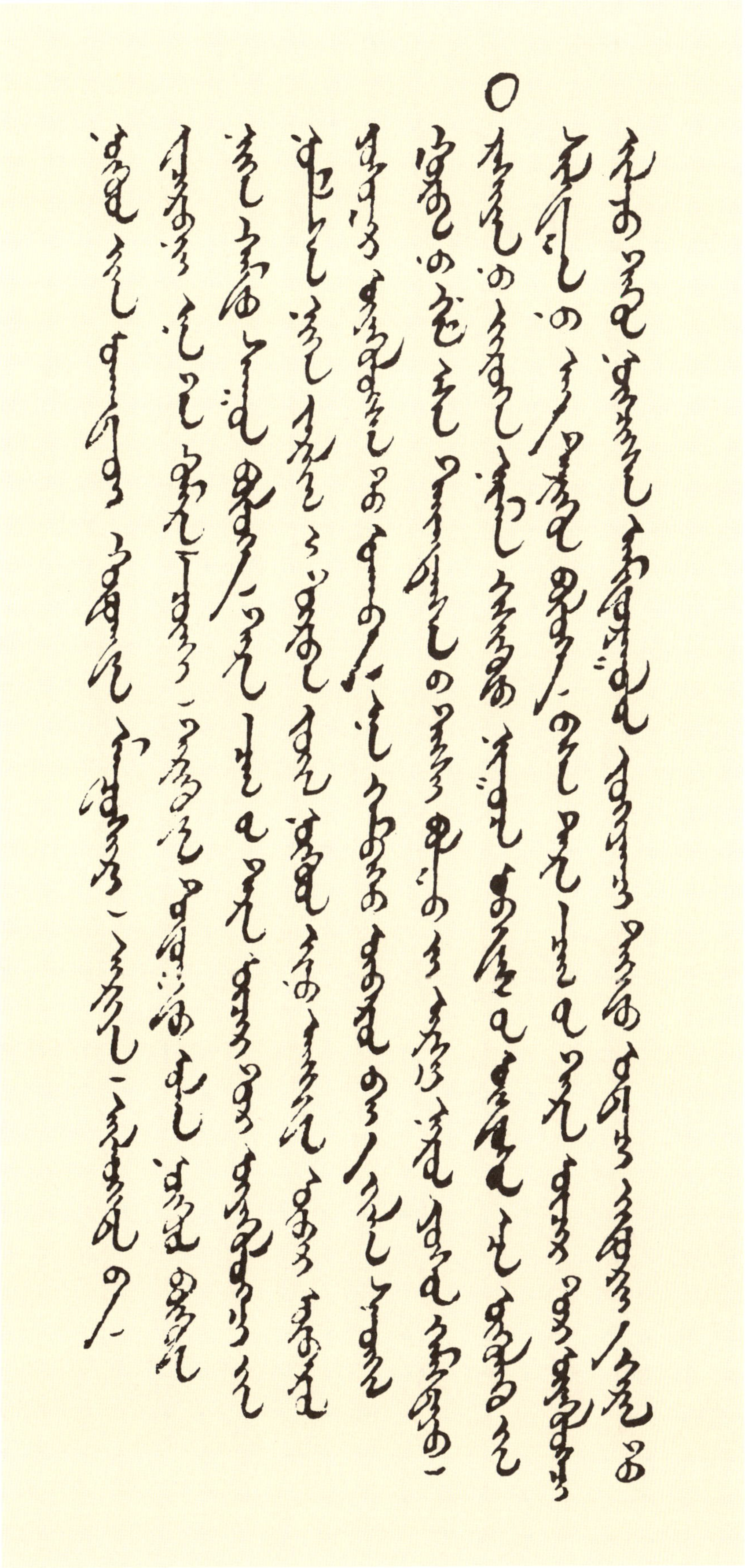

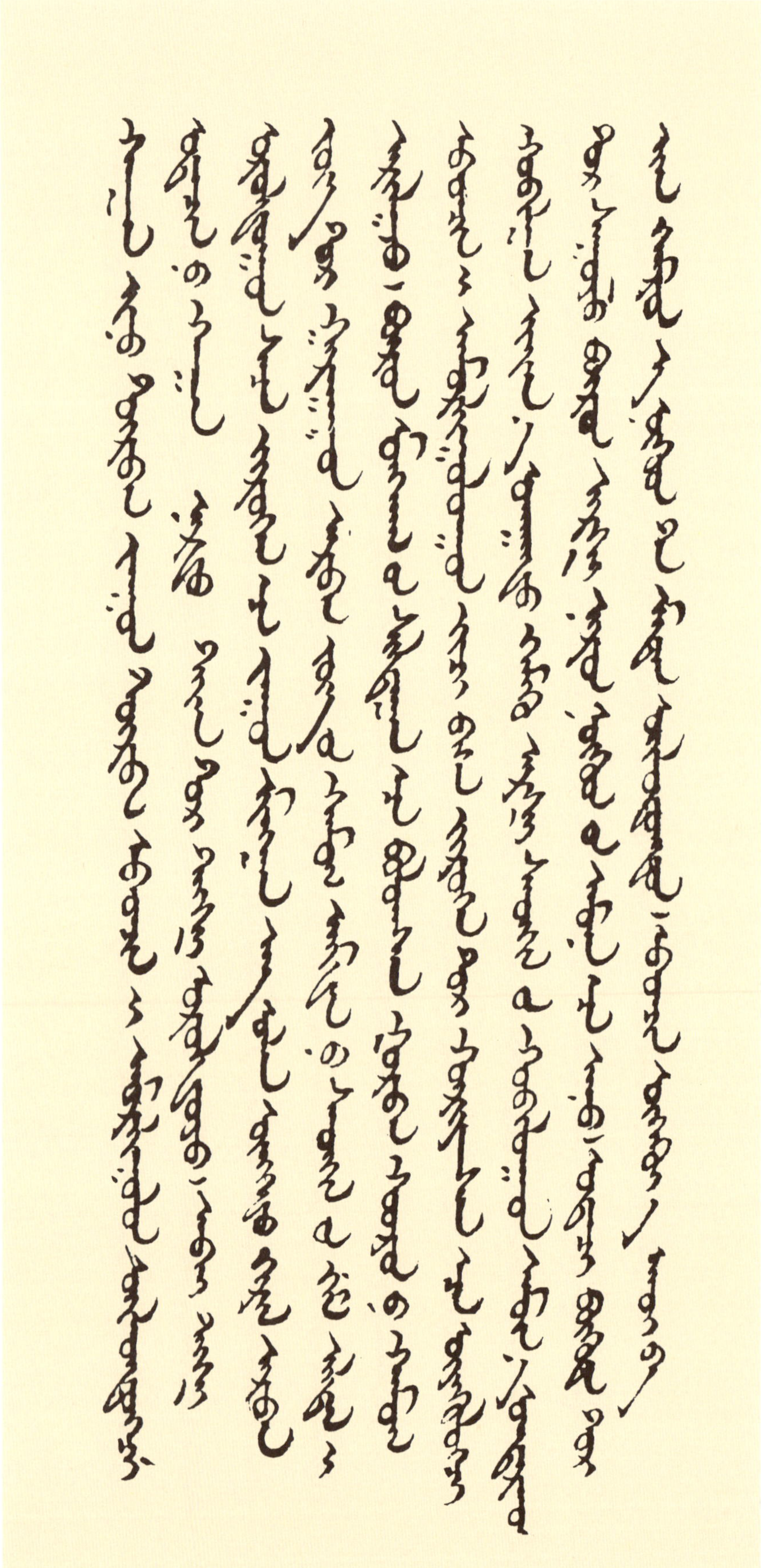

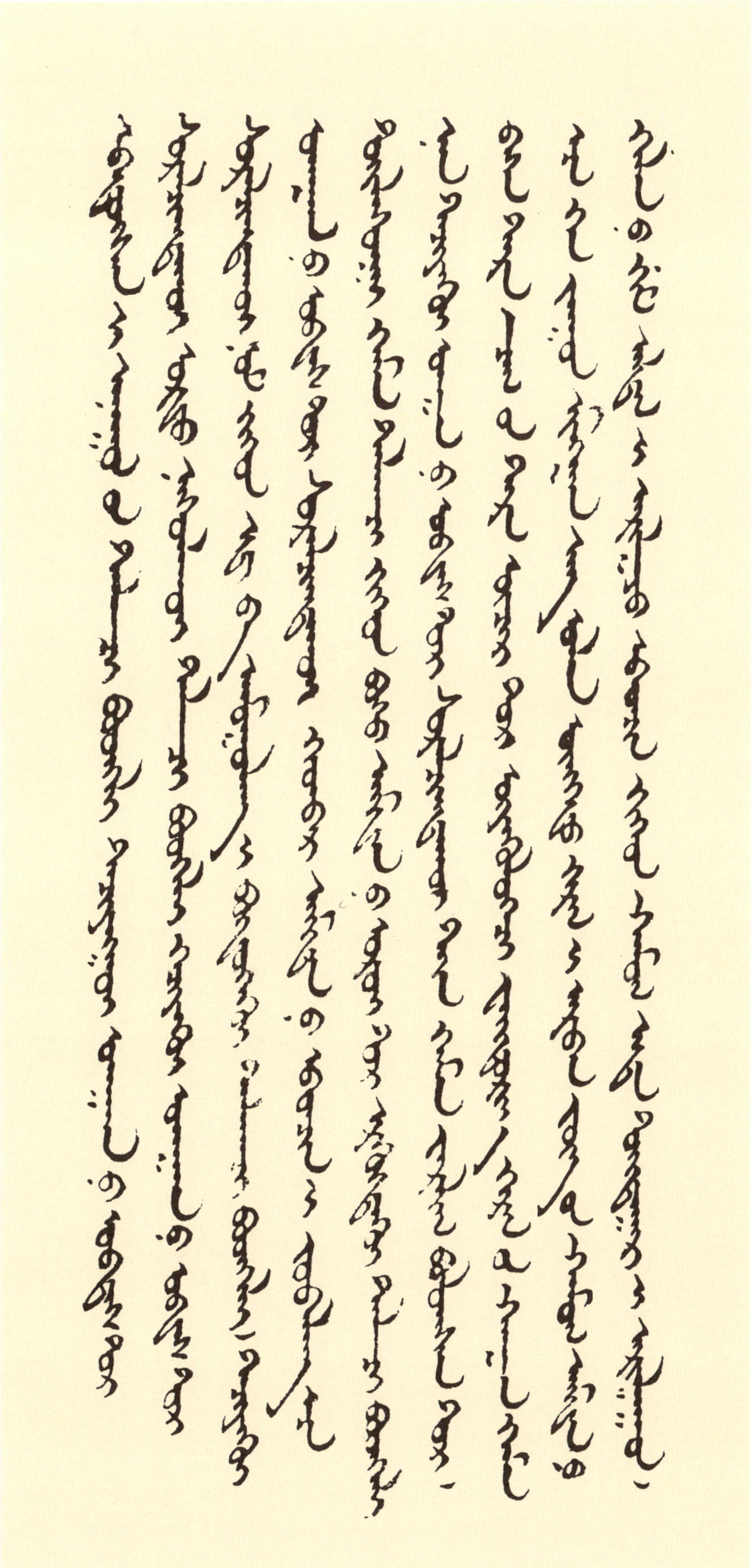

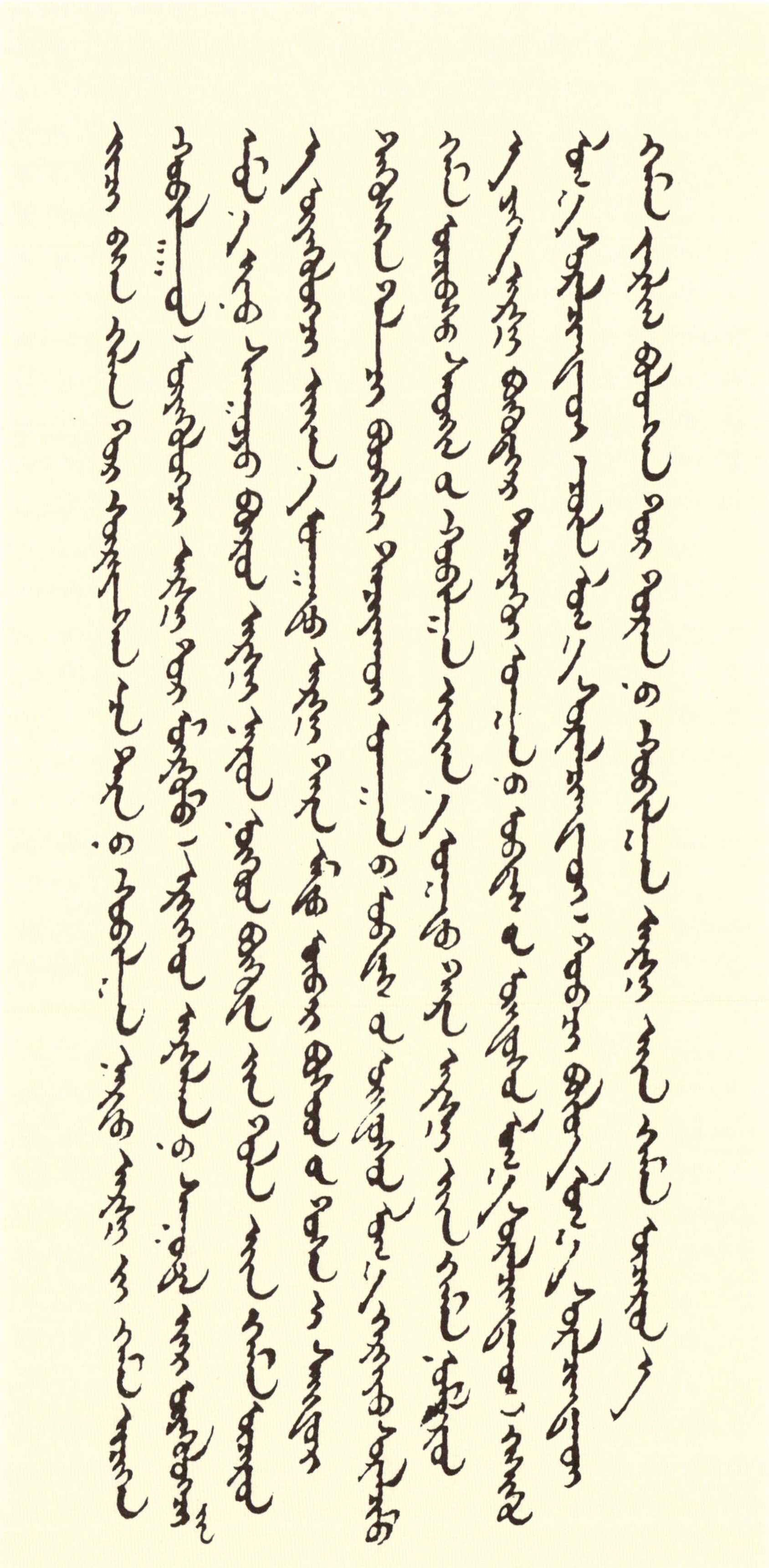

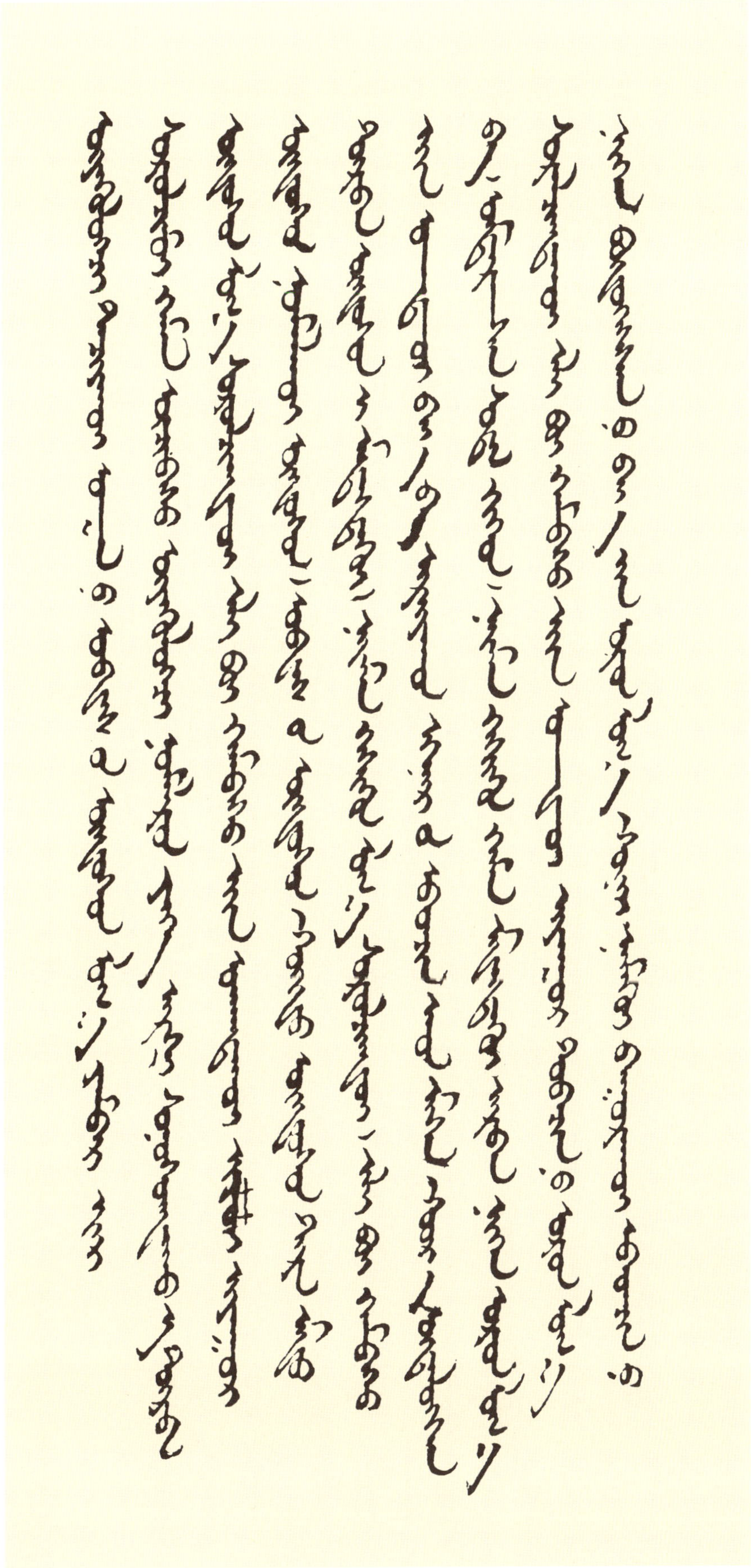

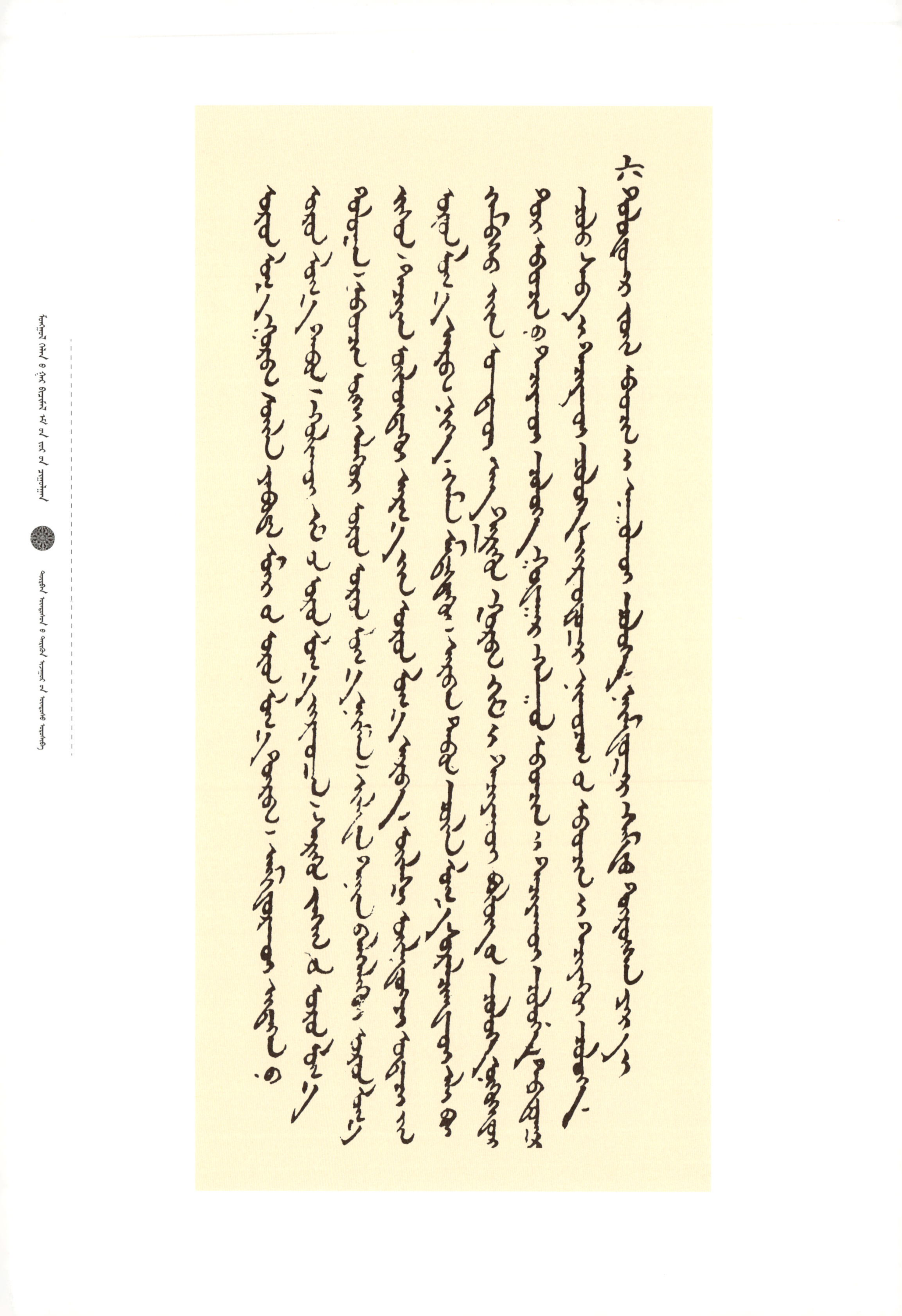

六

[illegible]

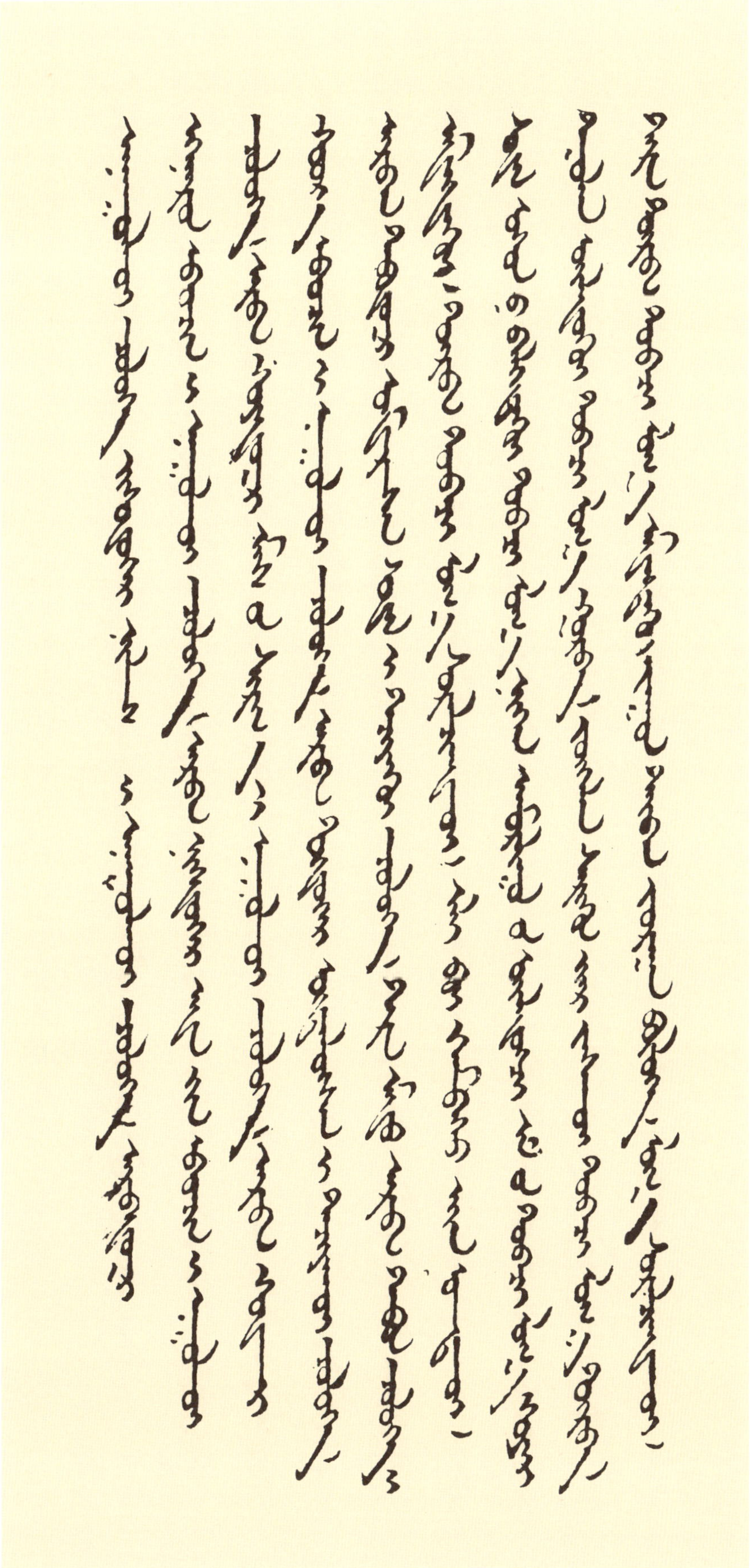

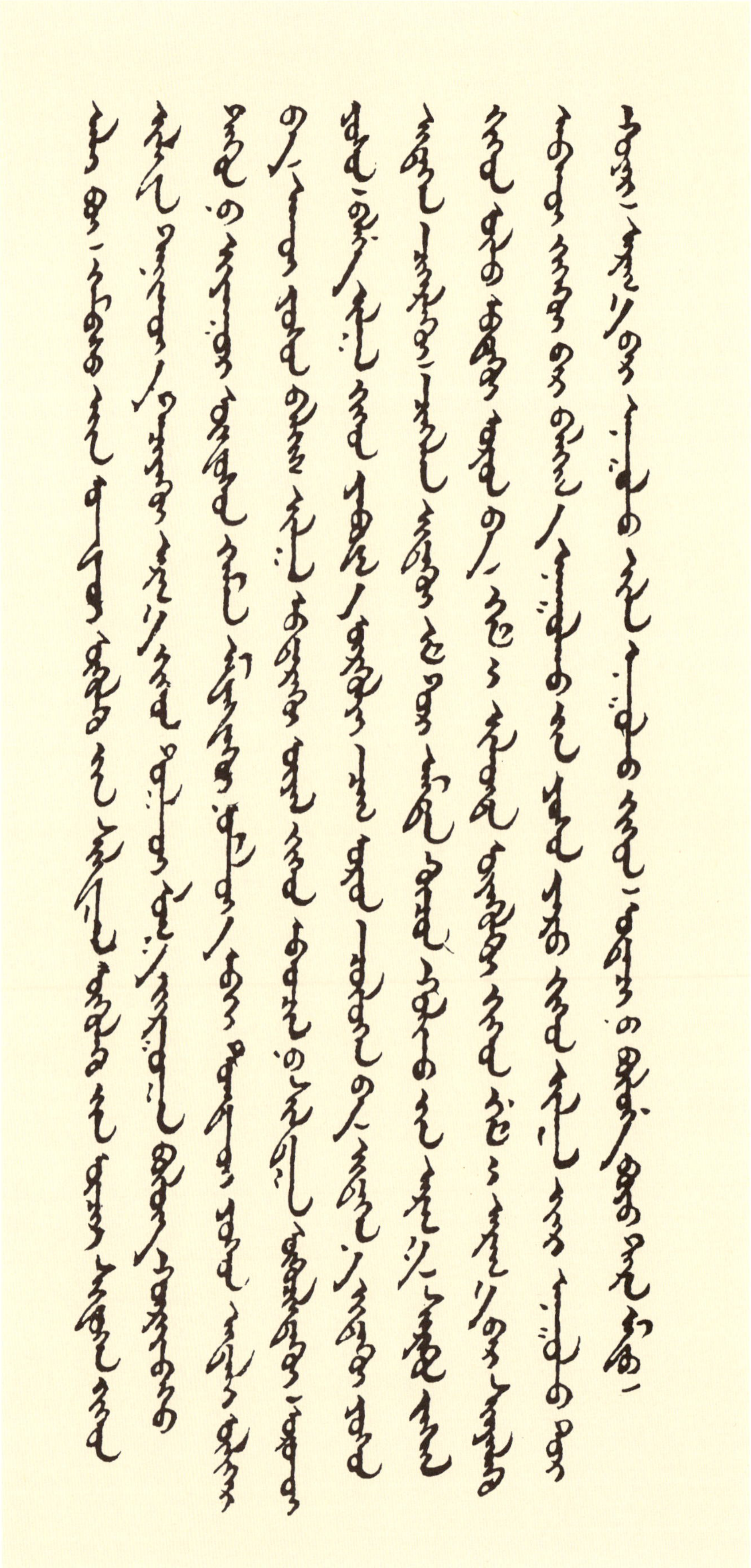

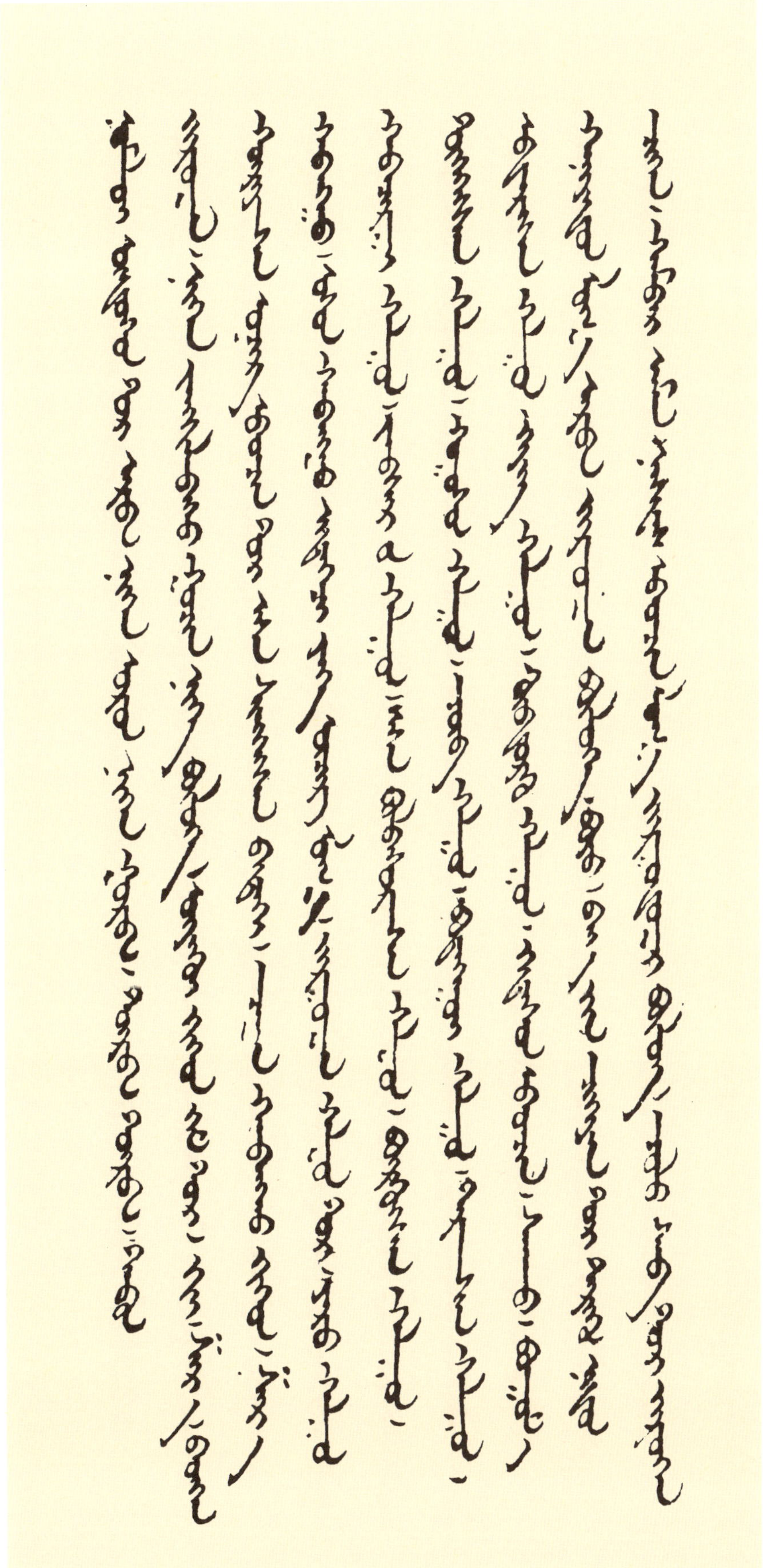

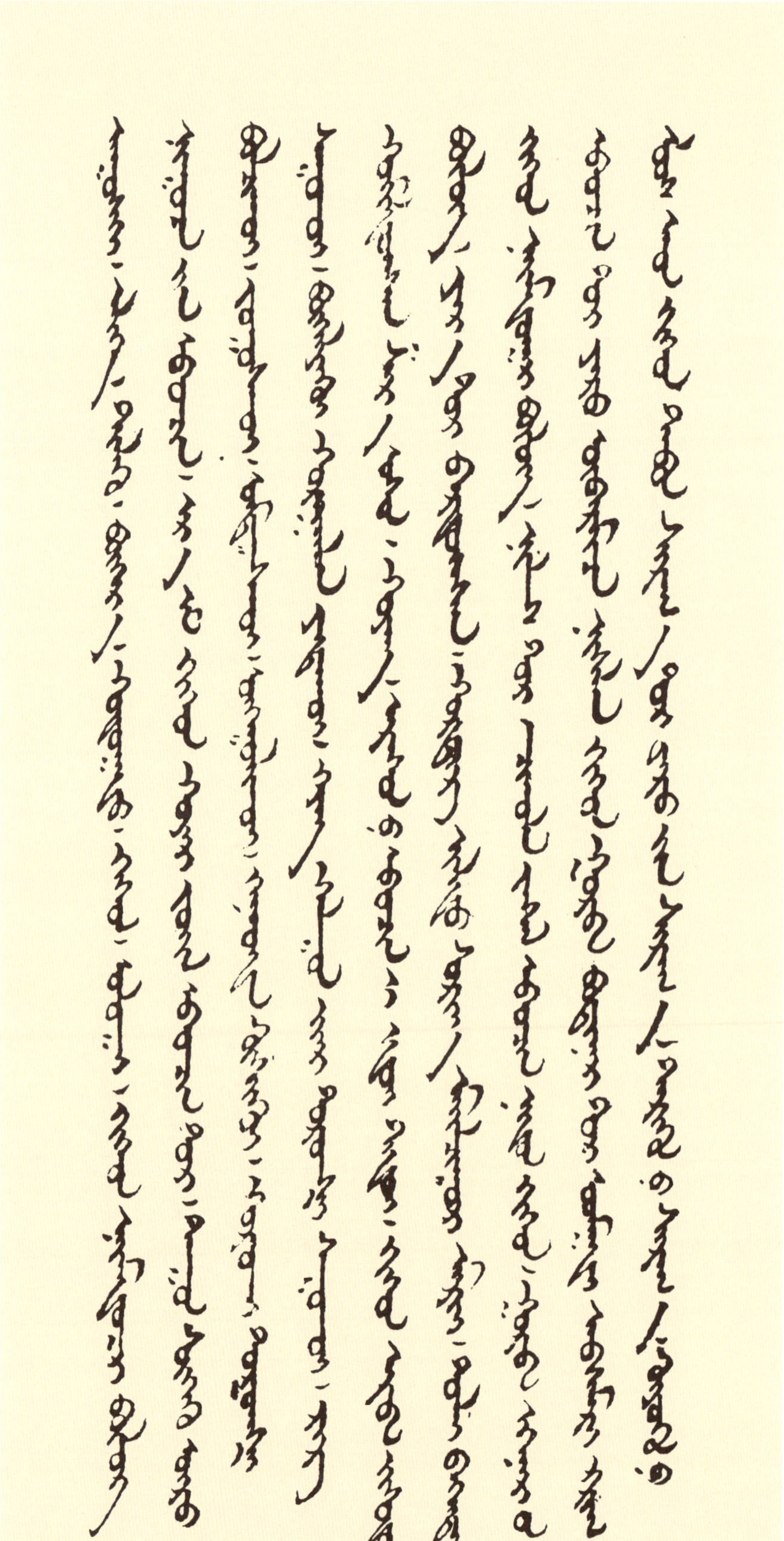

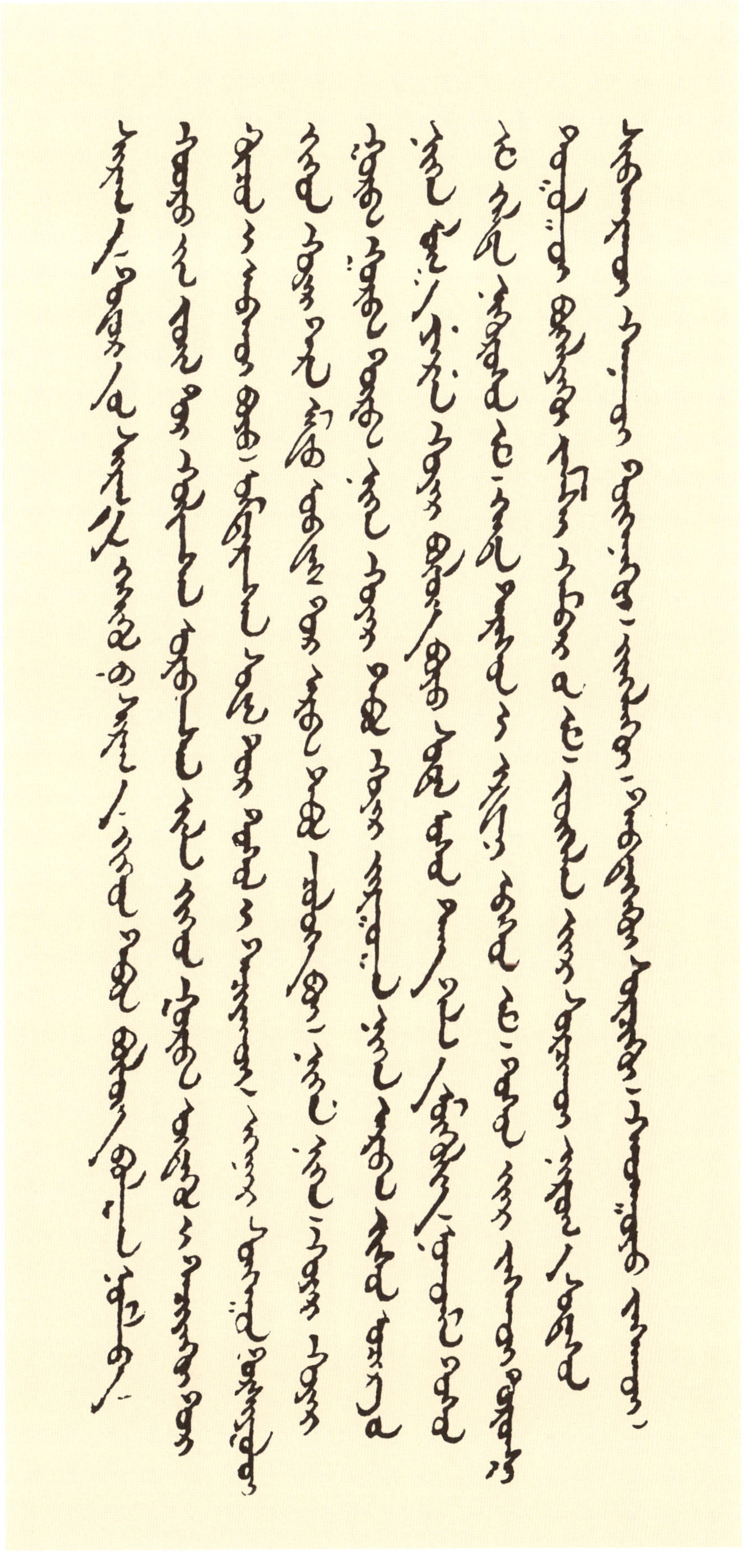

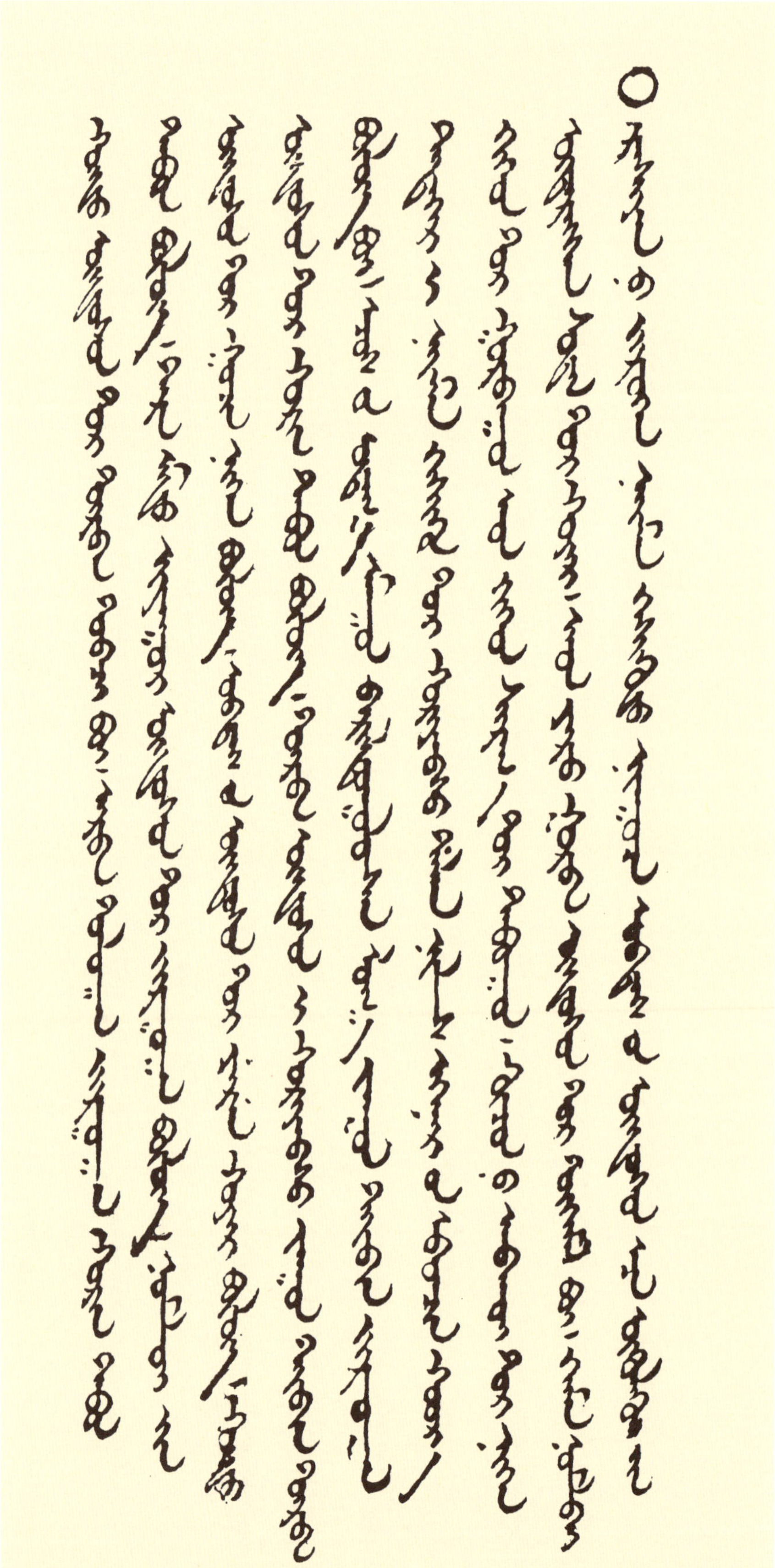

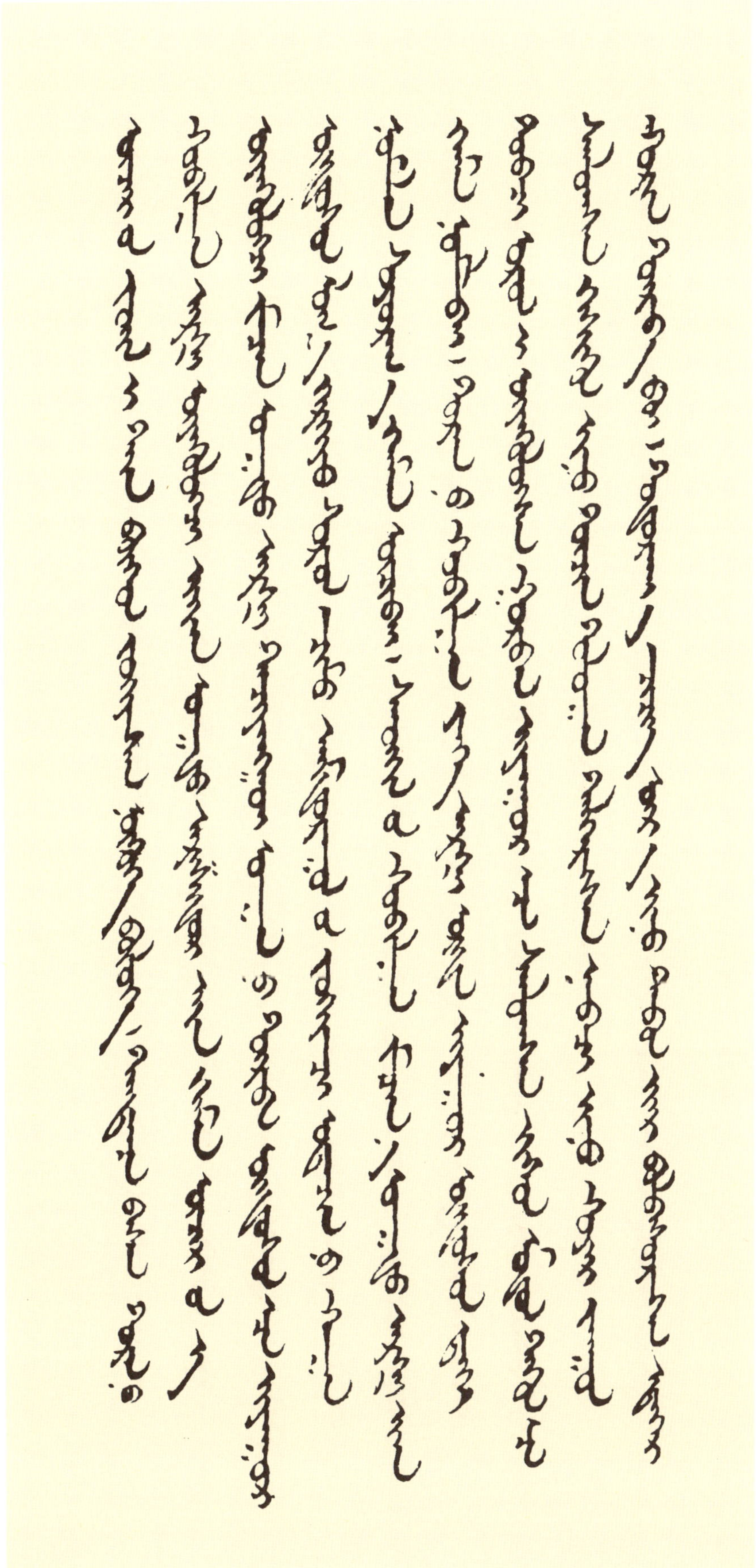

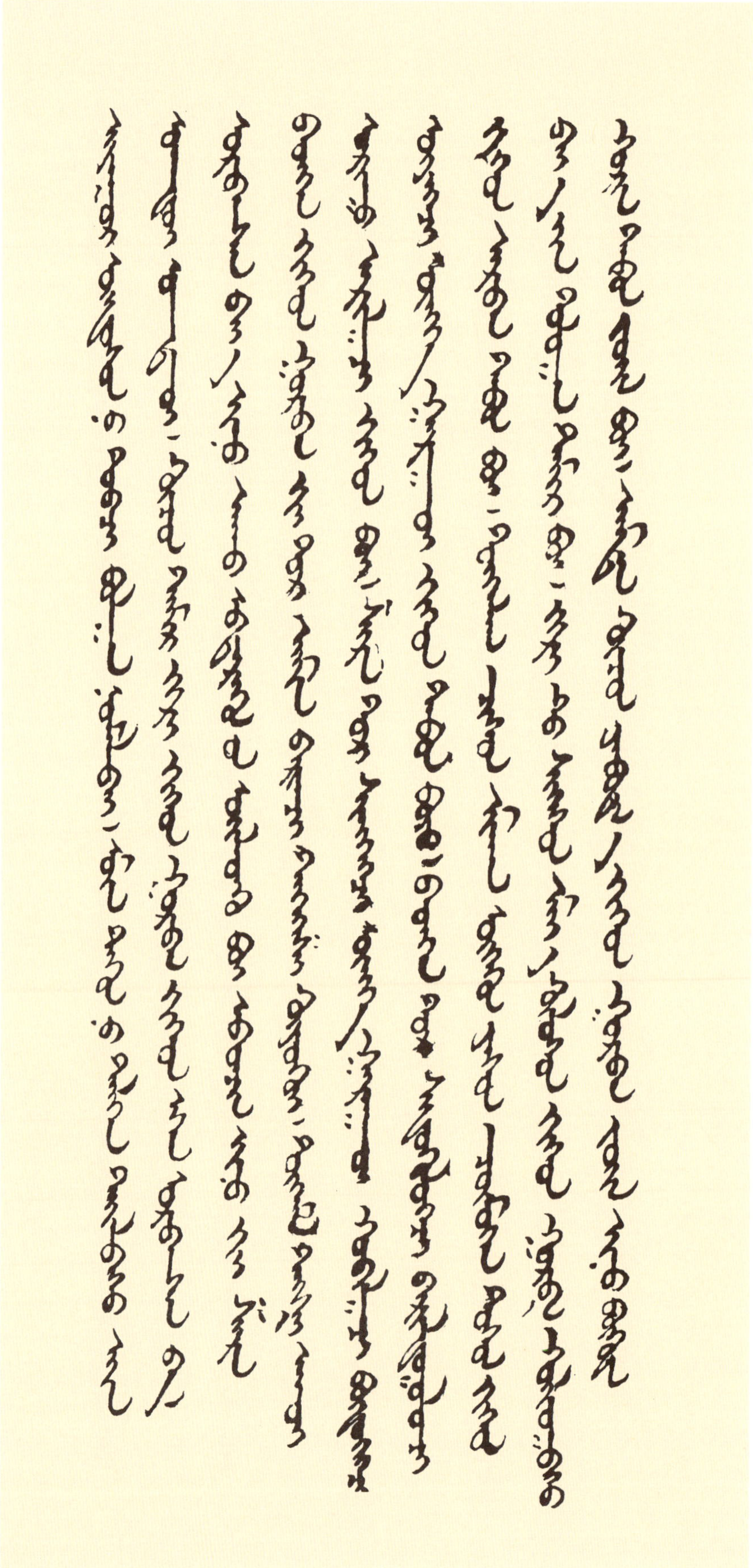

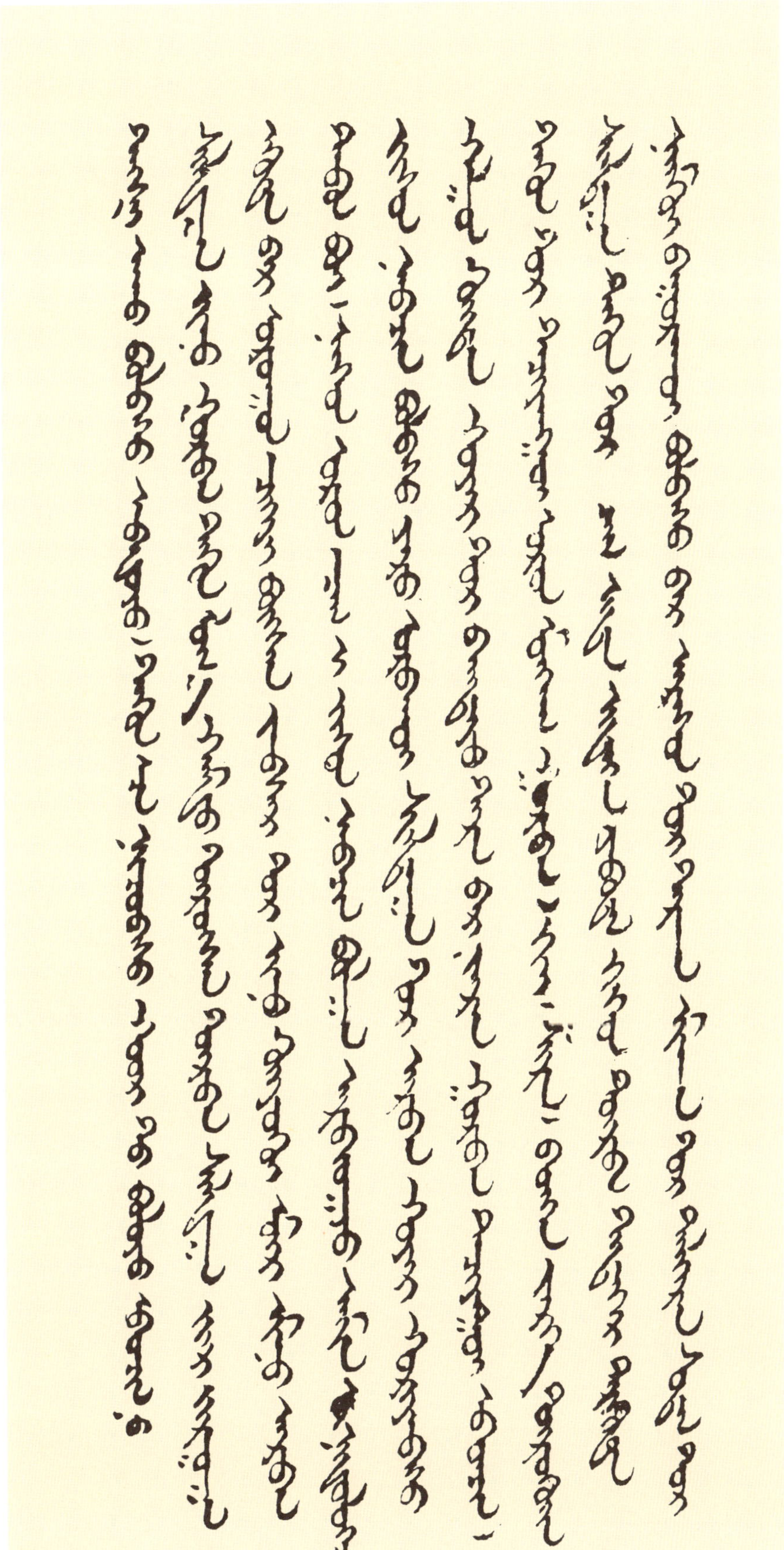

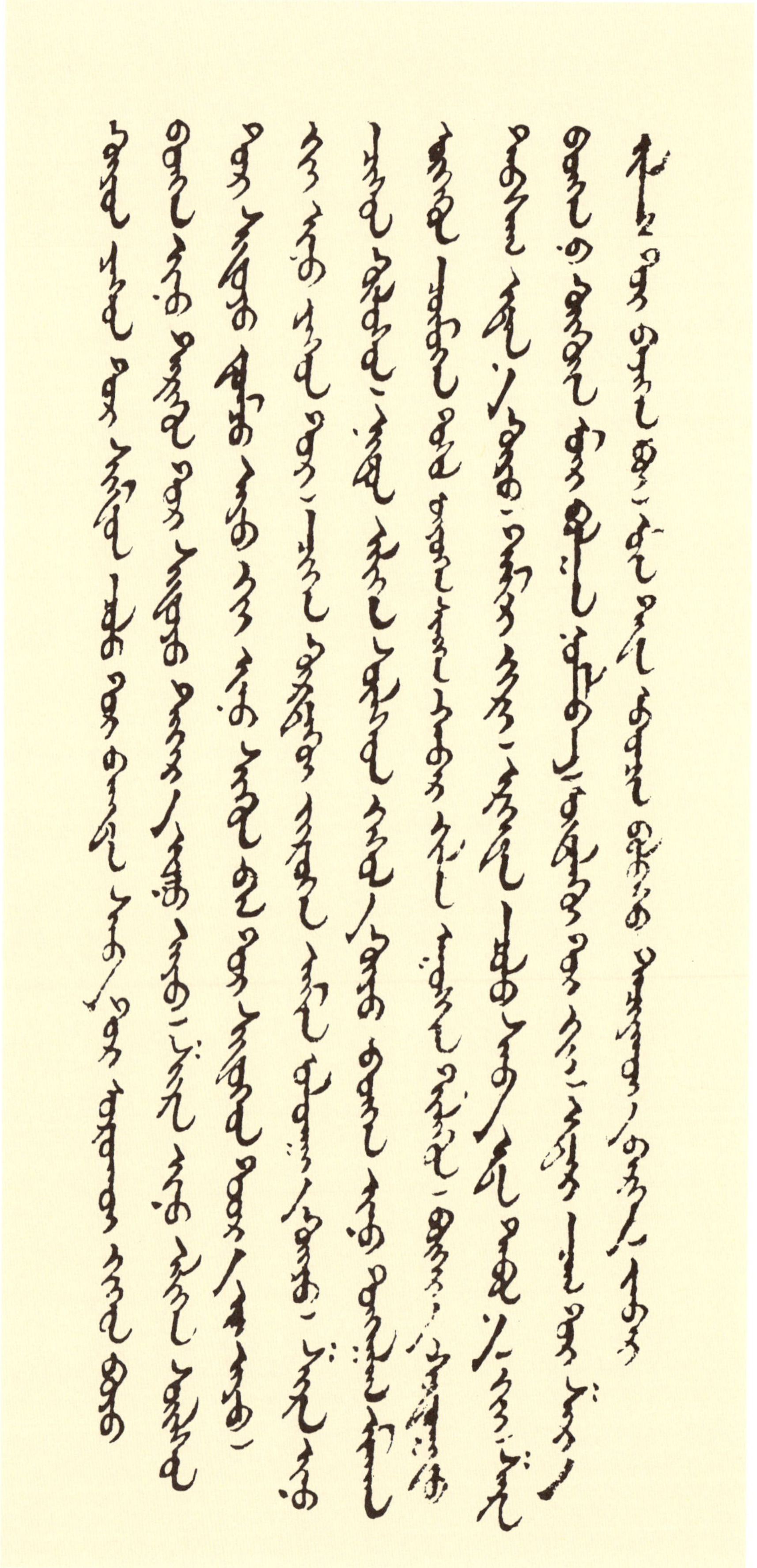

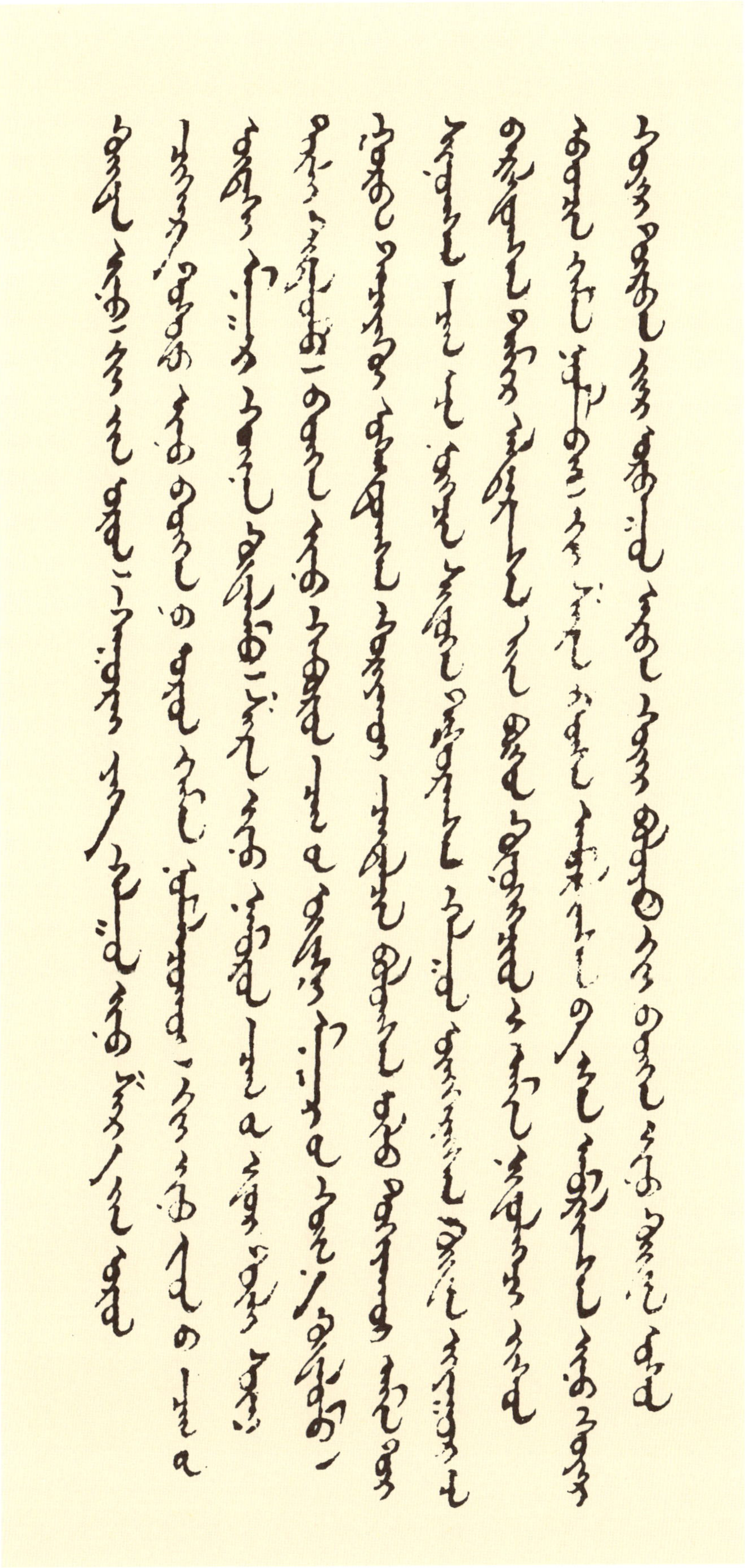

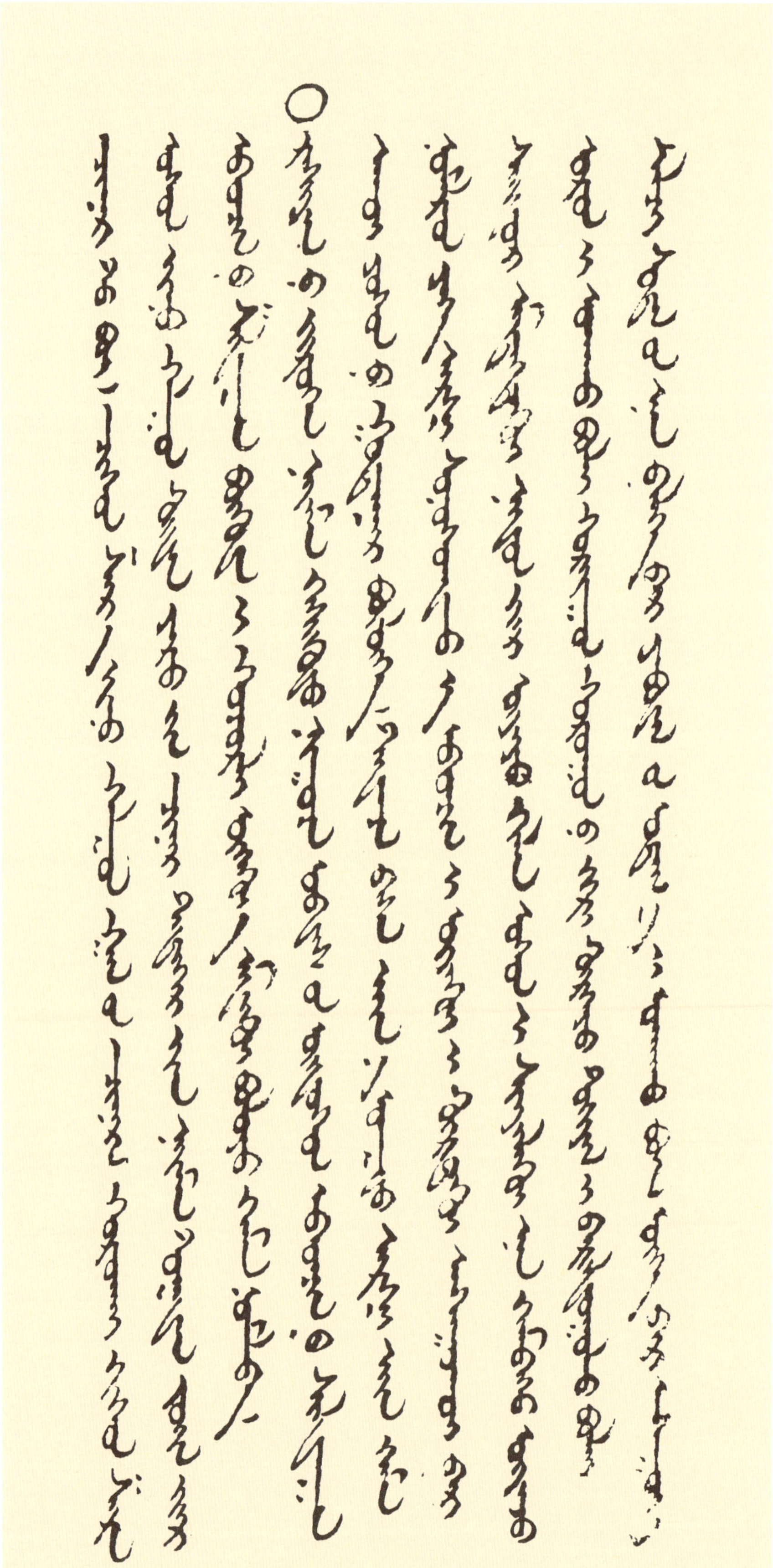

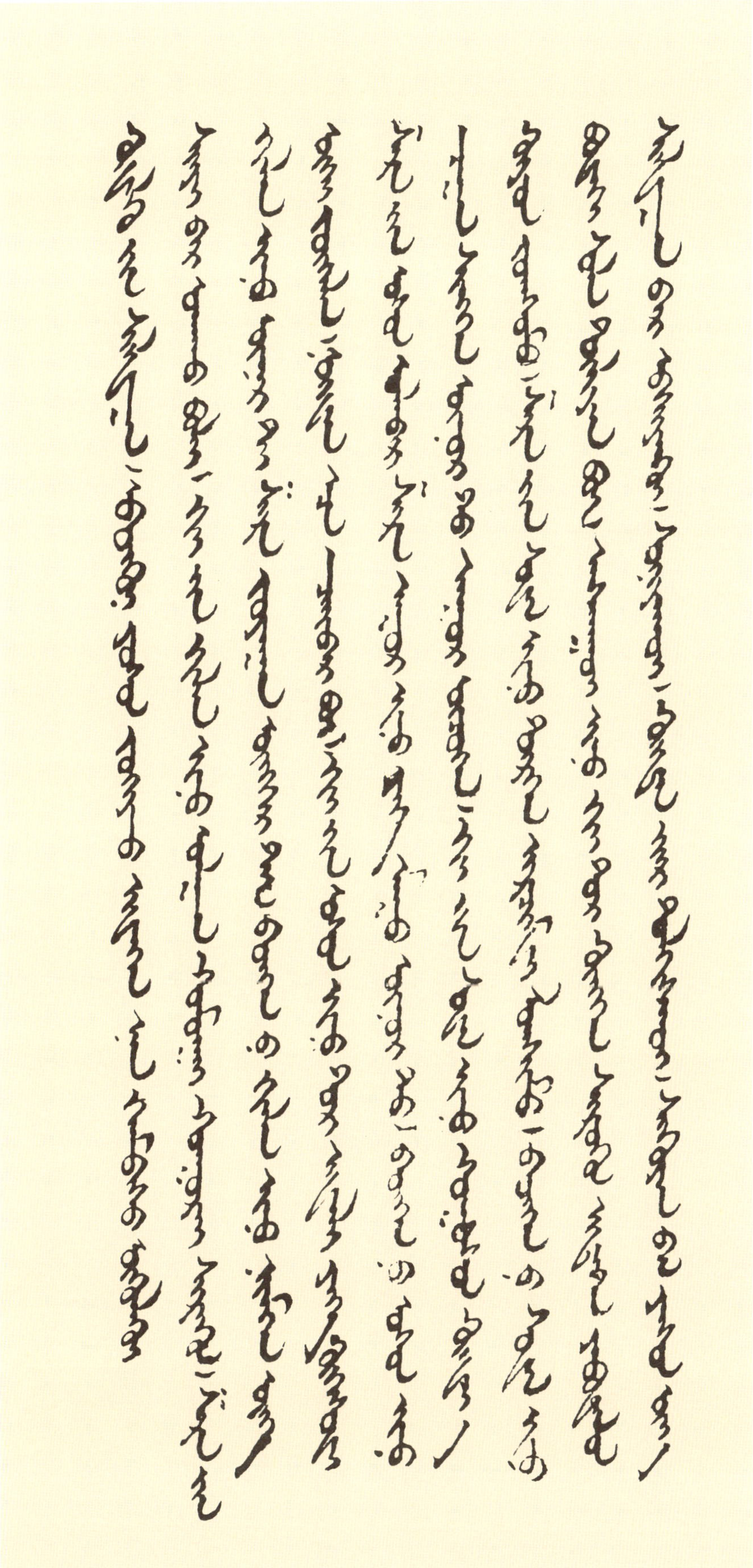

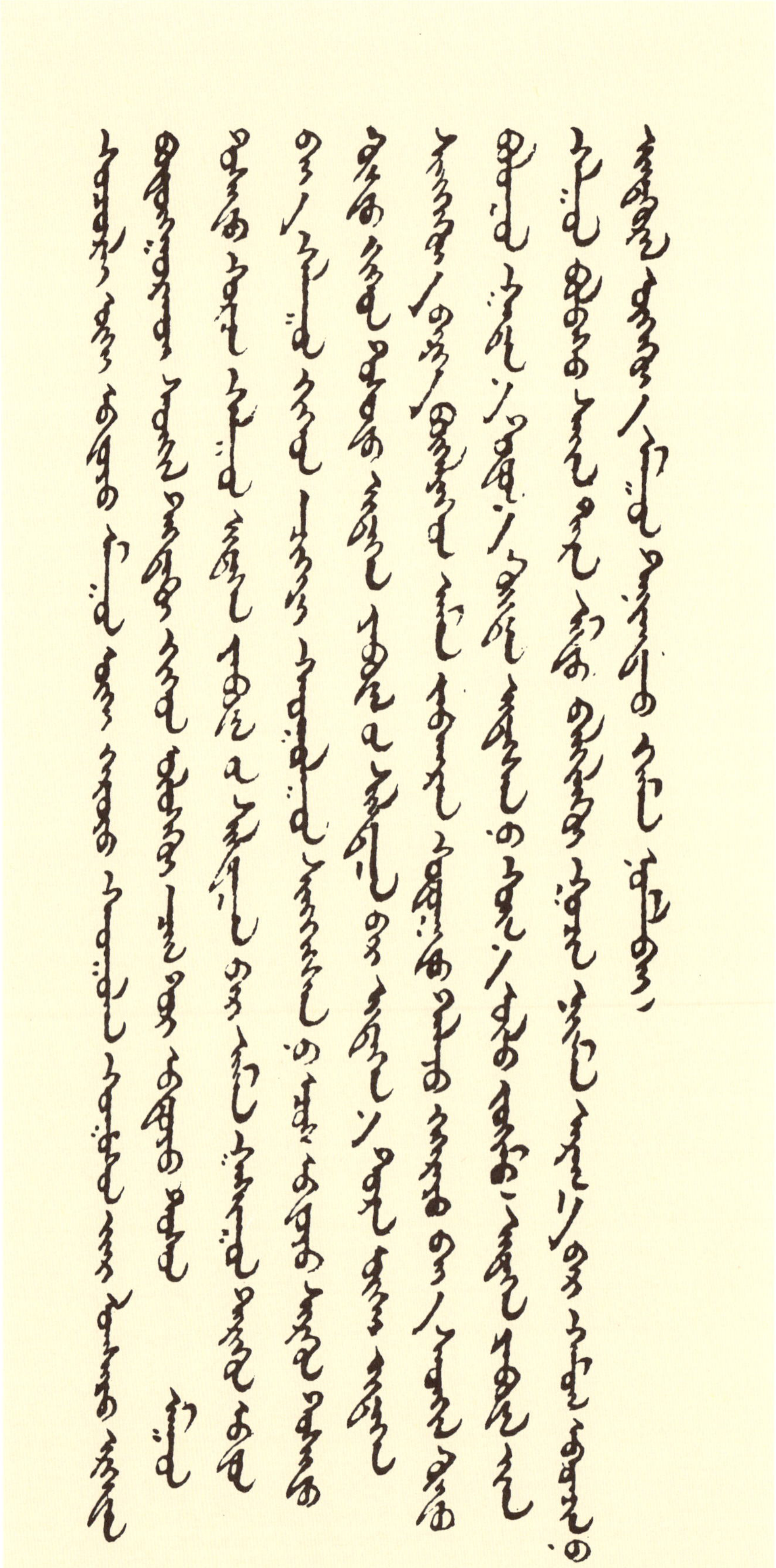

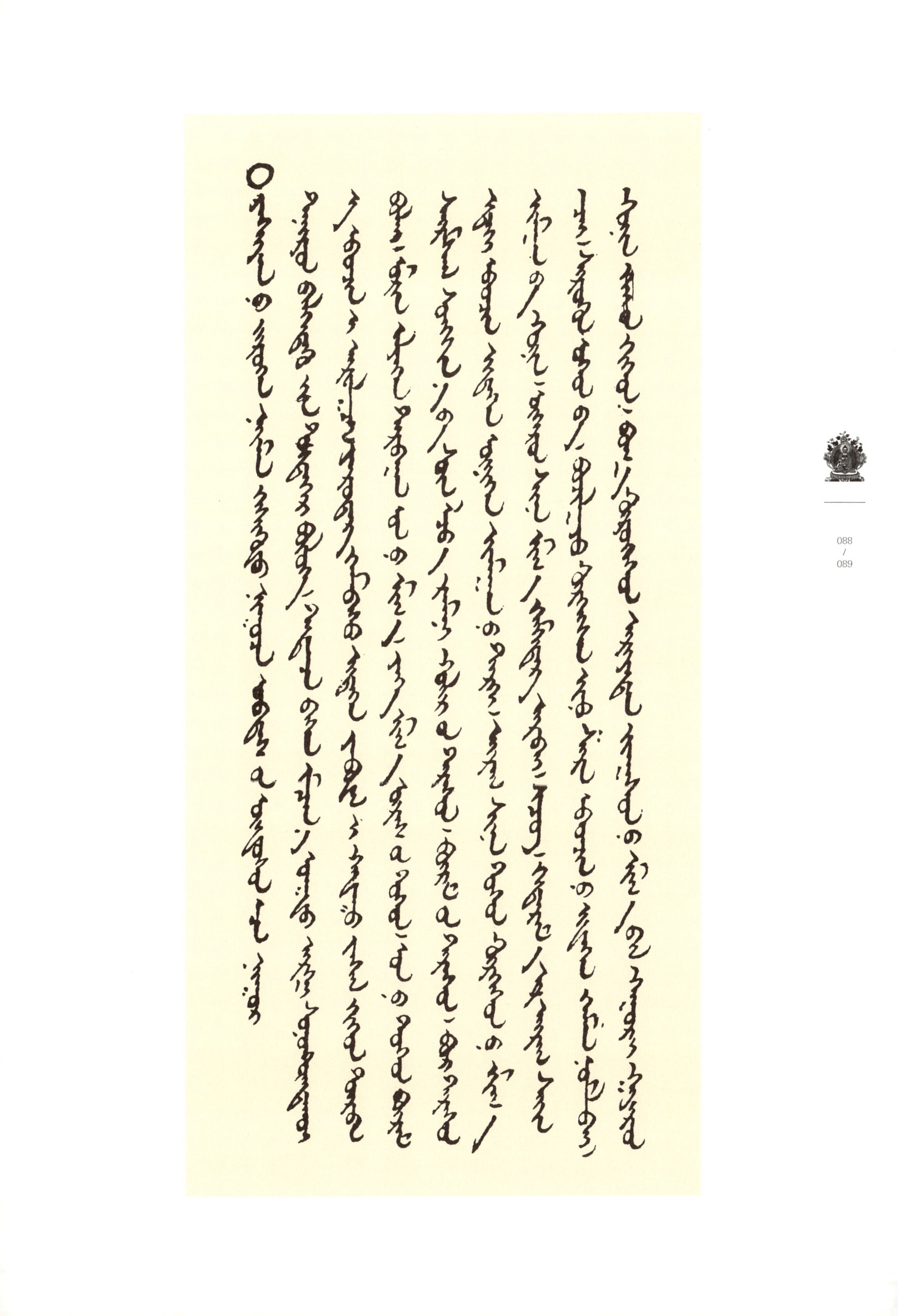

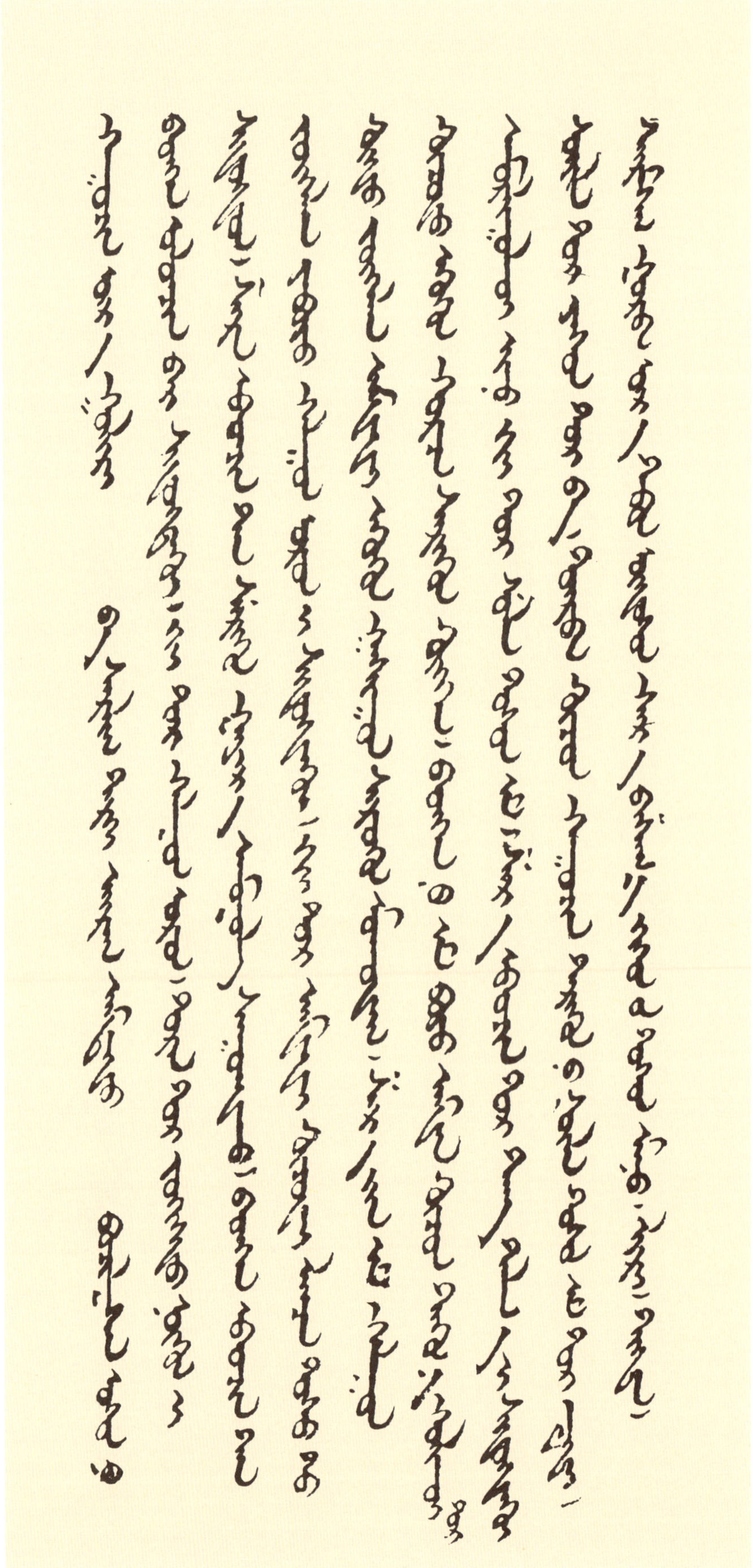

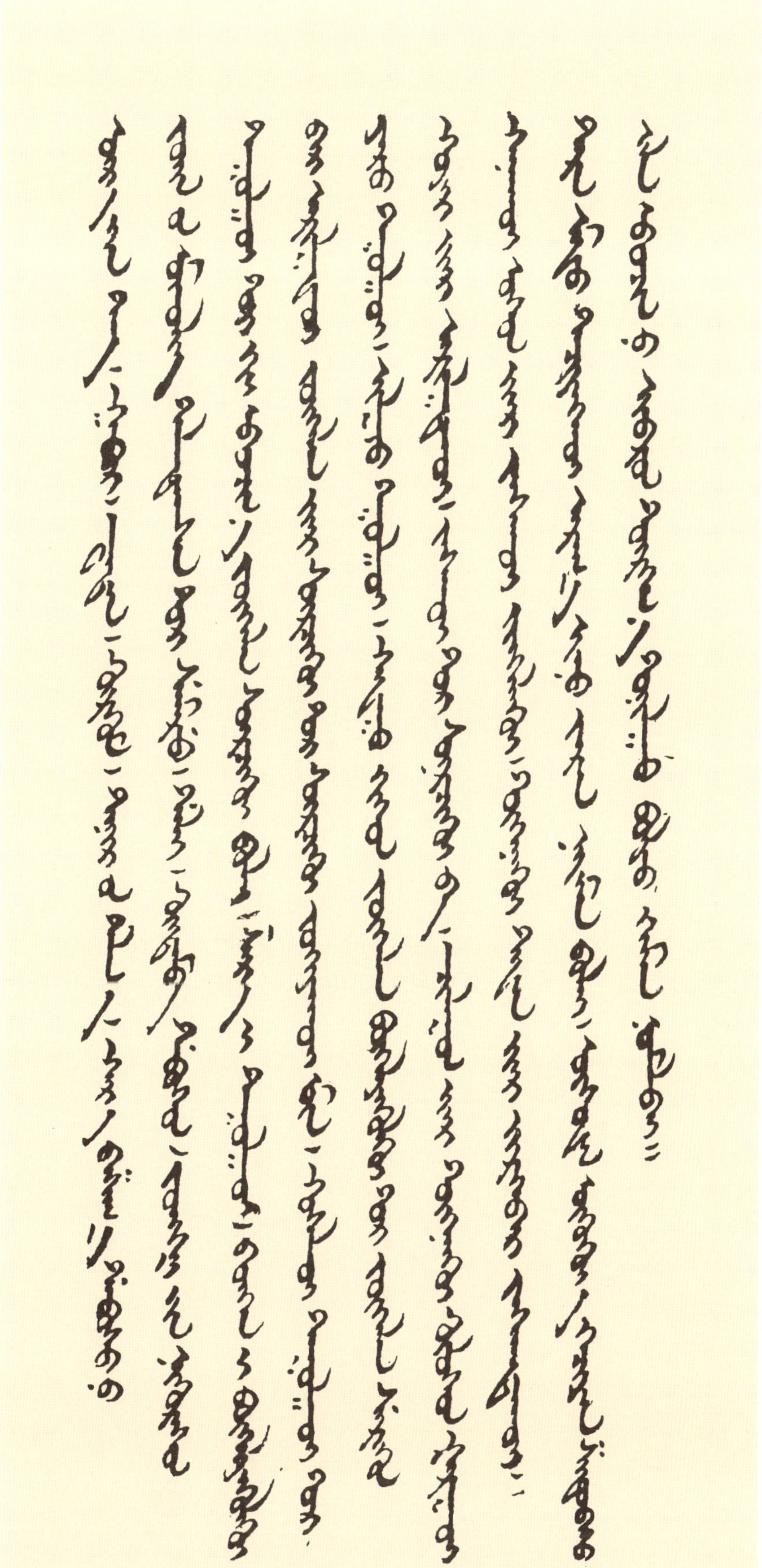

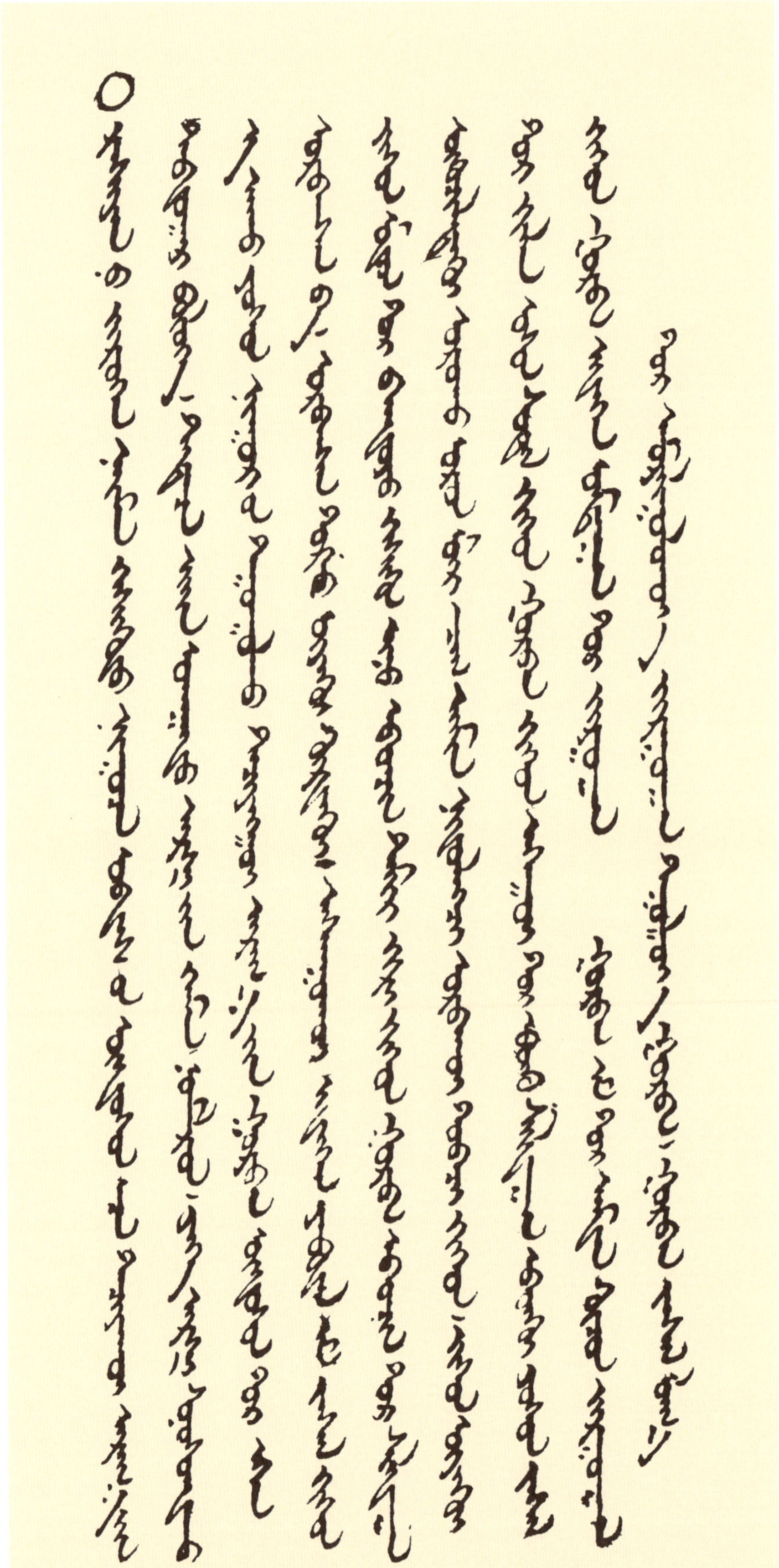

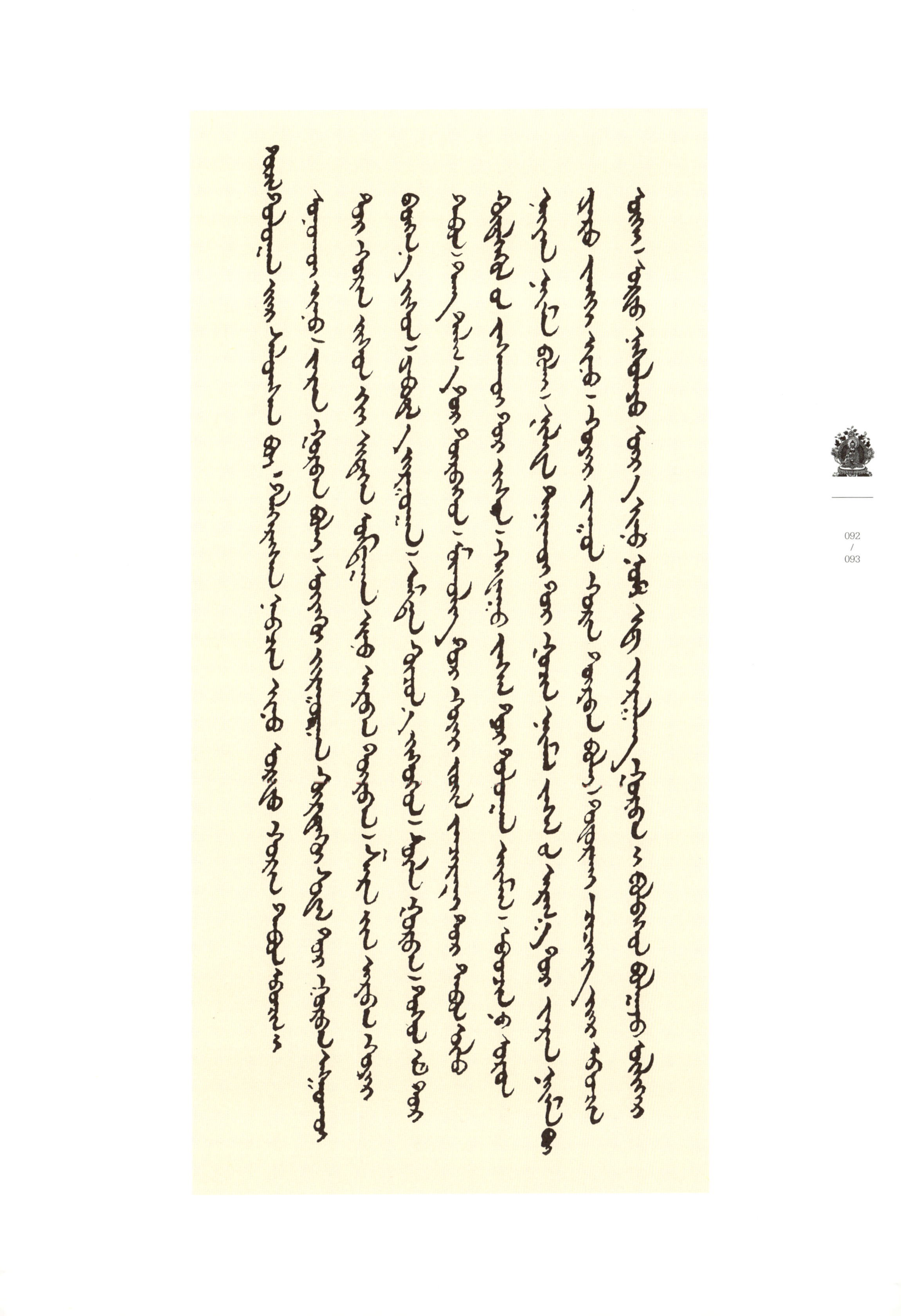

[illegible]

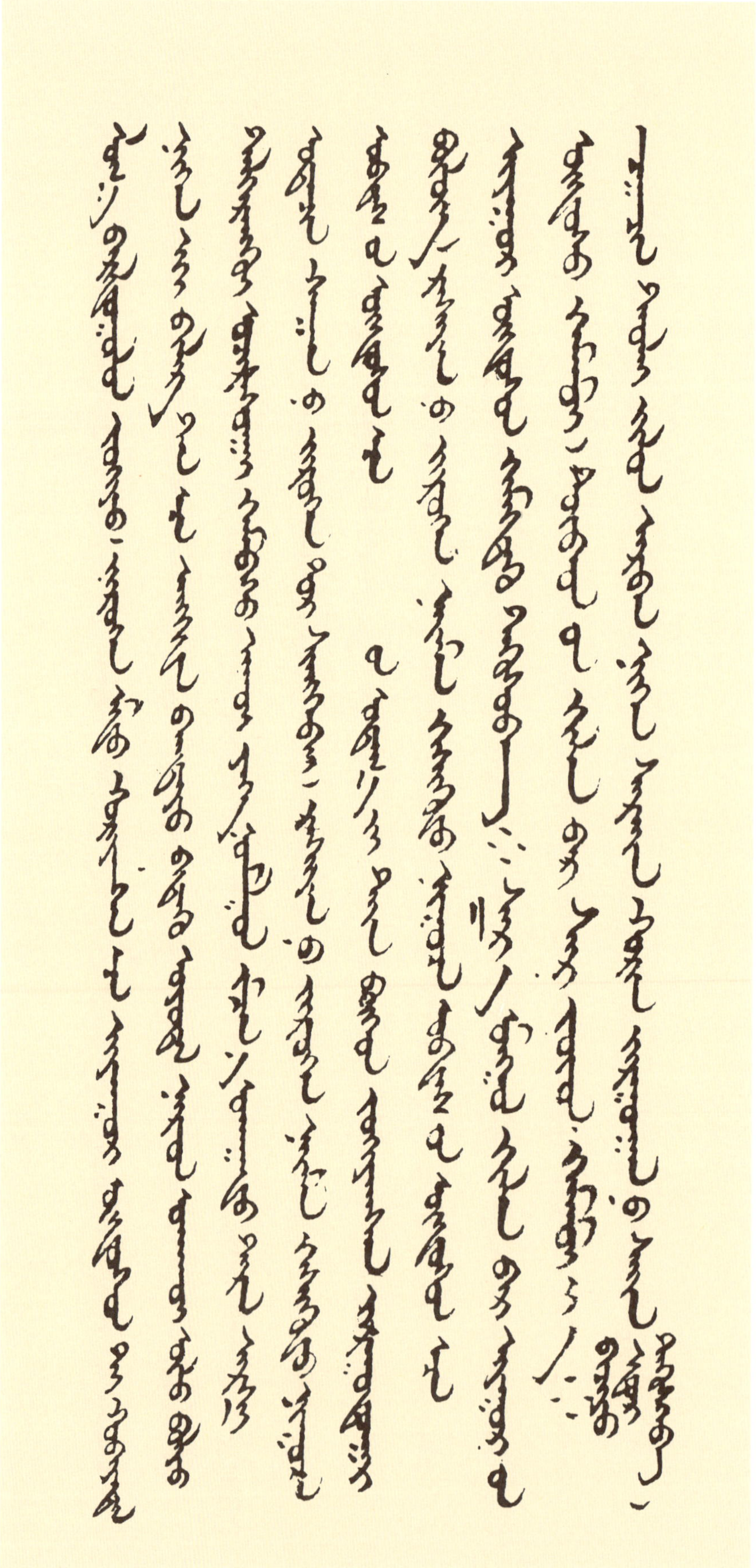

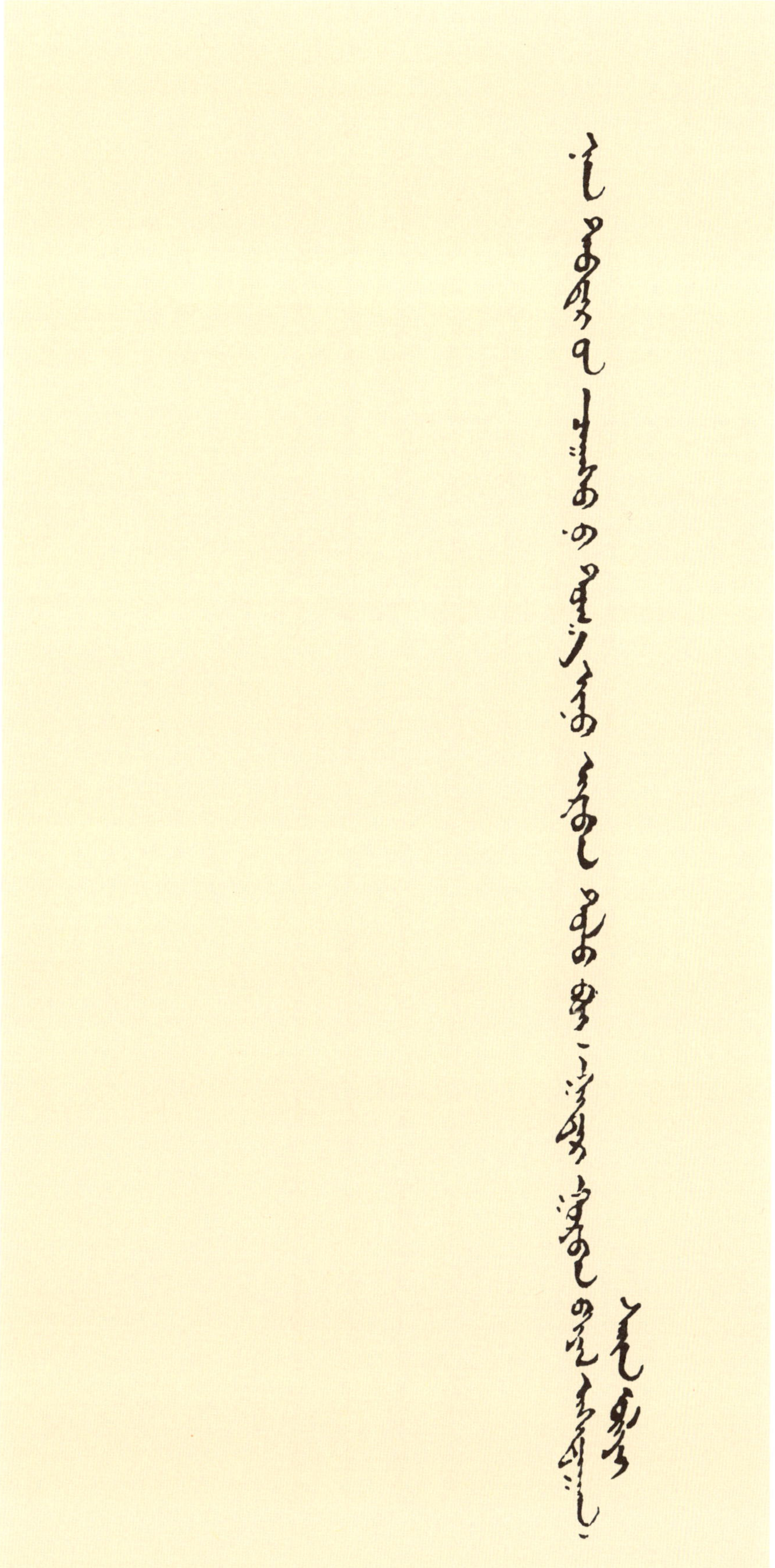

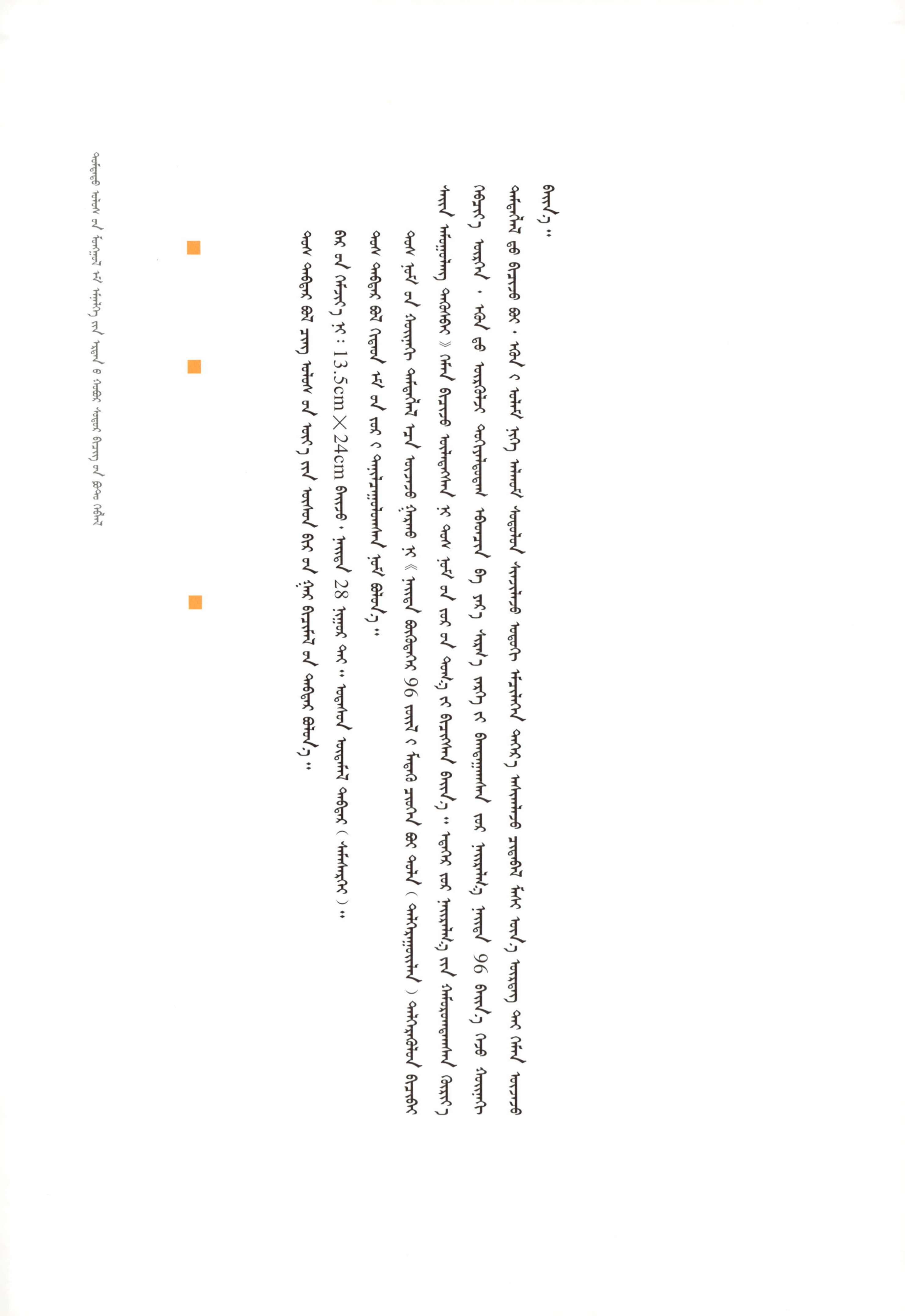

ᠪᠢᠴᠢᠭ ᠦᠨ ᠬᠡᠮᠵᠢᠶ᠎ᠡ ᠨᠢ : 13.5cm×24cm ᠪᠣᠯᠤᠭᠰᠠᠨ ᠂ ᠨᠡᠢᠲᠡ 28 ᠨᠢᠭᠤᠷ ᠲᠠᠢ :: ᠬᠠᠳᠠᠭᠠᠯᠠᠭᠰᠠᠨ ᠬᠠᠳᠠᠭᠠᠯᠠᠭᠴᠢ ᠣᠷᠣᠨ (ᠬᠣᠲᠠ) ::

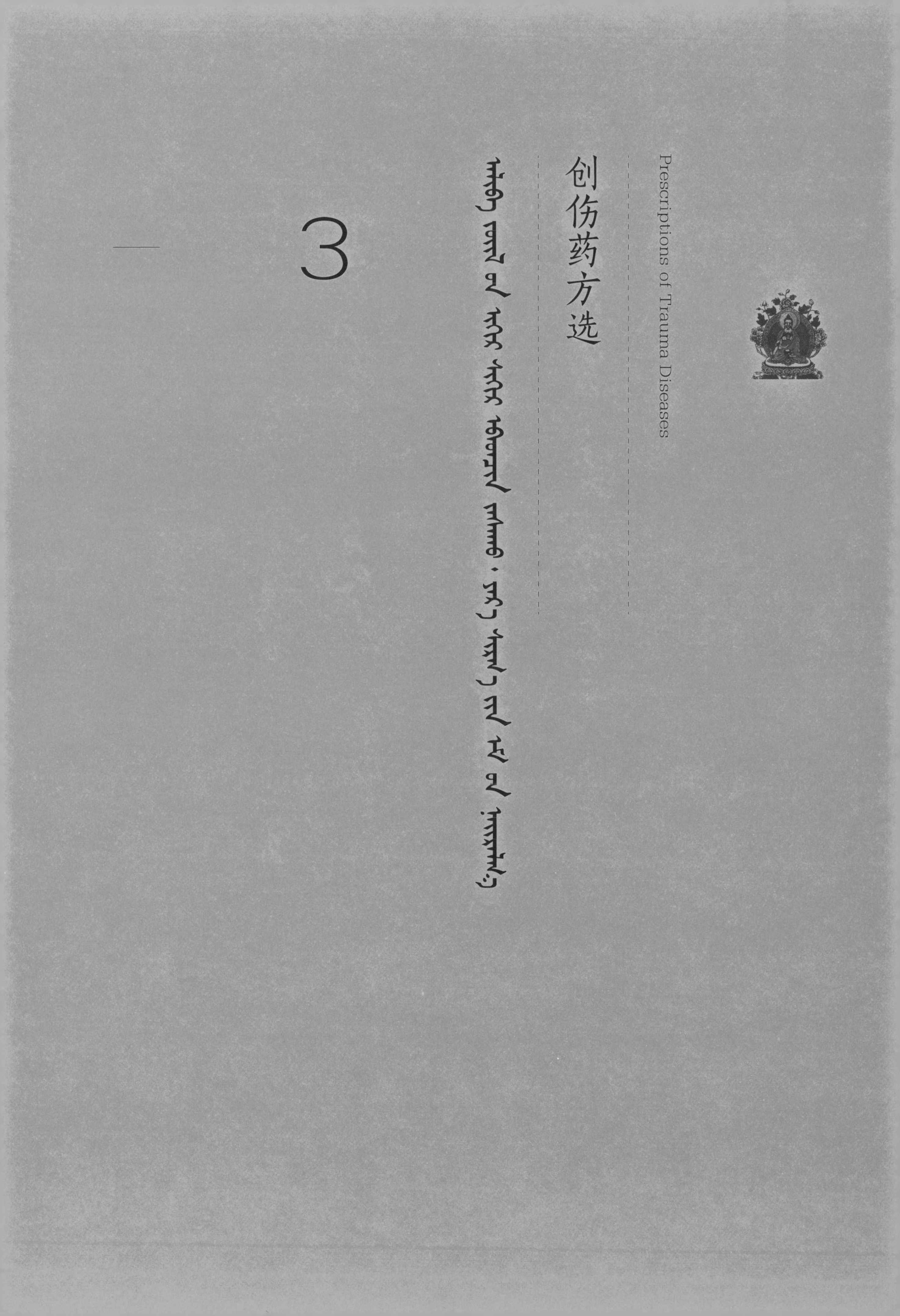

Prescriptions of Trauma Diseases

创伤药方选

3

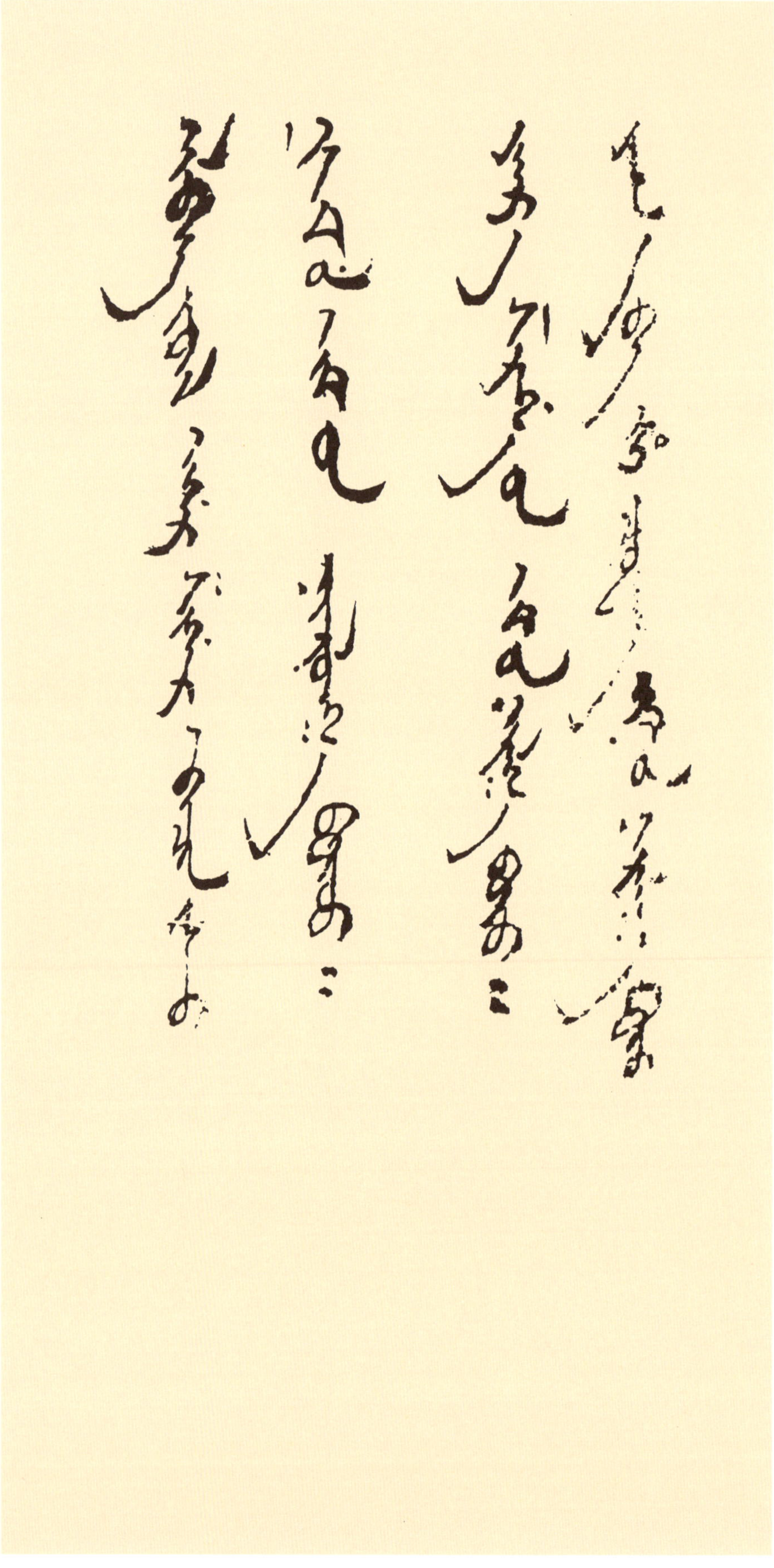

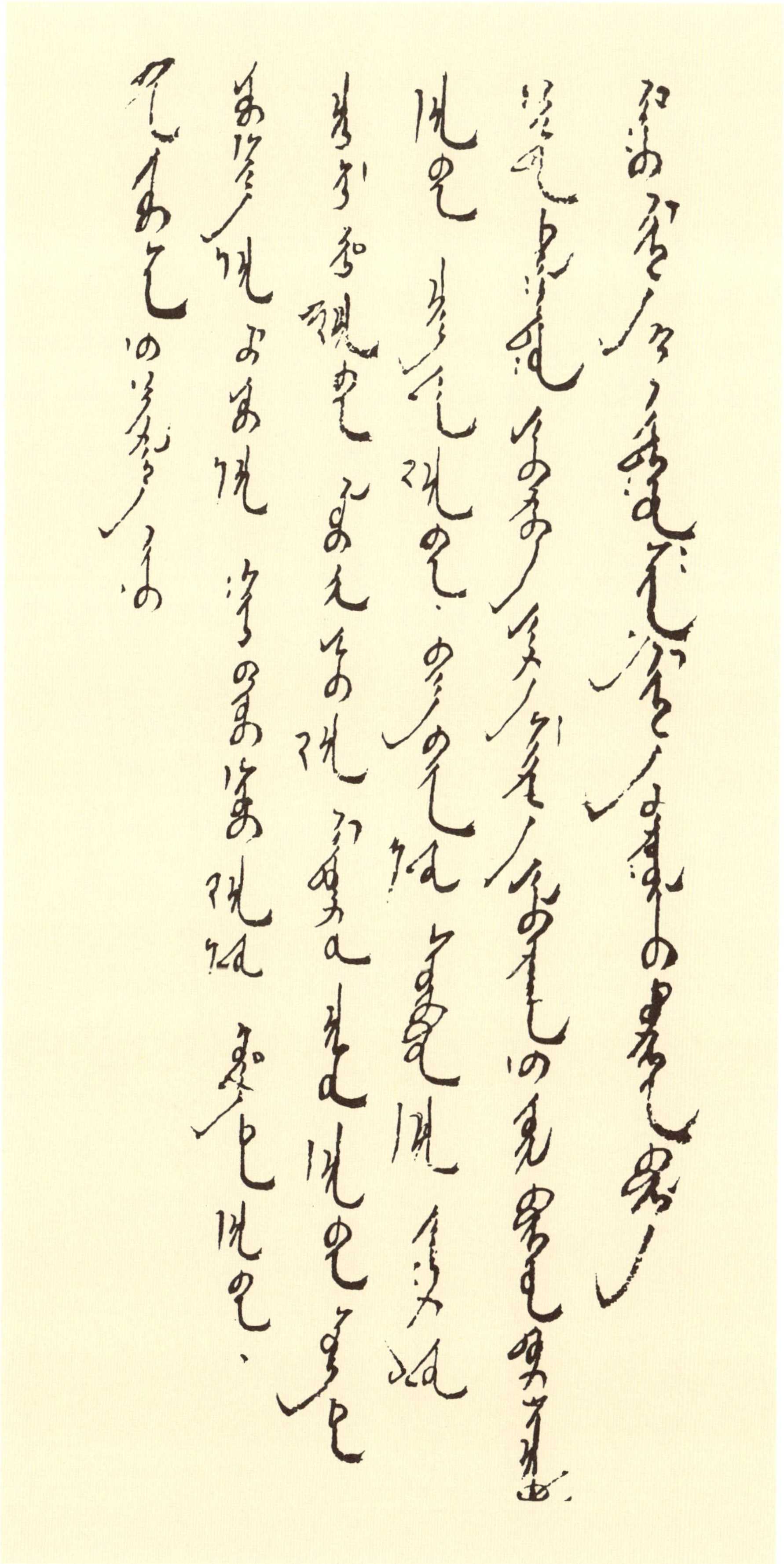

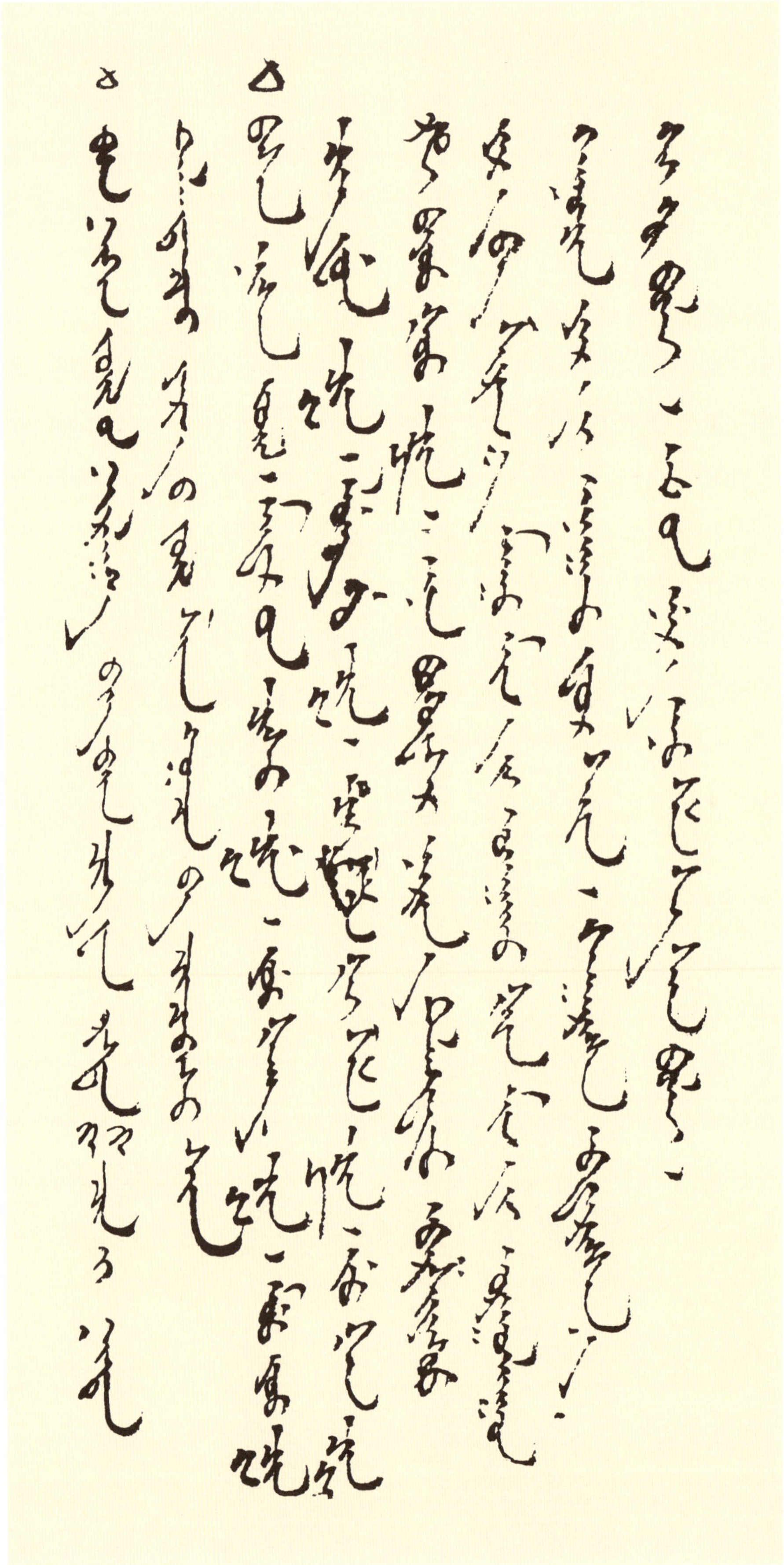

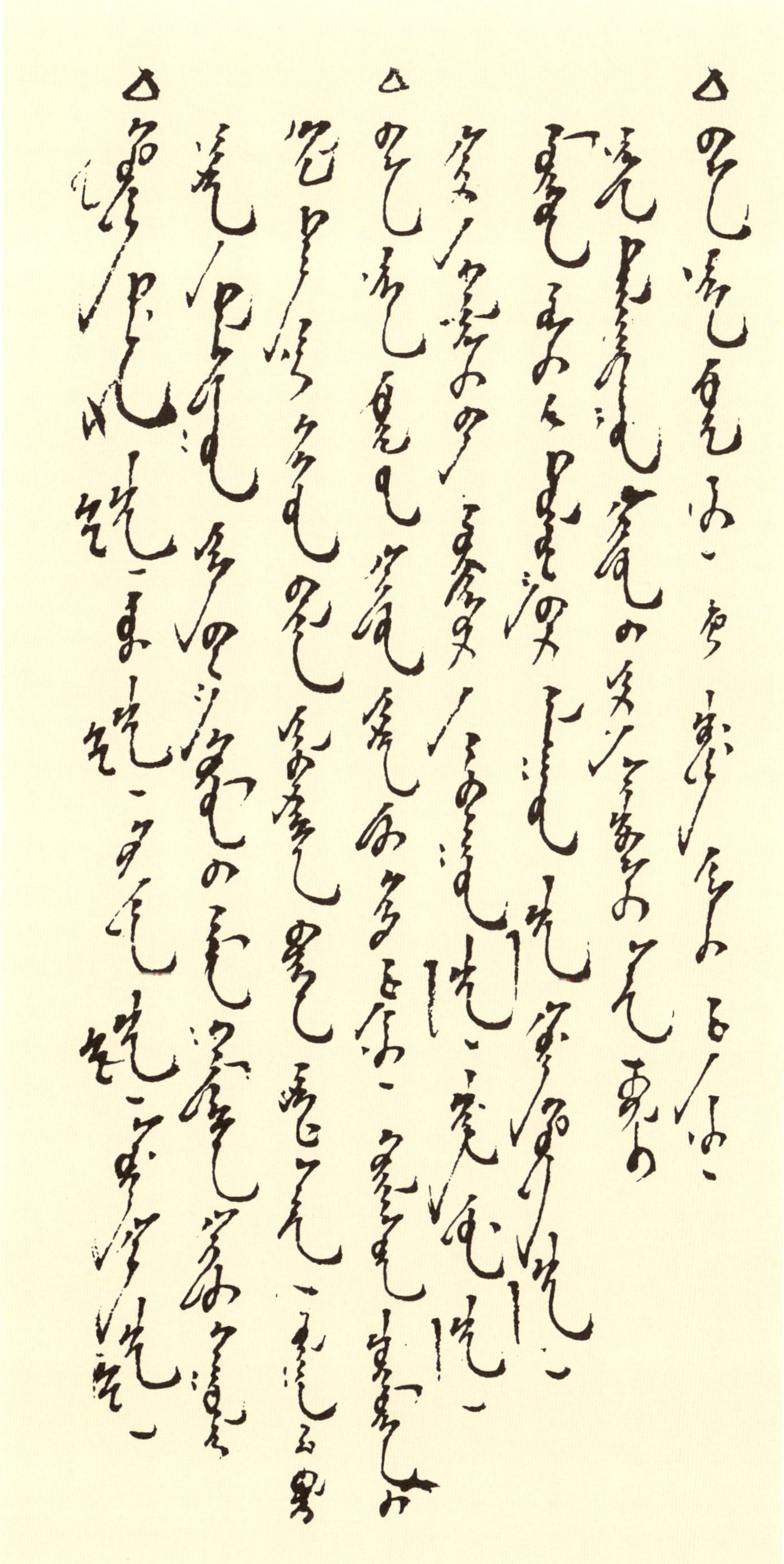

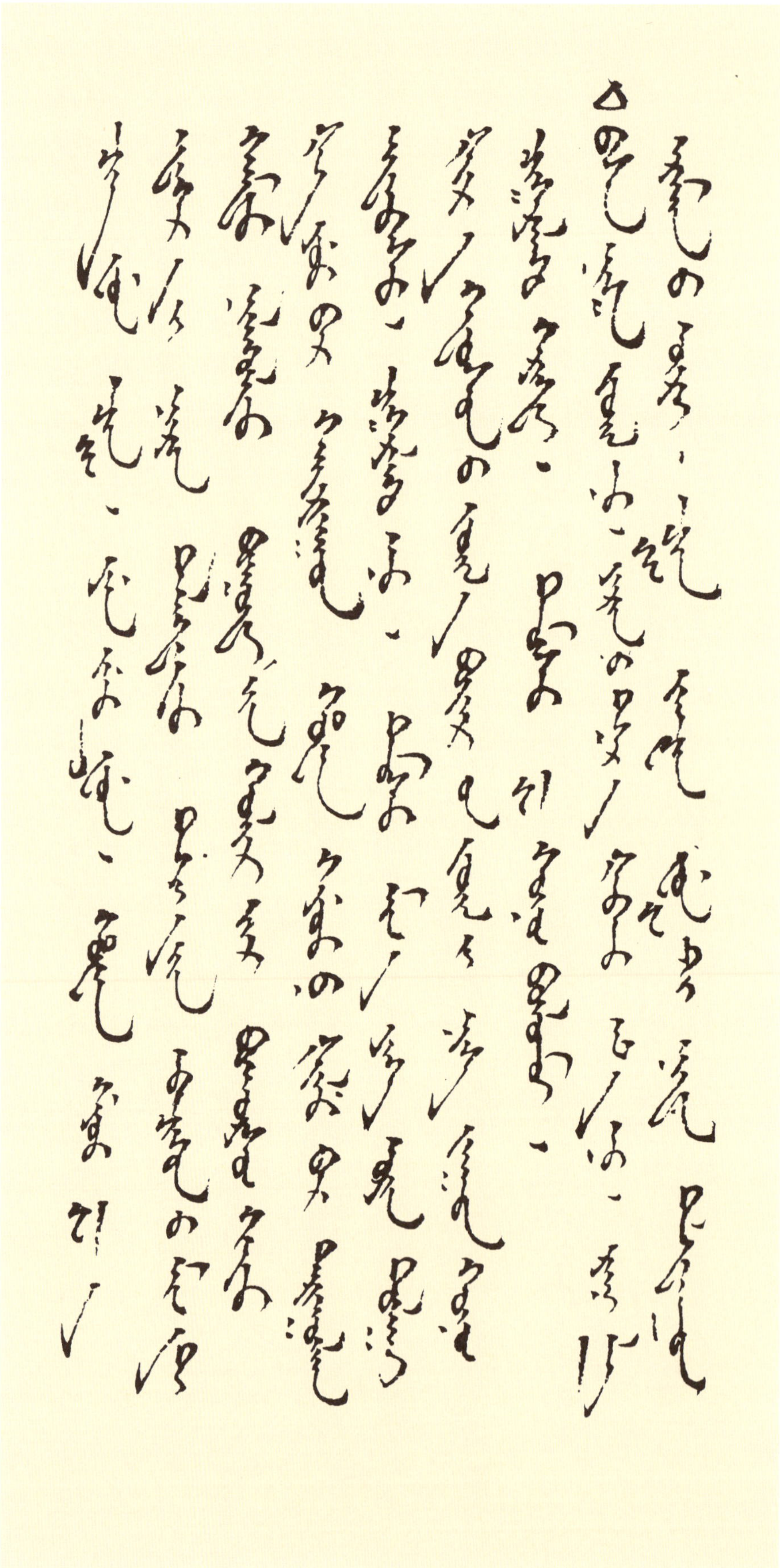

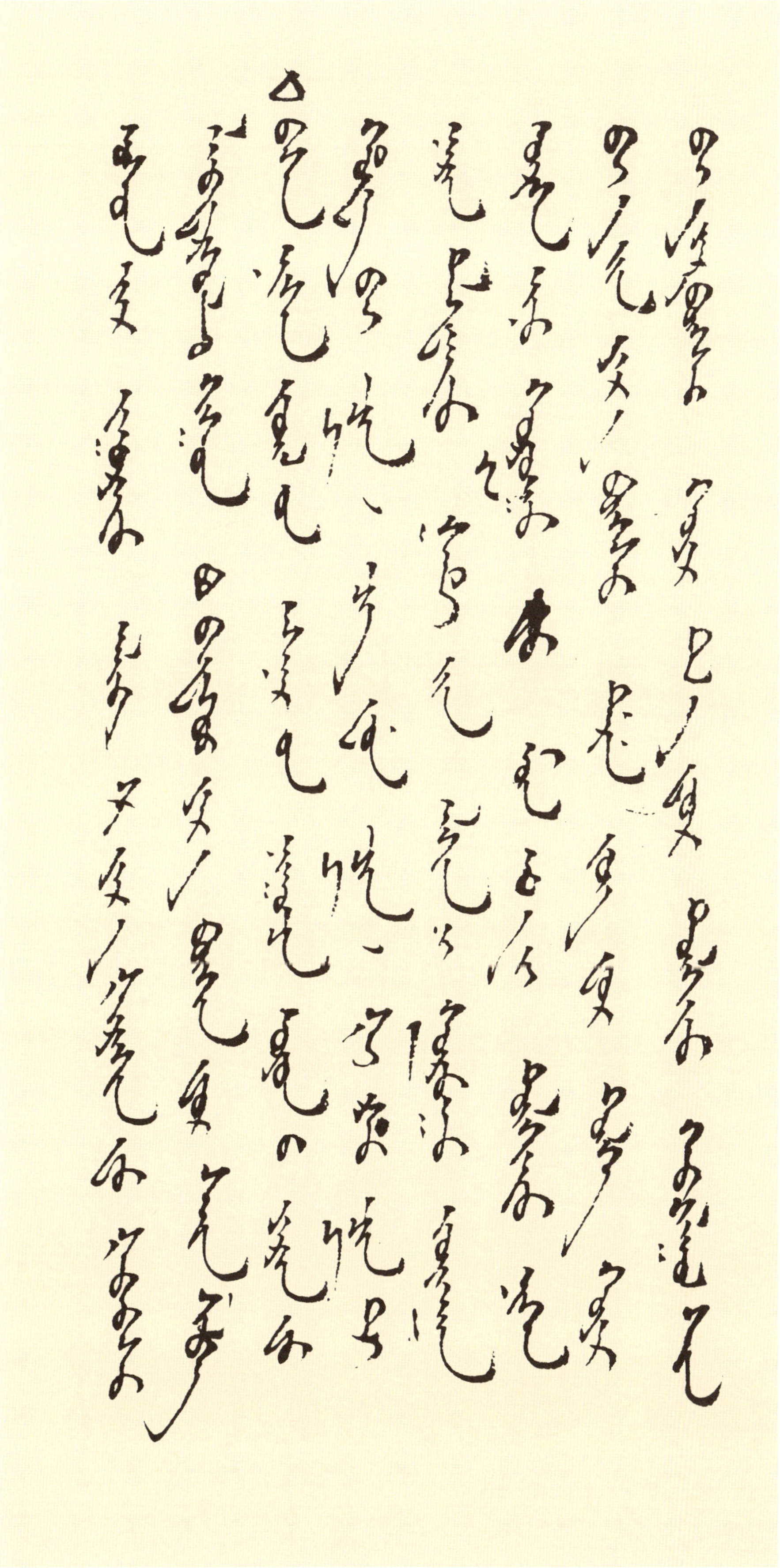

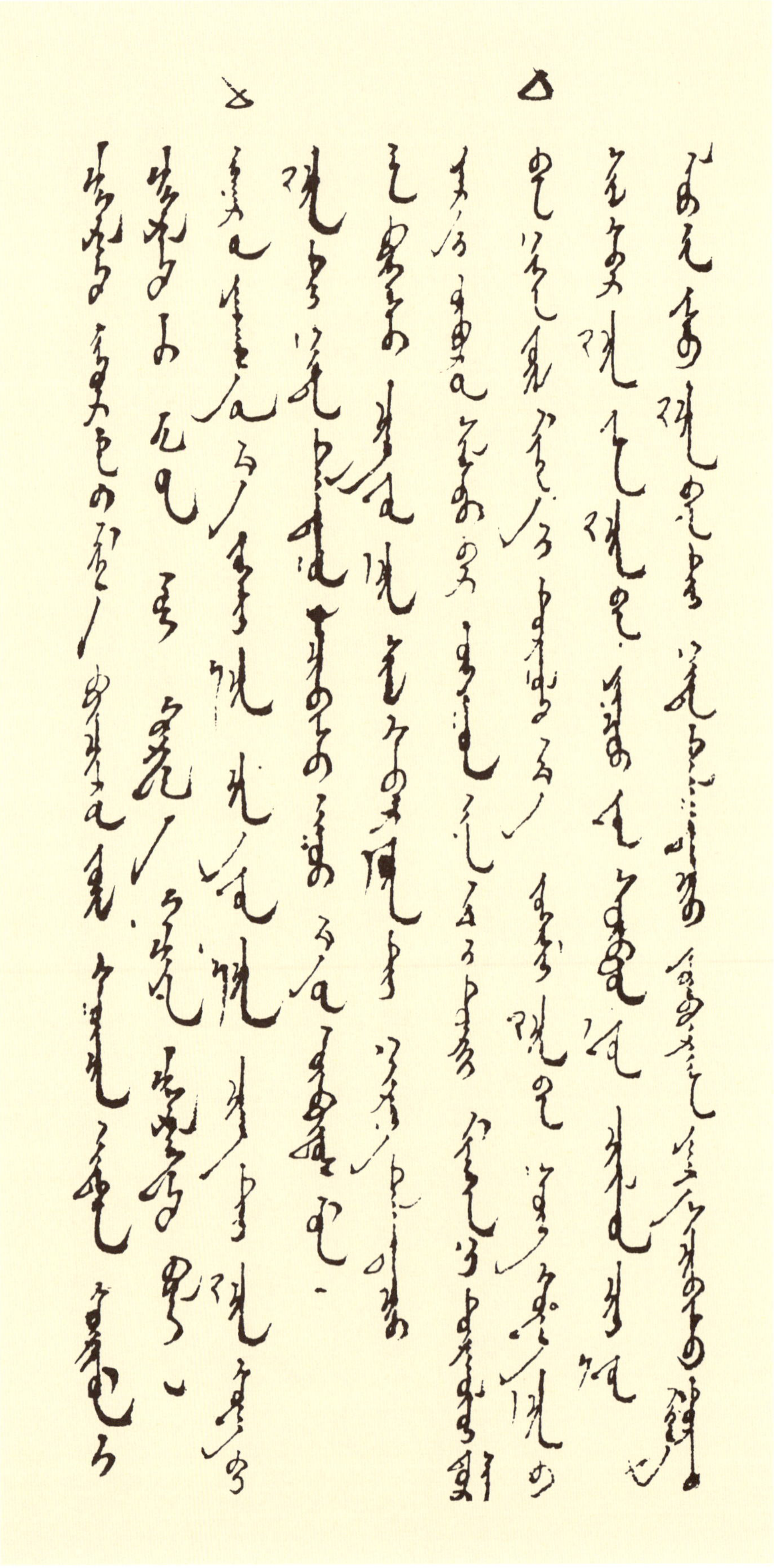

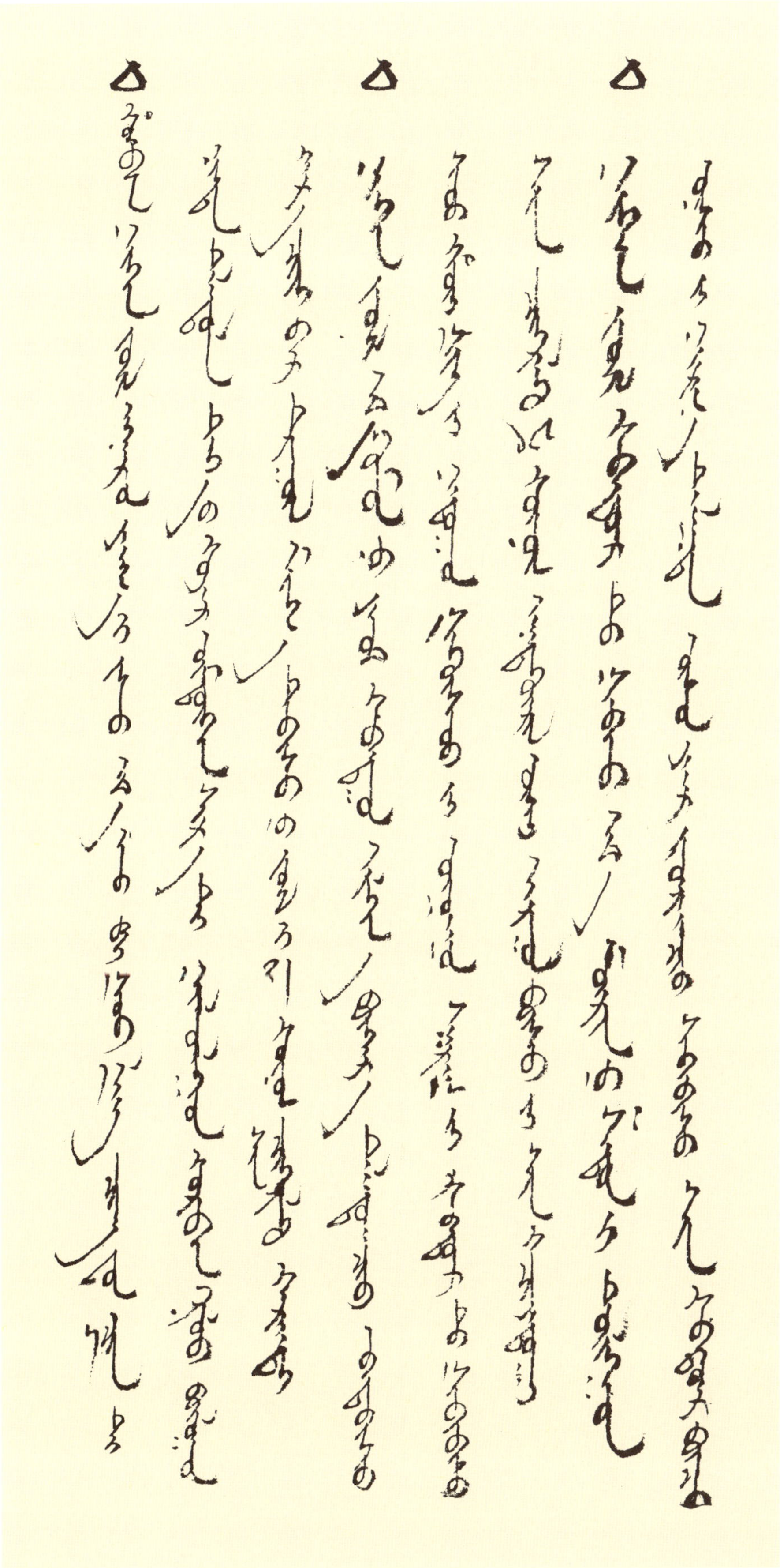

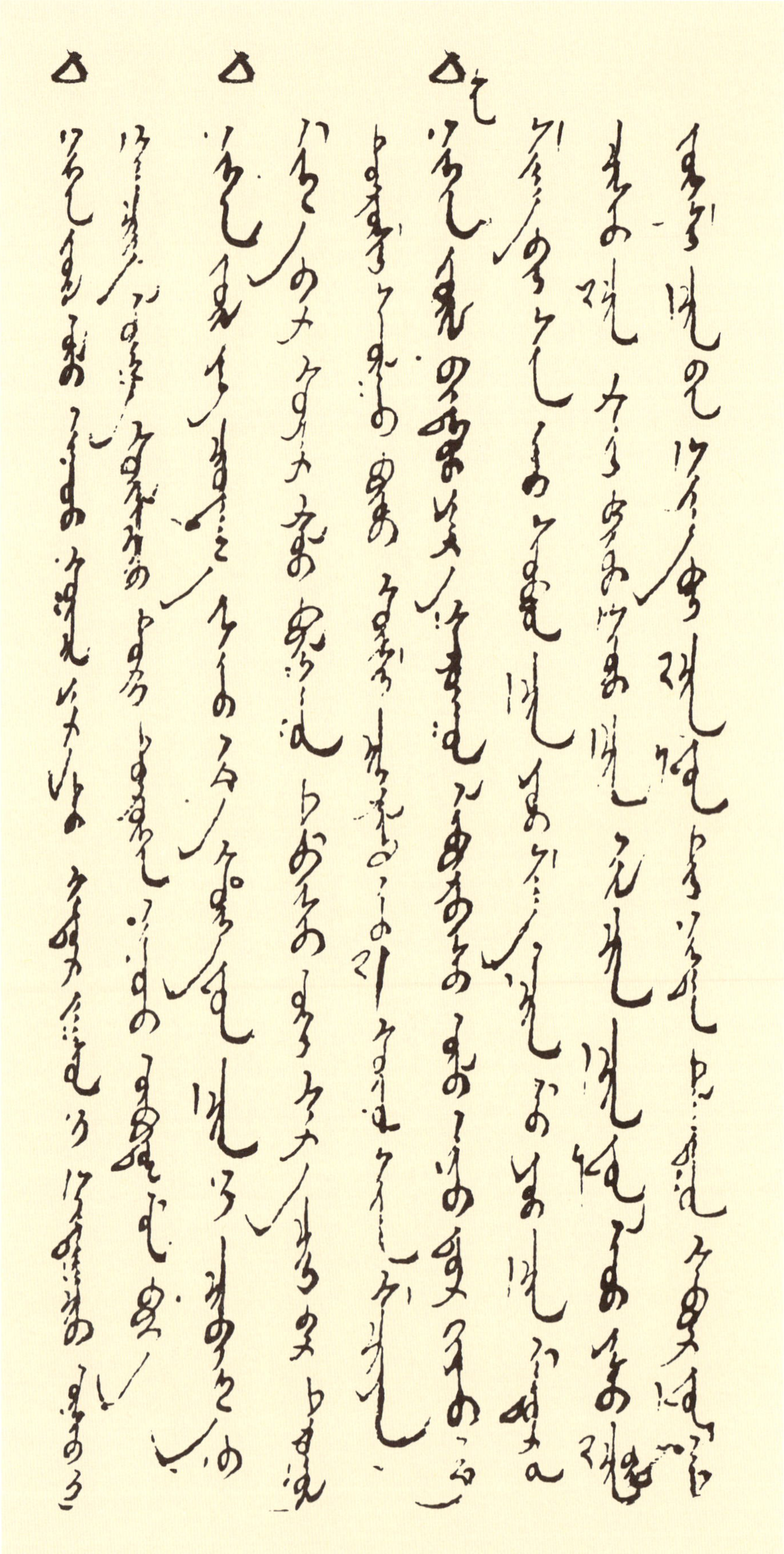

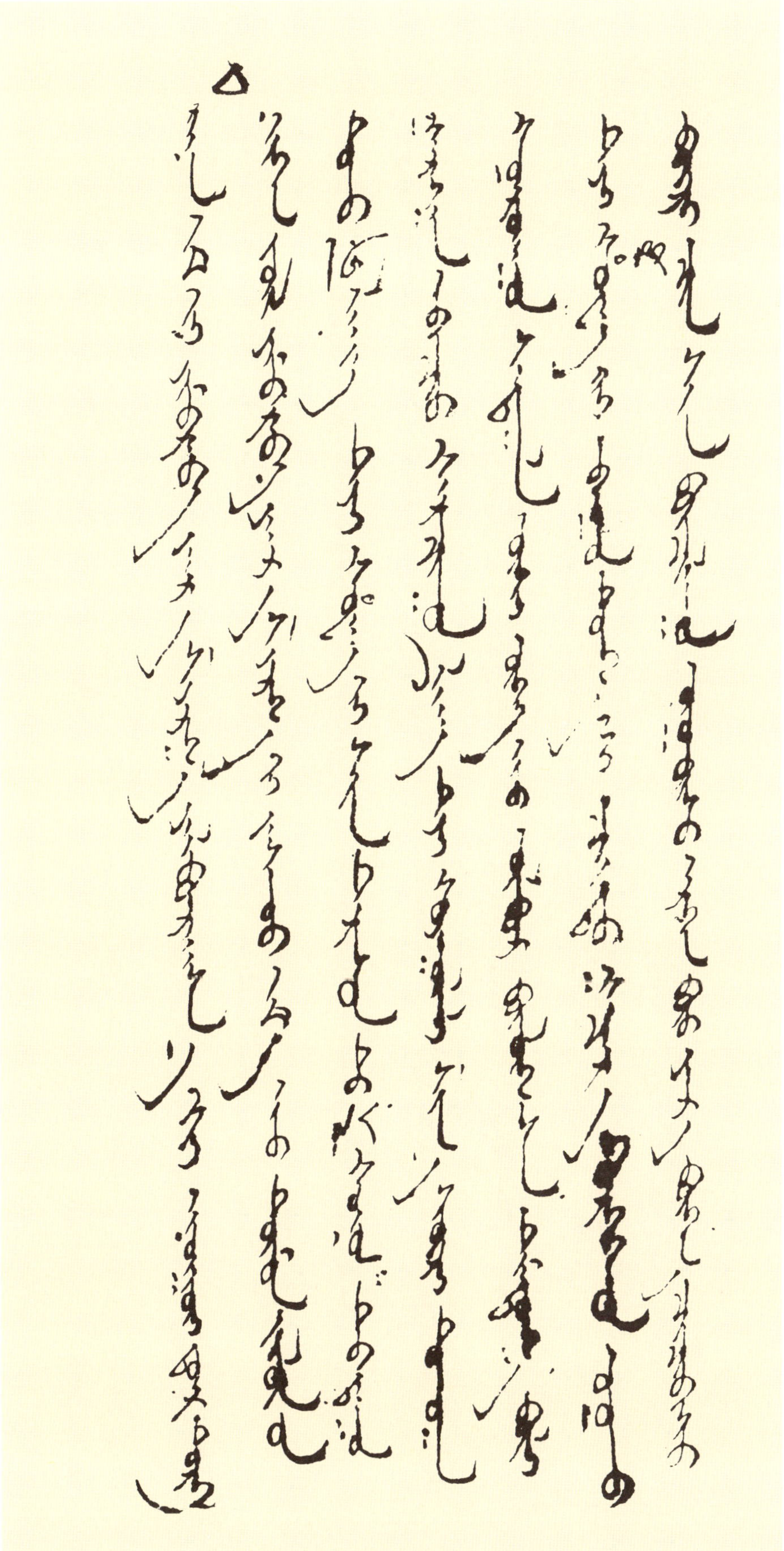

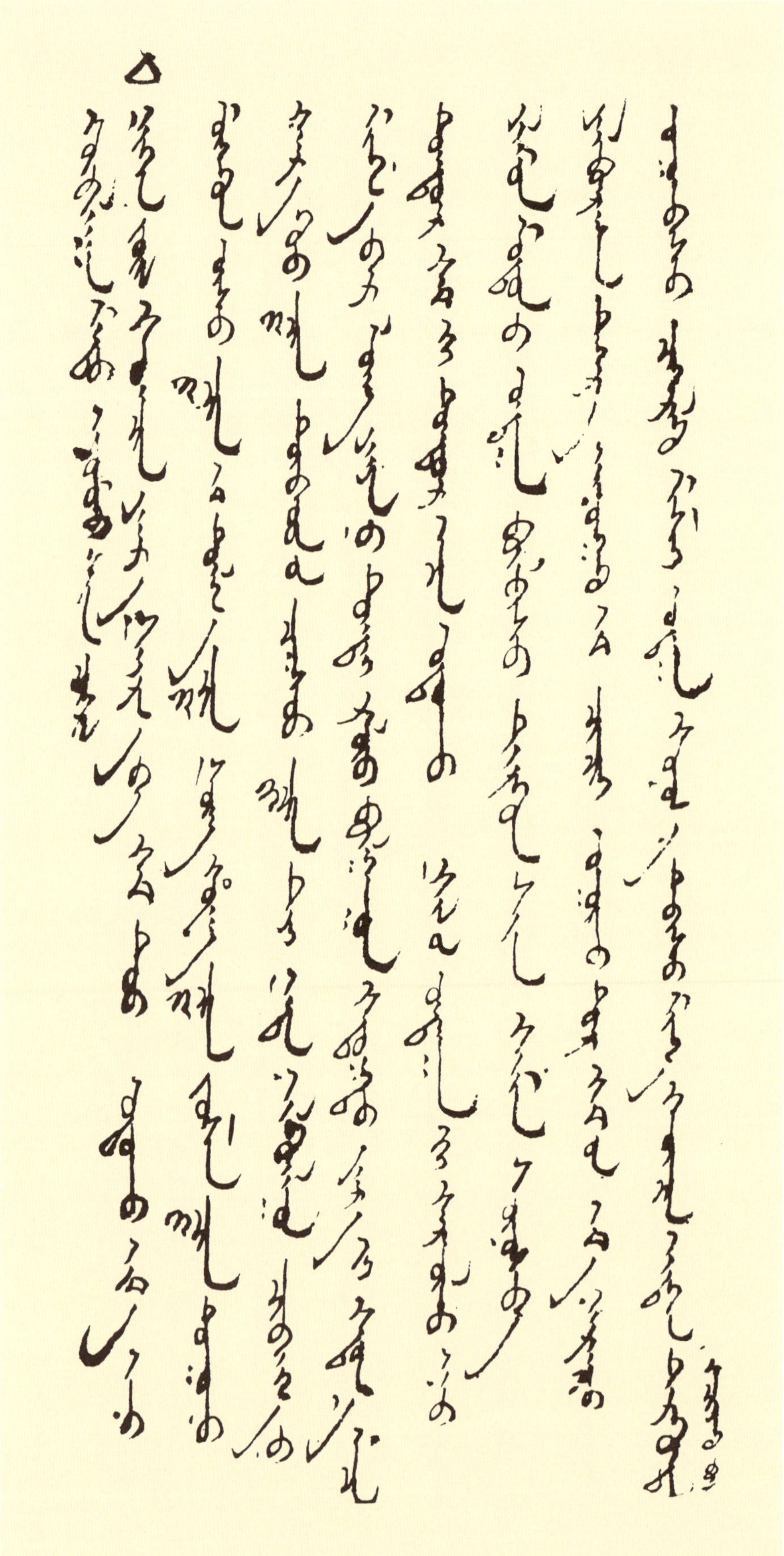

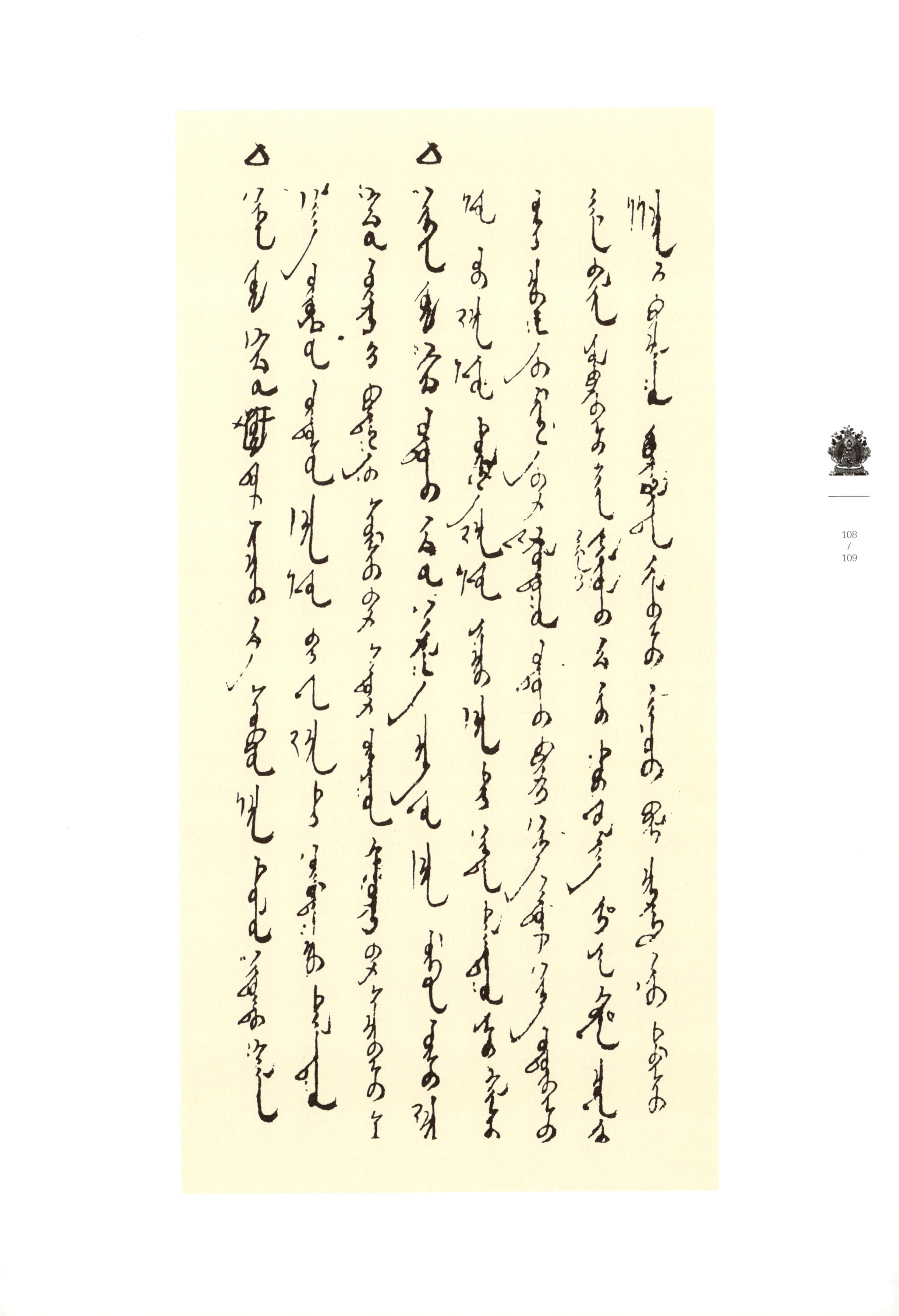

[illegible]

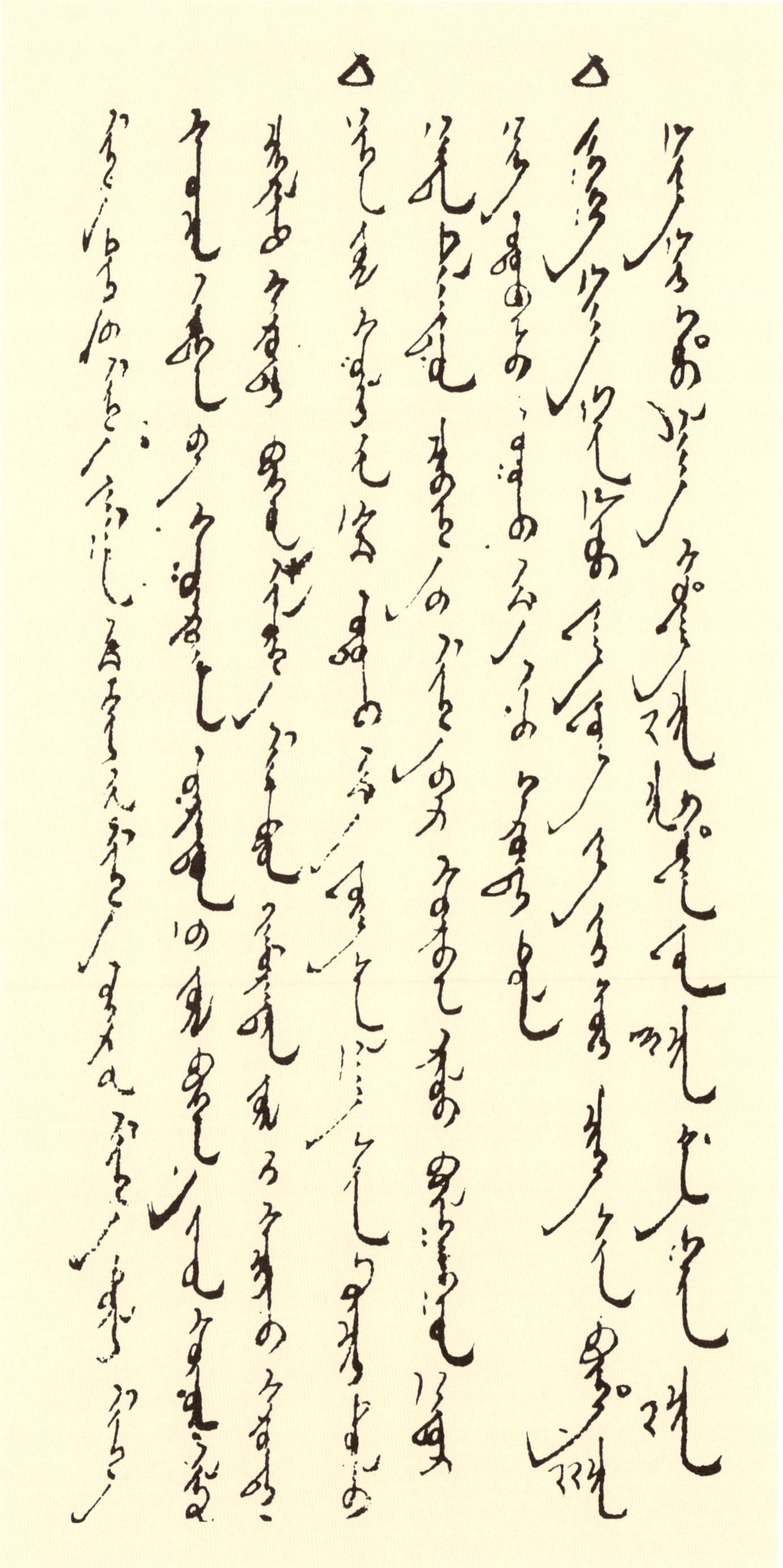

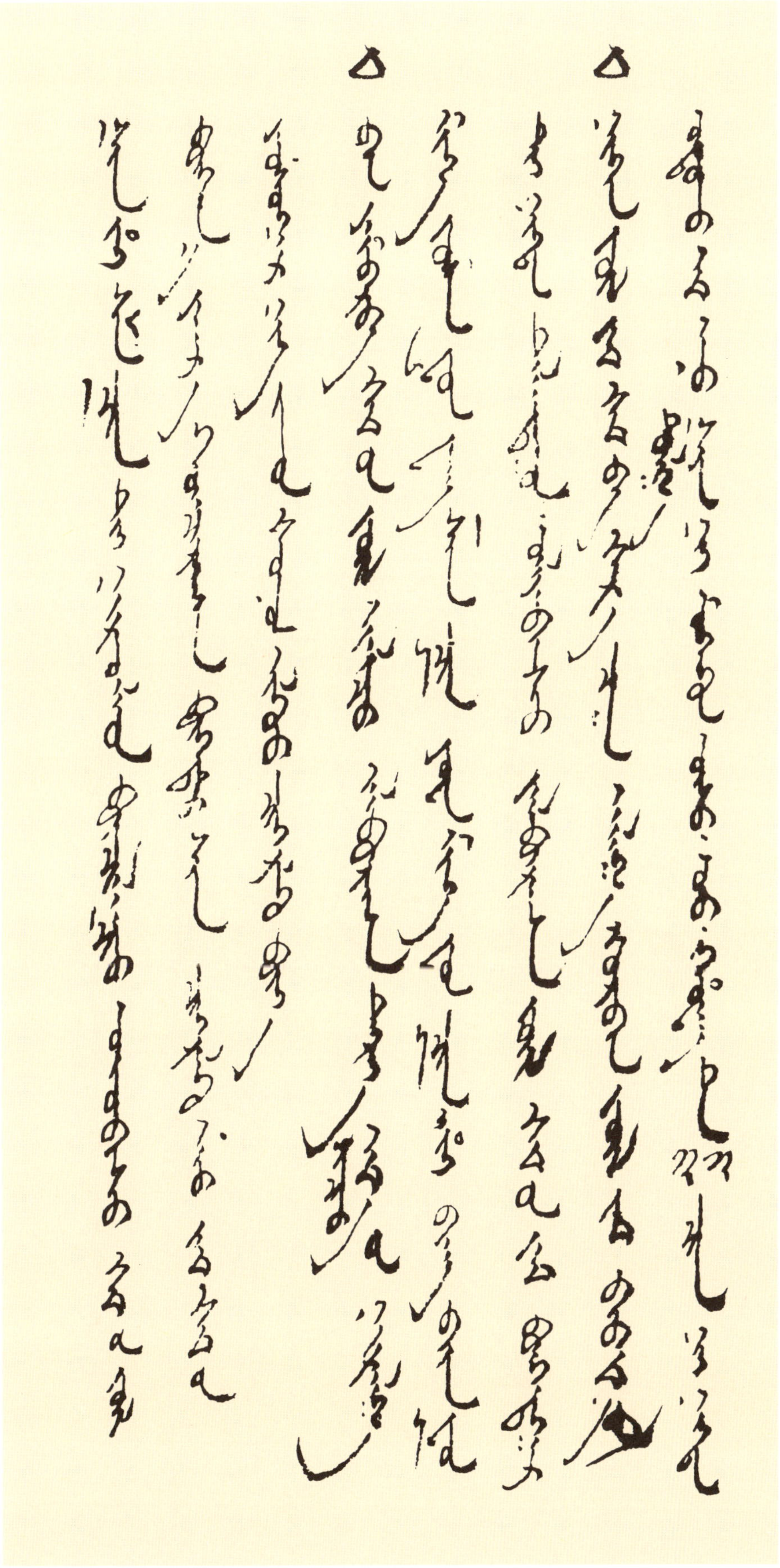

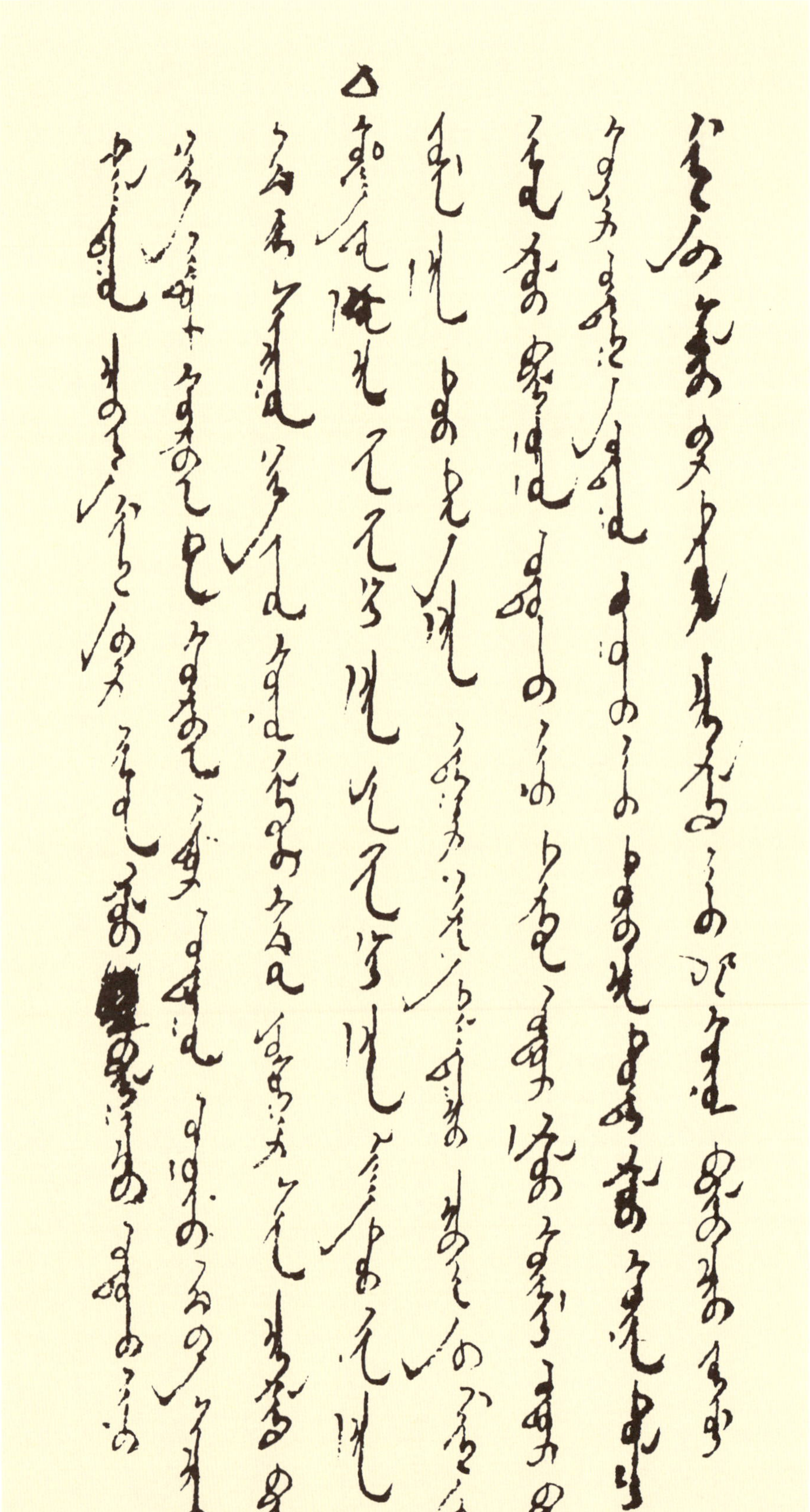

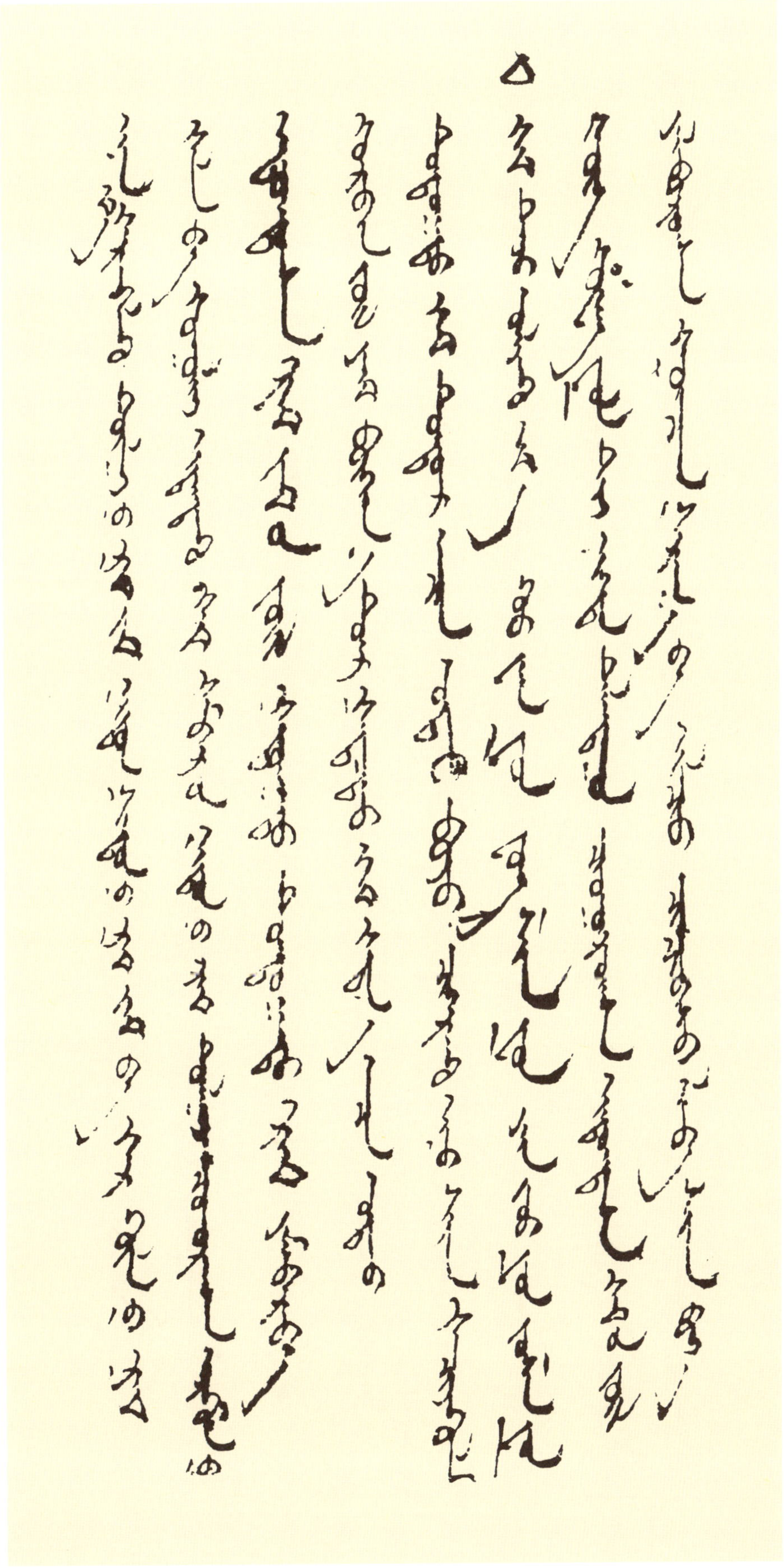

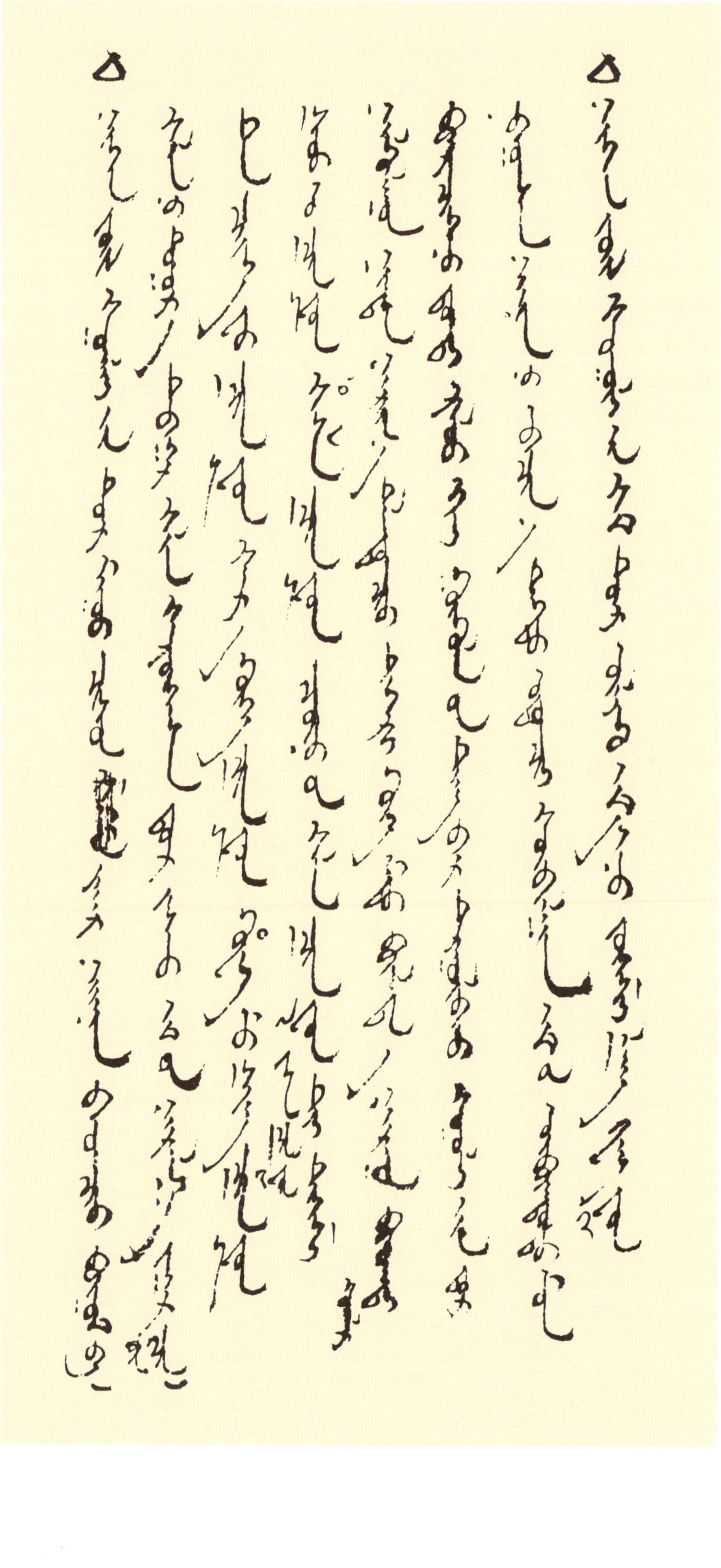

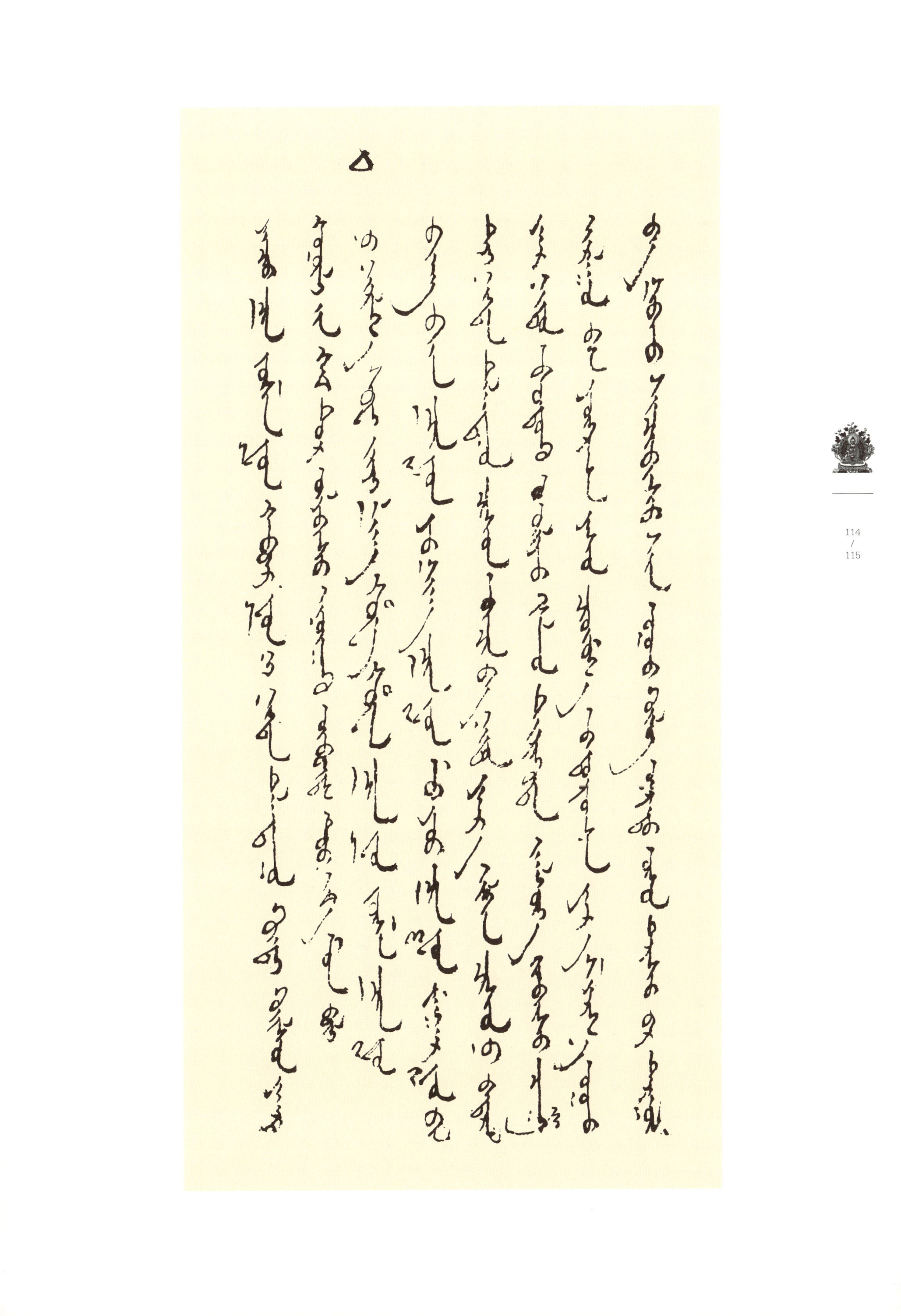

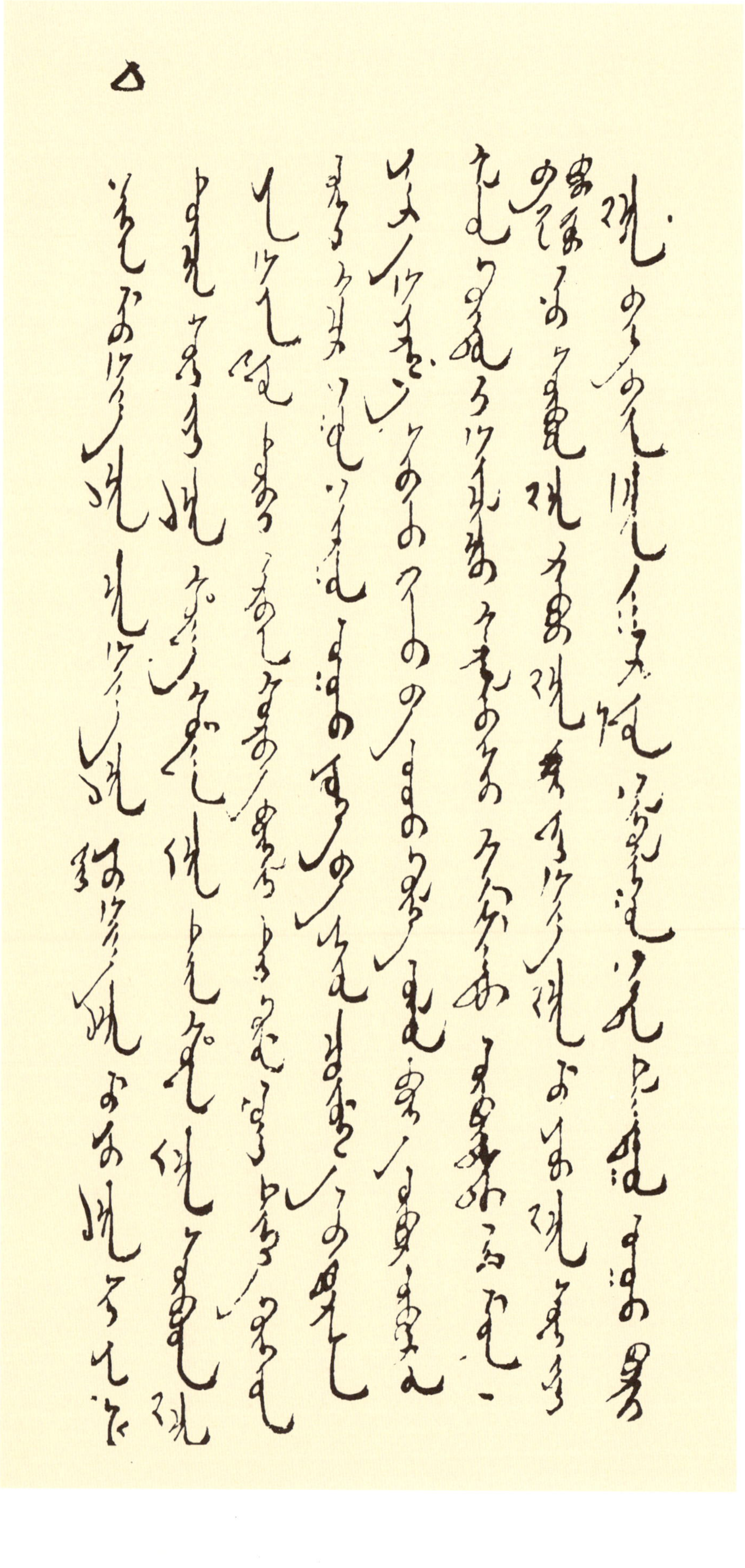

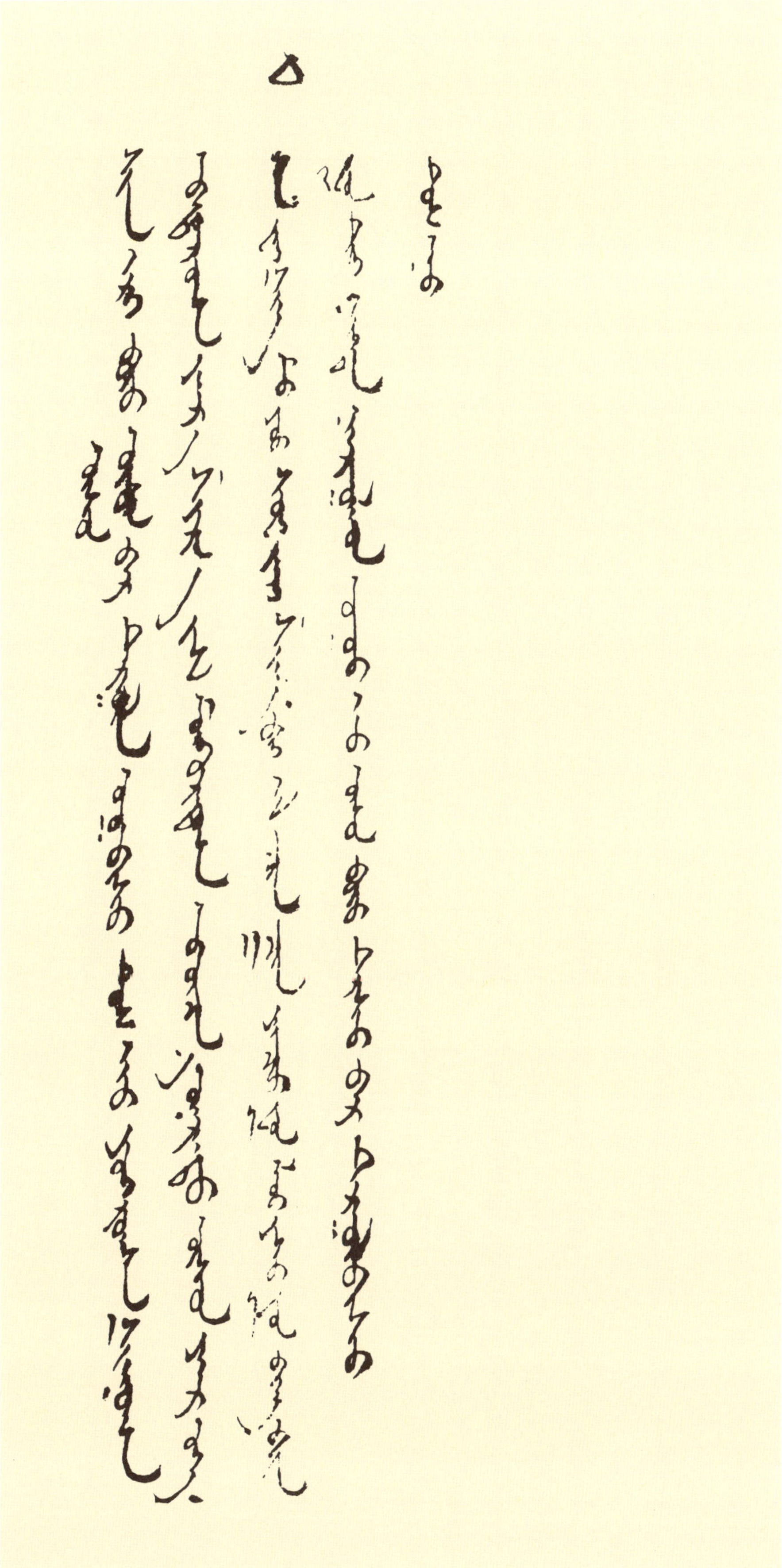

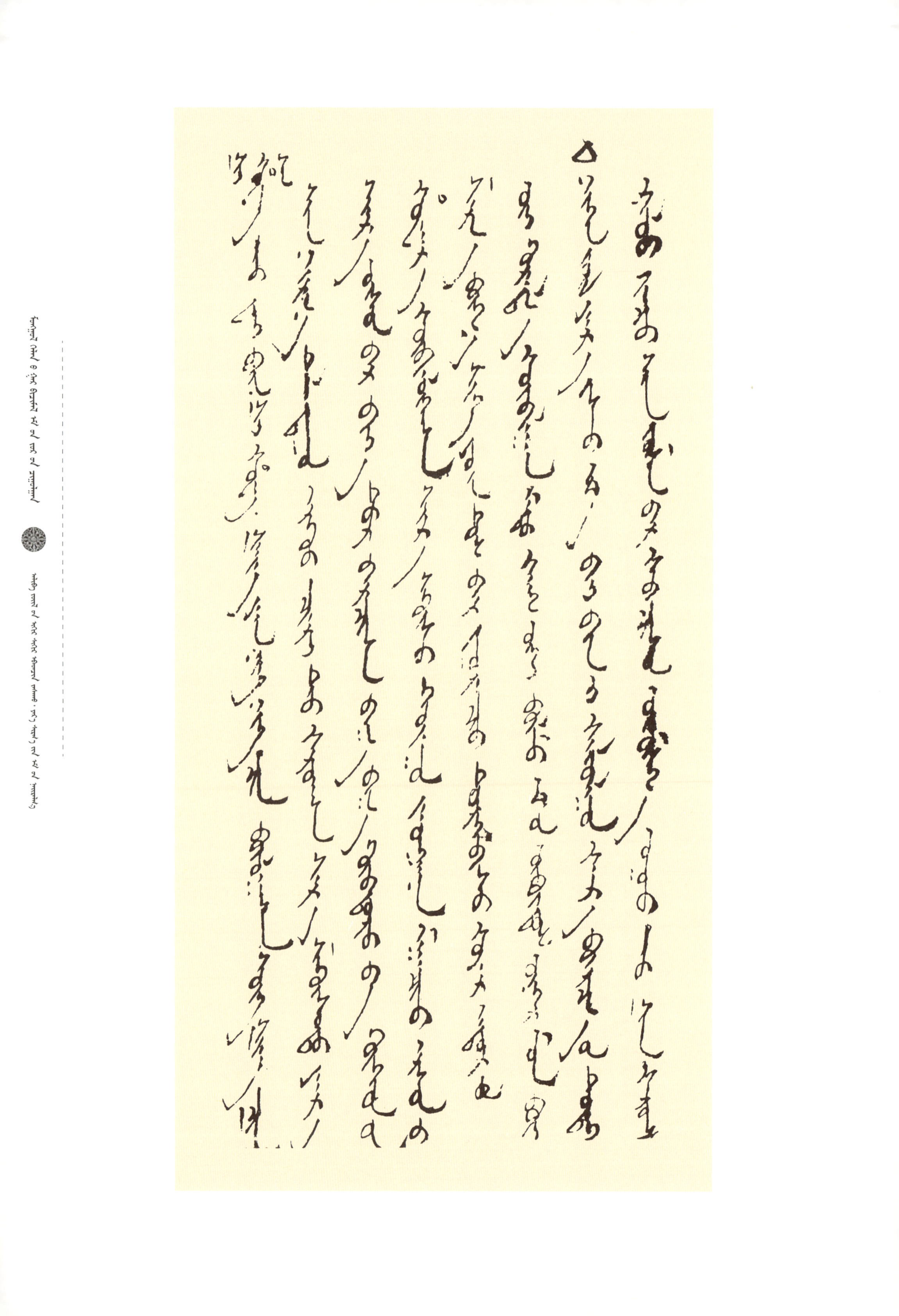

[illegible]

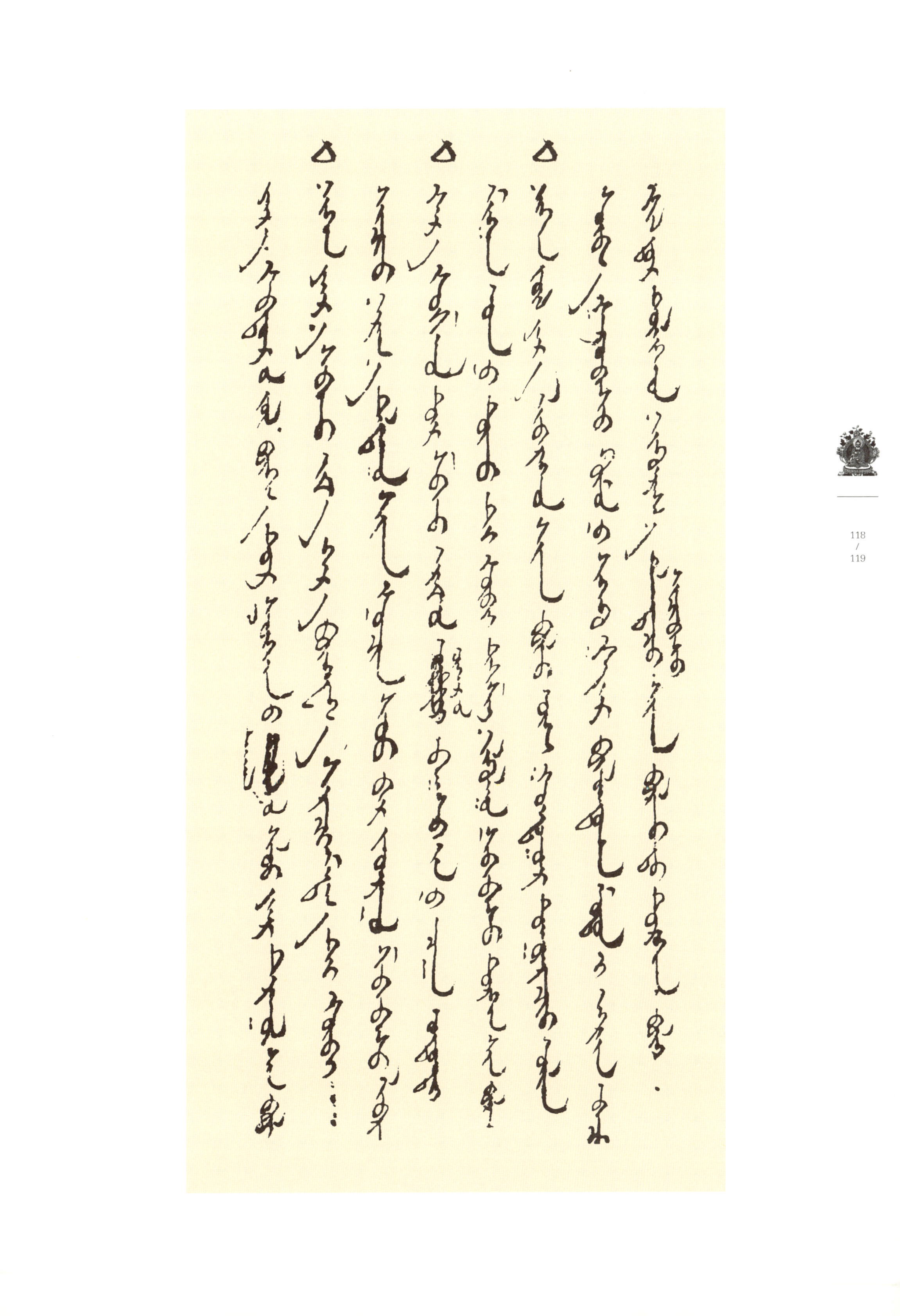

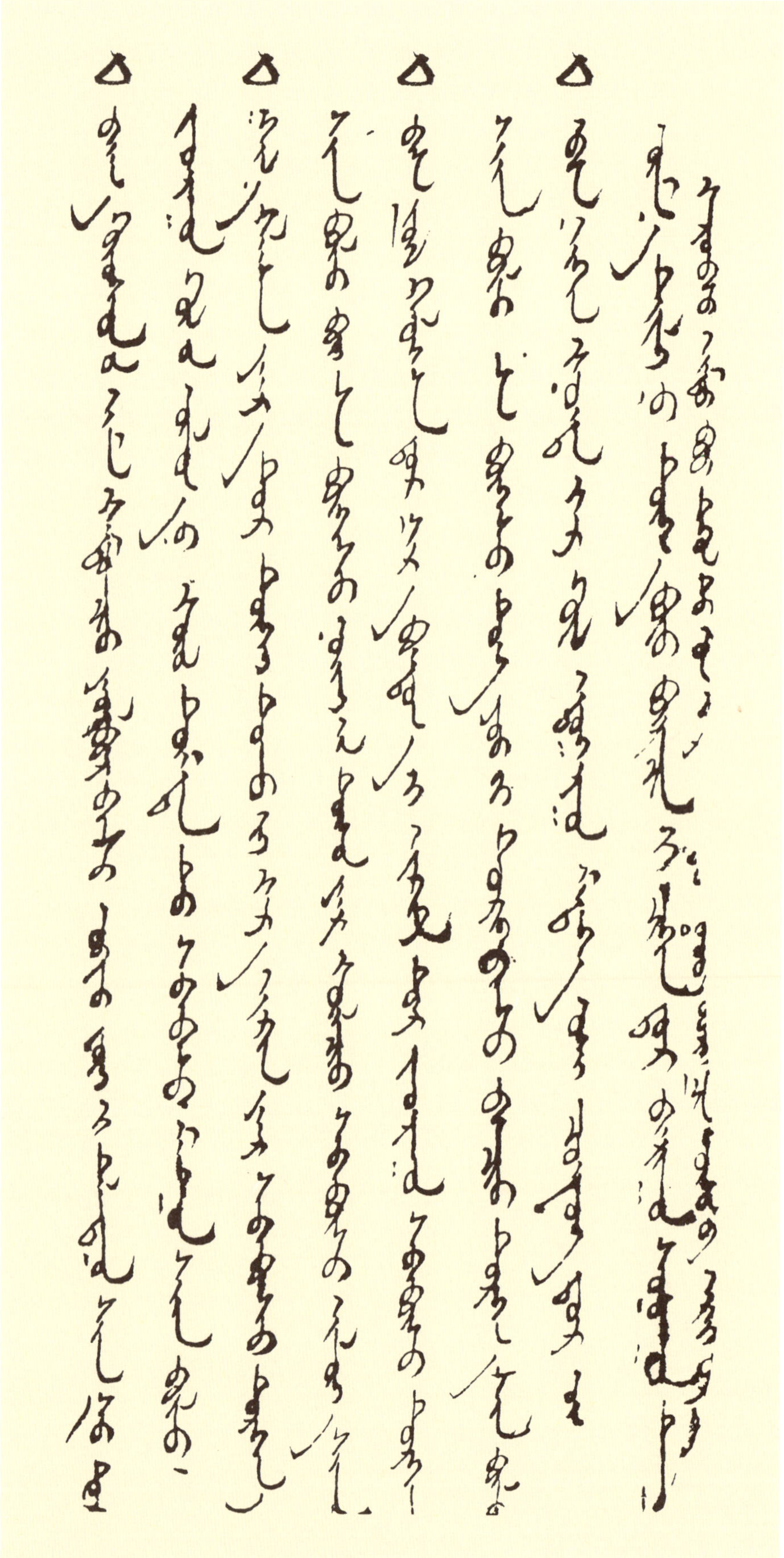

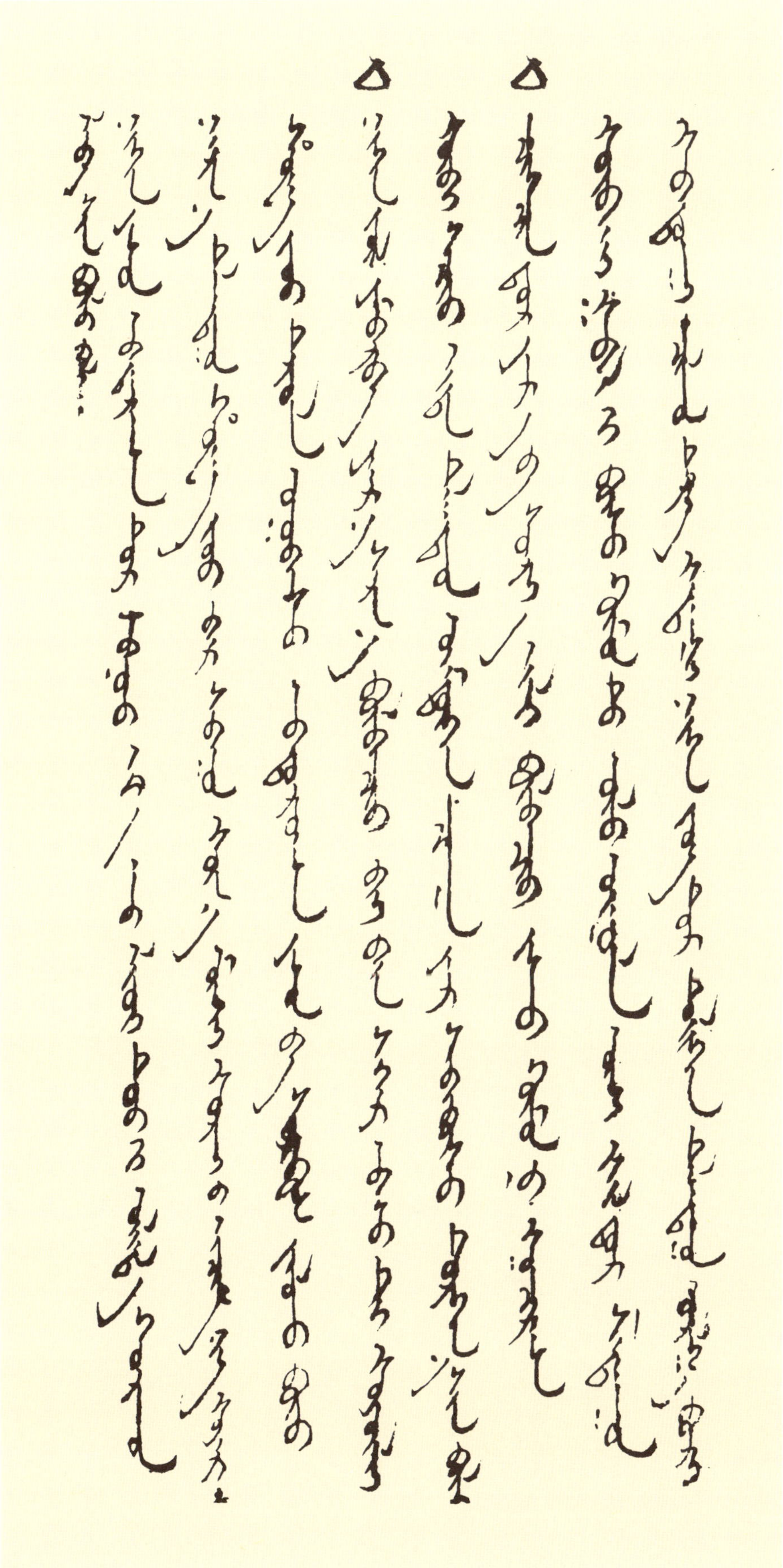

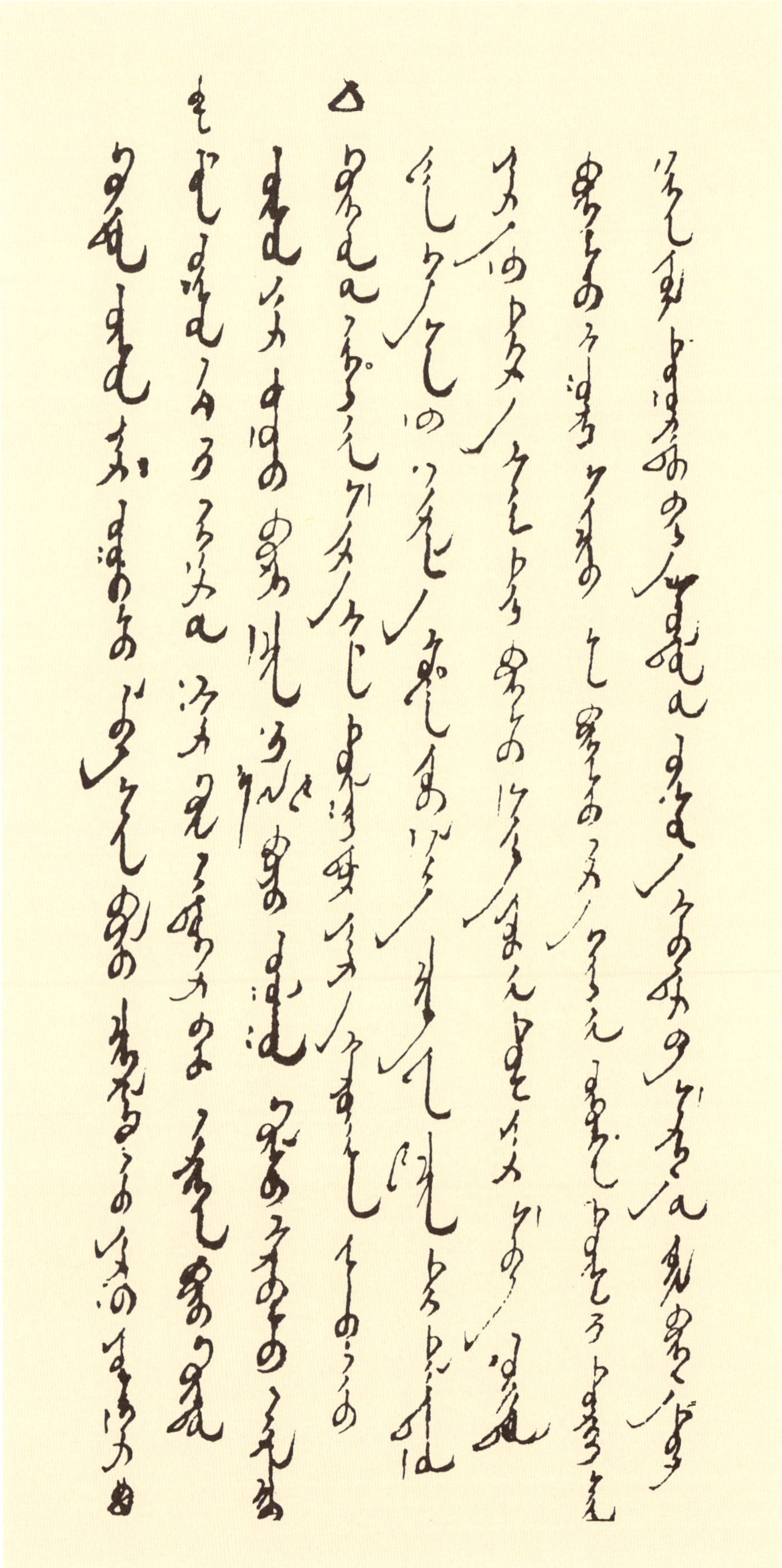

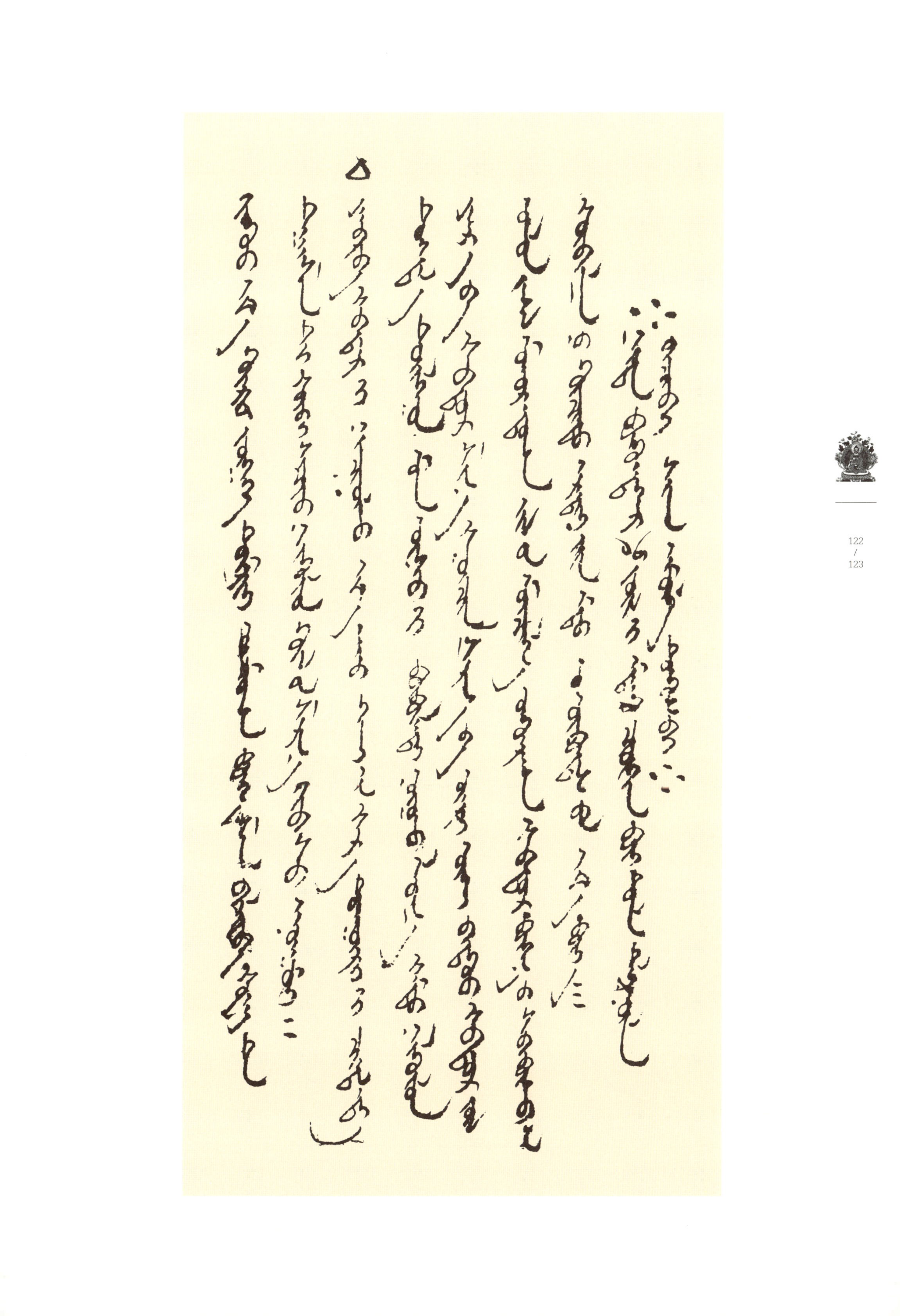

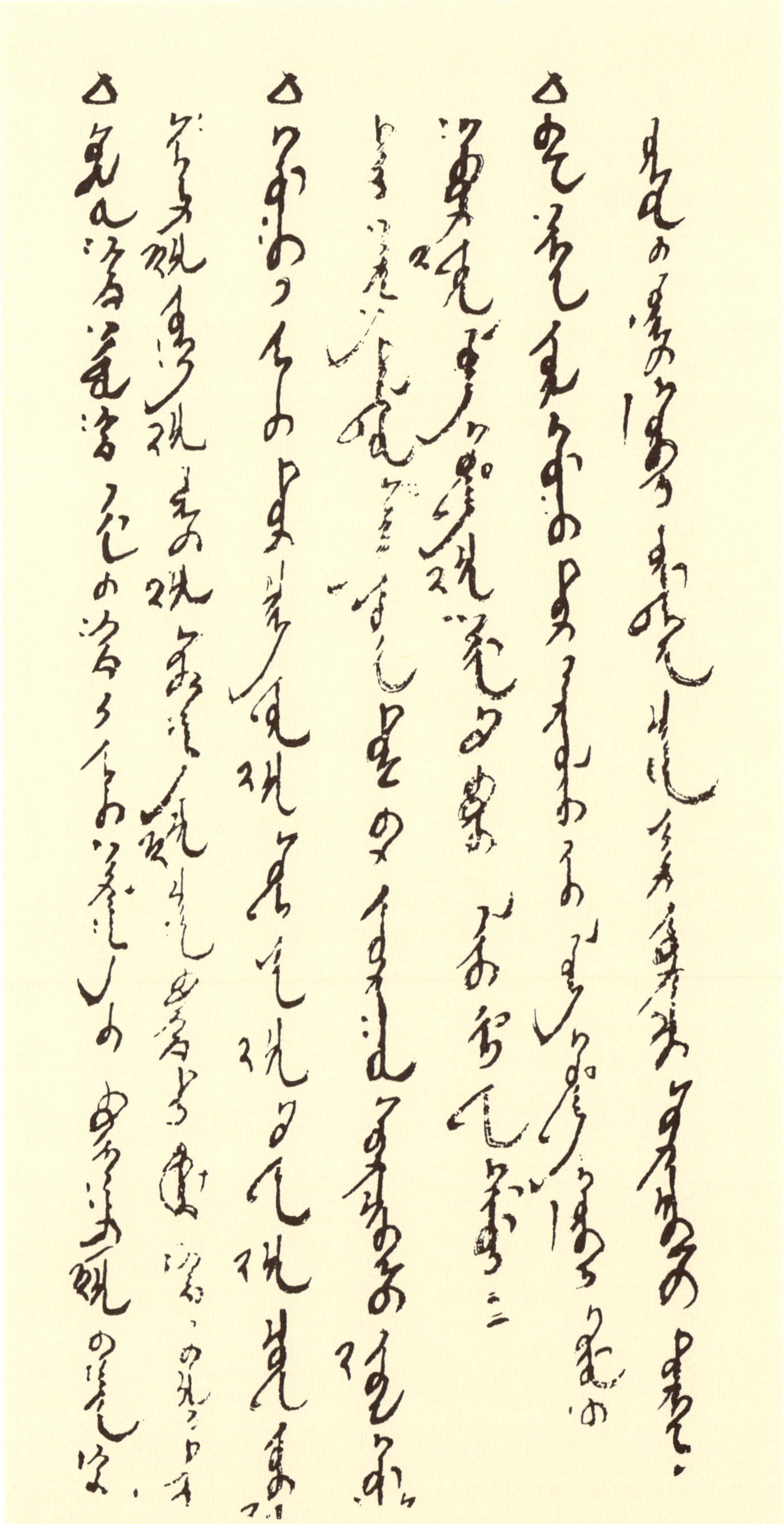

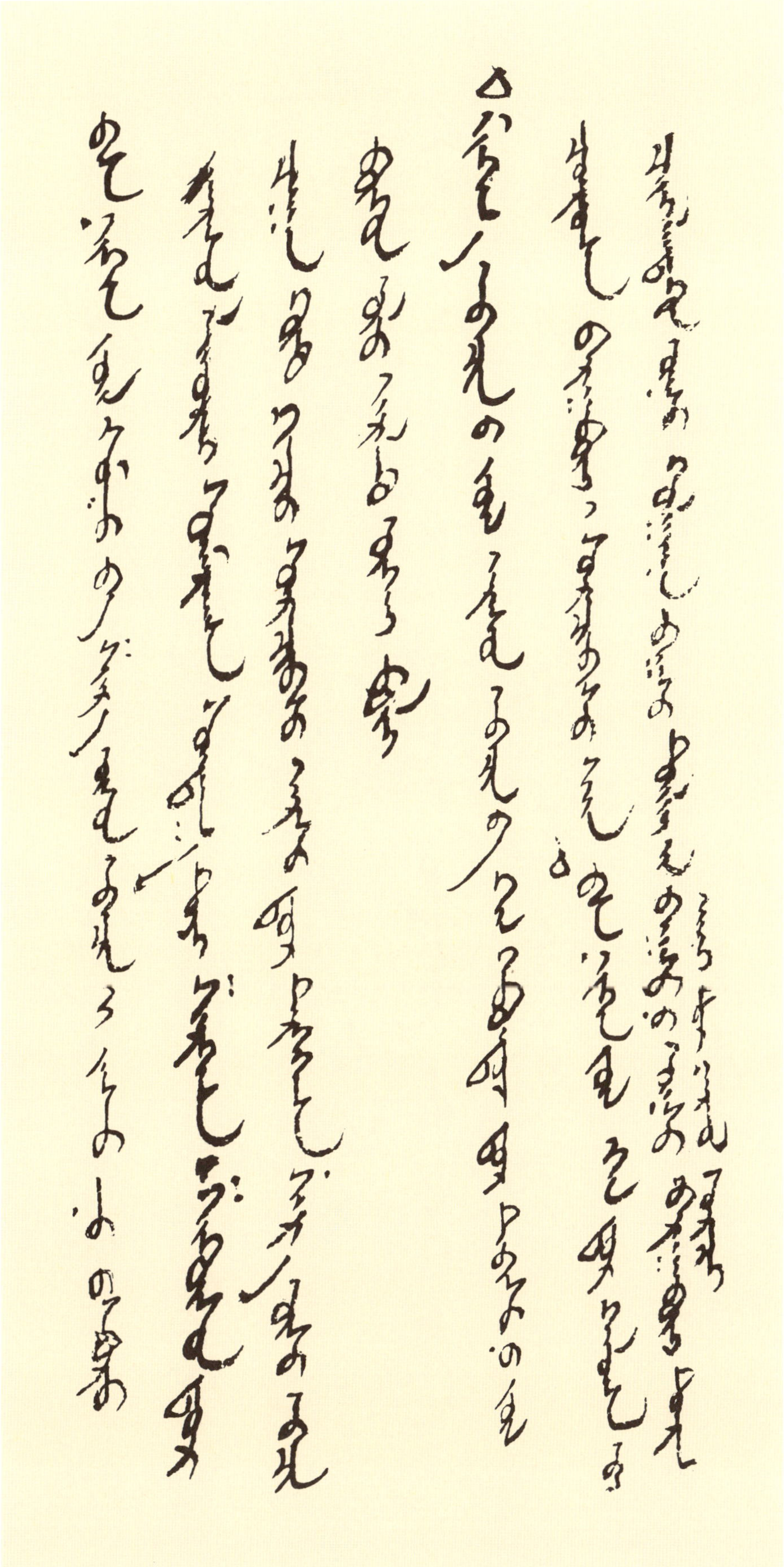

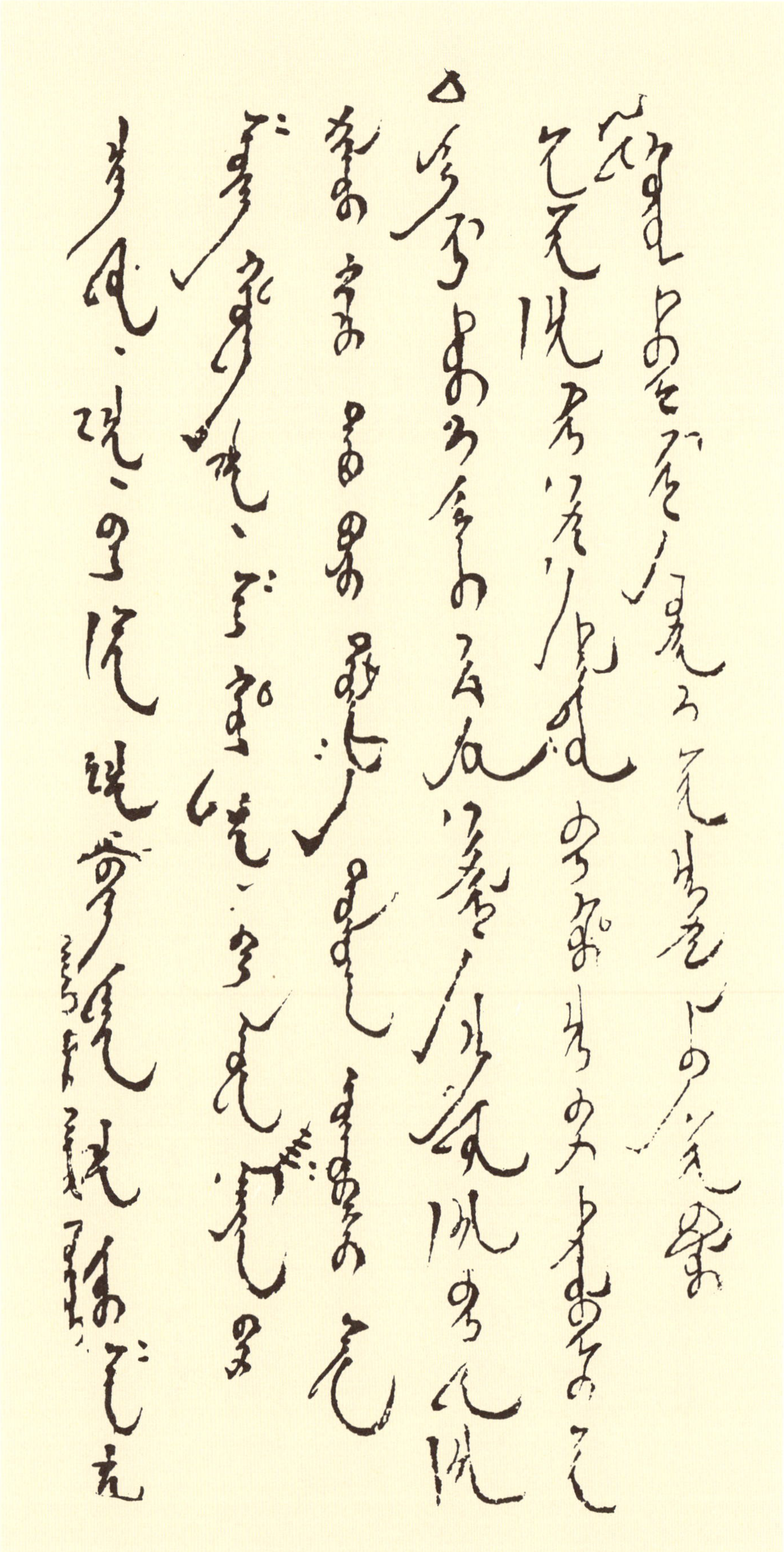

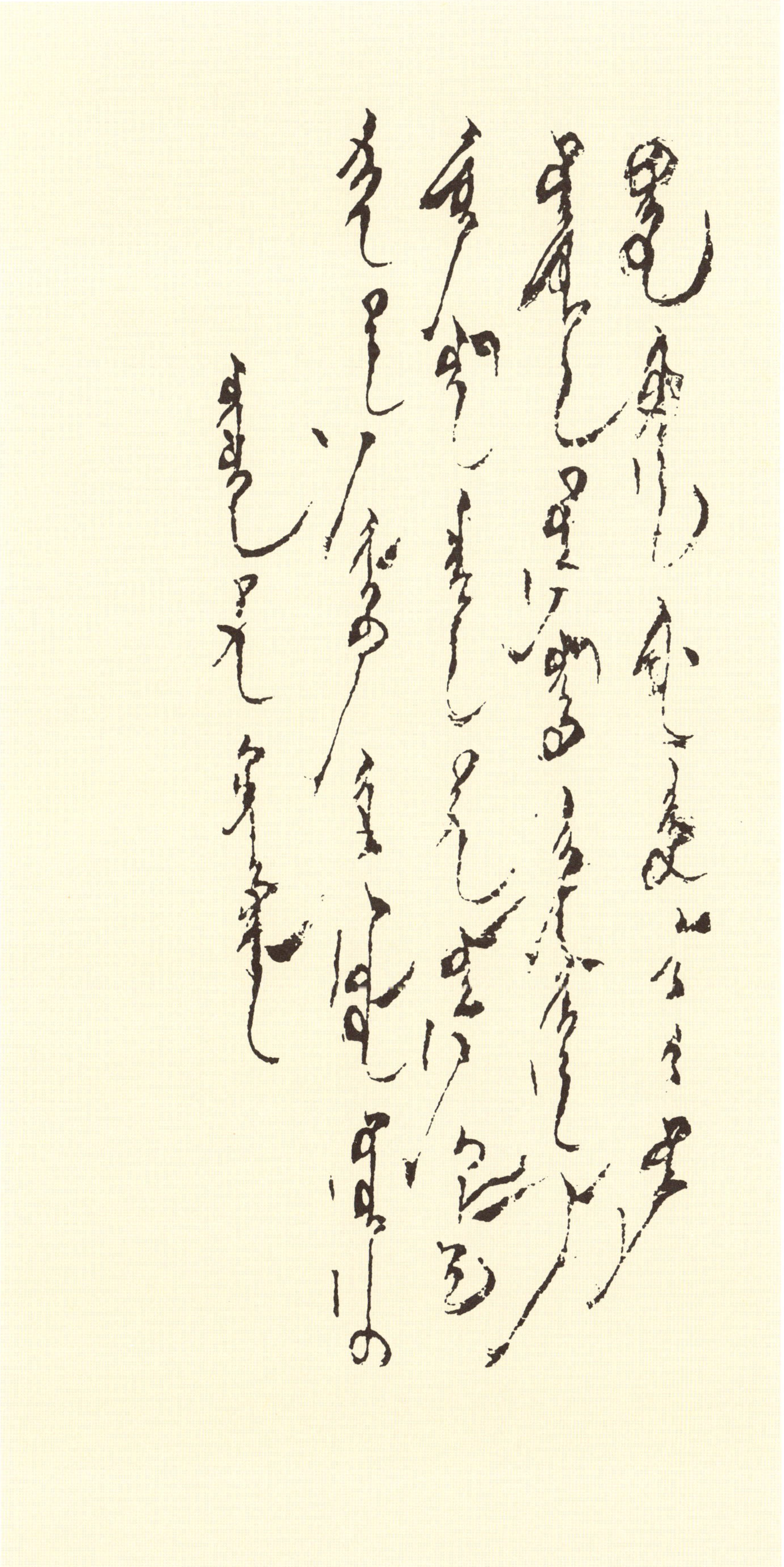

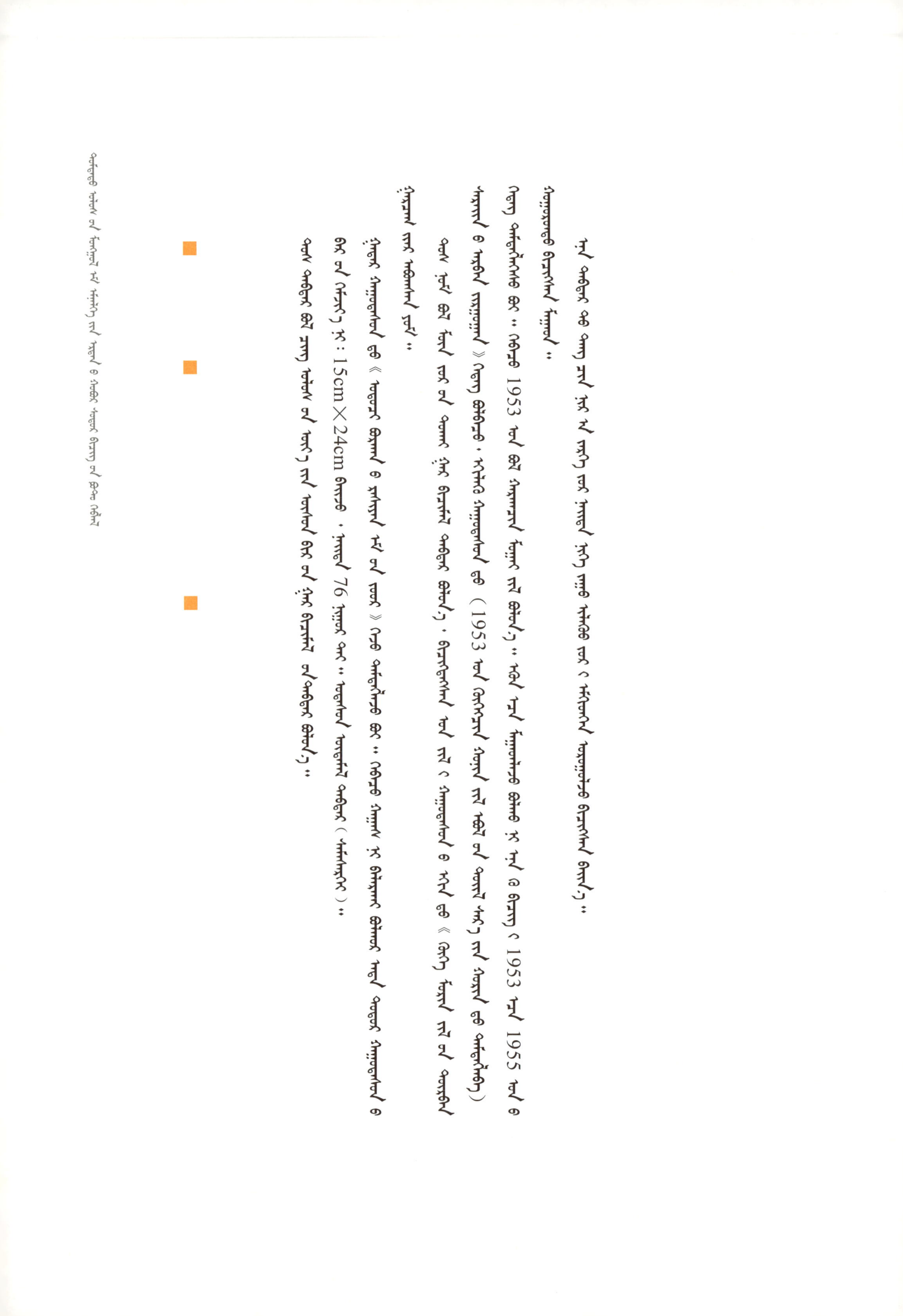

ᠪᠠᠷ ᠨᠢ ᠬᠡᠮᠵᠢᠶ᠎ᠡ ᠢ : 15cm×24cm ᠪᠣᠯᠤᠨ · ᠨᠢᠭᠤᠷ 76 ᠨᠢᠭᠤᠷ ᠲᠠᠢ :: ᠮᠣᠩᠭᠣᠯ ᠮᠣᠩᠭᠣᠯᠴᠤᠳ ᠬᠡᠪᠯᠡᠯ (ᠰᠢᠨᠵᠢᠯᠡᠬᠦ) ::

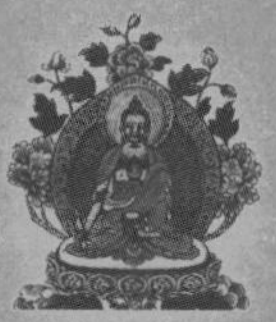

Yaowang Miraculous Prescriptions

药王灵丹药方

4

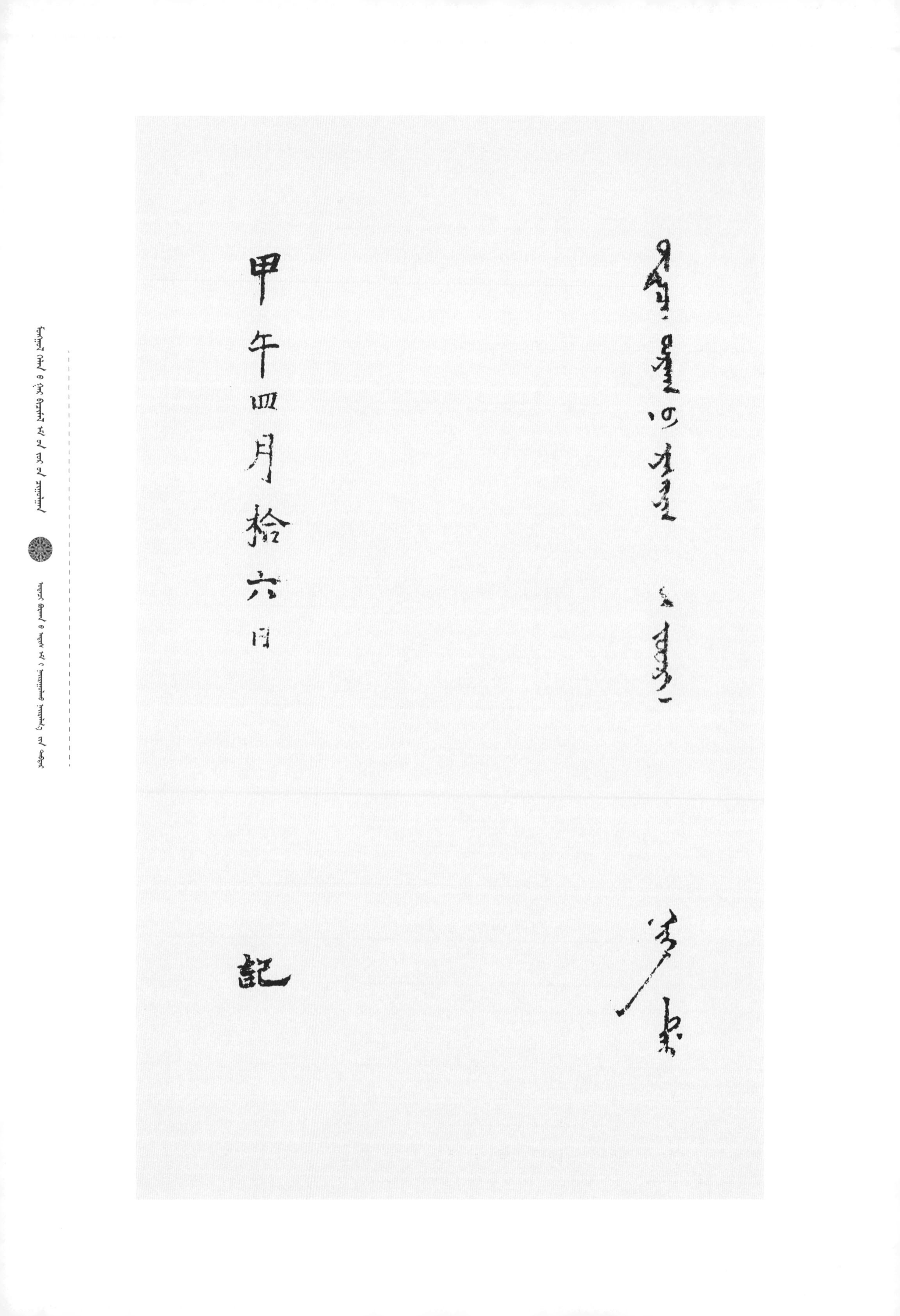

甲午四月拾六日

記

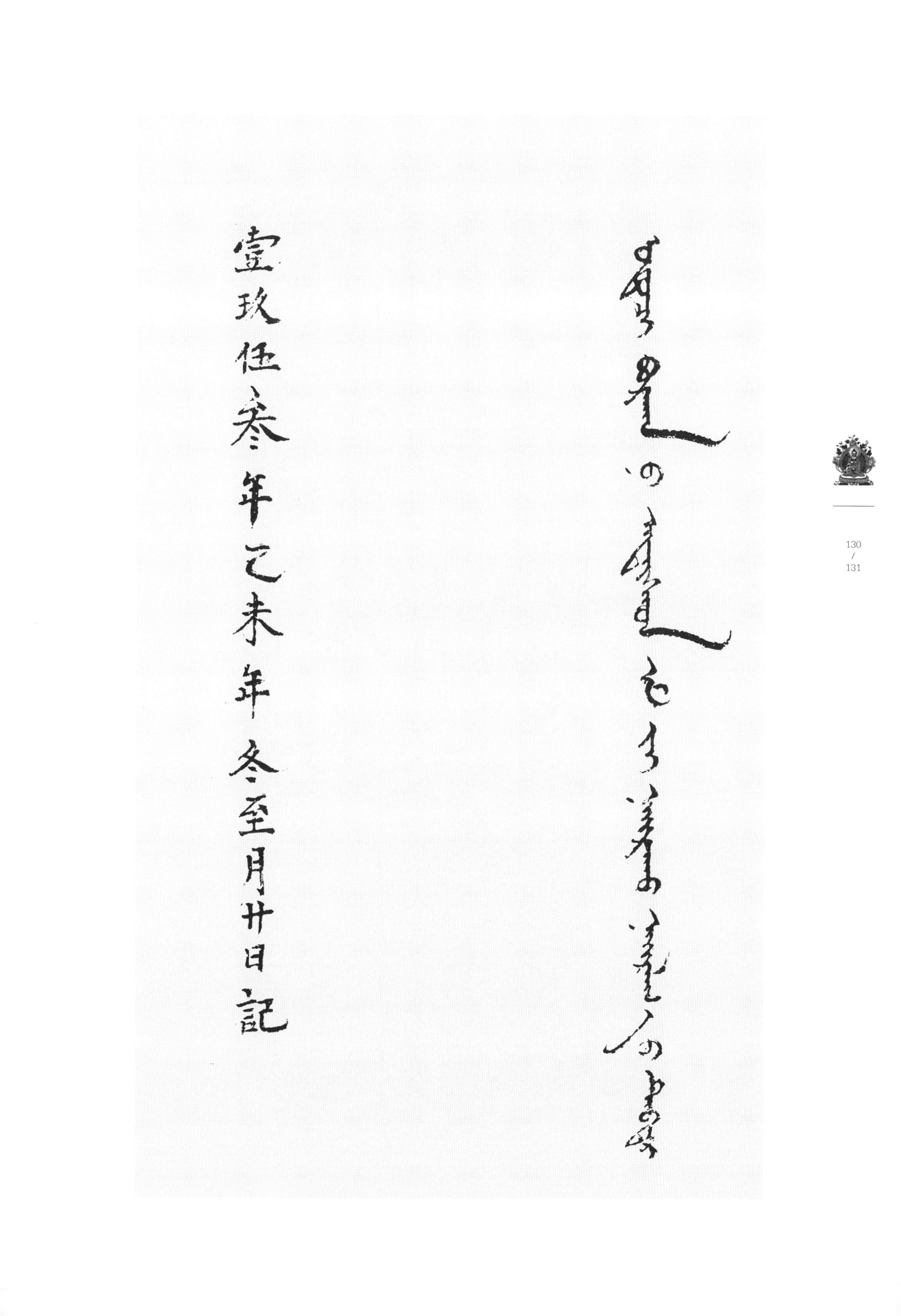

壹玖伍叁年乙未年冬至月廿日記

卅五

卅六

卅二

卅五

卅五

卅五

豆蔻、蓽撥、山奈、光明盐、胡椒、官桂、胡椒、草菓、訶子、商陸、

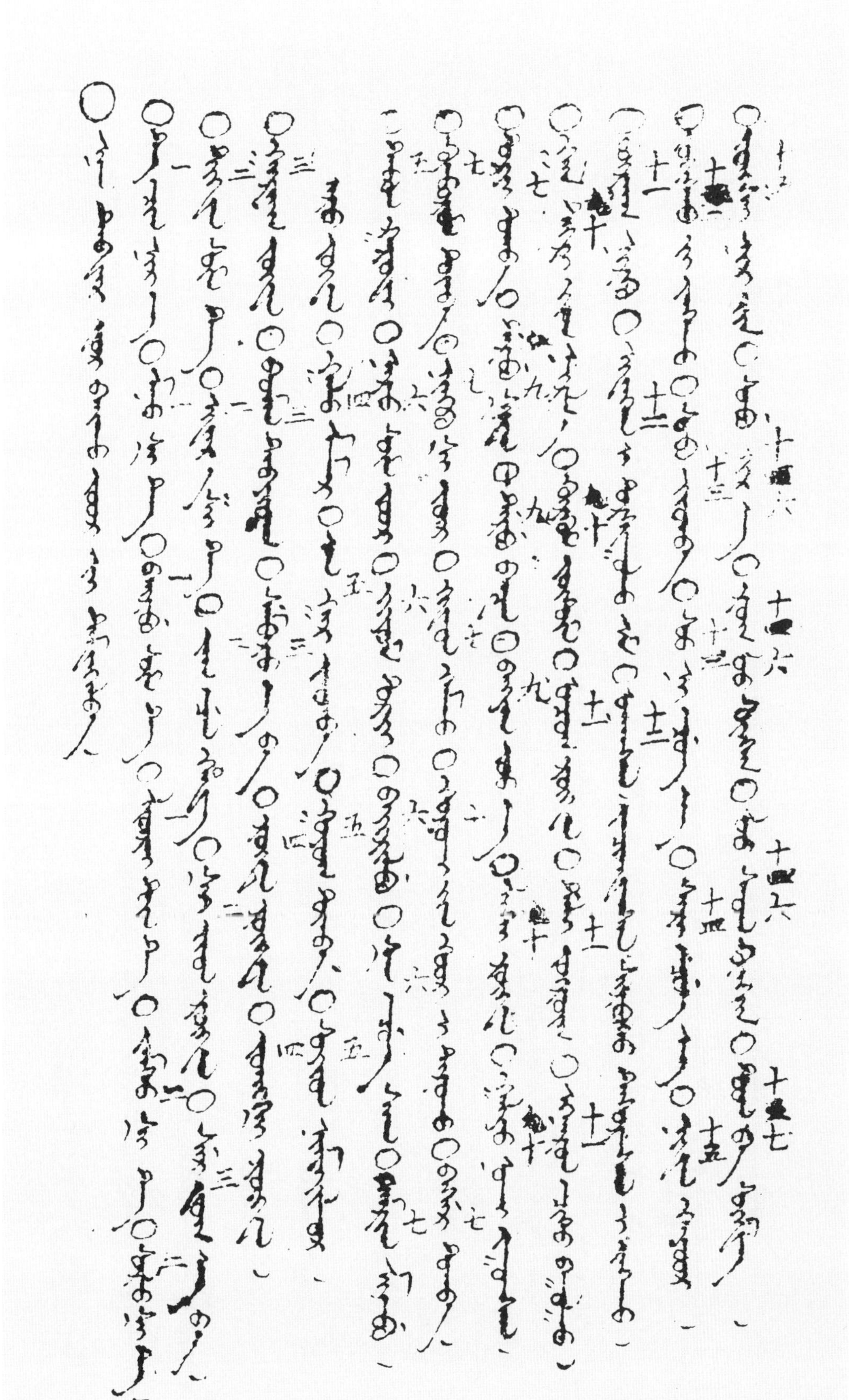

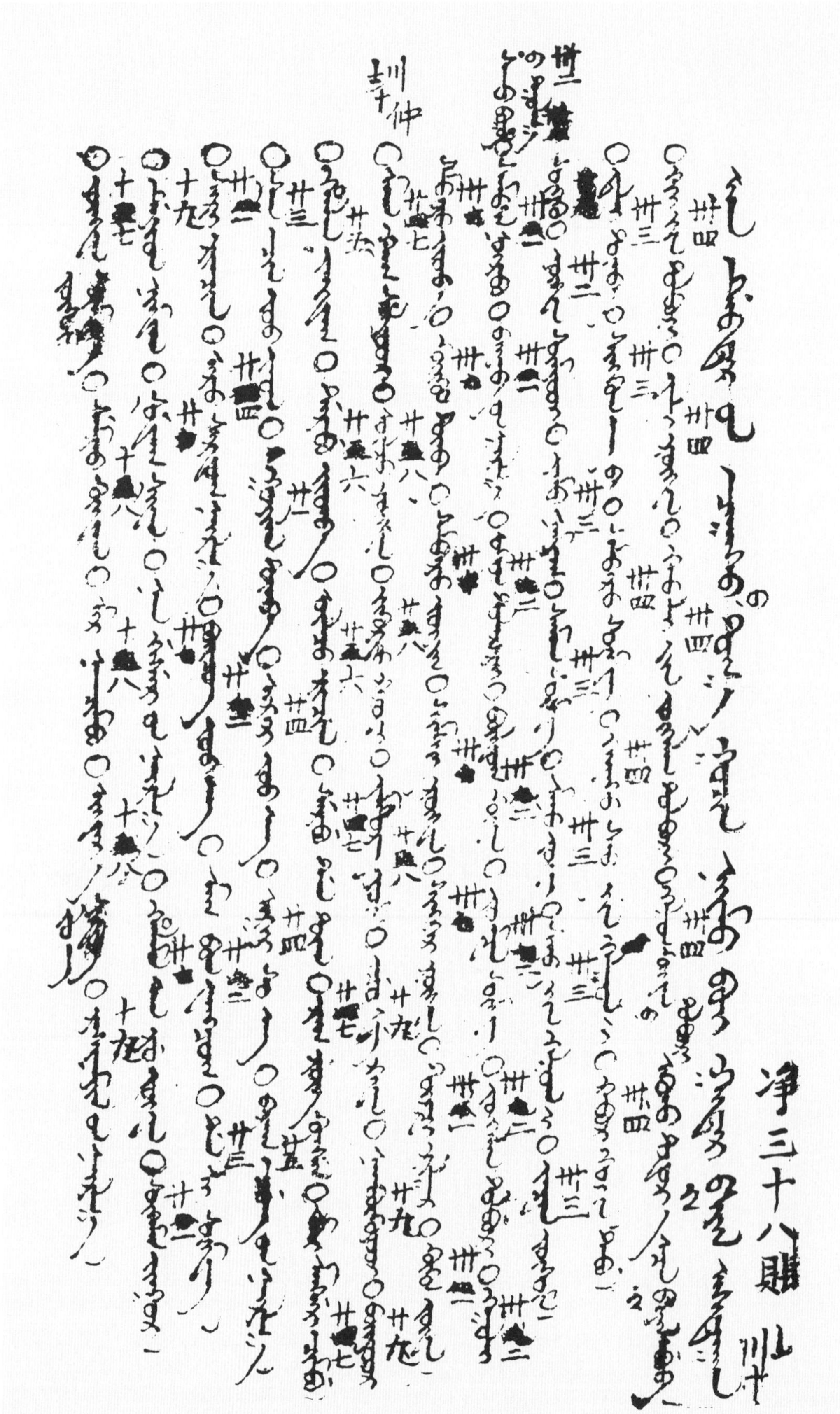
净三十八賬

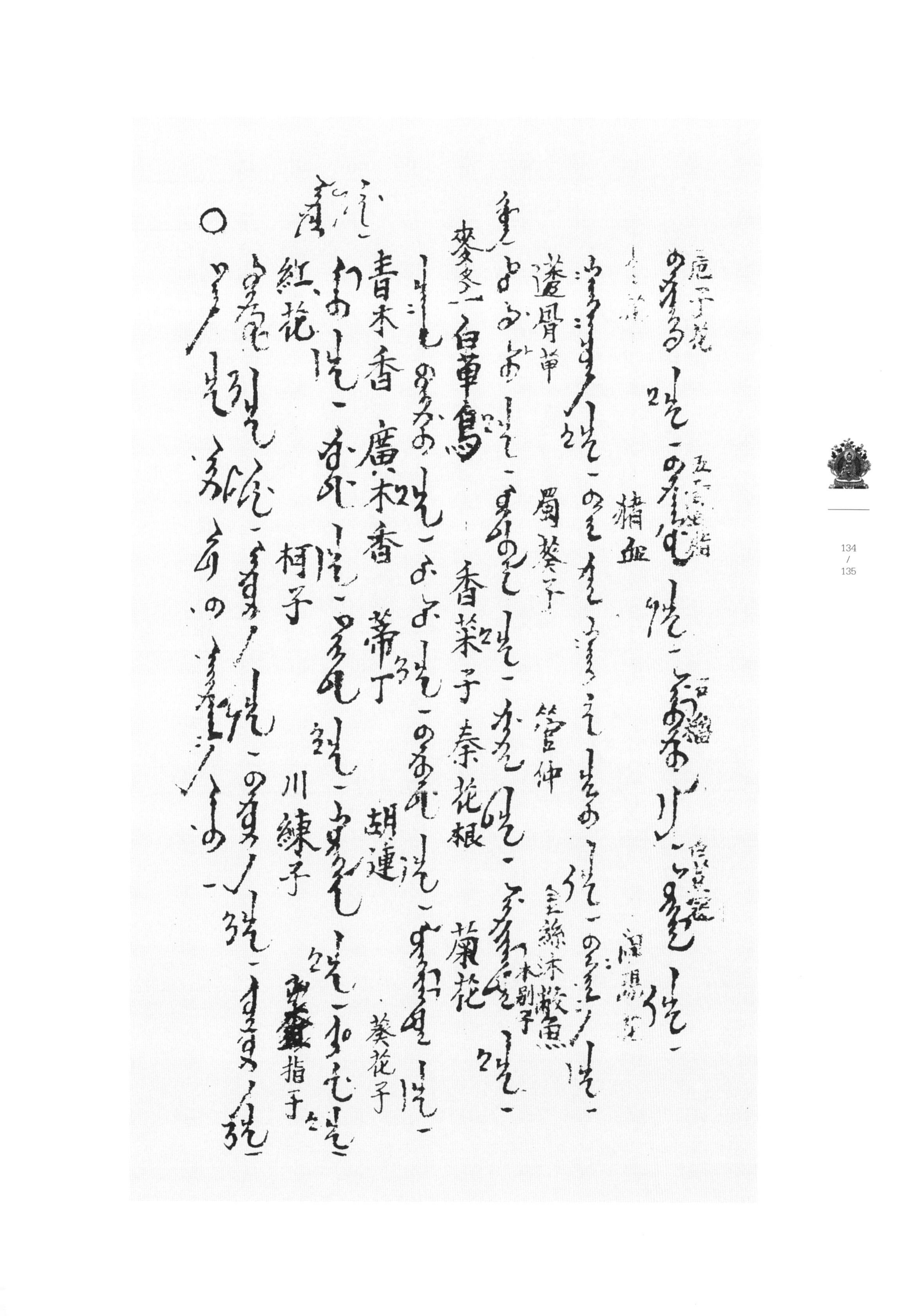

巵子花

精血

蓬骨單　蜀葵子　管仲　金絲沫　鱉魚　木別子

麥冬　白草烏　香菜子　秦花根　蘭花

青木香　廣木香　蓽丁　胡連　葵花子

紅花　柯子　川練子　指子

○

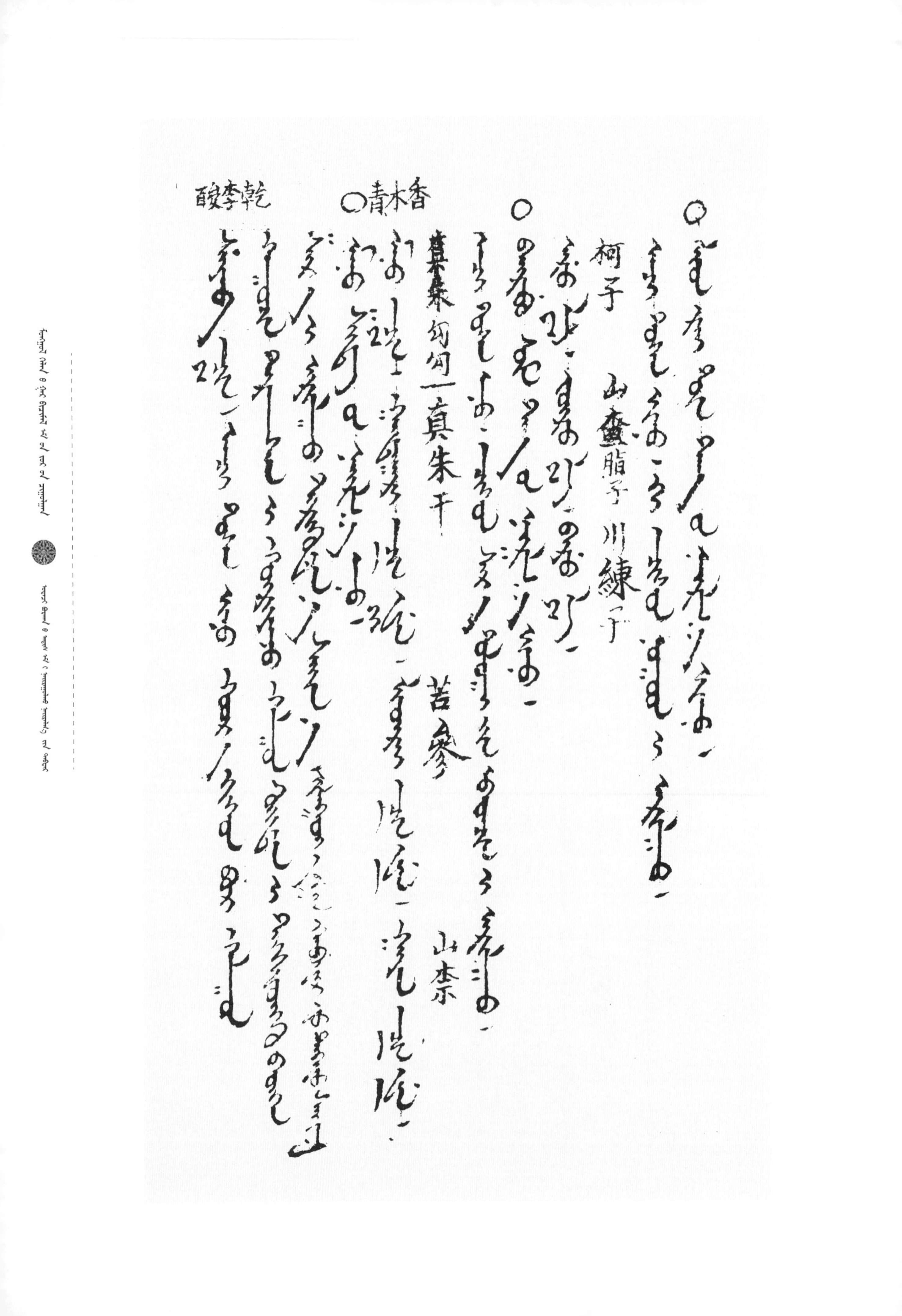

乾李酸

香木青

柯子

山鹽脂子

川練子

[illegible]

鉤一真朱干

苦參

山柰

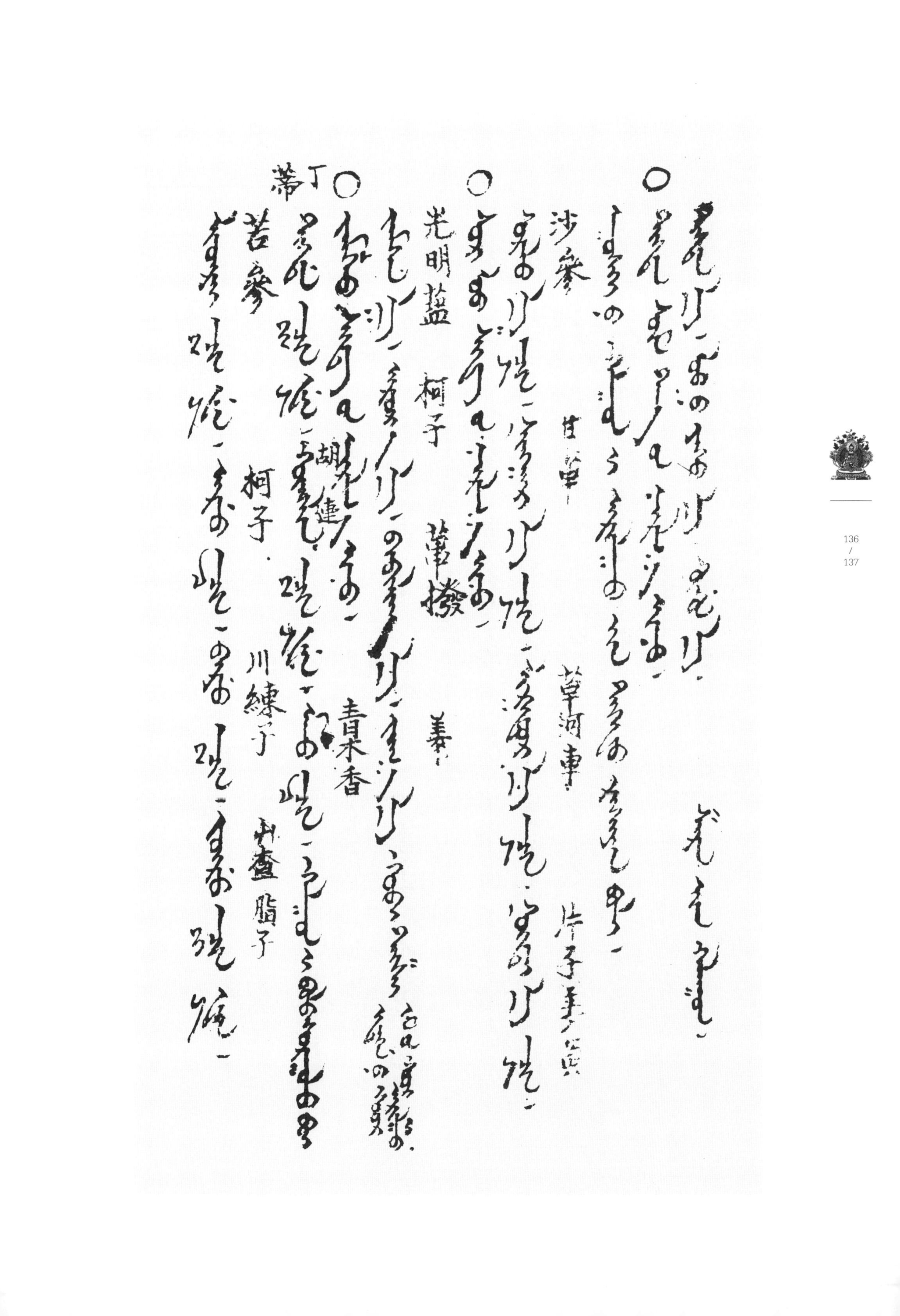

丁蒂
苦參 柯子 川練子 山查 脂子

胡連 青木香

光明鹽 柯子 蓽撥 姜

沙參 甘草 草河車 芐子黄

大黄 寒水石 硼

鐵末子 夏草冬蟲 栀子 川楝子 血竭

雀瓜 白草烏 麥冬 草河車 南硼砂

木通

蒂丁 龍膽 唵巴香

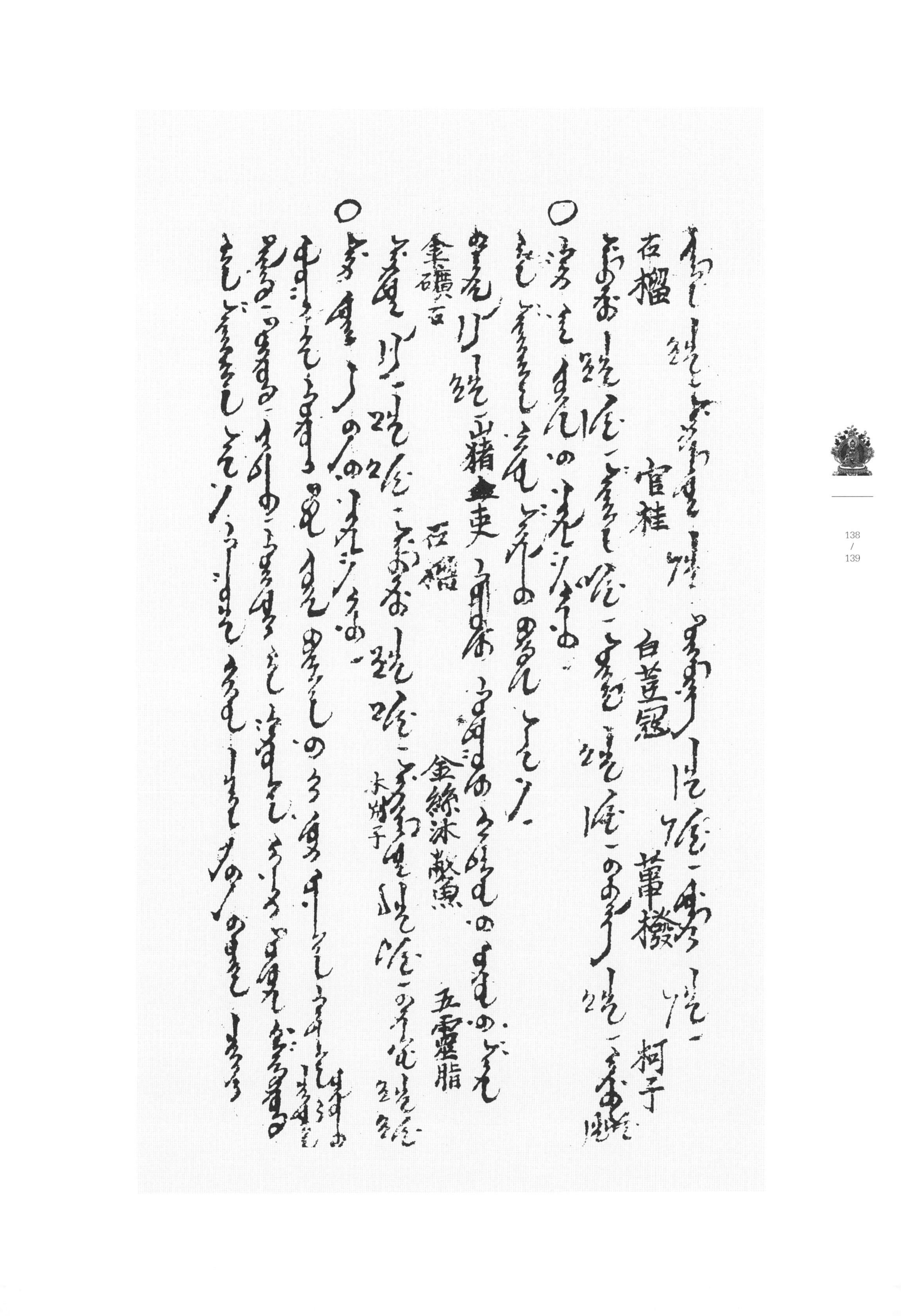

石榴 官桂 白荳冠 蓽撥 柯子

山豬糞

金礦石 石榴 金絲沐薰 五靈脂

木鱉子

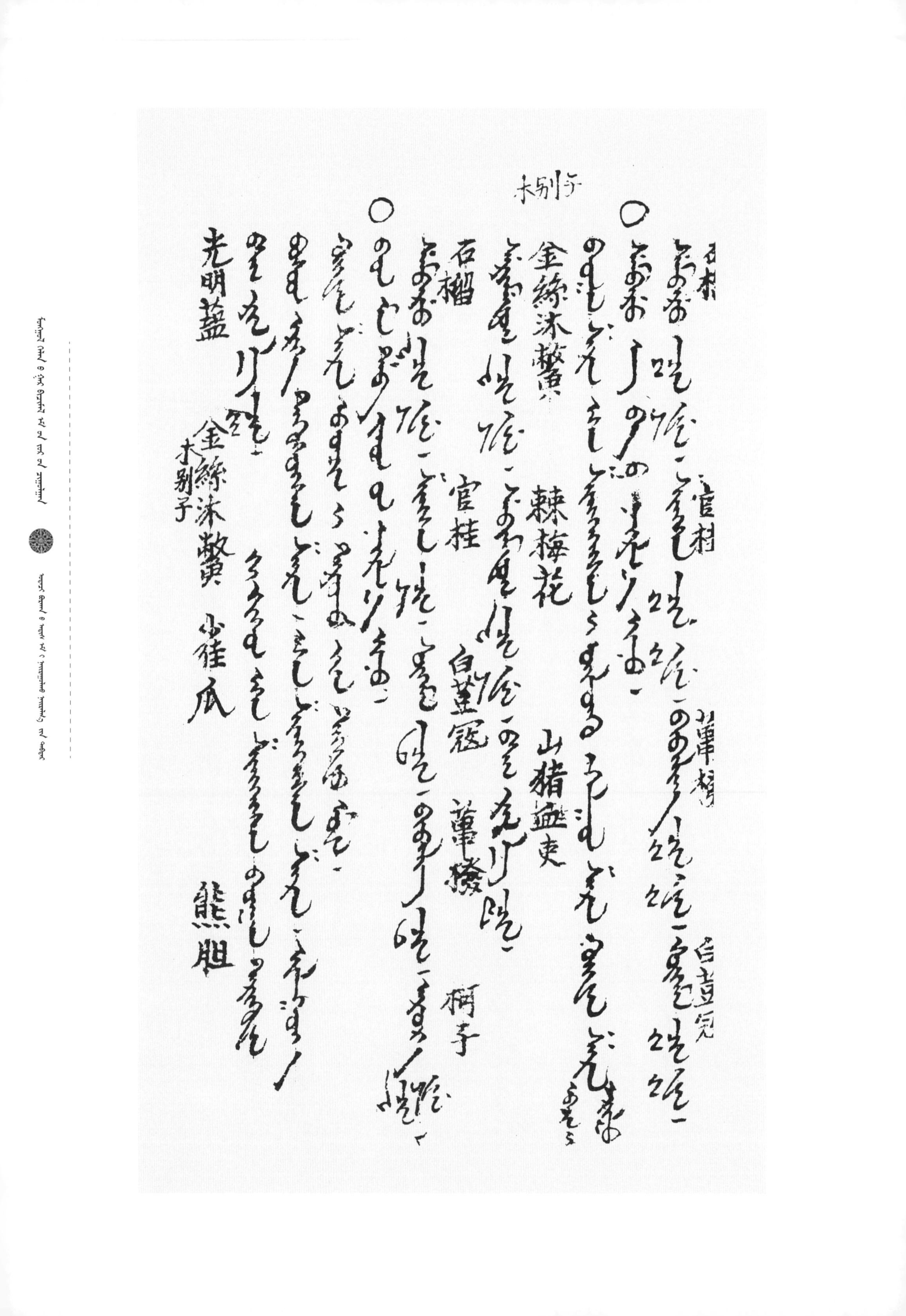

木別子

石榴 官桂 蓽撥 白荳蔻

金絲沐鼈 棘梅花 山豬血

石榴 官桂 白荳蔻 蓽撥 桐子

光明鹽 金絲沐鼈 木別子 倭瓜 熊膽

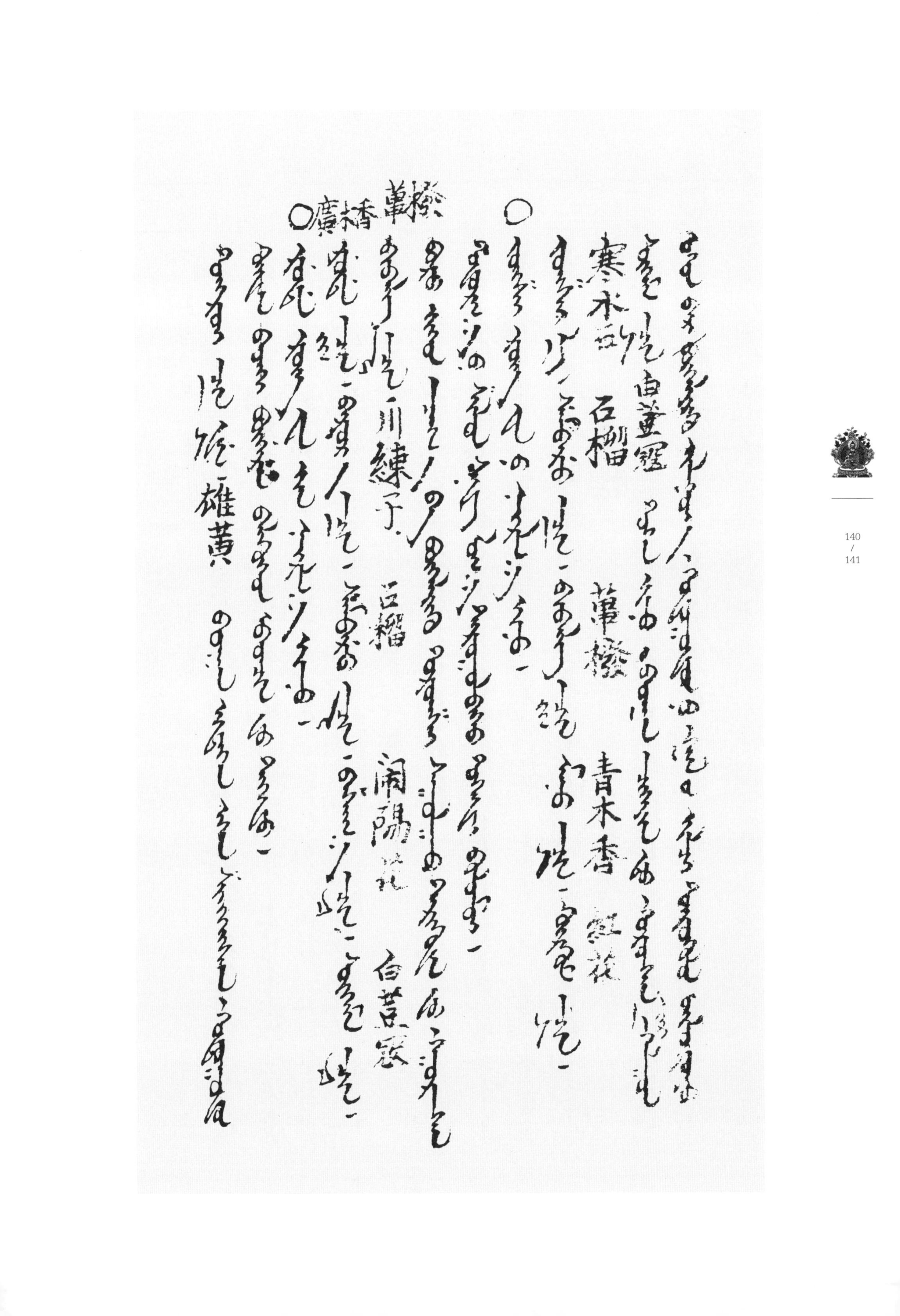

寒水石 白蓋鏡 石榴 蓽橙 青木香 紅花

蓽橙 香樟 廣

川練子 石榴 鬧陽花 白荳蔻

雄黃

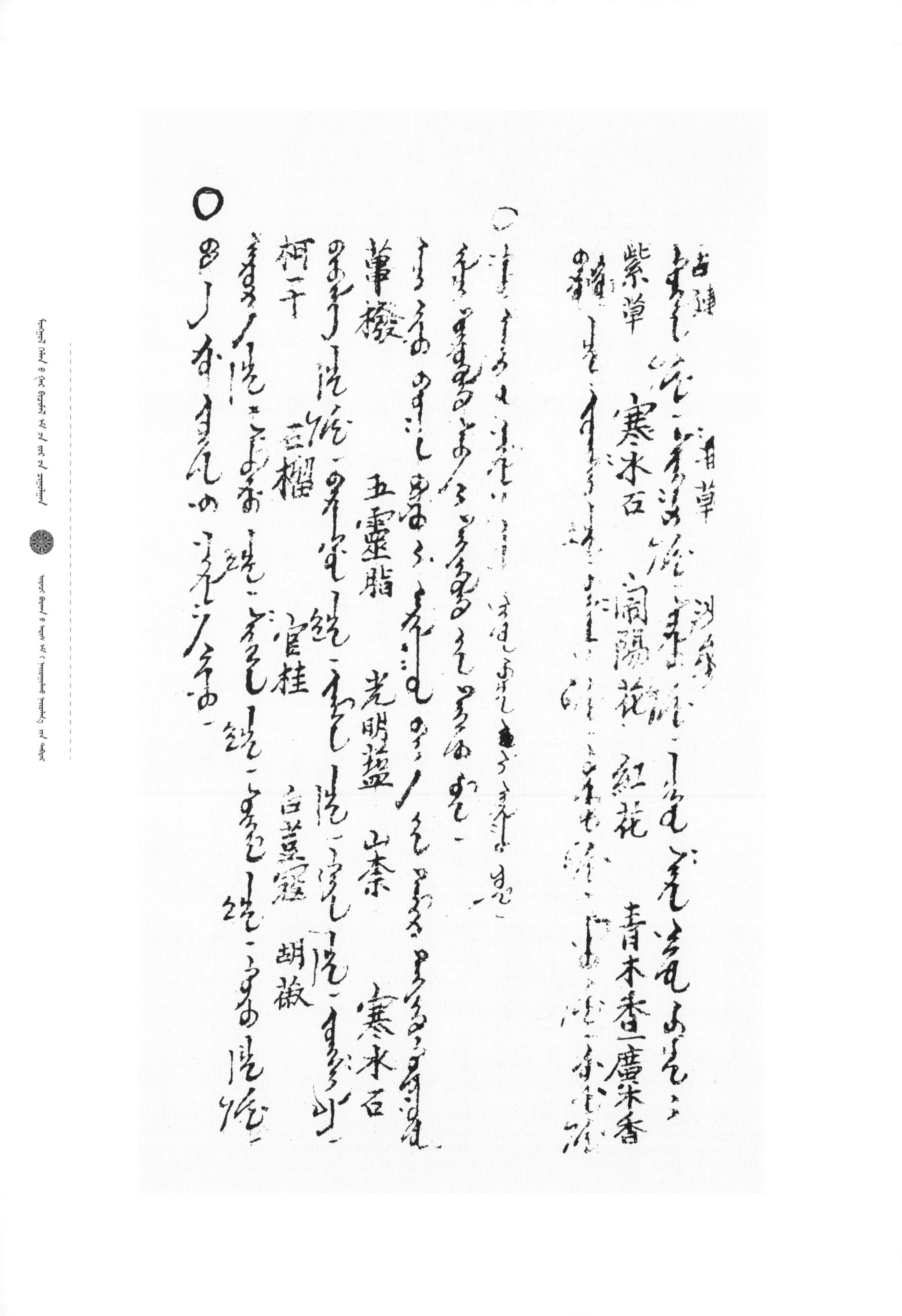

訶子　石榴　官桂　白荳蔻　胡椒

蓽撥　五靈脂　光明塩　山柰　寒水石

紫草　寒水石　閙陽花　紅花　青木香　廣木香

苦楝　甘草　沙參

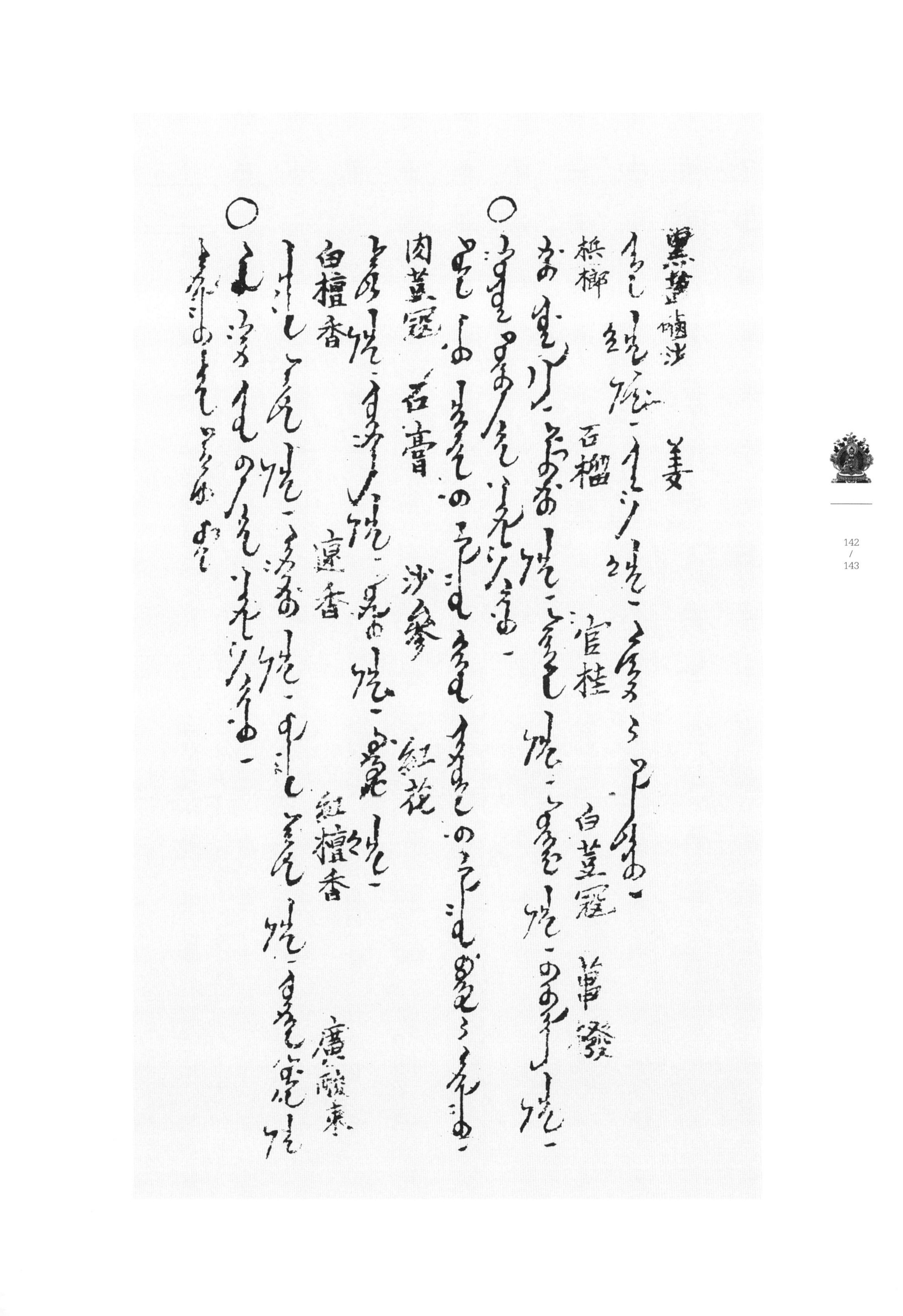

白檀香　速香　紫檀香　廣酸棗

肉荳蔻　石膏　沙參　紅花

檳榔　石榴　官桂　白荳蔻　蓽撥

黑荳　硇沙　姜

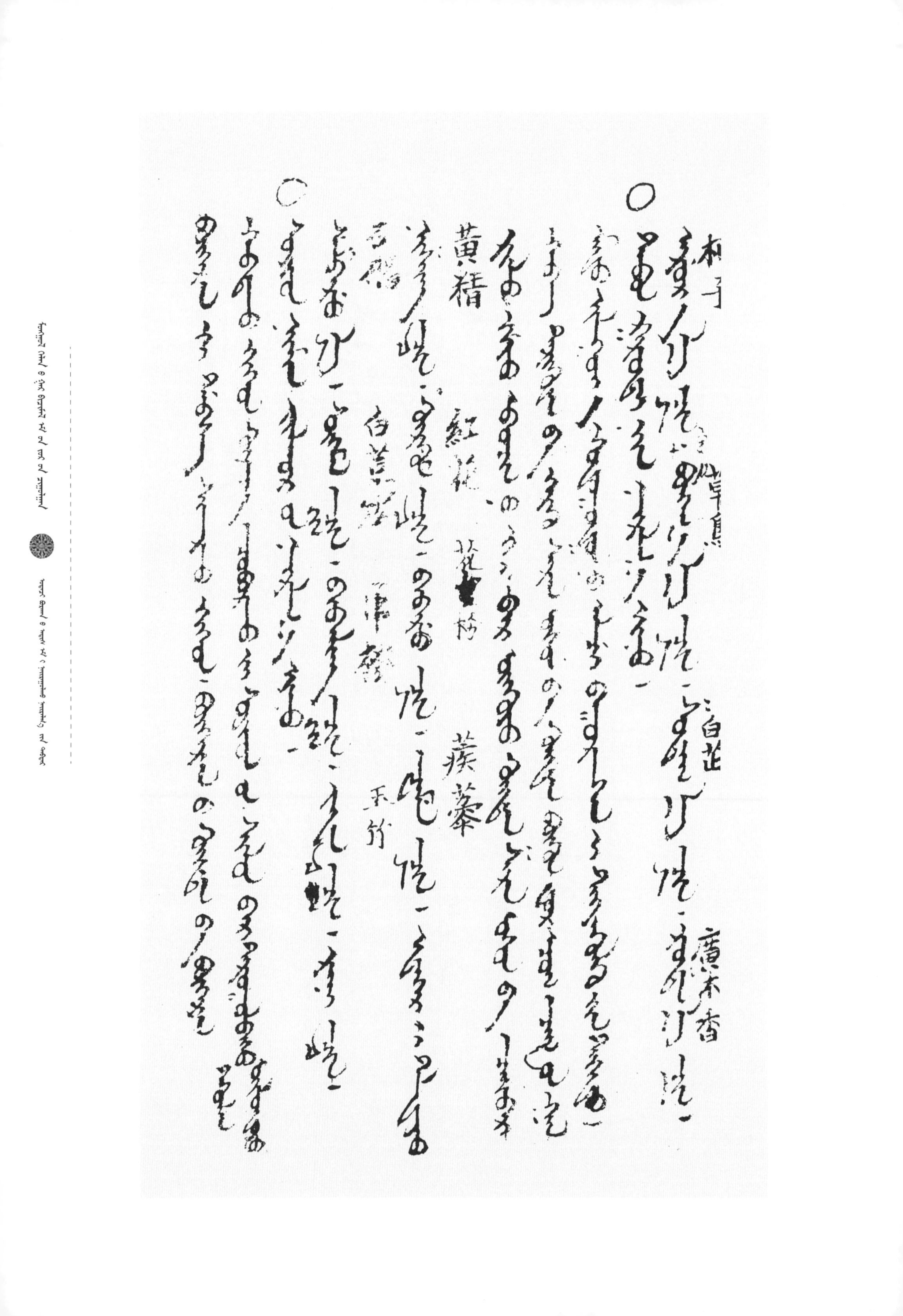

柯子 草烏 白芷 廣木香

黃精 紅花 花檳榔 蒺藜

白荳蔻 草荳蔻 天竹

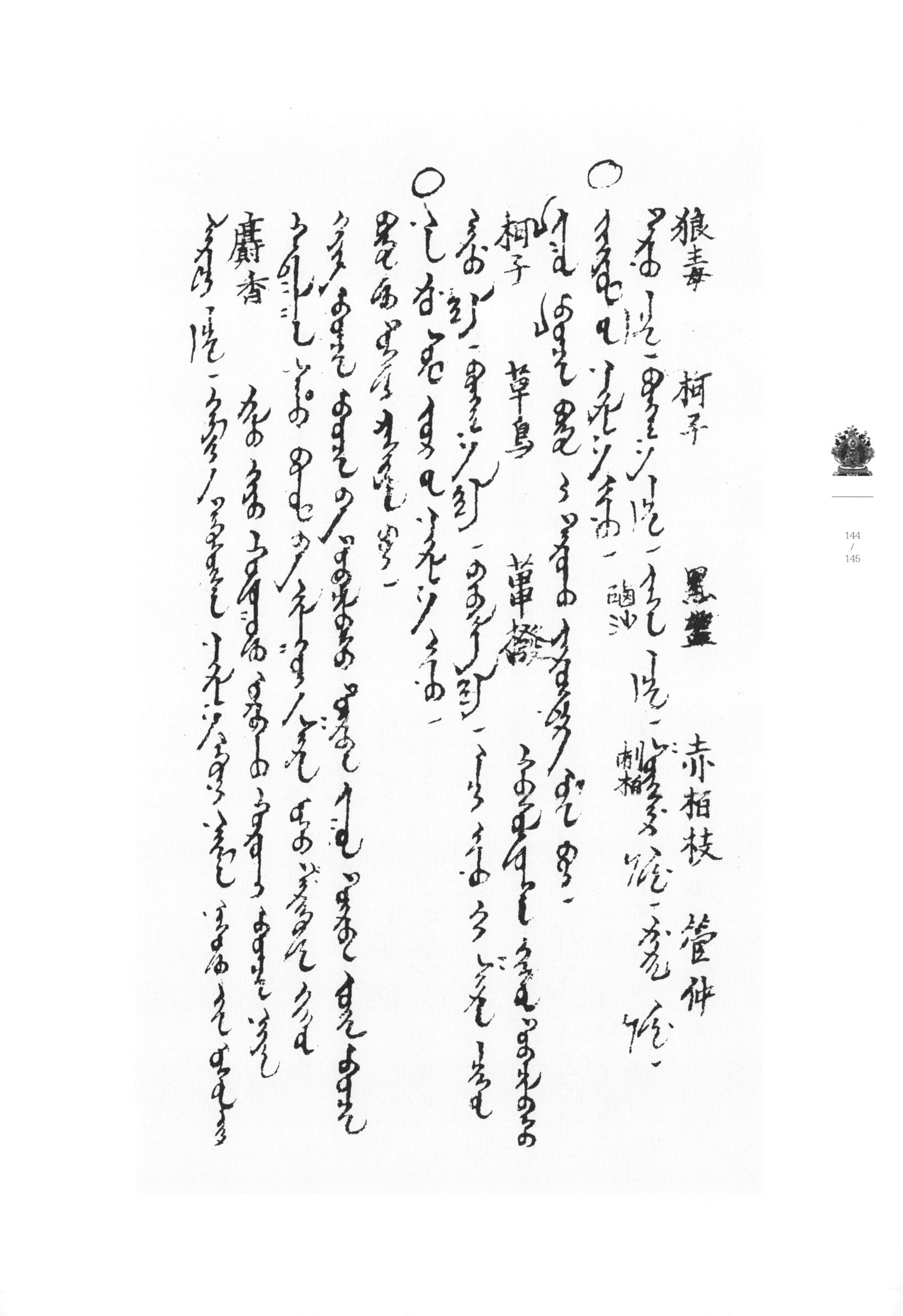

狼毒 柯子 黑鹽 赤柏枝 管仲

硇沙 刺柏

訶子 草烏 蓽撥

麝香

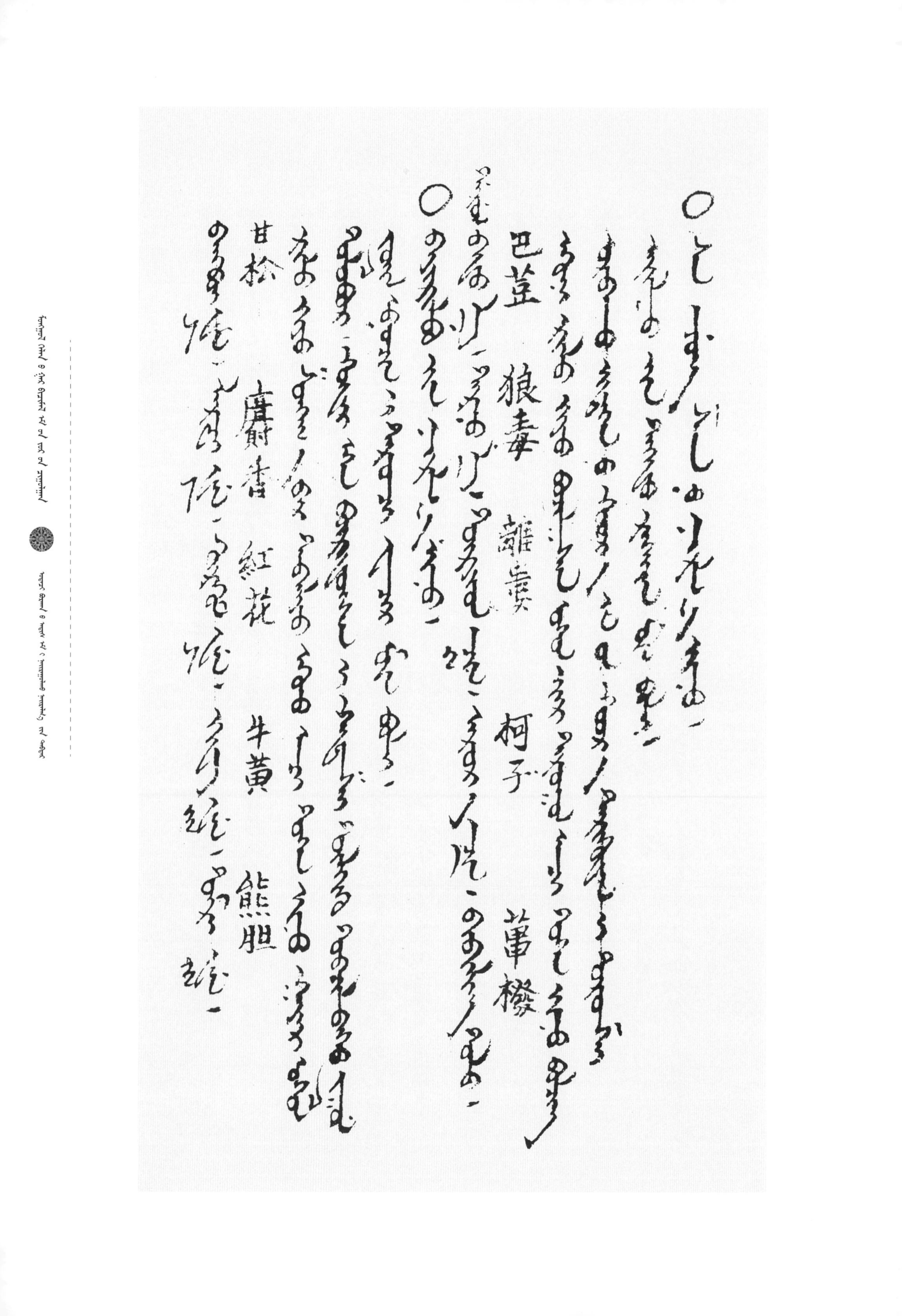

[illegible]

巴豆　狼毒　雌黄　訶子　蓽撥

[illegible]

甘松　麝香　紅花　牛黄　熊胆

[illegible]

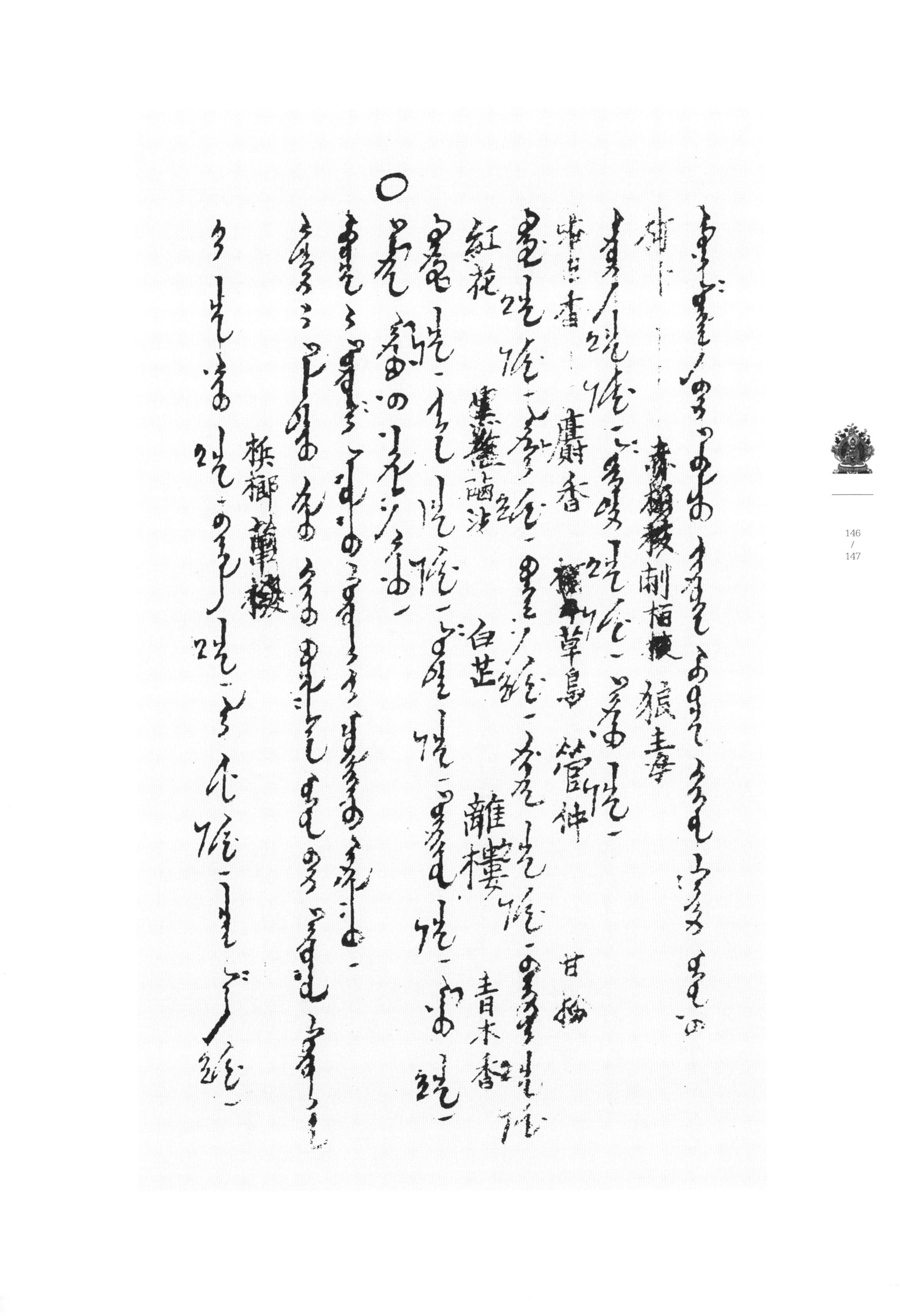

刺猬皮 刺栢皮 狼毒
麝香 草烏 管仲 甘松
紅花 硇砂 白芷 離樓 青木香
檳榔

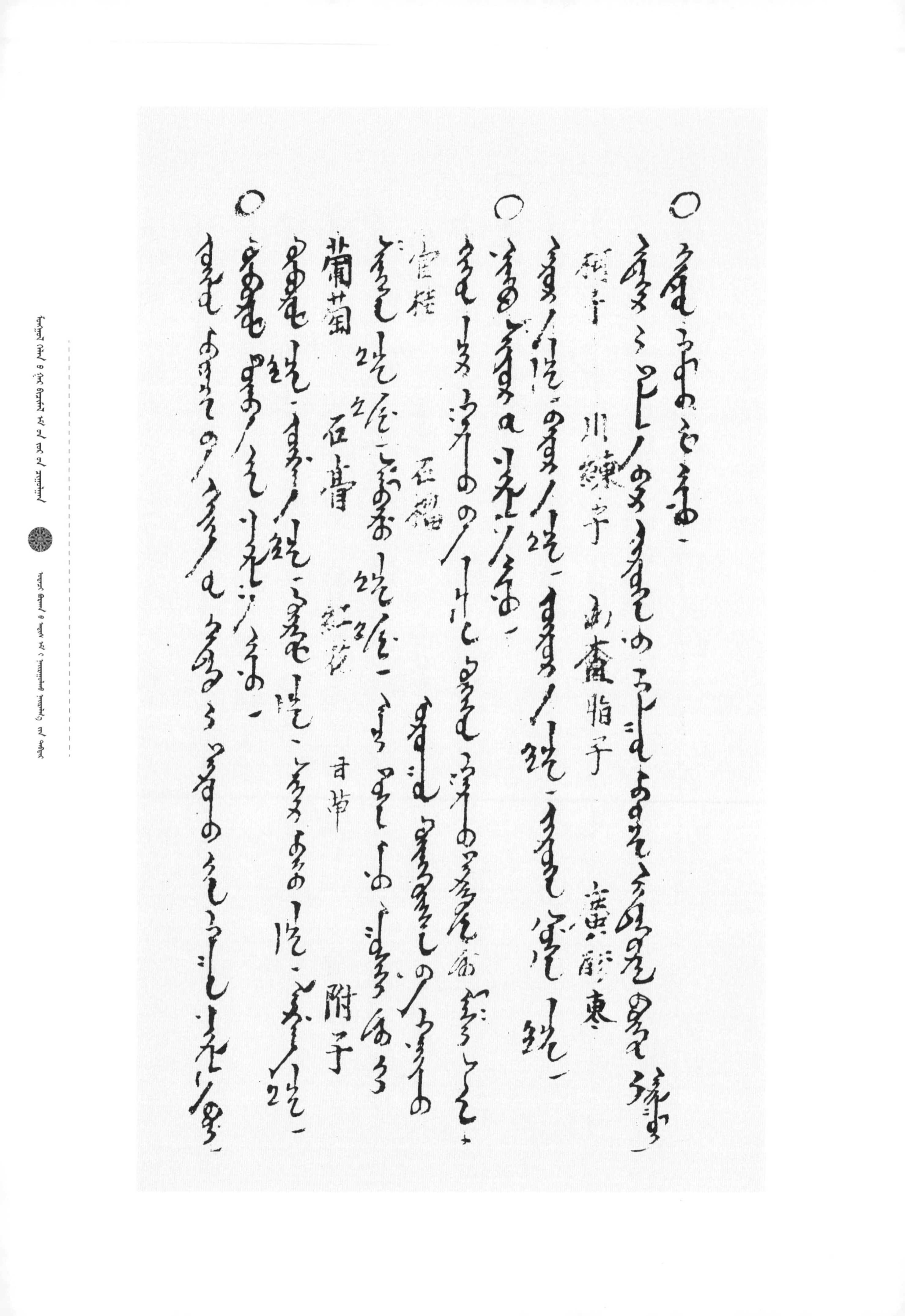

桅子 川楝子 山查 脂子 黄酸枣

官桂 石榴

葡萄 石膏 红花 甘草 附子

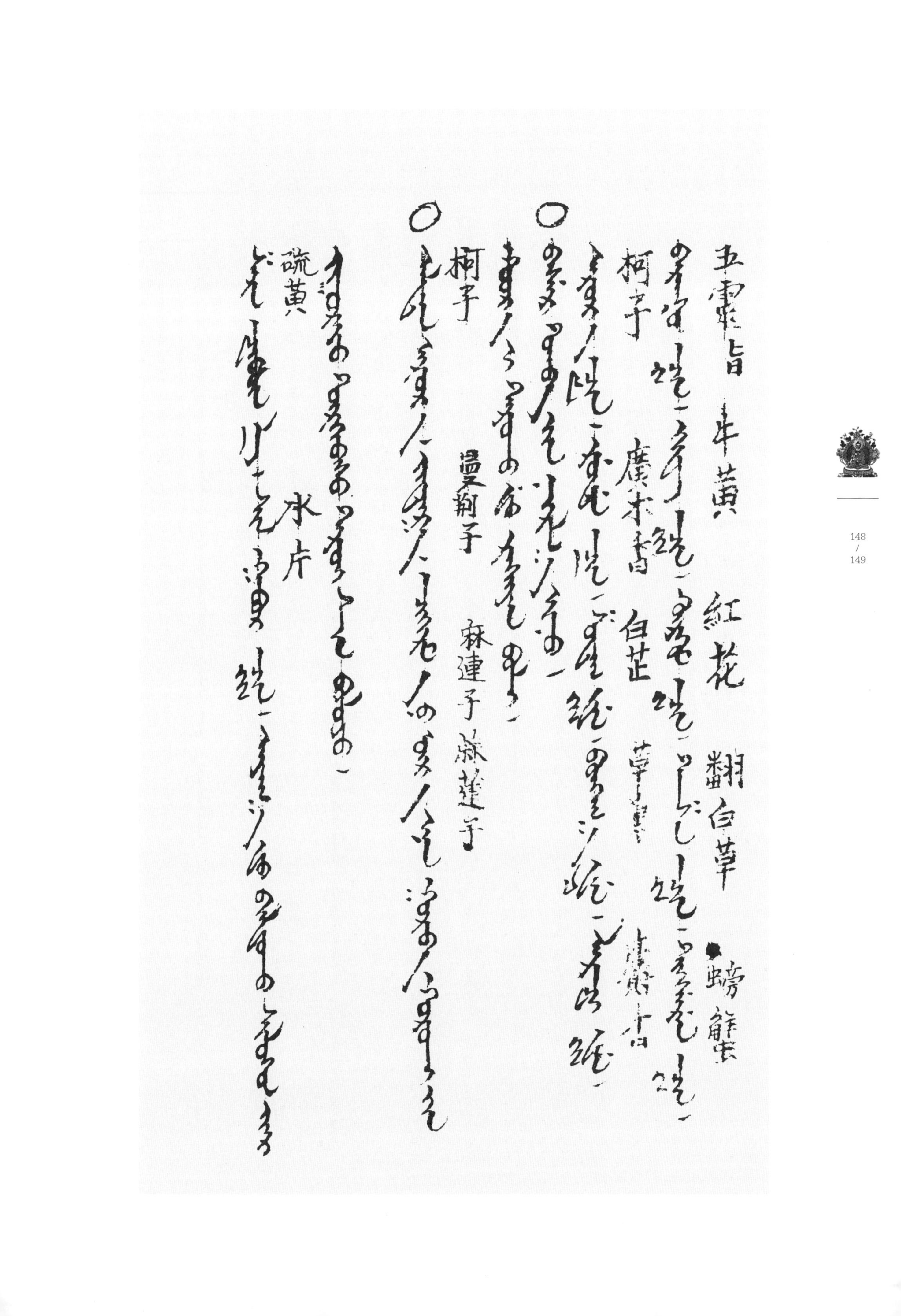

五靈脂 牛黃 紅花 翻白草 ●螃蟹

柯子 廣木香 白芷 草豆蔻 [illegible]

柯子 蔓荊子 麻連子 麻蓮子

硫黃 水片

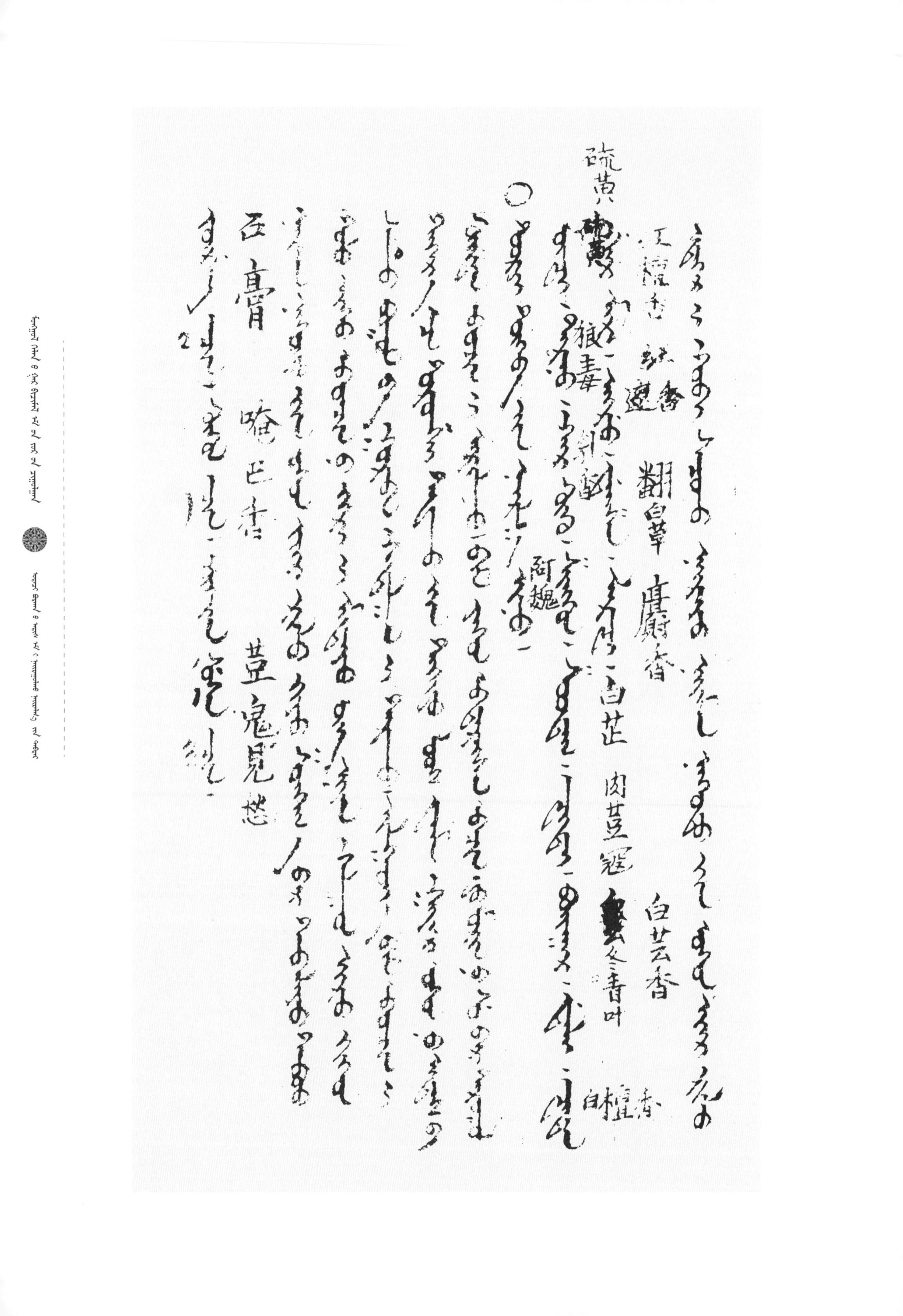

白芸香 白檀香 翻白草 麝香 白芷 肉荳蔻 青叶 狼毒 阿魏 硫黄

石膏 哈巴香 荳鬼兒愁

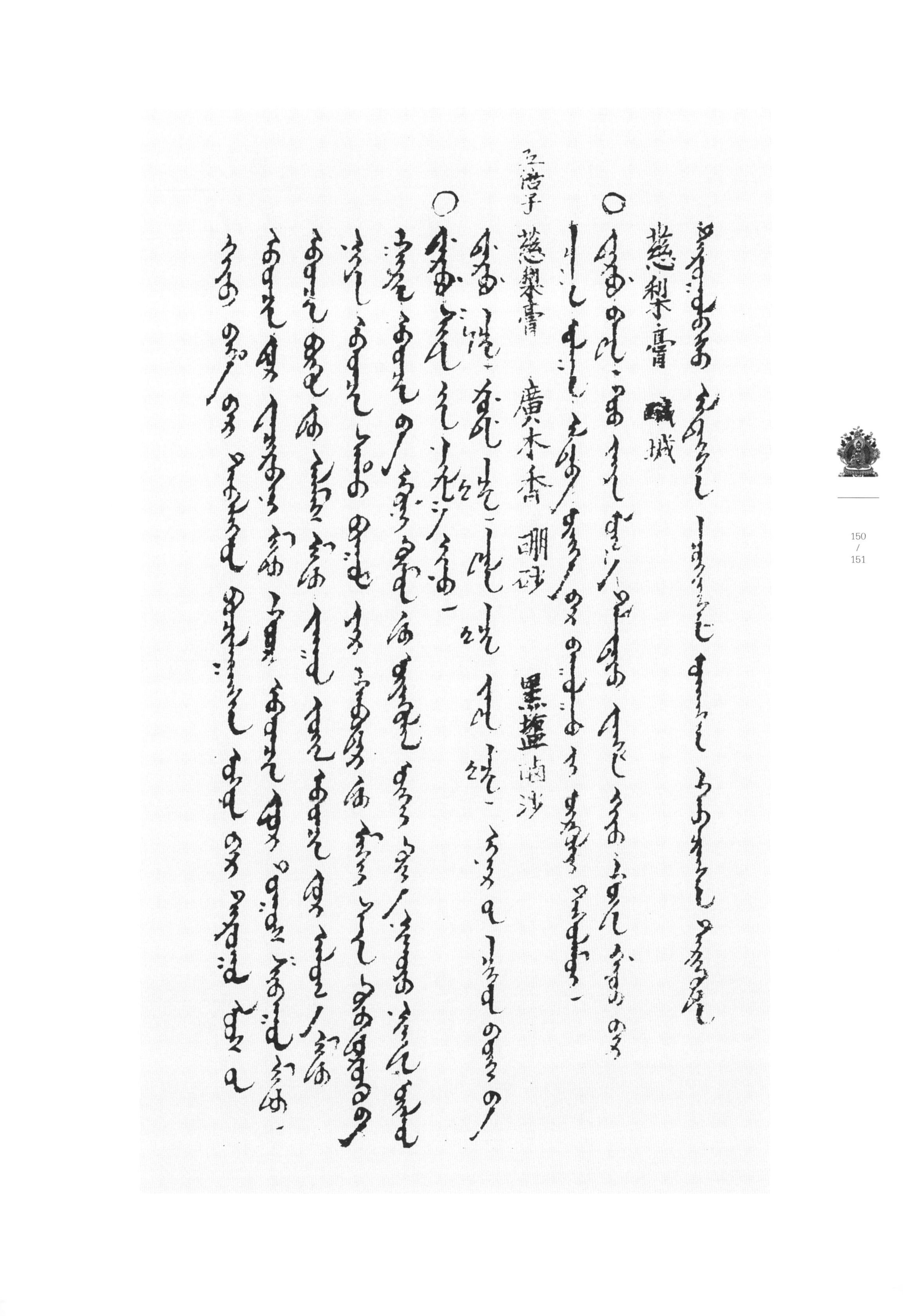

[illegible]

[illegible]

[illegible]

[illegible]

[illegible]

○ [illegible]

[illegible]

五倍子 蕊梨膏 廣木香 硼砂 黑鹽 硇沙

[illegible]

○ [illegible]

蕊梨膏 鹹城

[illegible]

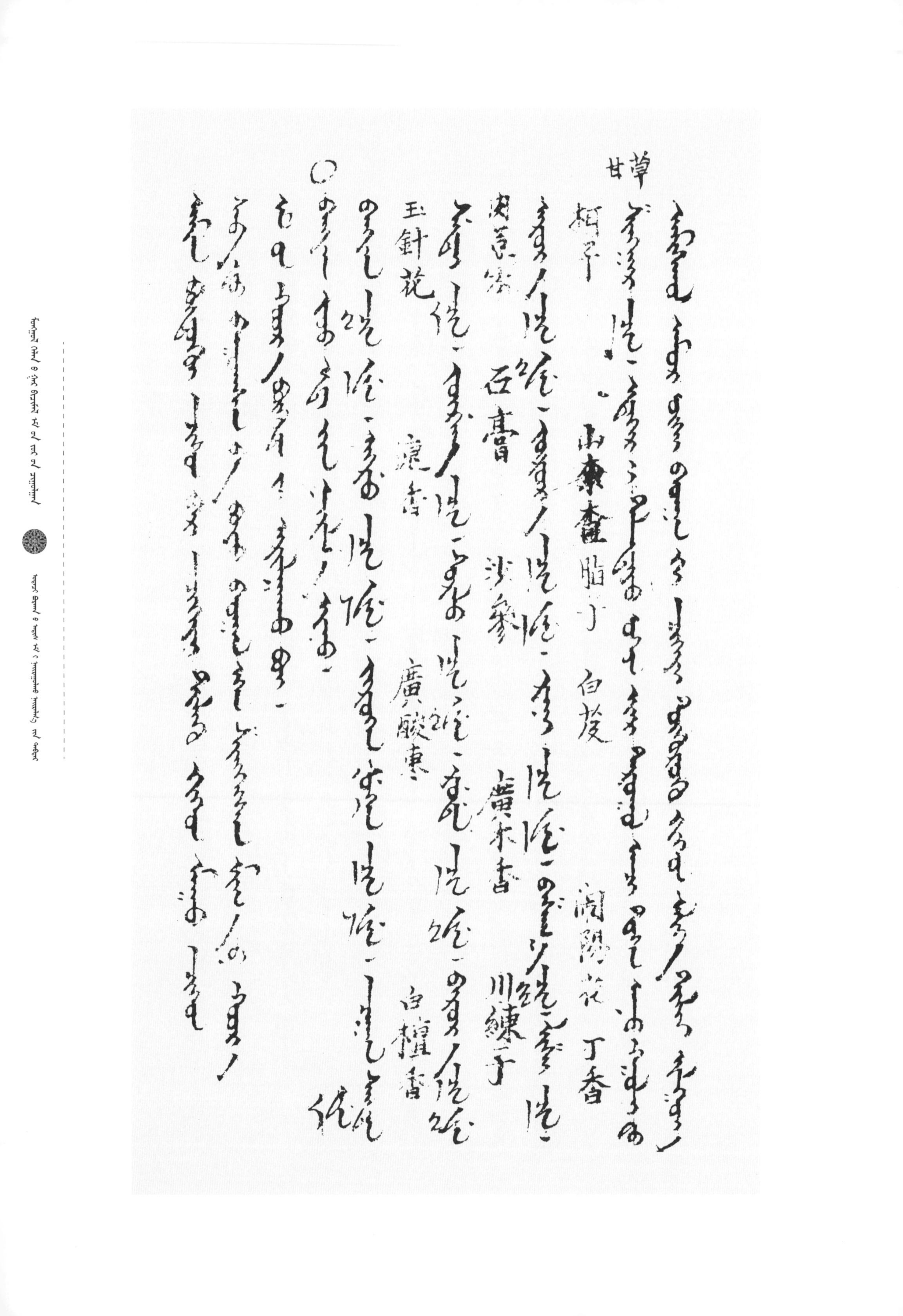

甘草

柯子 山柰 臙脂 白芨 鬧陽花 丁香

肉荳蔻 石膏 沙參 廣木香 川練子

玉針花 麝香 廣酸棗 白檀香

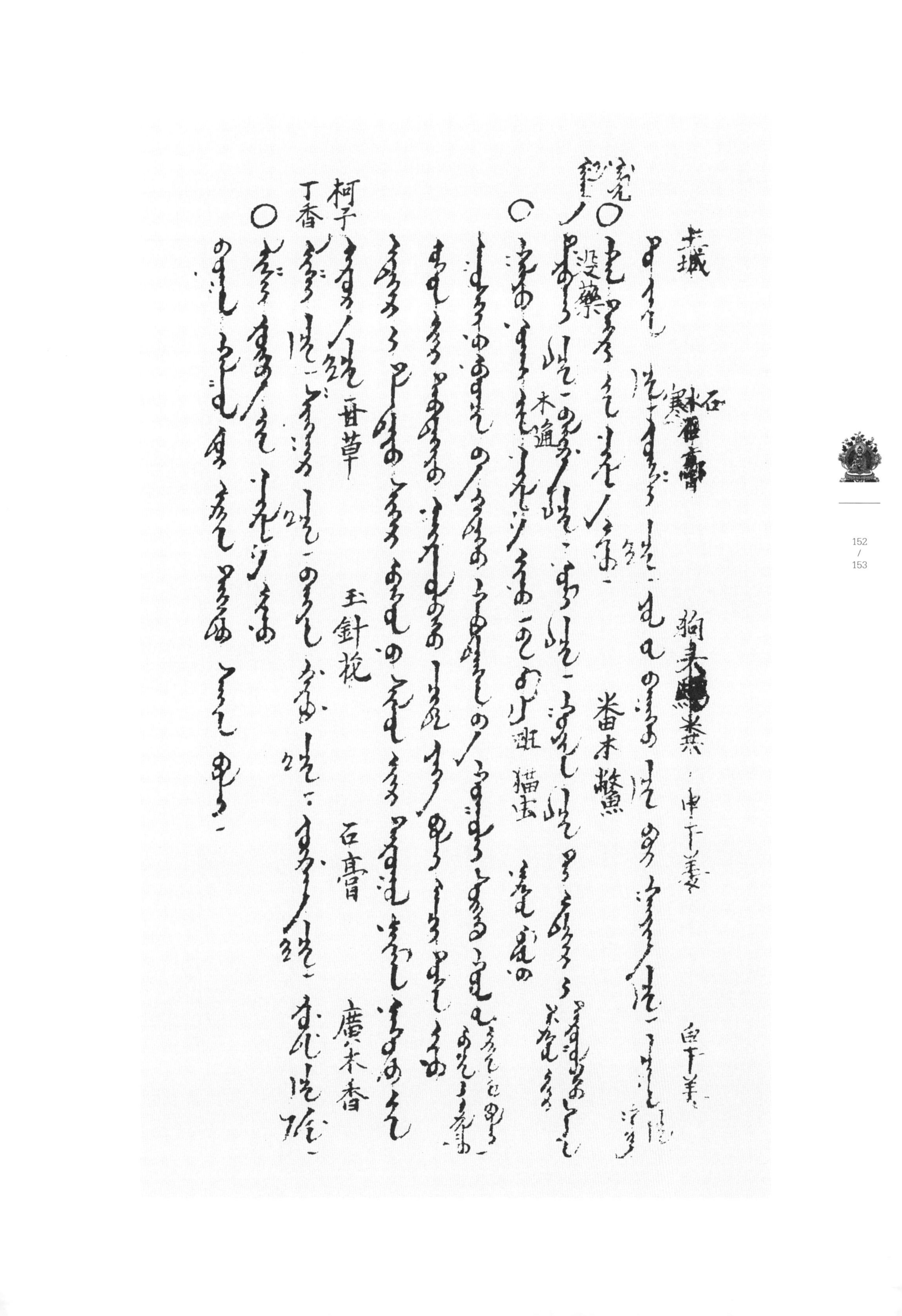

沒藥 木通 番木鱉 斑猫 柯子 丁香 石膏 廣木香

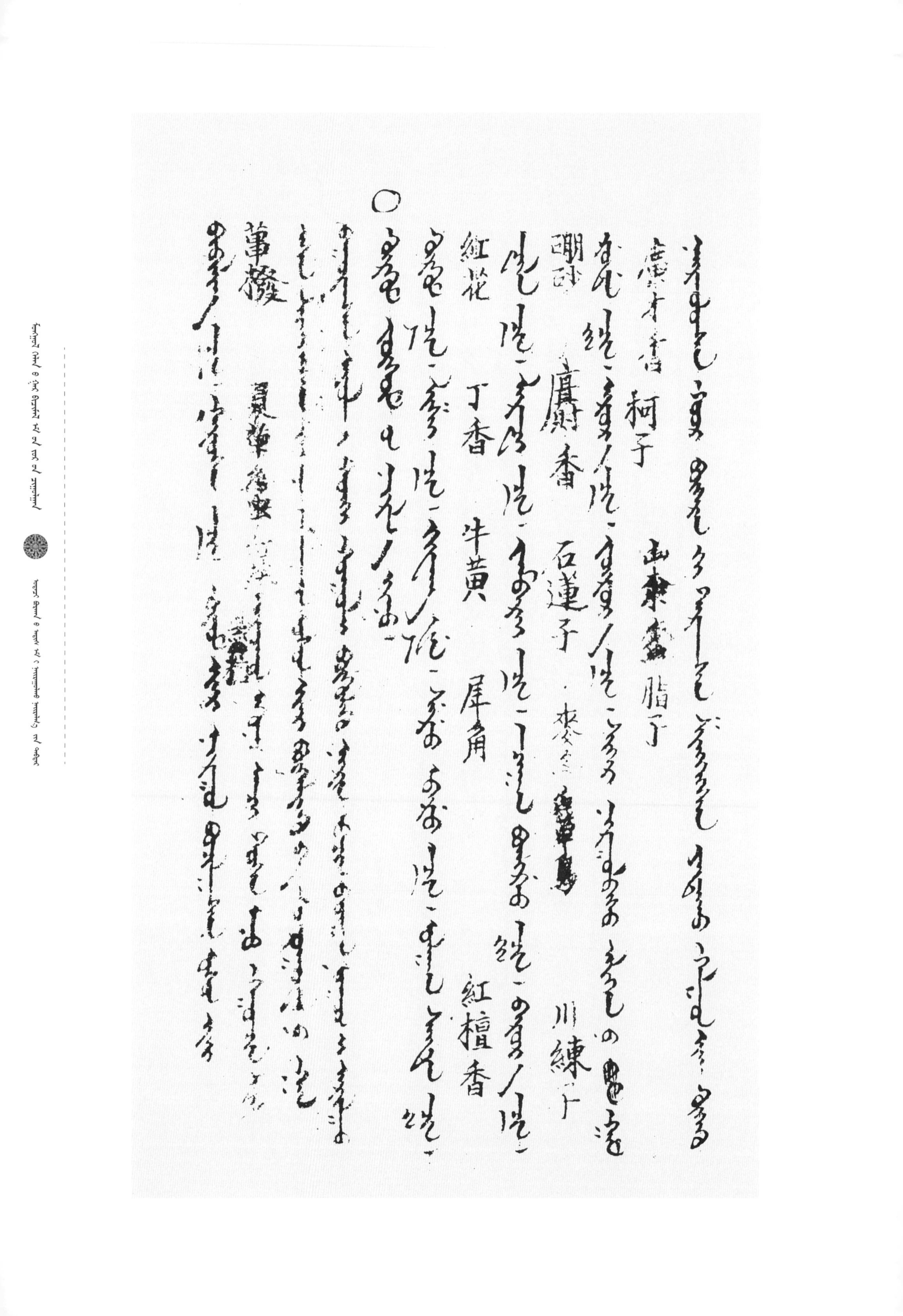

廣木香 訶子 山柰 益脂子

珊瑚 麝香 石蓮子 川楝子

紅花 丁香 牛黃 犀角 紅檀香

○

蓽撥 夏草冬虫

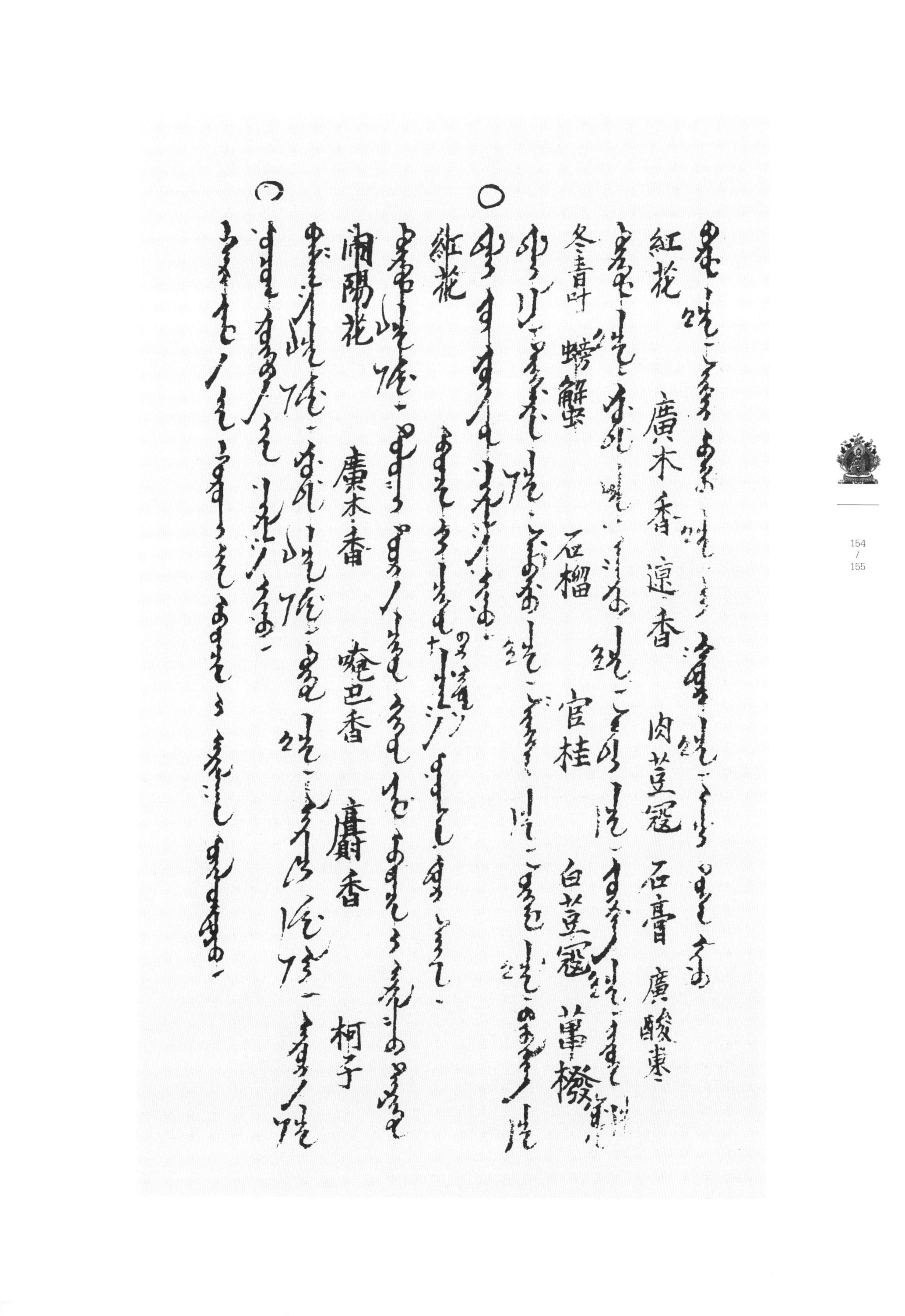

紅花 廣木香 遠香 肉荳蔻 石膏 廣酸棗

冬青叶 螃蟹 石榴 官桂 白荳蔻 蓽撥

紅花

鬧陽花 廣木香 唵巴香 麝香 柯子

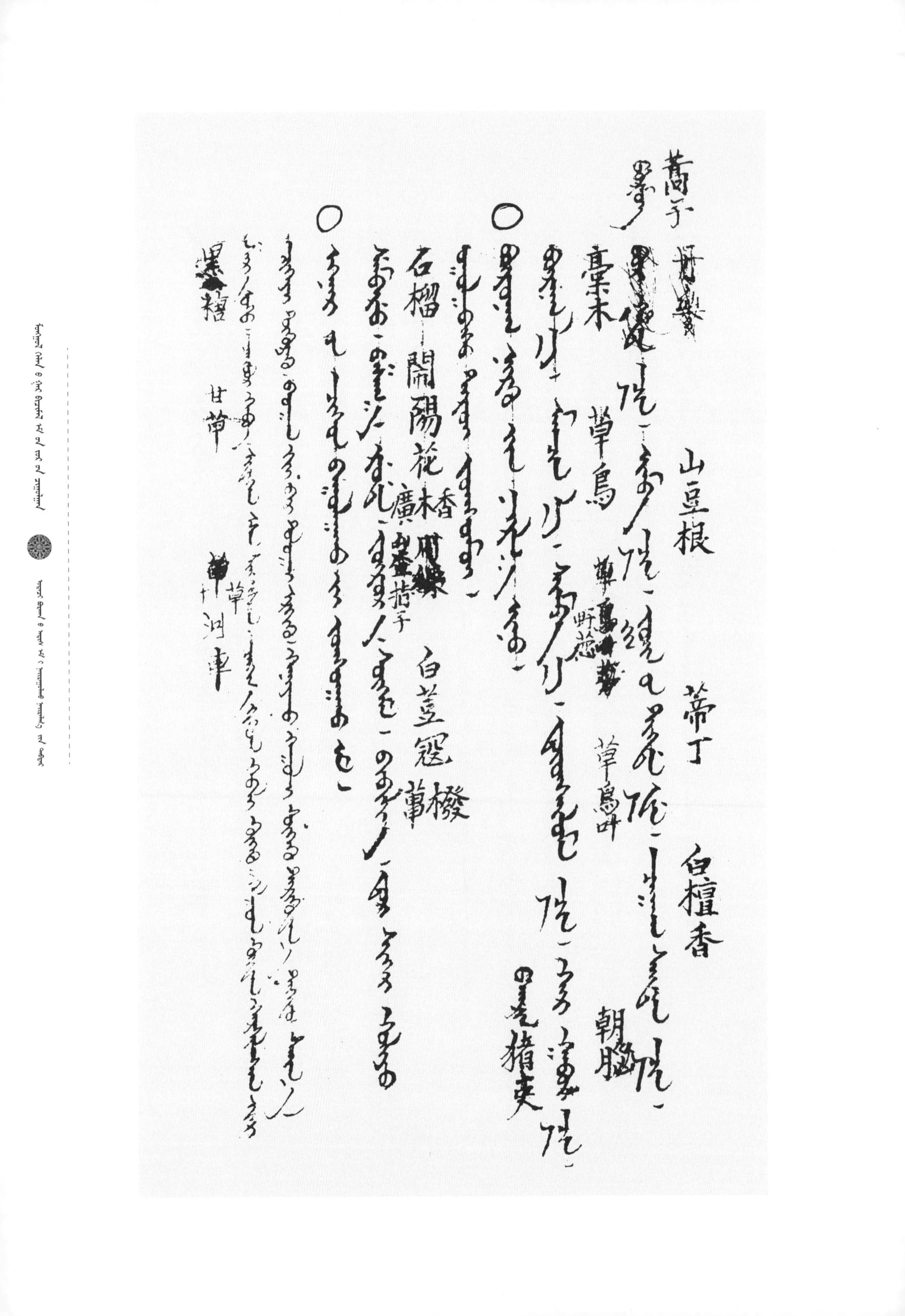

蒿子 山豆根 蒂丁 白檀香

朝腦

藁木 草烏 草烏葉 野葱 草烏叶

猪夷

石榴 鬧陽花 木香 廣 指子 白荳蔻 蓽撥

墨糖 甘節 草 十洲車

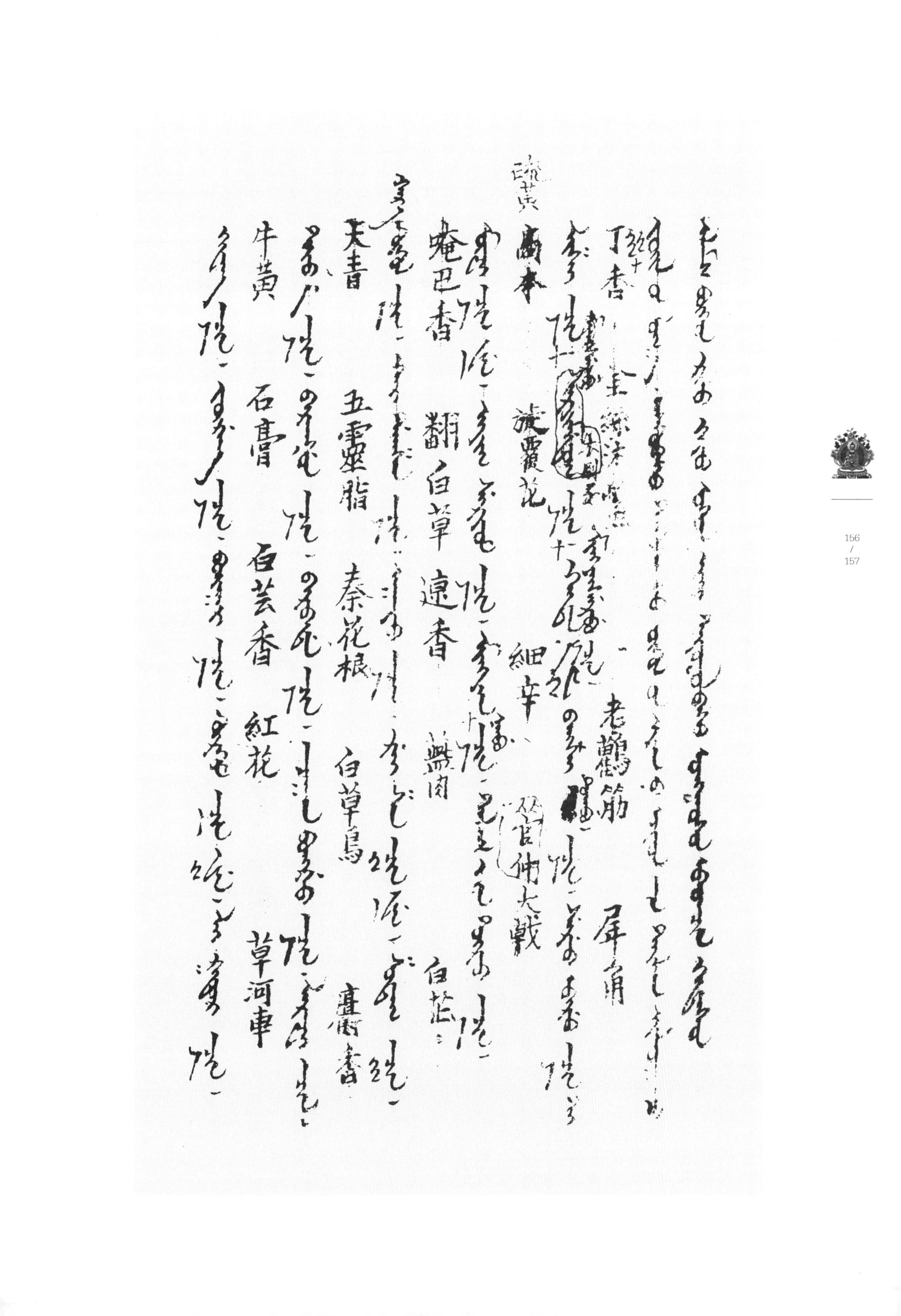

琉黄

丁香 老鸛筋 犀角

南本 旋覆花 細辛 [illegible]大戟

菴巴香 翻白草 遠香 燕肉 白芷

天青 五靈脂 秦花根 白草烏 [illegible]

牛黄 石膏 白芸香 紅花 草河車

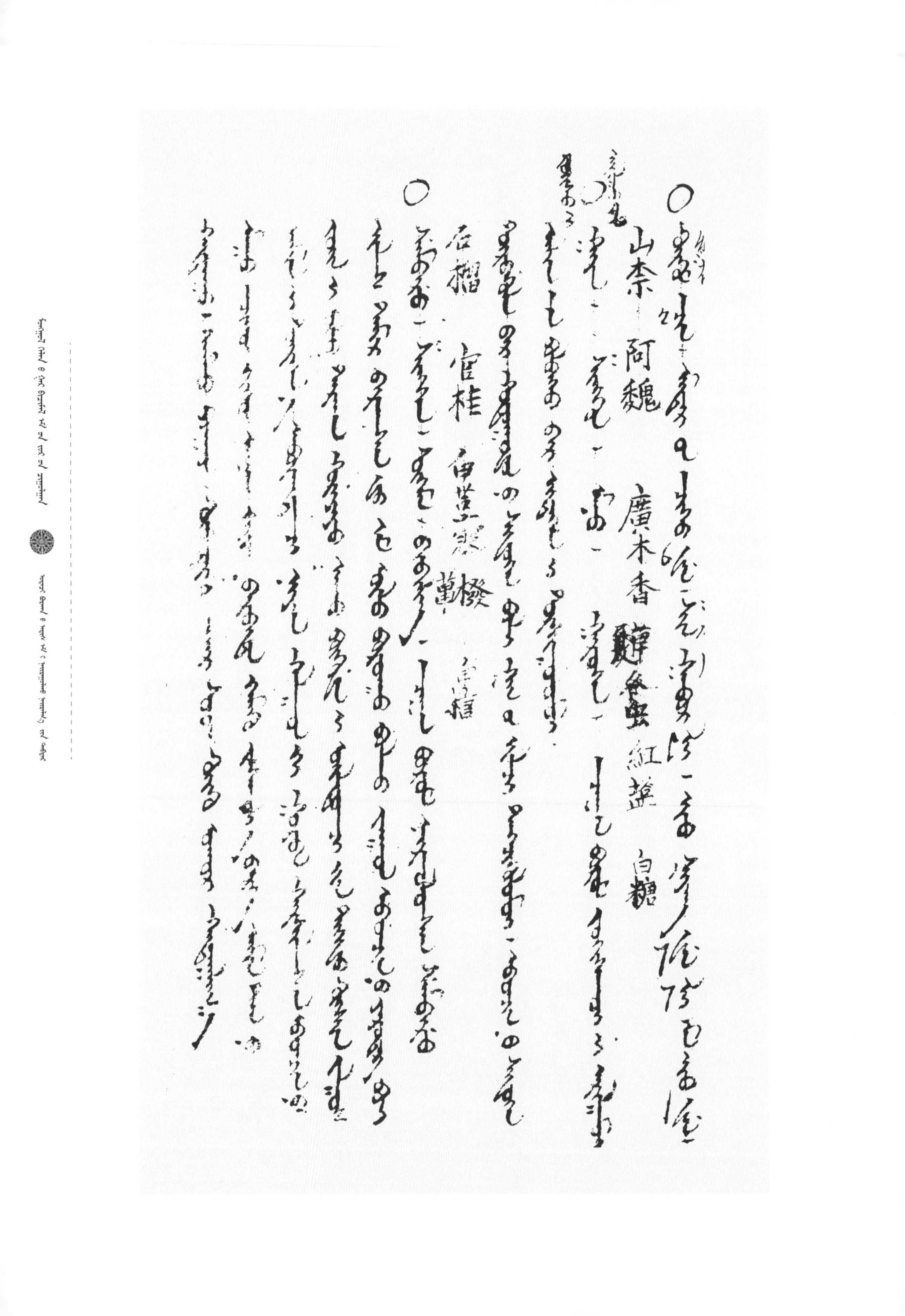

山柰 阿魏 廣木香 [illegible] 紅藍 白糖

石榴 官桂 白荳蔻 蓽撥

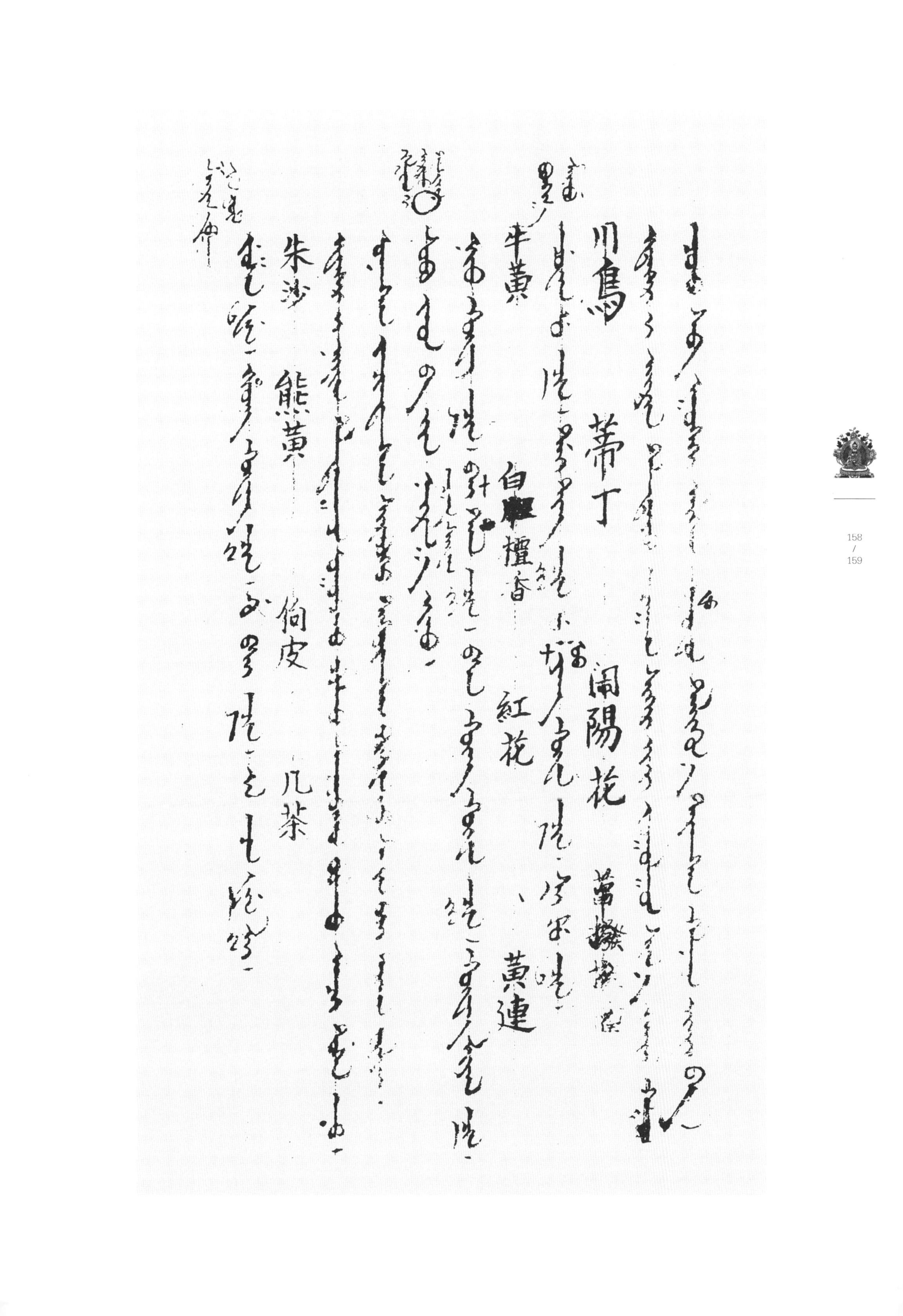

朱沙 熊黃 倘皮 几茶

牛黃

白檀香 紅花 黃連

川烏 蒂丁 鬧陽花 蓽撥

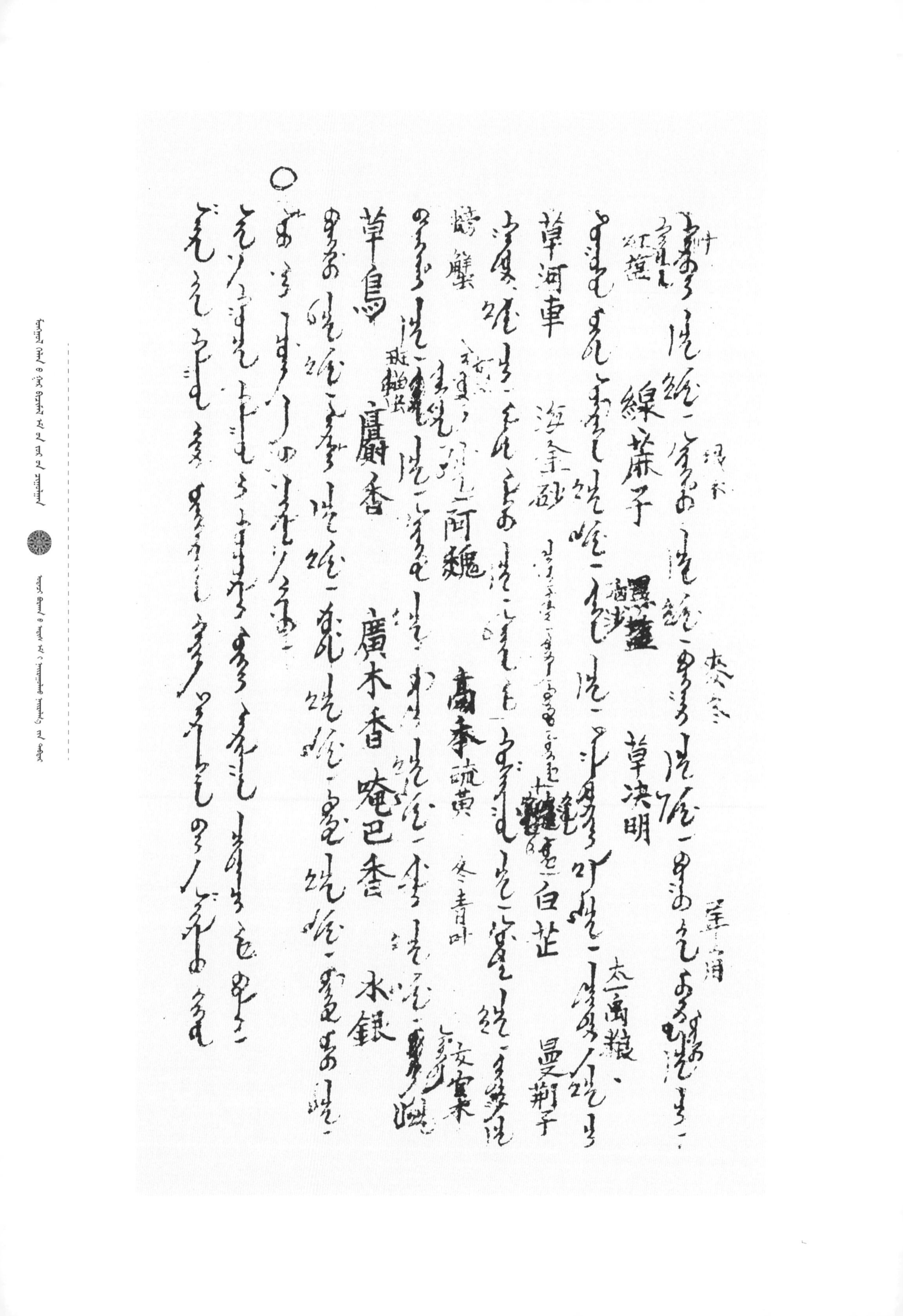

線麻子

草決明

太一禹粮

草河車

海金砂

白芷

蔓荊子

鱉

阿魏

高

硫黃

冬青葉

文官果

斑蝥

草烏

廣木香

唵巴香

水銀

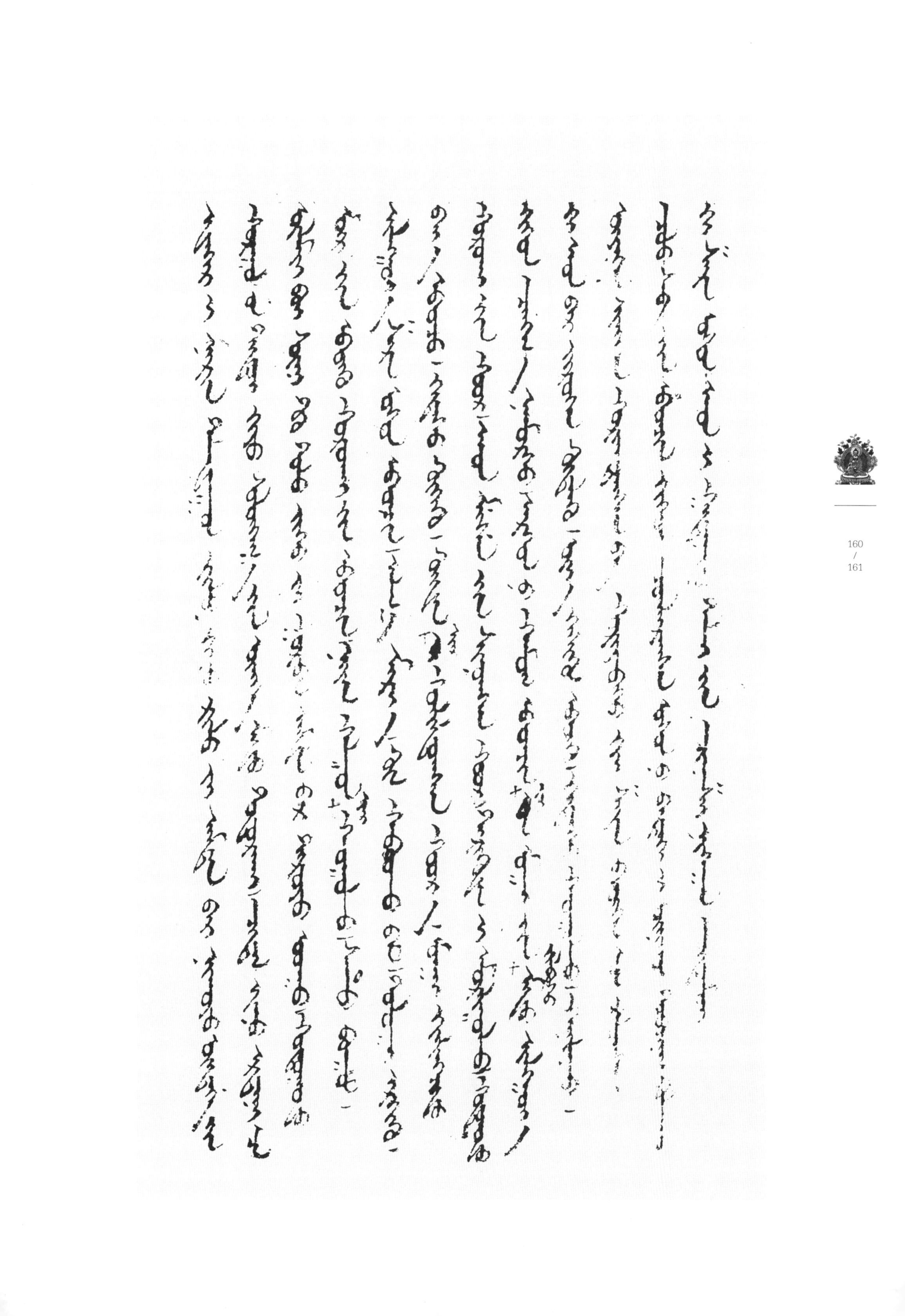

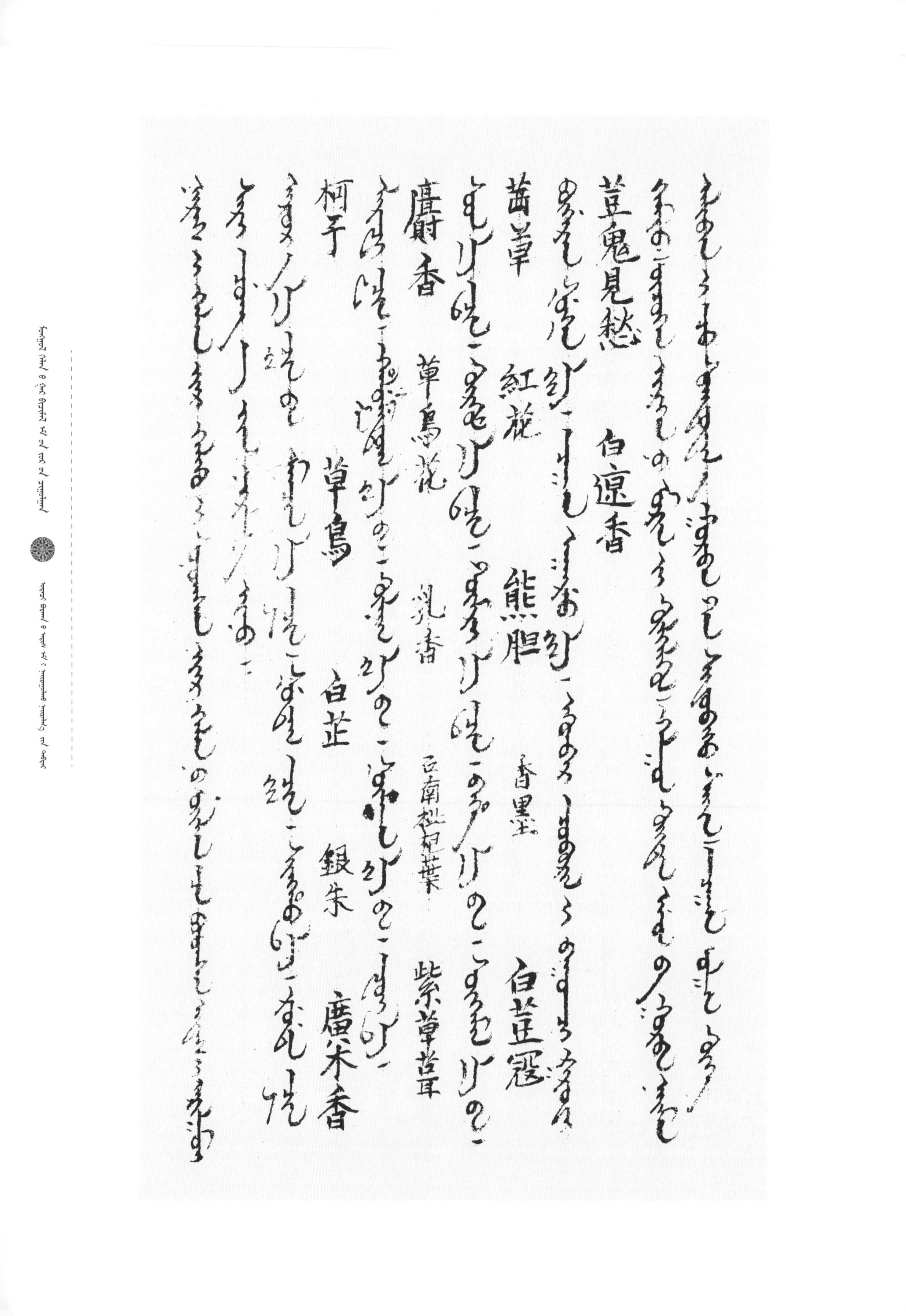

荳鬼見愁　白遼香

茜草　紅花　熊膽　香墨　白荳蔻

麝香　草烏花　乳香　雲南松柏葉　紫草茸

柯子　草烏　白芷　銀朱　廣木香

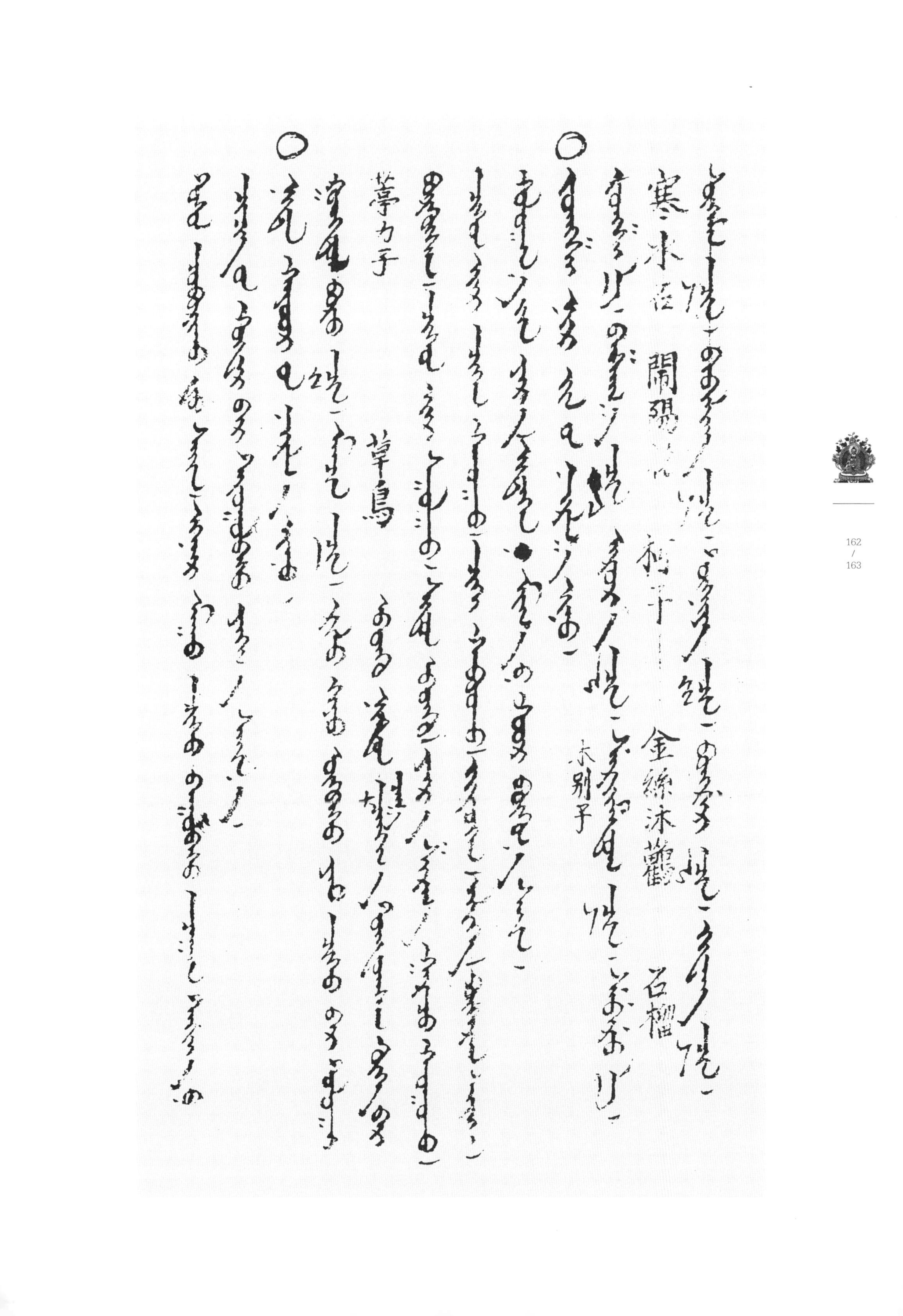

寒水石 閙羊花 秋千 金絲沐鶴 石榴

木別子

葶力子 草烏

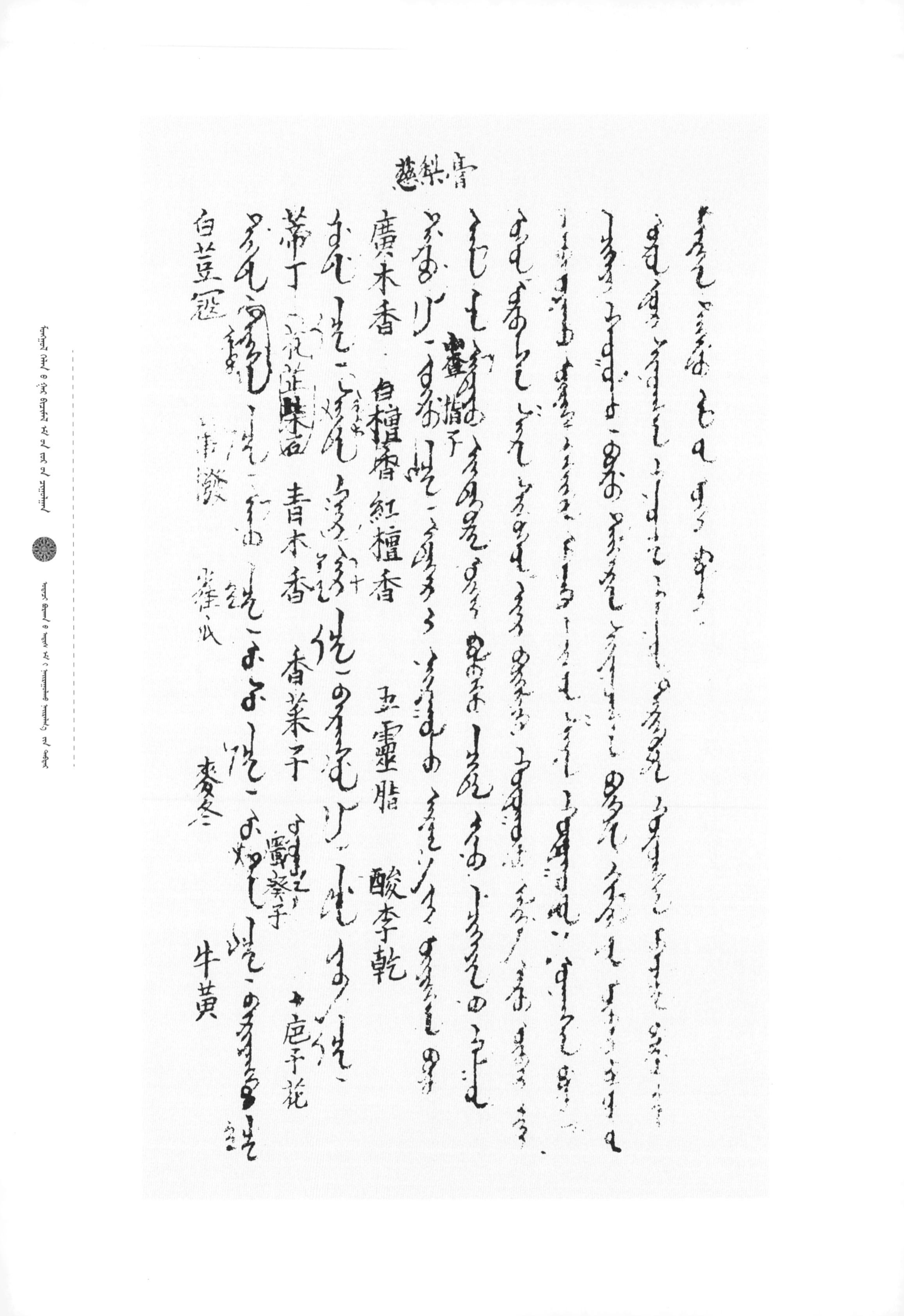

膏料藥

蠶指子

廣木香 白檀香 紅檀香 五靈脂 酸李乾

蒂丁 青木香 香菜子 劉寄子 庖子花

白荳蔻 蓽撥 麥冬 牛黃

叶業酸

草烏叶 訖柏

蓽澄車 夜宮木 玉針花 大麥 茵陳

鬧陽花 真朱干肉肉 山柰 葱梨膏 蒲蘭

麥冬 柯子 川練子 蠻指子 青木香 苦參

廣木香 白檀香 石膏 紅花 蓽丁 胡連

○

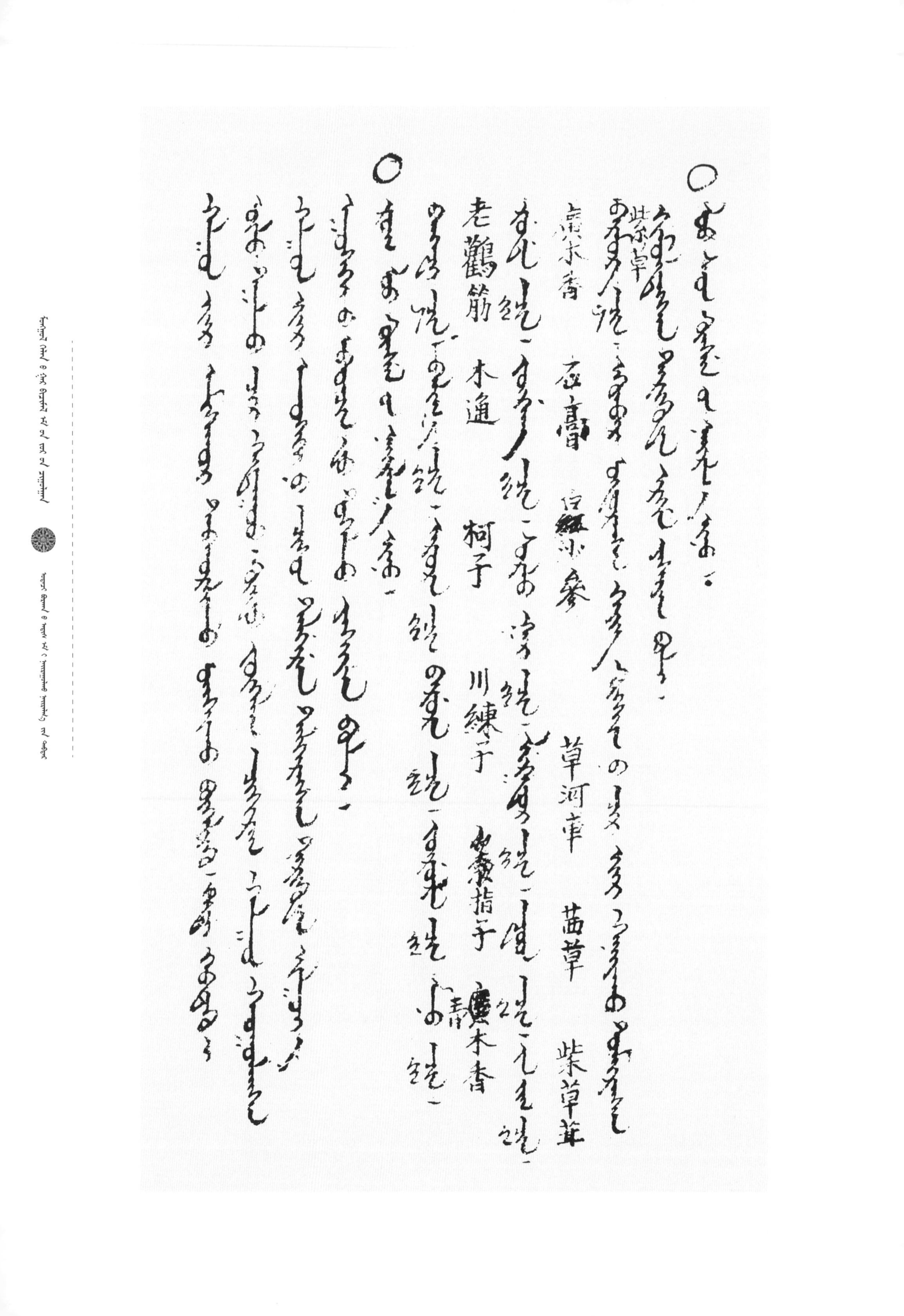

紫草

廣木香　石膏　白沙參　草河車　茜草　紫草茸

老鸛筋　木通　柯子　川楝子　鹿指子　廣木香　青

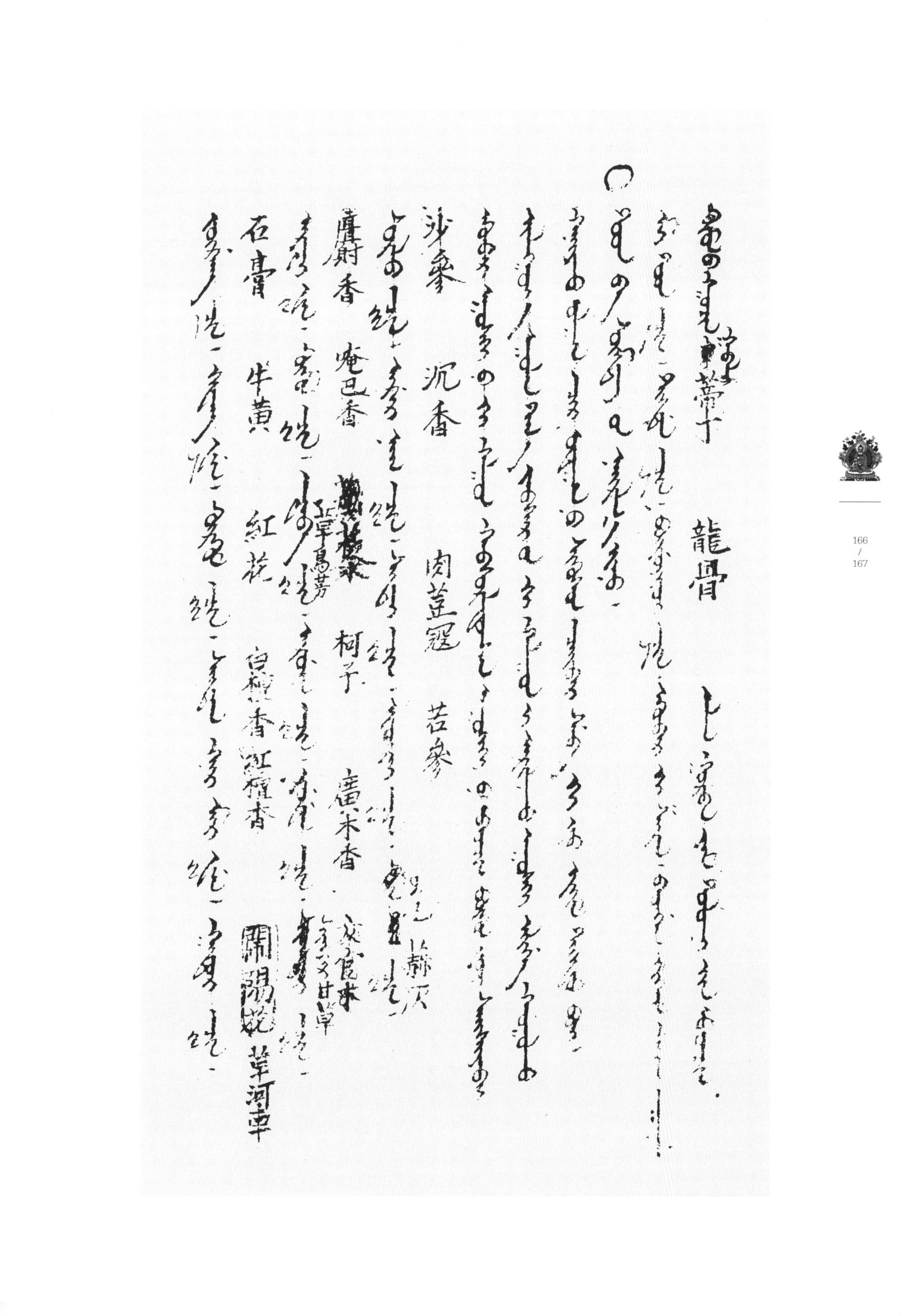

龍骨

沙參　沉香　肉苁蓉　苦參　[illegible]

麝香　庵巴香　[illegible]　柯子　廣木香　官桂　甘草

石膏　牛黄　紅花　白檀香　紫檀香　[illegible]　草河車

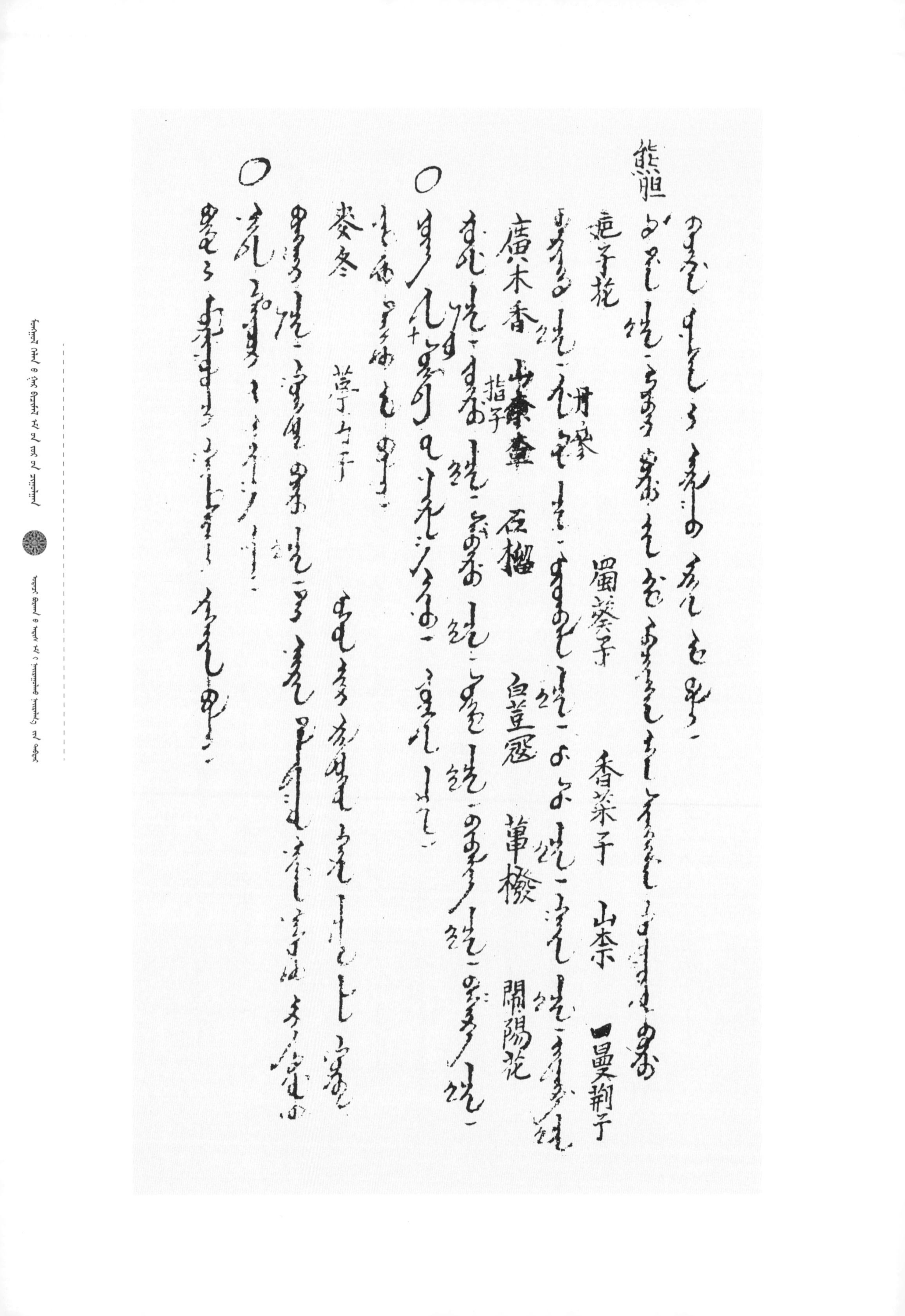

熊胆

巵子花

蜀葵子　香菜子　山柰　蔓荆子

丹參

廣木香　山柰　指甲　石榴　白荳蔻　蓽橃　鬧陽花

麥冬　葶苈子

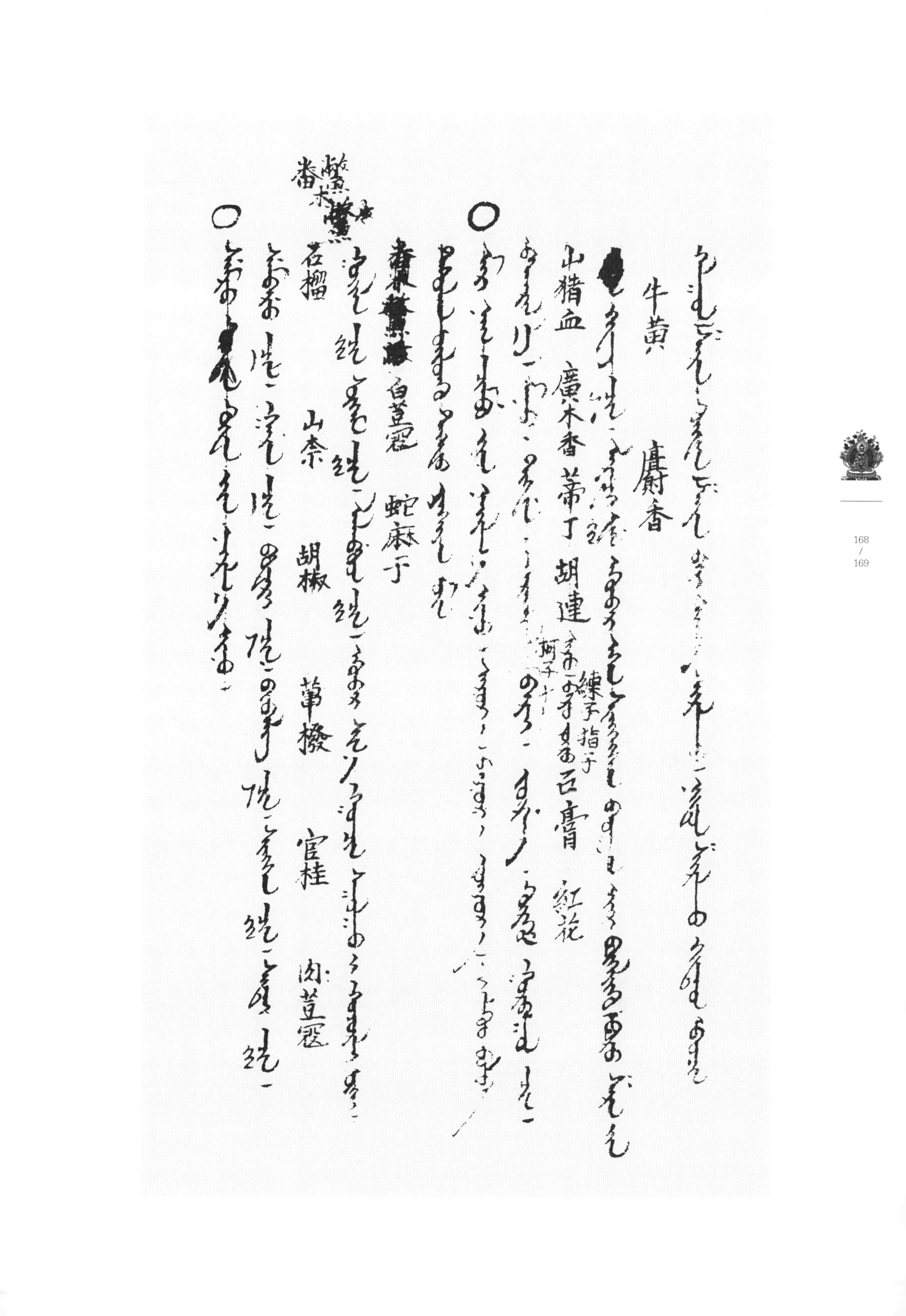

牛黄 麝香

山猪血 廣木香 蔕丁 胡連 練子 指子 石膏 紅花

訶子

白荳蔻 蛇麻子

石榴 山柰 胡椒 蓽撥 官桂 肉荳蔻

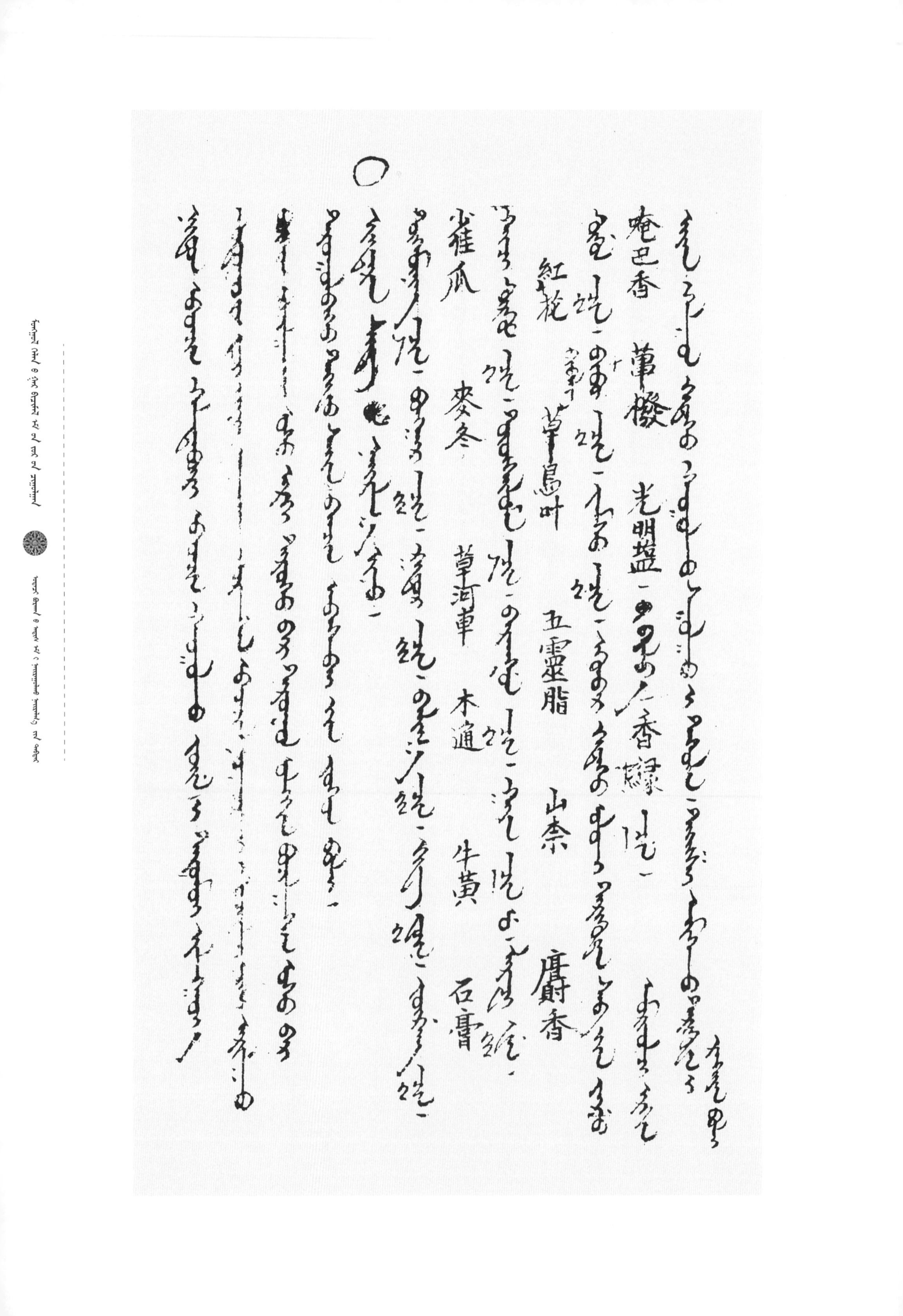

○

雀瓜　麥冬　草河車　木通　牛黄　石膏

紅花　草烏叶　五靈脂　山柰　麝香

唵巴香　蓽撥　光明鹽　香櫞

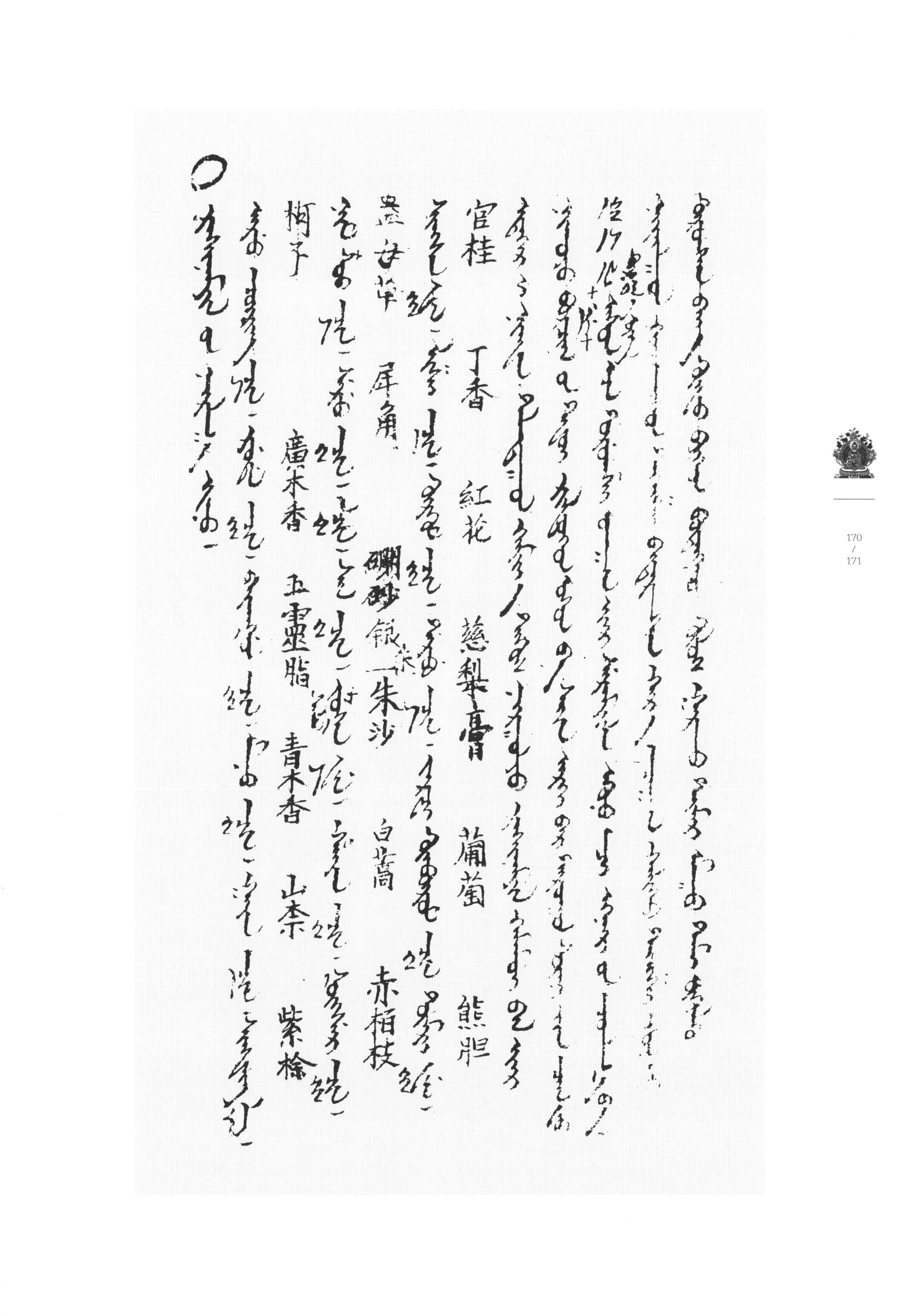

梔子　廣木香　五靈脂　青木香　山柰　紫檜

益母草　犀角　硼砂　銀朱　白蒿　赤柏枝

宮桂　丁香　紅花　葱梨膏　葡萄　熊胆

官桂
草菓
寒水石 〇

白檀香 列当
山柰 蓽茇 胡椒 冬青叶 赤石脂
石膏 石膏 紅花 丁香 肉荳蔻 白荳蔻

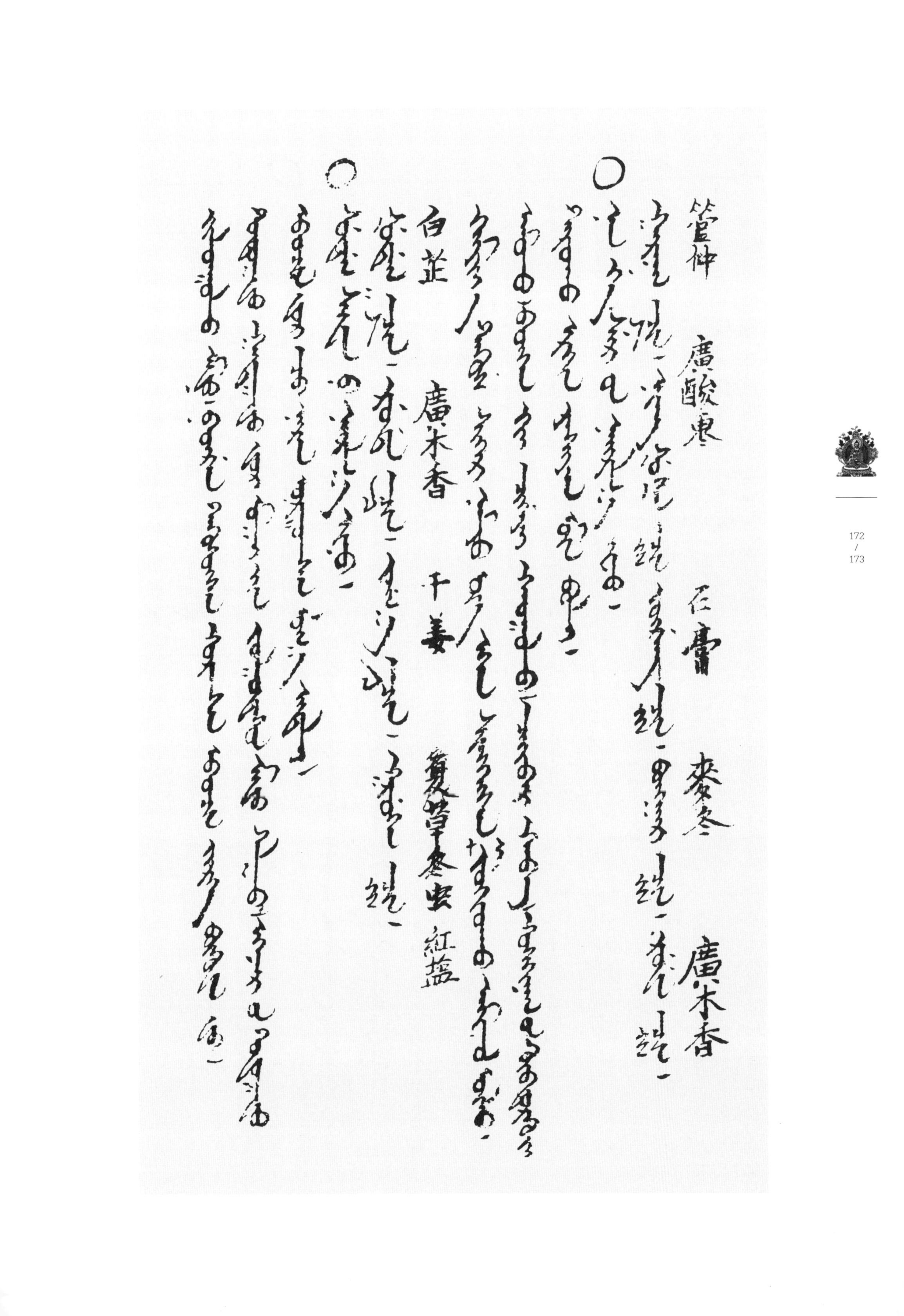

[illegible]

[illegible]

[illegible]

○ [illegible]

[illegible]

白芷 廣木香 干姜 夏草冬虫 紅鹽

[illegible]

[illegible]

[illegible]

○ [illegible]

[illegible]

管仲 廣酸棗 茌當 麥冬 廣木香

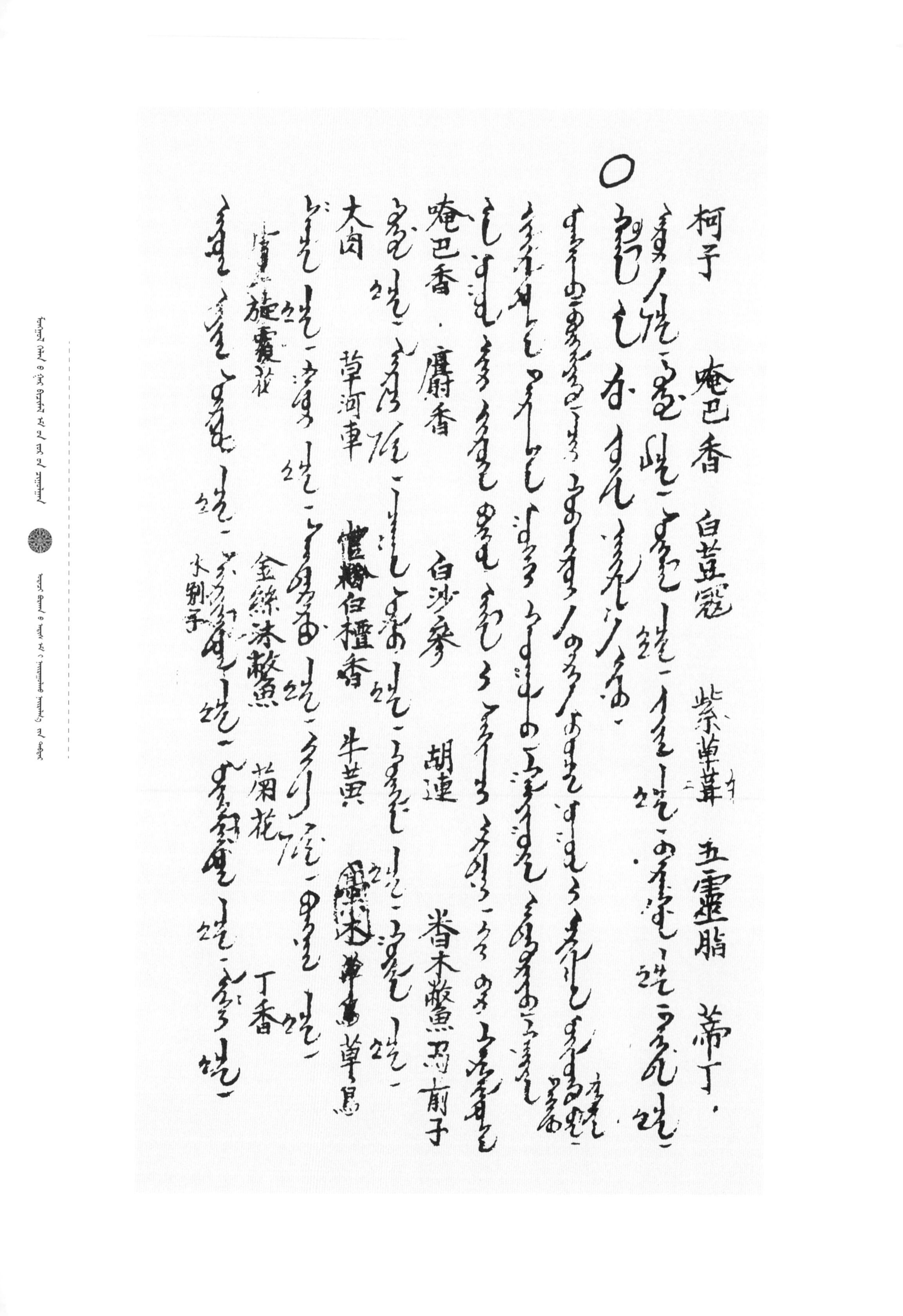

○

柯子 唵巴香 白荳蔻 紫草茸 五靈脂 蓽丁

唵巴香 · 麝香 白沙參 胡連 番木鱉 羽前子

大肉 草河車 白檀香 牛黄 木 草烏

旋覆花 金絲沐鱉魚 菊花 丁香

水別子

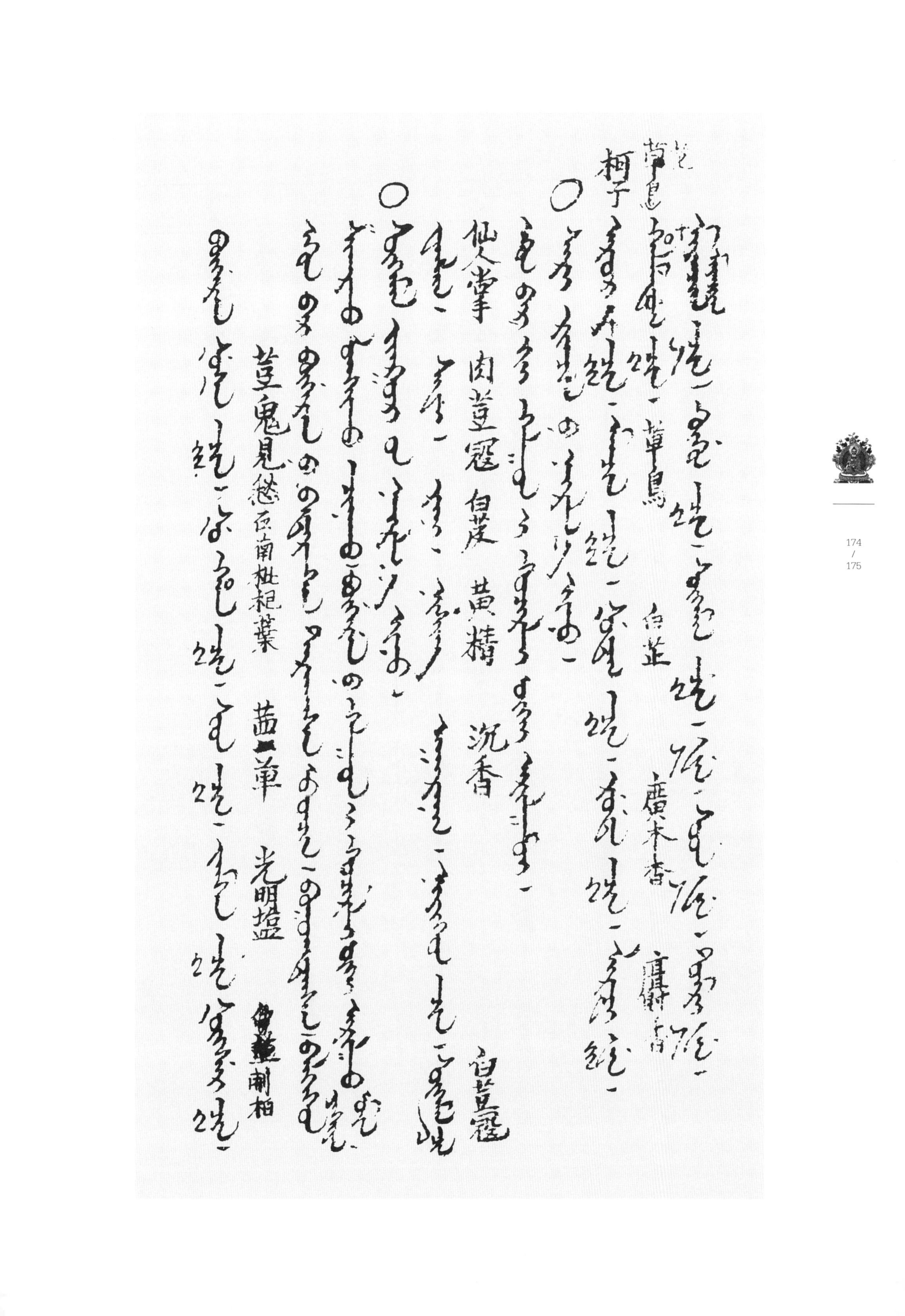

背鳥 柯子

草烏 白芷 廣木香 麝香

仙人掌 肉荳蔻 白茇 黃精 沉香 白荳蔻

荳蔻 鬼見愁 西南柑杞葉 茜草 光明鹽 刺柏

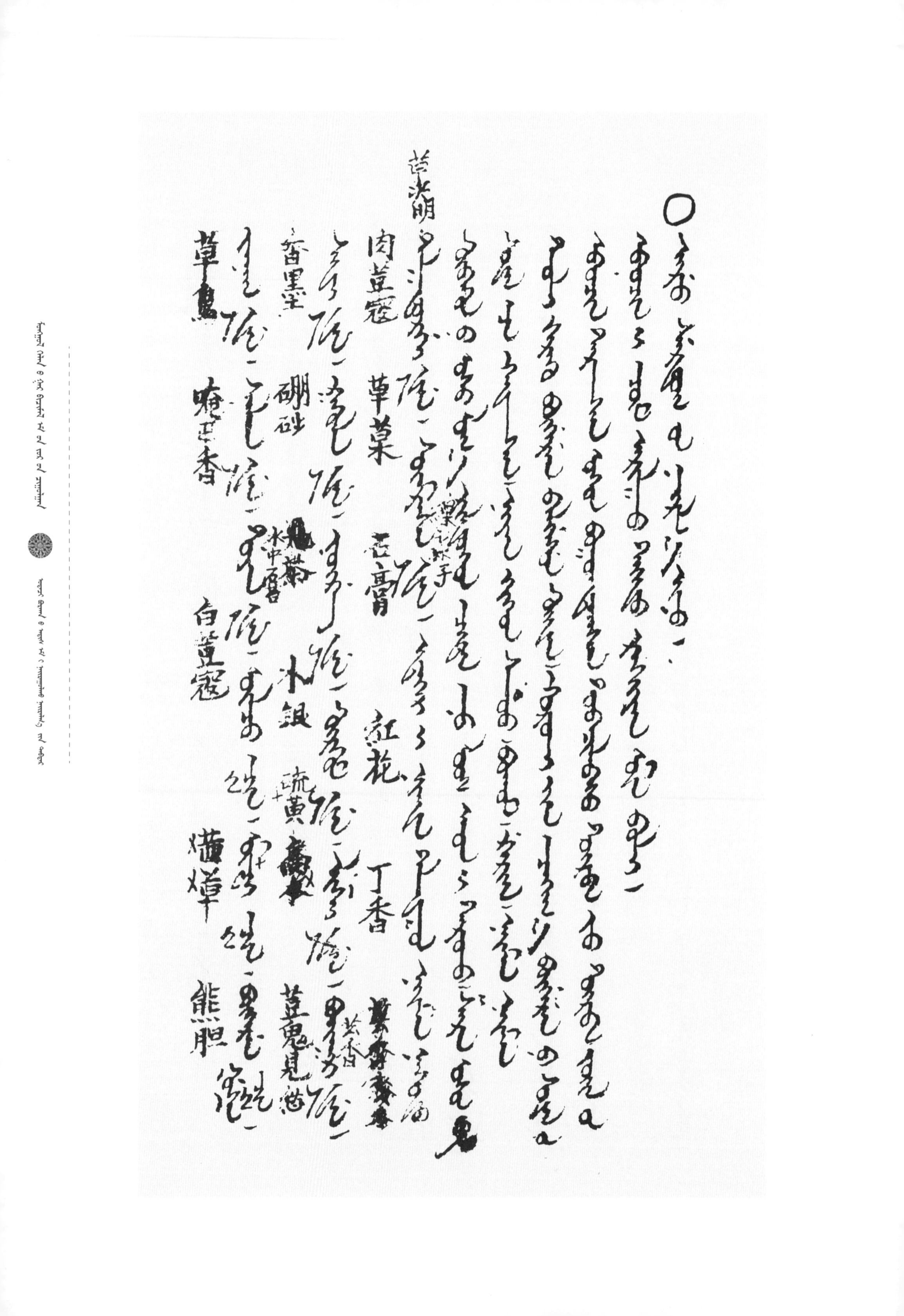

草烏 嚩芷香 白荳蔻 燈草 熊胆

香墨 硼砂 鬼臉 水中鹽 水銀 硫黃 蟾酥 荳蔻見湿

肉荳蔻 草菓 石膏 紅花 丁香 紫蘇 紫香白

荳蔻 决明 紫花杏子

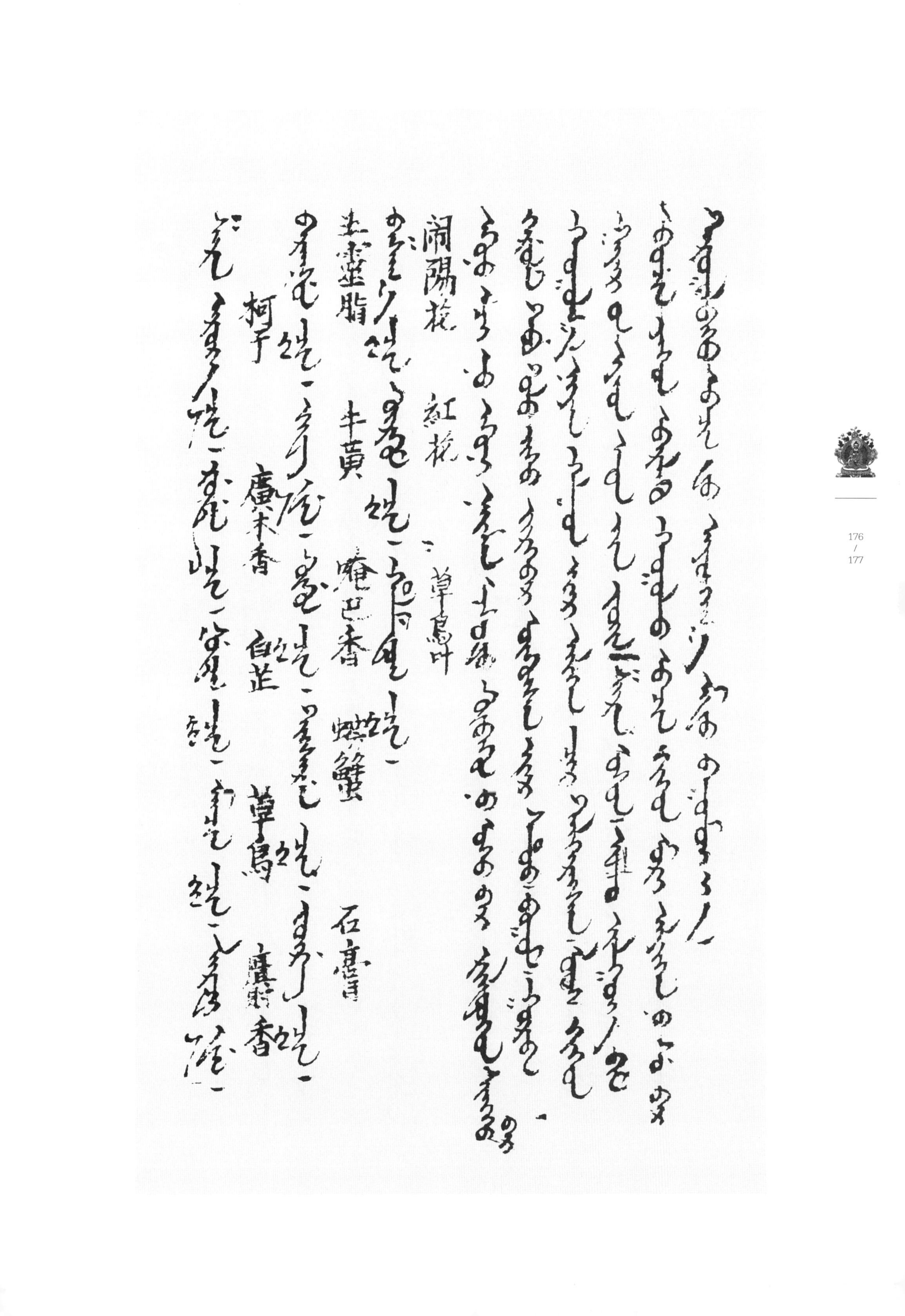

鬧陽花 紅花 草烏叶

土蜜脂 牛黄 唵巴香 螃蟹 石膏

柯子 廣木香 白芷 草烏 廣藿香

唵巴香 五味藥用 巴豆 麝香 硇

麥狼

蓽撥 廣木香

◯ 白芷 柯子 草烏

紅花 唵巴香 茴香

蘆薈指子 苦參 五靈脂 草烏 白芷 麝香

沙參 蒂決明 線蔴子 廣木香 柯子 川練子

◯

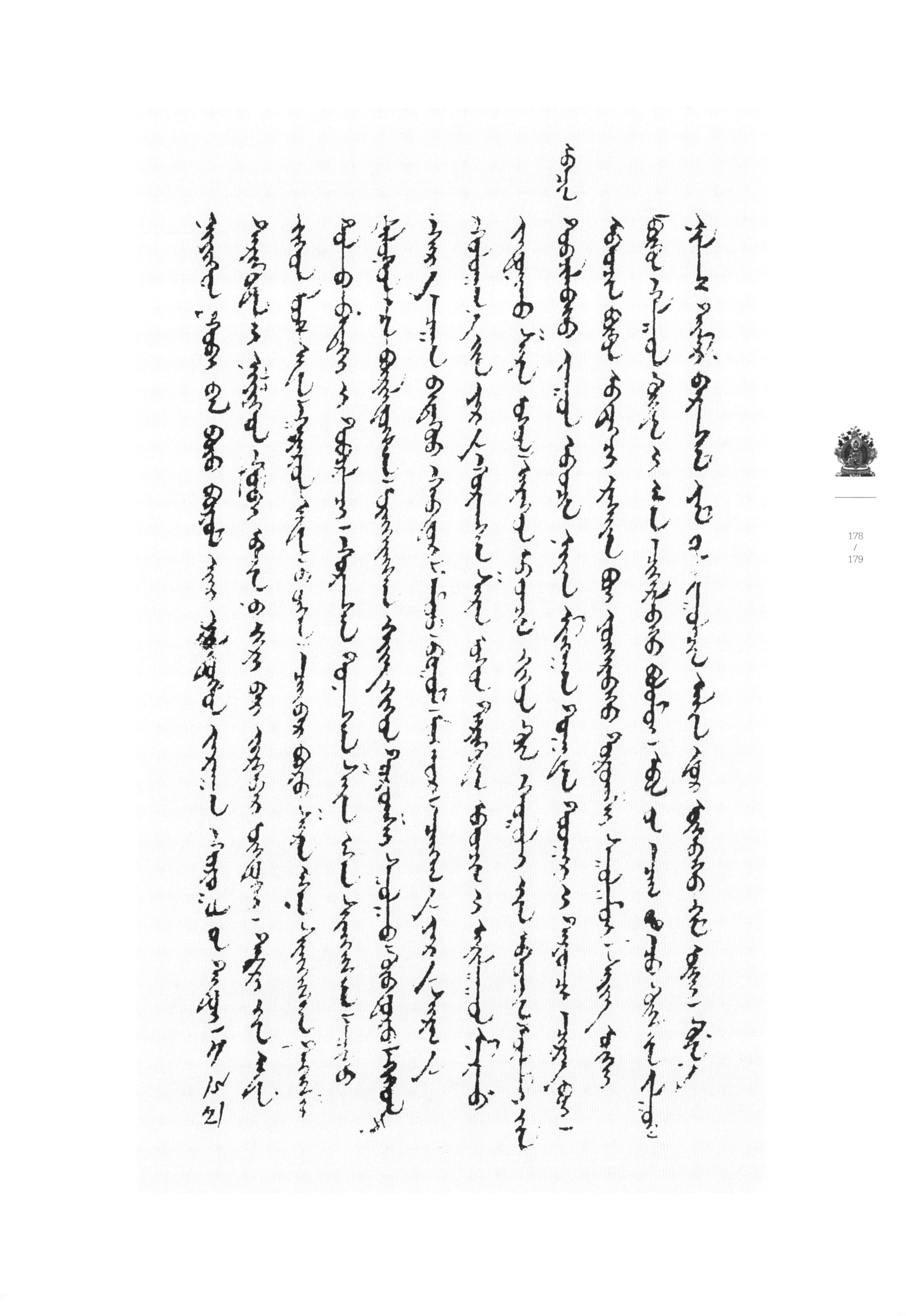

安硝 斷白草 丁香 沙參 川練子 附子 萆鬼見愁

大楓 柯子 蘆薈指子 黑礬 白礬 冰片

冬青叶 白芷霜 山柰

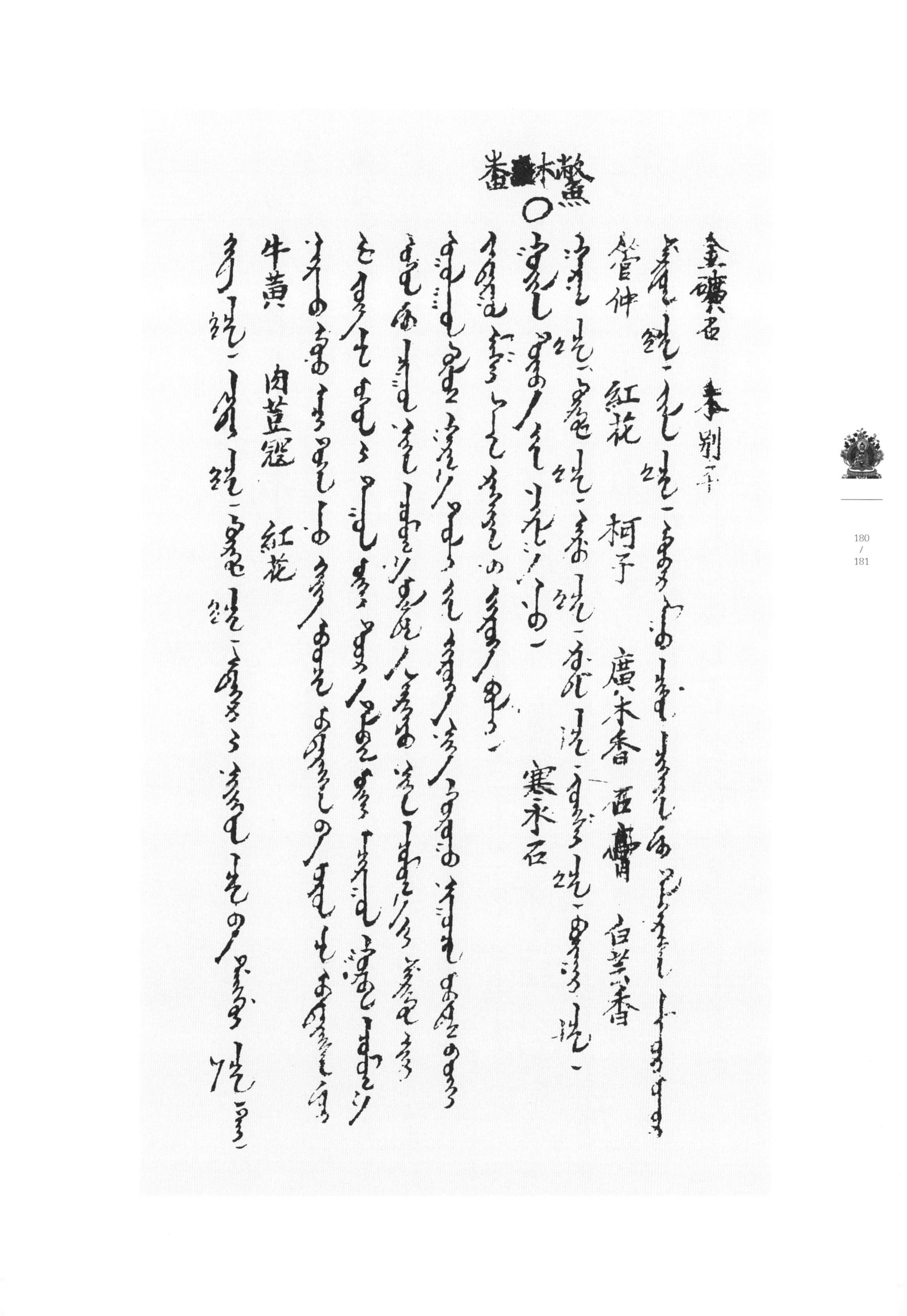

鱉木散

金礞石　李別一斗

管仲　紅花　柯子　廣木香　西[illegible]　白芷香

寒水石

牛黃　肉荳蔻　紅花

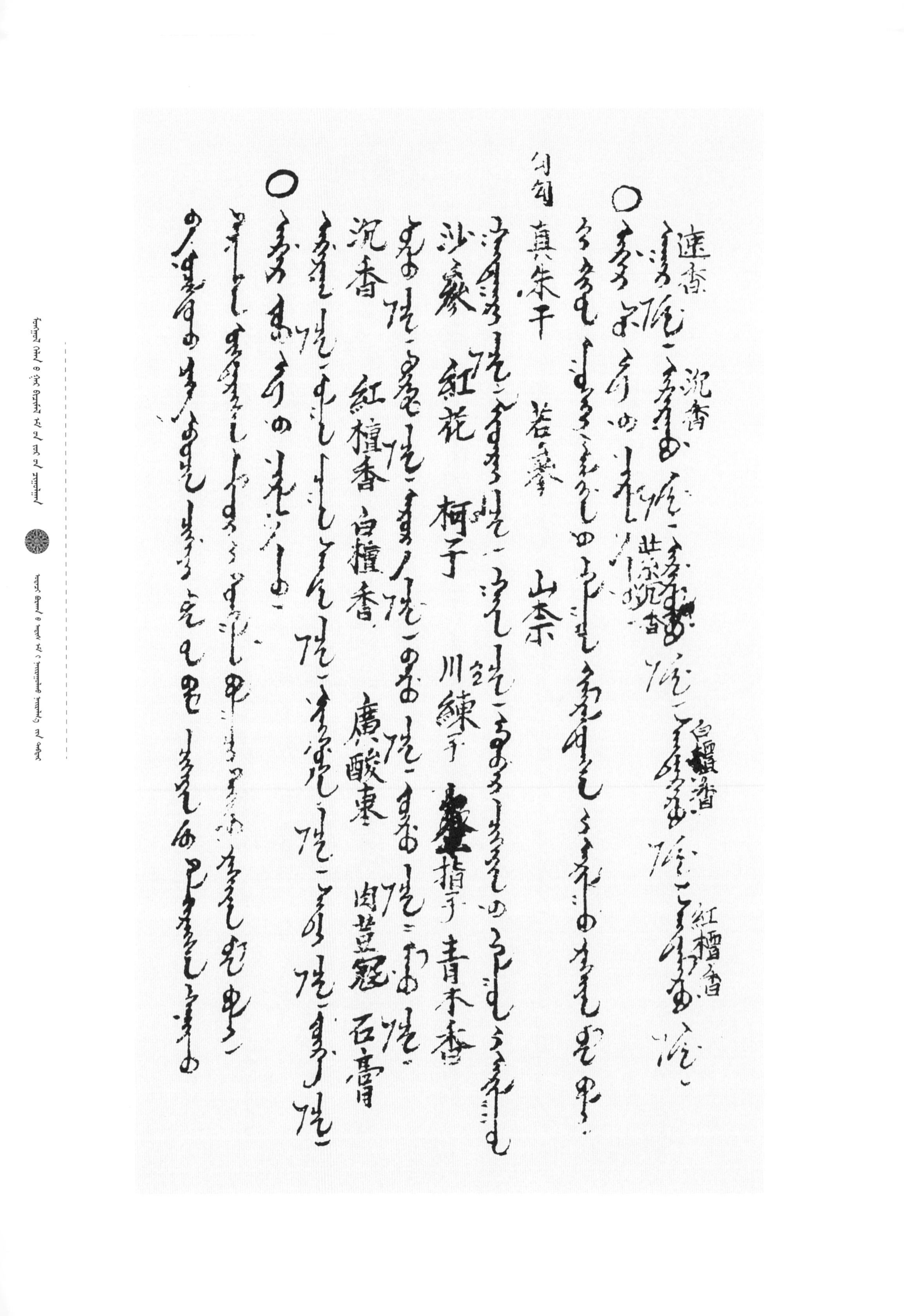

速香 沉香 紫沉香 白檀香 紅檀香

眞朱干 苍□ 山柰

沙參 紅花 柯子 川練子 □□指子 青木香

沉香 紅檀香 白檀香 廣酸棗 肉豆蔻 石膏

廣酸棗

石榴 青木香 劉发 勾勾一 若參 山柰

廣木香 白芸香 廣木香 沙參 金櫻子 番木鱉

闹陽花 蒂丁 草烏 萸肉 麝香 俺巴香

草菓 柯子 線子 指子 旋覆花 旋覆根 細辛

石膏 肉豆蔻 丁香 紅花 白豆蔻

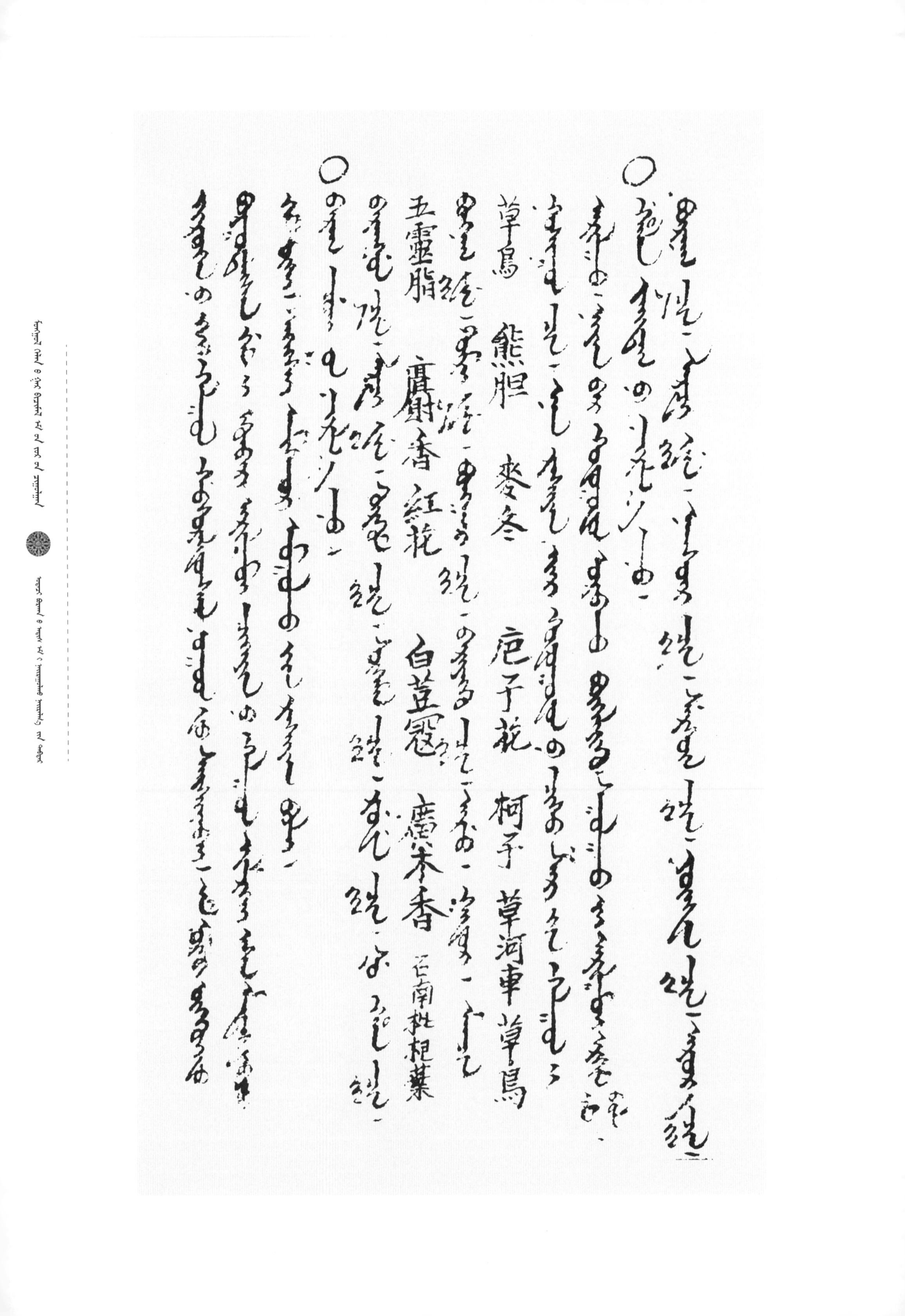

草烏 熊胆 麥冬 卮子花 柯子 草河車 草烏

五靈脂 廣麝香 紅花 白豆蔻 廣木香 江南枇杷葉

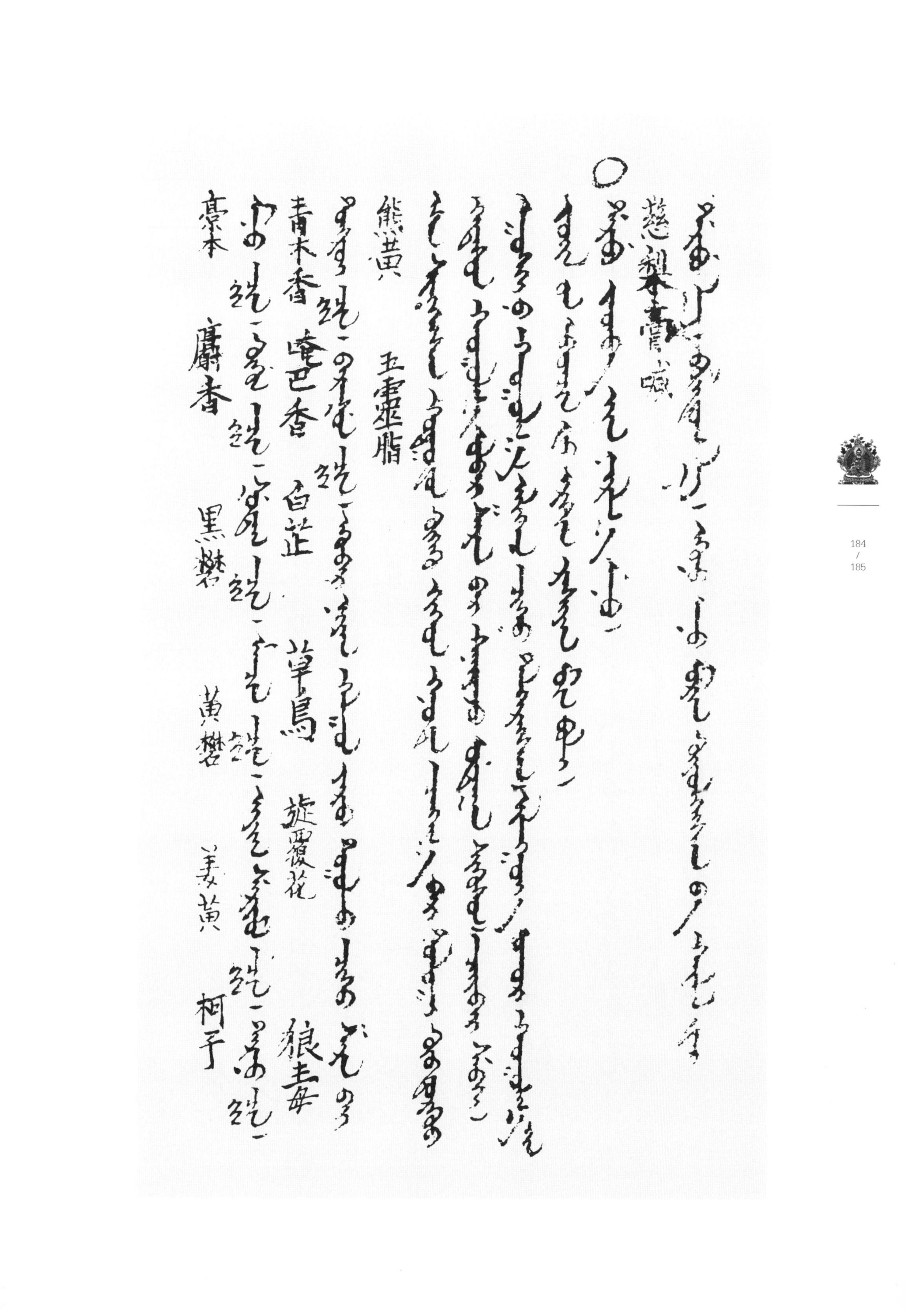

慈梨膏嗽

熊黄 五靈脂

青木香 唵巴香 白芷 草烏 旋覆花 狼毒

藁本 麝香 黑礬 黄礬 姜黄 柯子

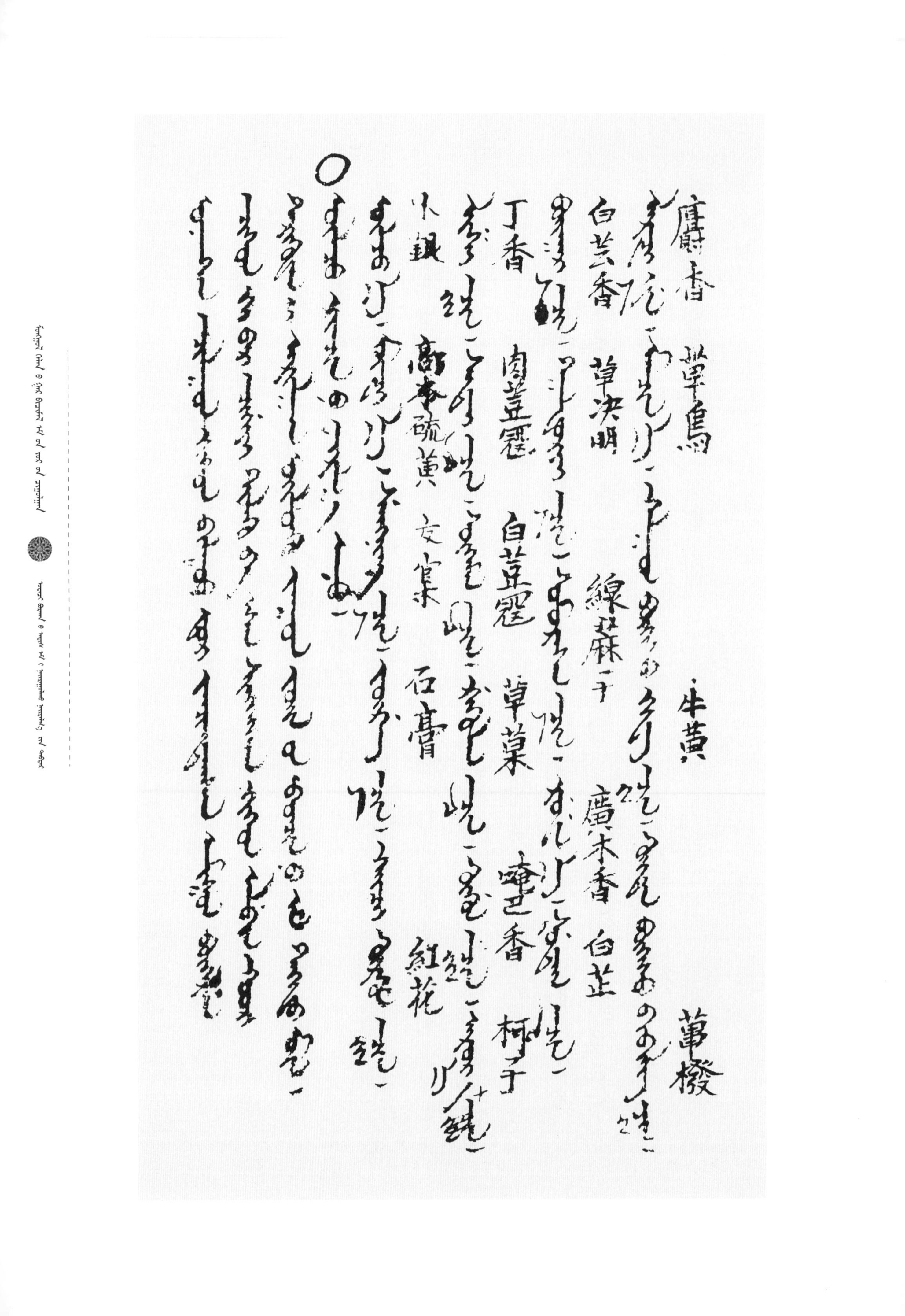

麝香 草烏 牛黄 蓽撥

白芸香 草决明 線麻子 廣木香 白芷

丁香 肉荳蔻 白荳蔻 草菓 嗱香 柯子

小鎖 高本 疏黄 安泉 石膏 紅花

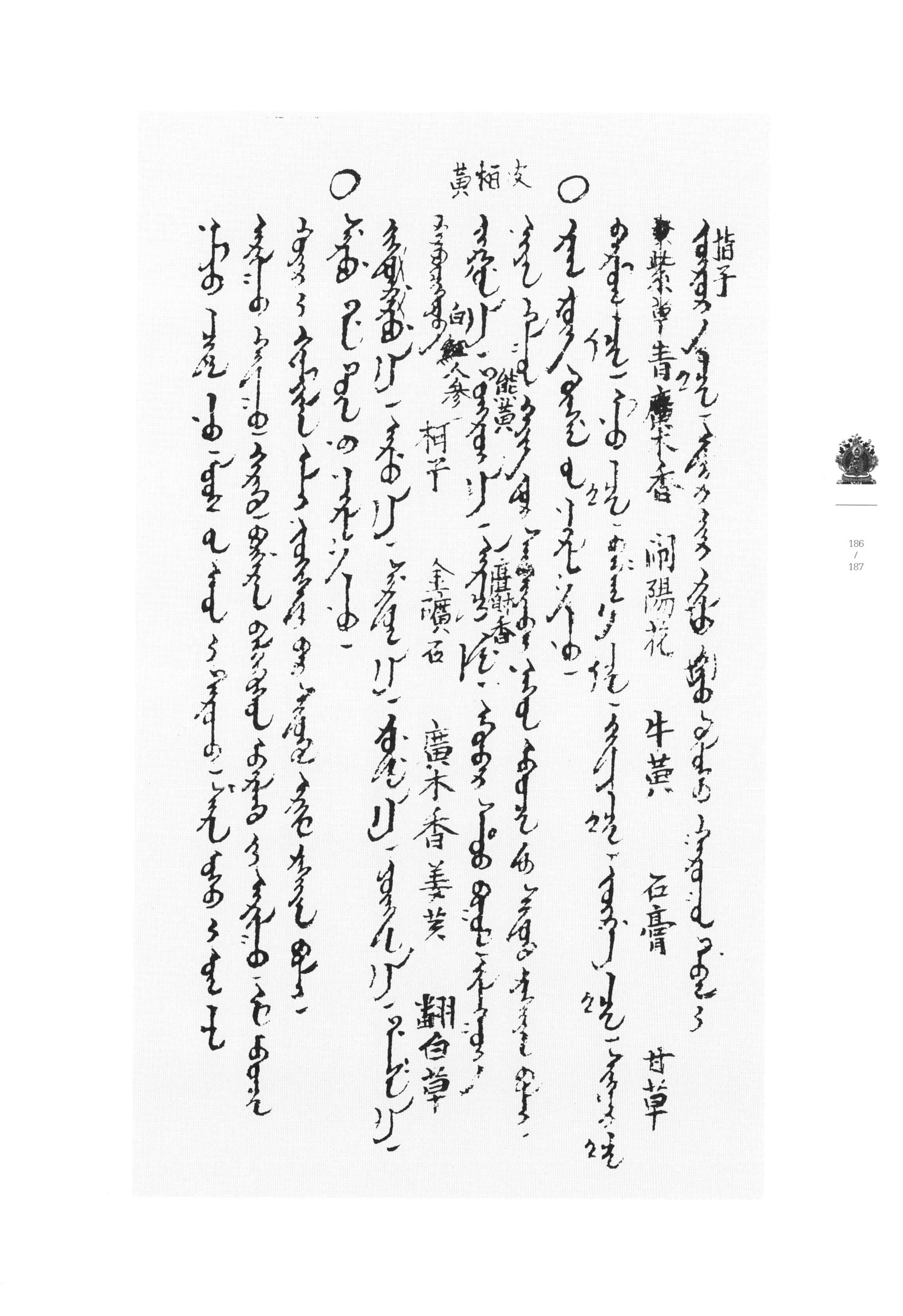

黄栢皮

指子 紫草 青黛 木香 朝陽花 牛黄 石膏 甘草

熊黄 麝香 白鮮 人参 栢子 金礦石 黄木香 姜黄 翻白草

白檀香 牛黃 石膏 紅花 五靈脂

麥冬 廣蔚香 乳香 翻白草 劉葱

草烏 槀木 狼毒

白/紅檀香　紅檀香　牛黄　訶子

金絲沐鱉（木鱉子）　訶子　白荳蔻　石膏

蜀葵子

草菓　丁香　紅花　肉荳蔻　赤石脂　麝香

蒂丁　雀爪　蓽撥　廣木香　[illegible]指子

麥冬　石榴　寒水石

訶子
紅花
廣木香
草烏
訶子
熊膽
紫草茸
乳香
廣木香
白芷
五靈脂
草烏
訶子

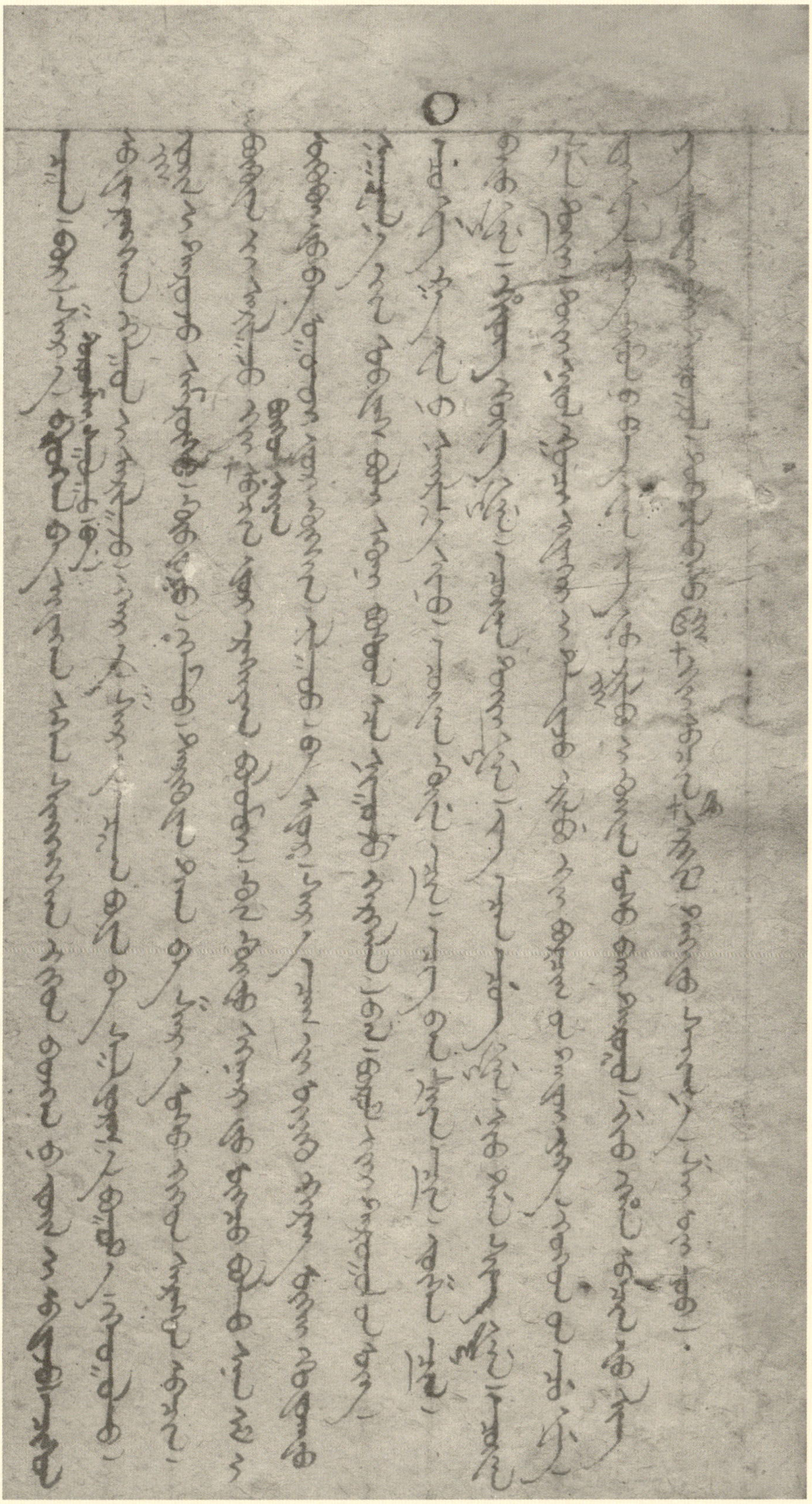

石榴
官桂
白荳蔻
大肉
麝香
冰片
青木香
石膏
丁香
白荳蔻
紅花
蟾酥
沉香
速香
牛黃
乳香
芸香
白檀香
紅檀香
硫黃
乳香
麝香
白芷
牛黃
銀朱
阿魏
訶子
墨

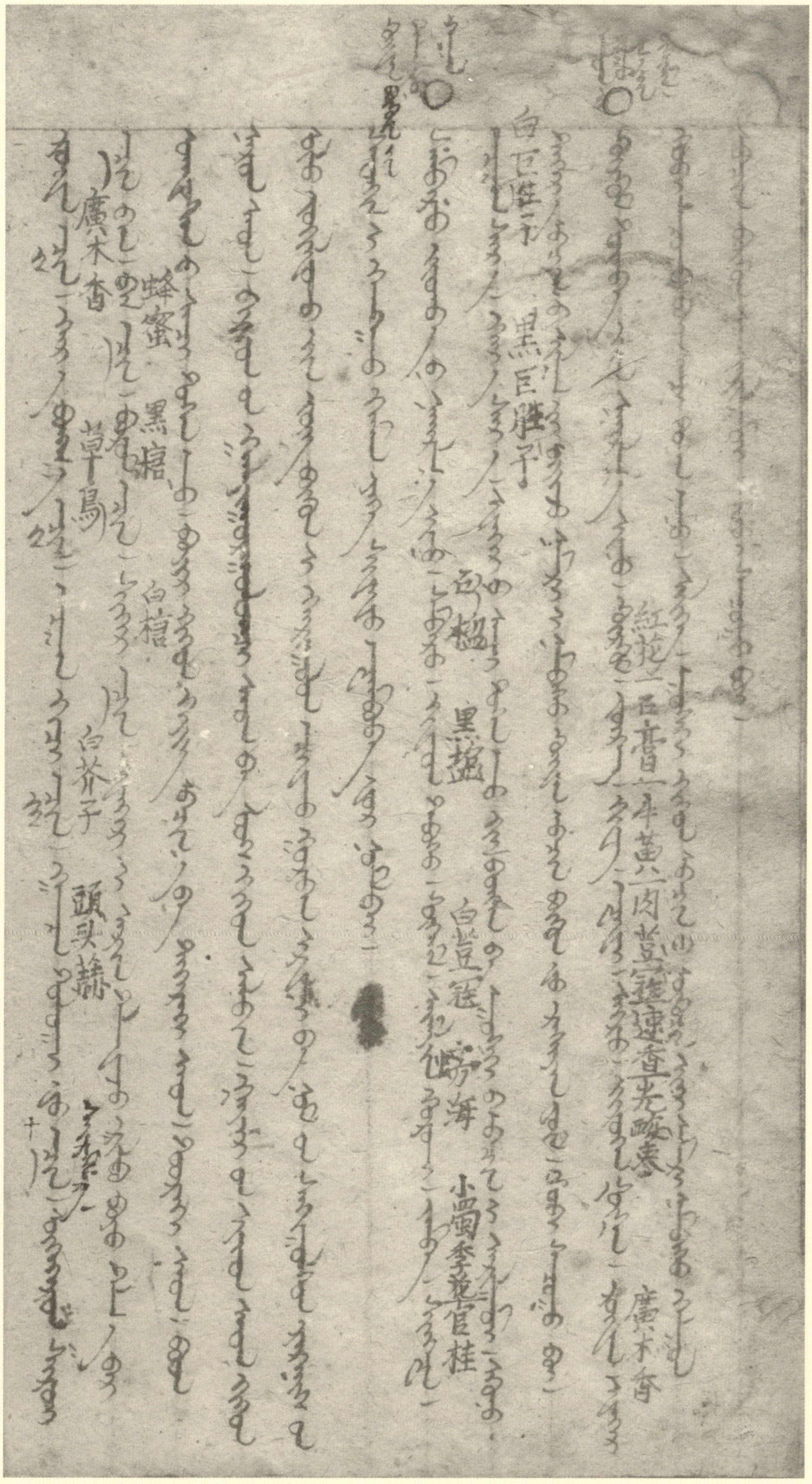
廣木香
黑巨胜子
官桂
蜂蜜
草烏
白芥子

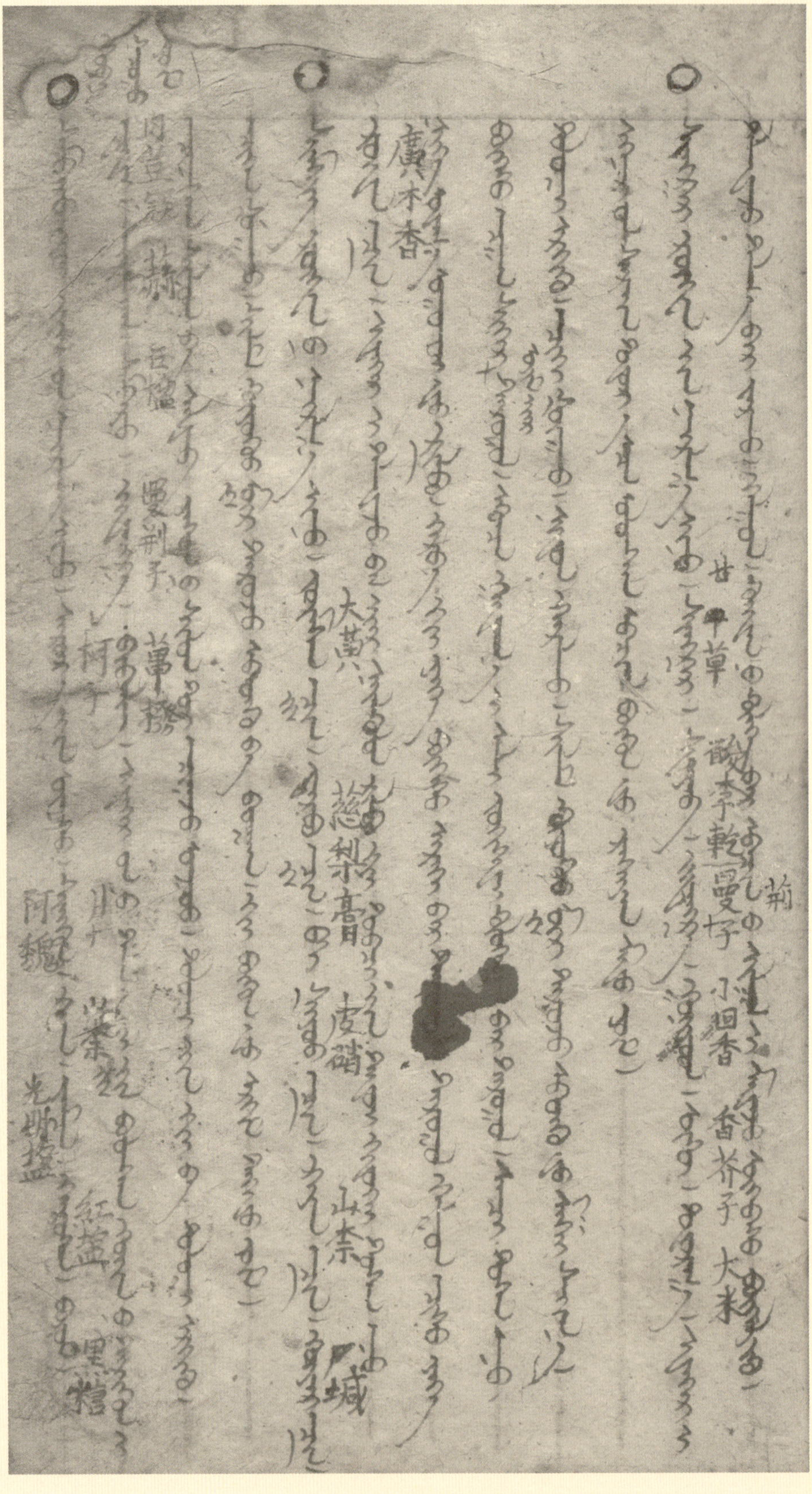

小茴香
香芥子
大米
廣木香
大黃
皮硝
山柰
紅鹽
黑鹽
光明鹽

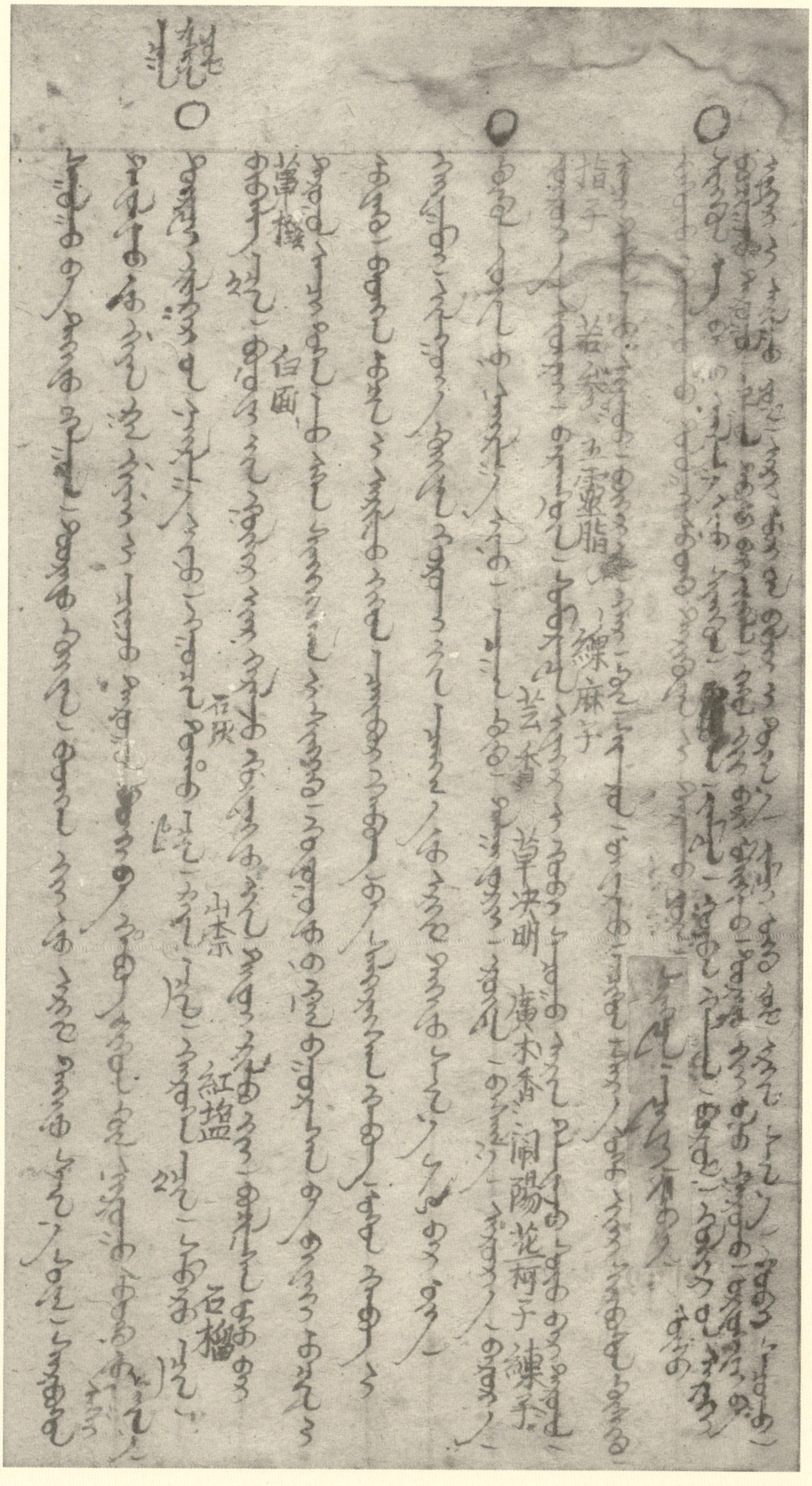
指子
苦參
五靈脂
練麻子
芸香
草決明
廣木香
鬧陽花
訶子
練子
蓽撥
白面
石灰
山柰
紅鹽
石榴

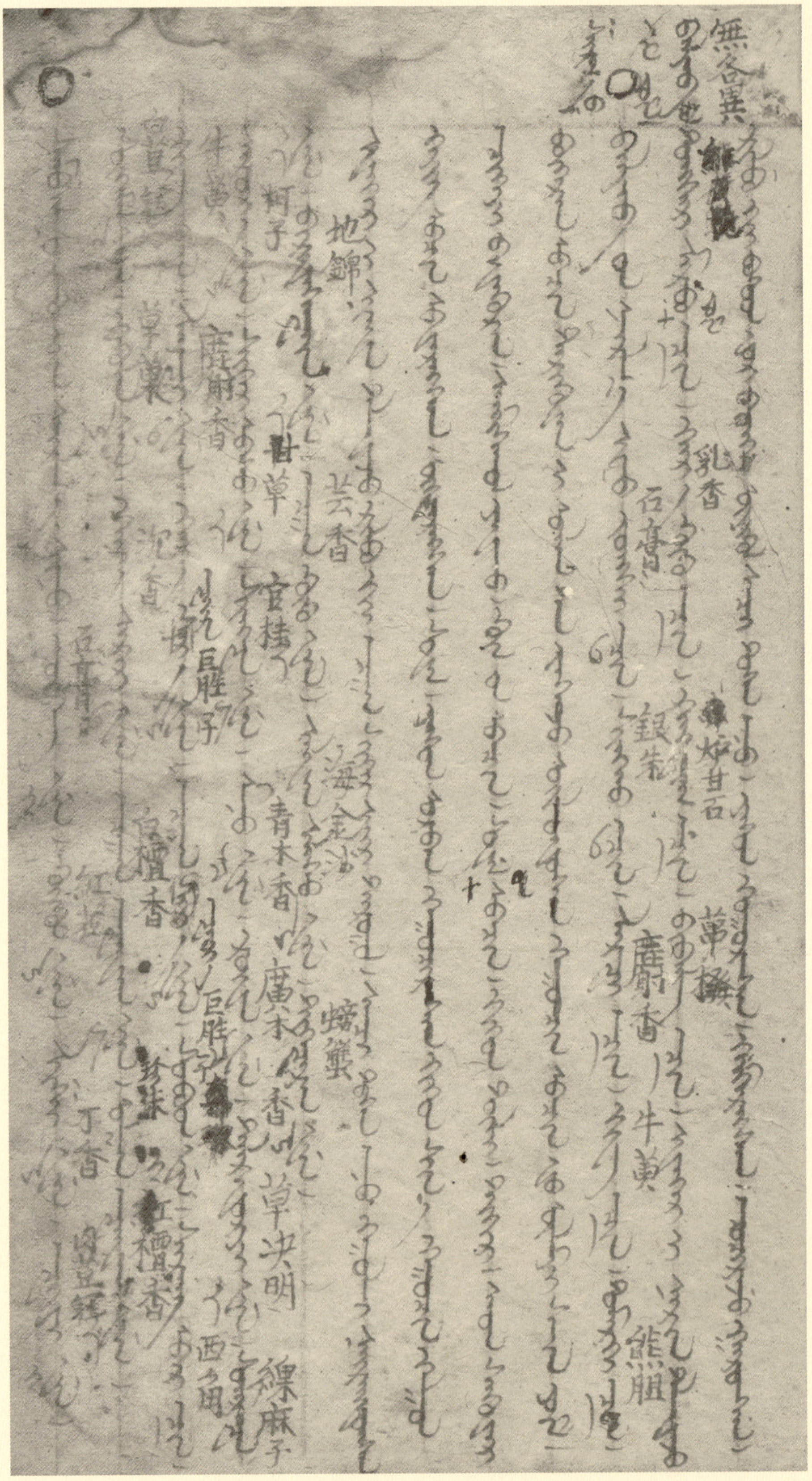

無名異
乳香
石膏
爐甘石
銀朱
麝香
牛黄
熊膽
地錦
芸香
海金沙
螃蟹
訶子
甘草
官桂
青木香
廣木香
草決明
巨勝子
沉香
白檀香
紅檀香
紅花
丁香

大黄　柯子　牛膝　紫桒膏　蟹肉　山柰　城　柯子　寒水石　硇砂　麝香　海金沙　螃蟹　小蜀李　香芥子

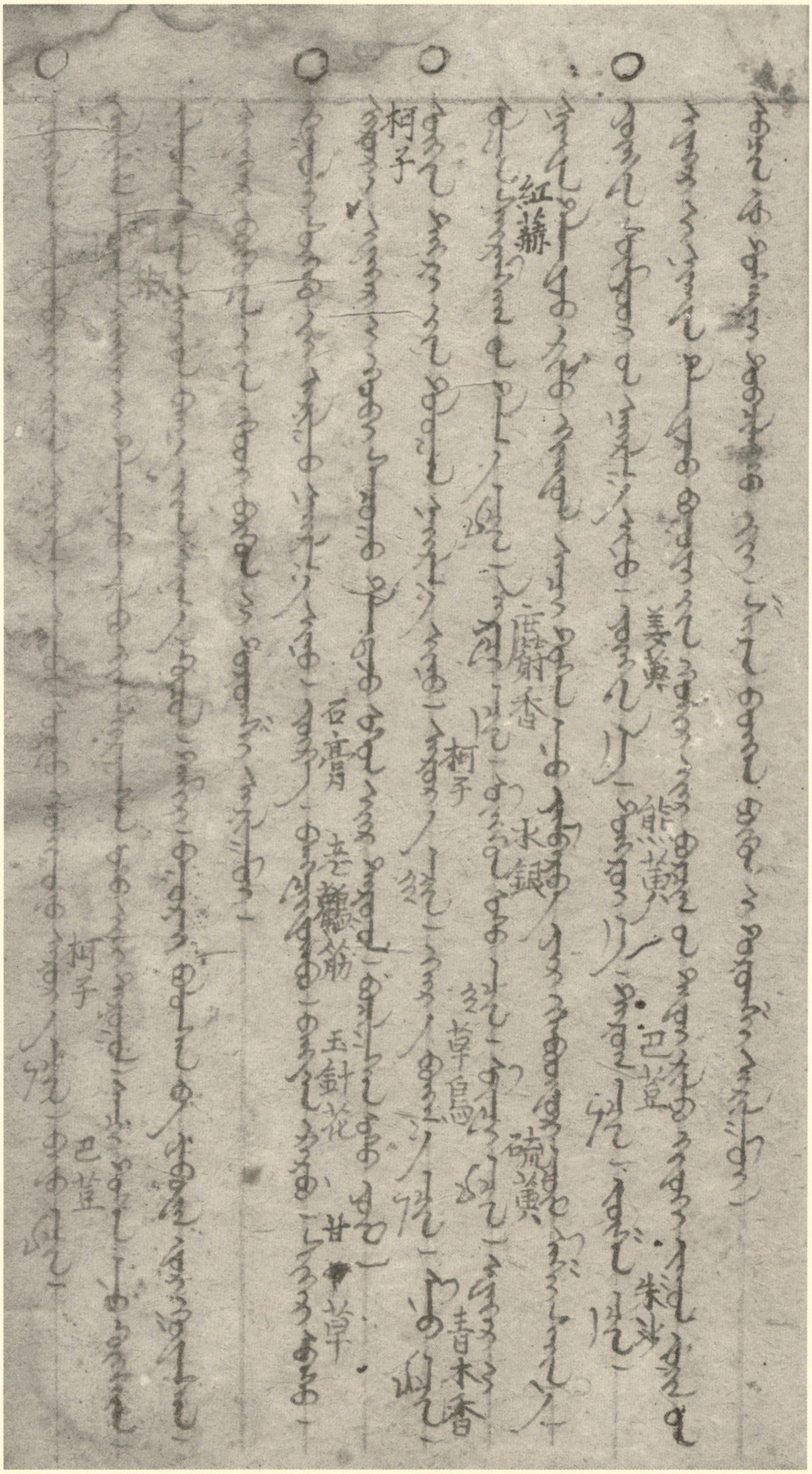
柯子
巴荳
椒
石膏
老鸛筋
玉針花
甘草
柯子
柯子
草烏
青木香
紅藤
麝香
水銀
硫黃
姜黃
熊黃
巴荳
朱砂

商陸

菴巴香

可瓜

水銀

硫黃

白檀香叶

丁香

白芨

蓯蓉

花芬

薫精

龍骨

青木香

勾勾

苦參

山奈

木別子

棘梅花

柯子

帝丁

京芝

川烏

番瓜

木通

帝丁

蔓荊子

射干

阿魏 青木香 廣木香 訶子 牙皂

冬青叶 官桂 白荳蔻 草菓 巨胜子 胡椒 蓽撥

甘草

珊瑚子 石綠 丁香 肉荳蔻 沉香 太一禹粮 磁鉄石

珍珠 訶子 草烏 白芷 廣木香

麝香

97

黄連 胡 花 線麻子

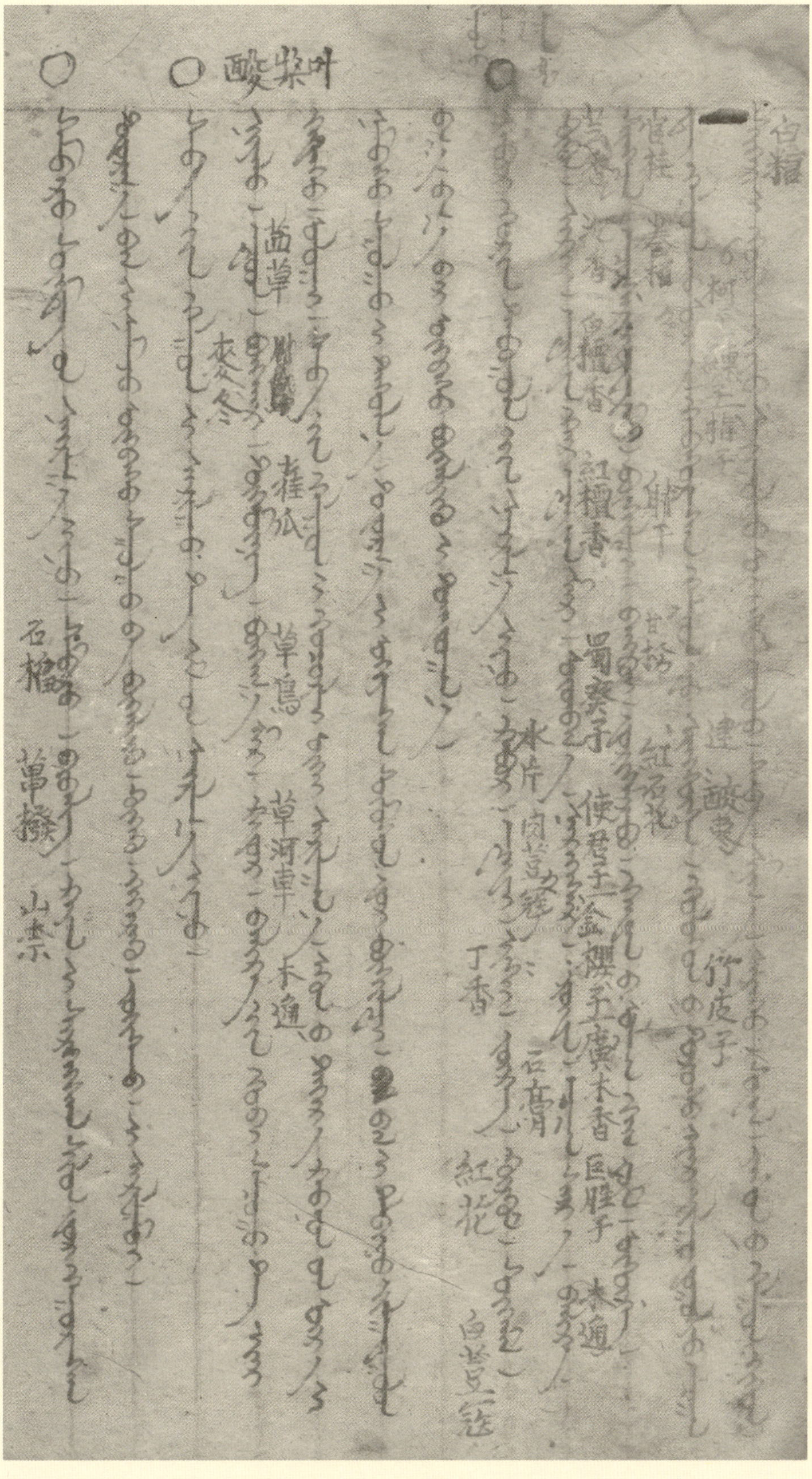
竹皮子
使君子
廣木香
蜀葵子
丁香
紅花
石膏
草河車
木通
山柰

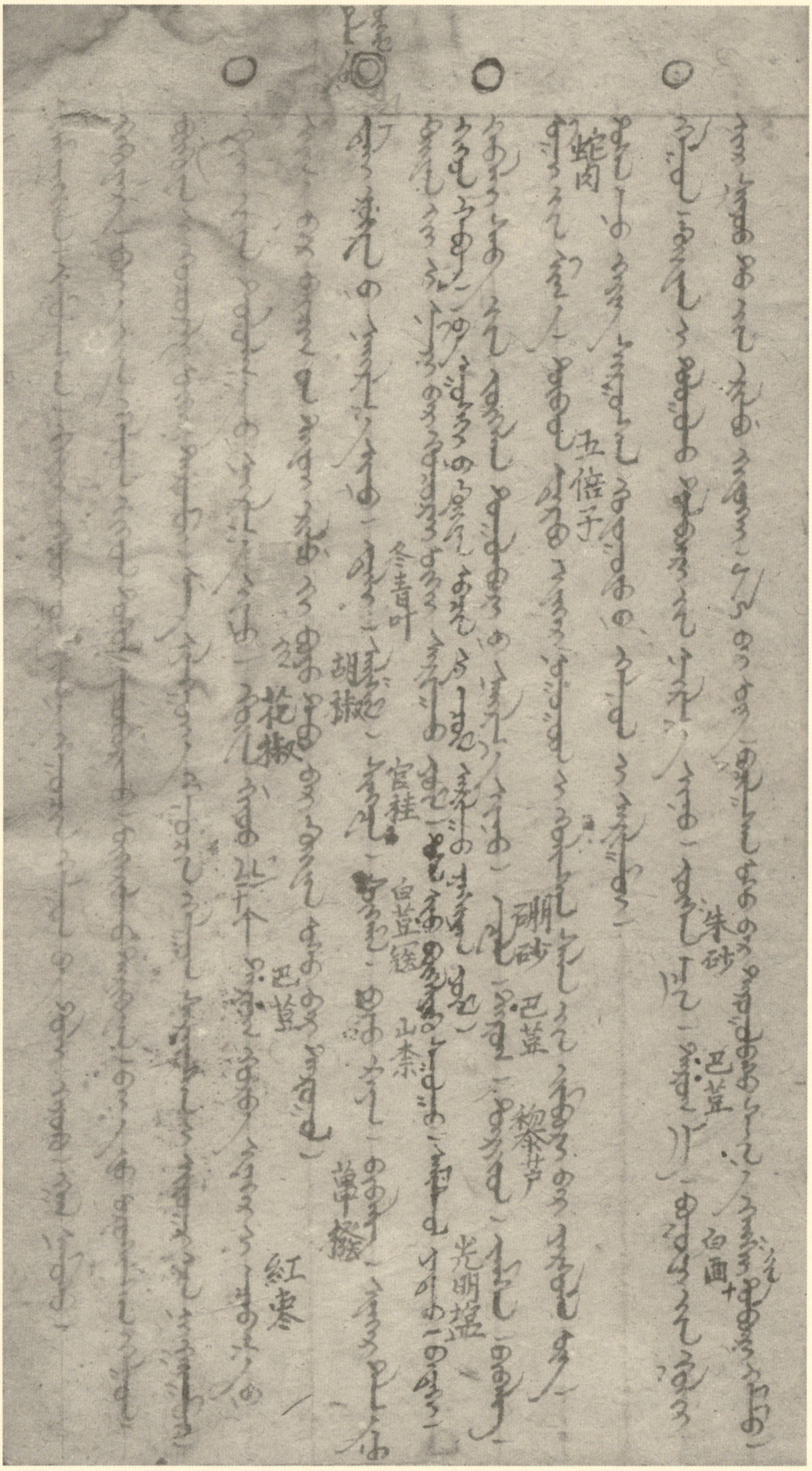
朱砂
巴豆
白面
蛇肉
五倍子
硼砂
巴豆
黎芦
冬青叶
胡椒
官桂
白豆蔻
山柰
光明塩
蓽撥
花椒
巴豆
紅棗

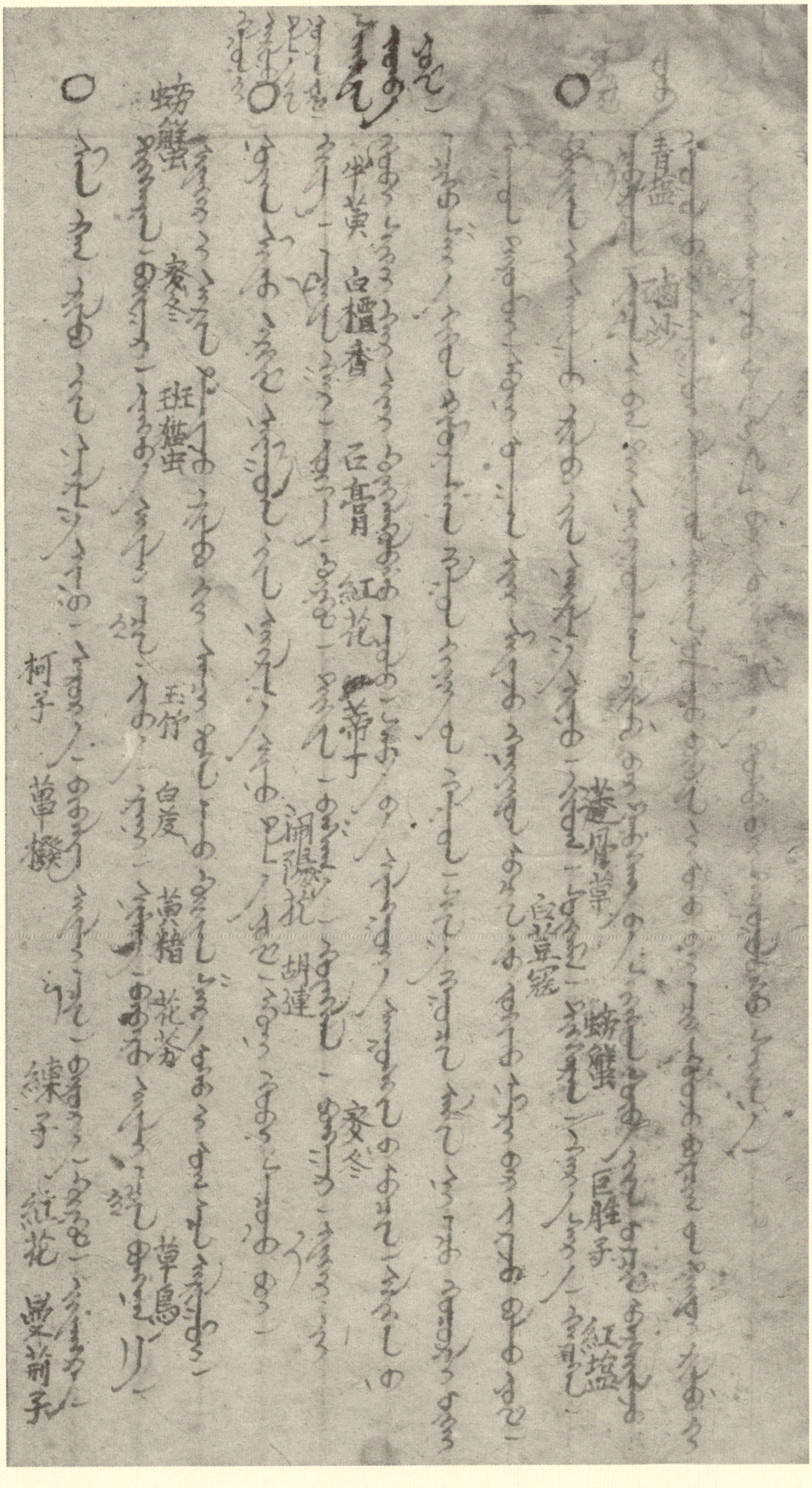
青塩
硇砂
螃蟹
紅塩
牛黄
白檀香
紅花
麥冬
螃蟹
斑蝥
麥冬
玉竹
草烏
柯子
楝子
紅花
蔓荊子

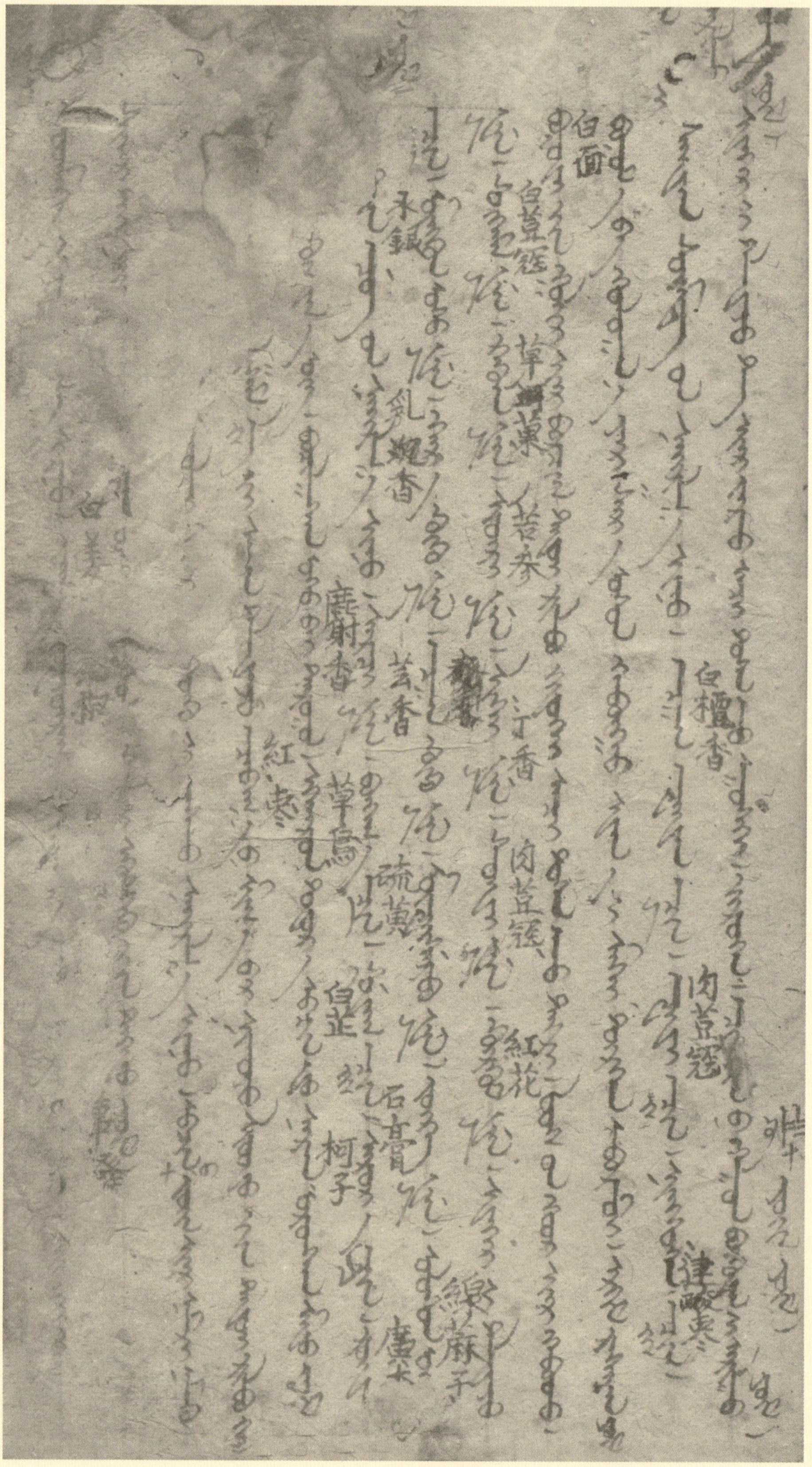

白檀香 肉苁蓉 白面 白豆蔻 草果 苦参 丁香 肉苁蓉 紅花 線麻子 水銀 乳香 芸香 麝香 草烏 白芷 石膏 訶子 紅棗 白姜

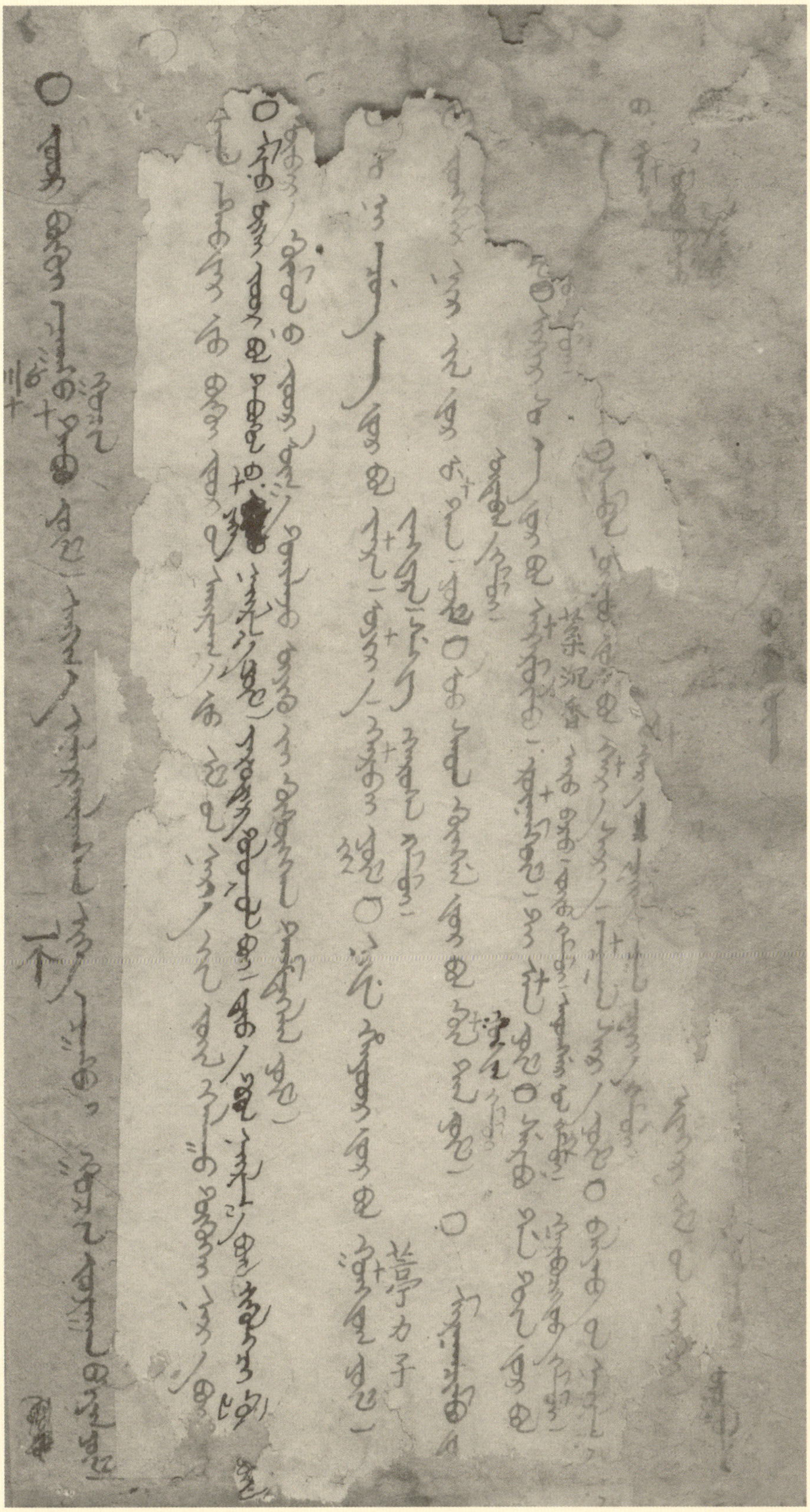

[illegible] ::
[illegible]
[illegible]
[illegible] ([illegible]) [illegible] :: ᠡᠨᠡ ᠨᠣᠮ
ᠤᠨ ᠬᠡᠮᠵᠢᠶ᠎ᠡ ᠨᠢ : 26.5cm × 14cm ᠪᠣᠯᠤᠨ᠎ᠠ᠂ ᠨᠡᠢᠲᠡ 28 ᠨᠢᠭᠤᠷ ᠲᠠᠢ ::
[illegible] ::

5

治疗天花秘诀方法

Secret Cures for Smallpox

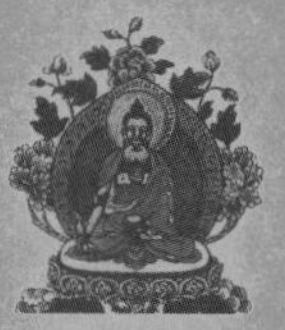

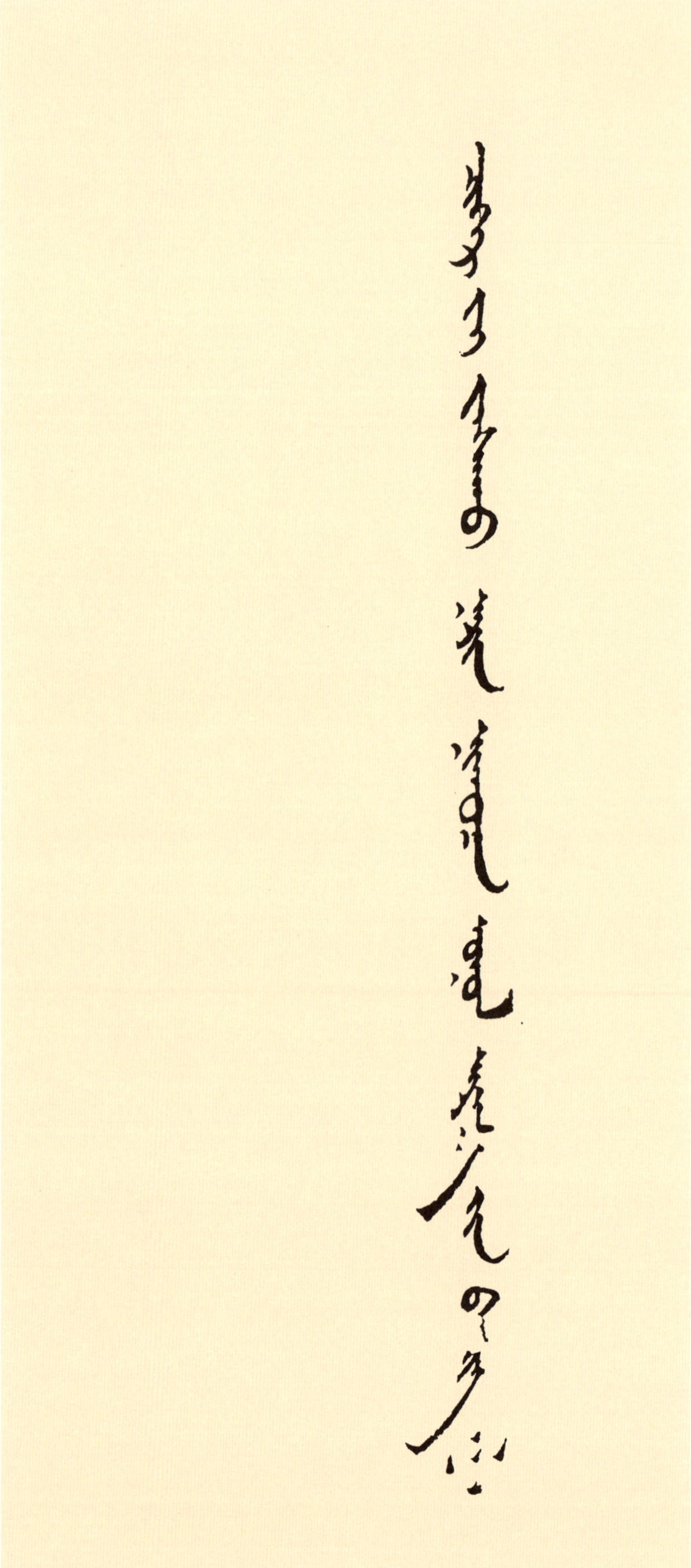

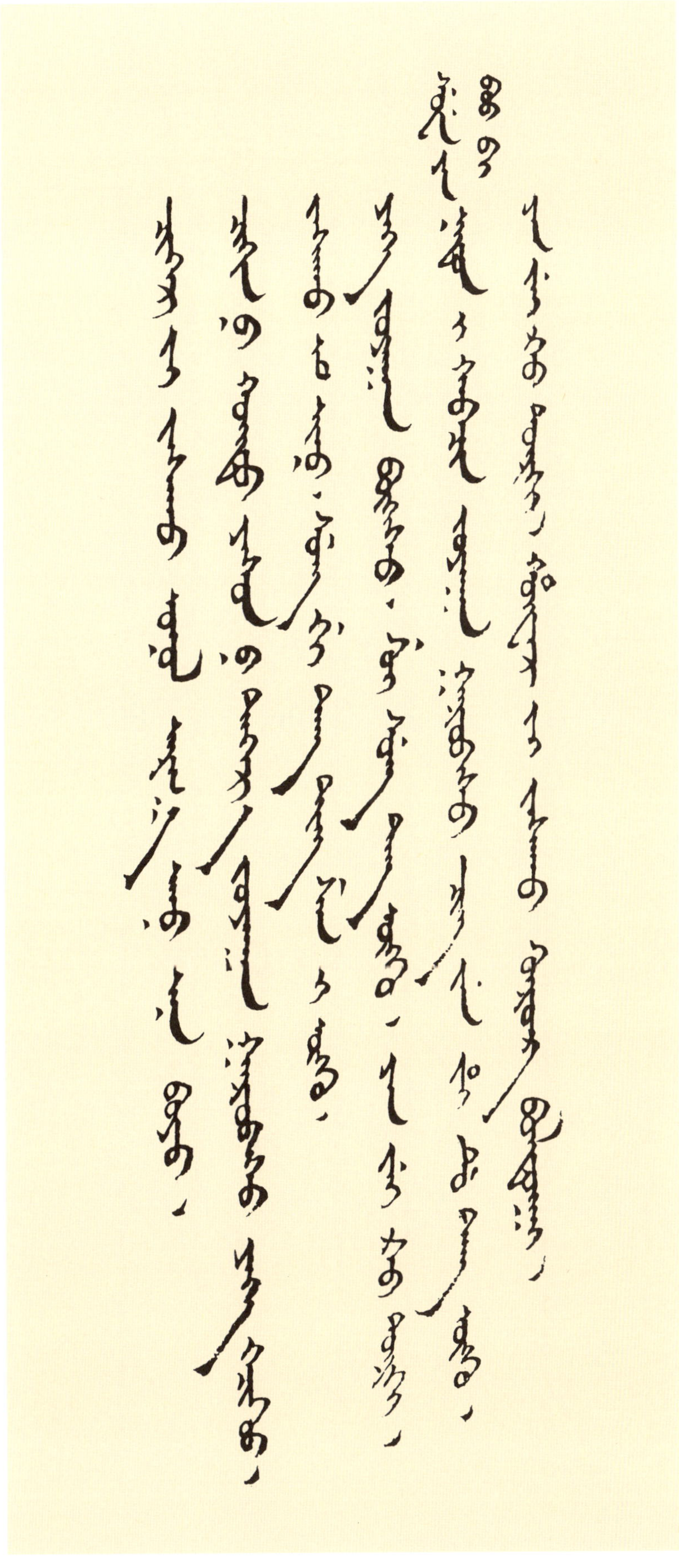

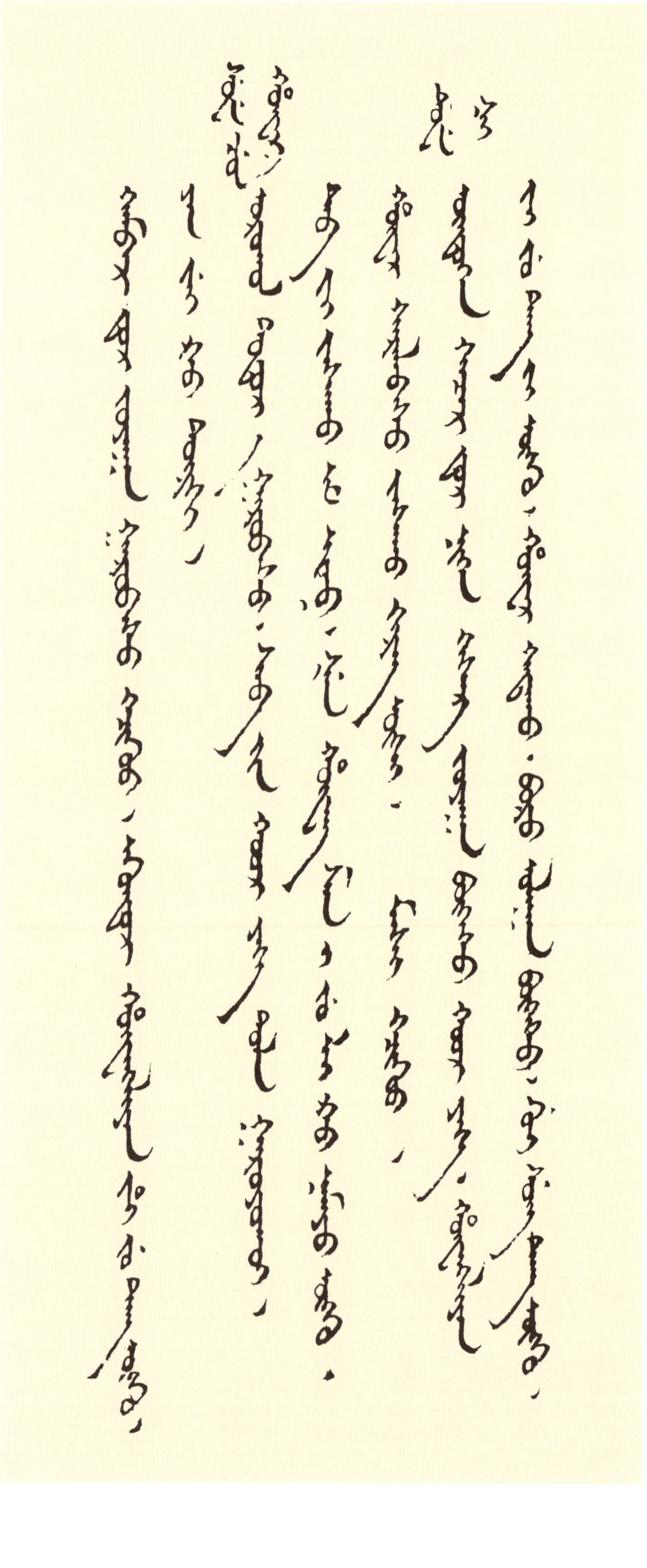

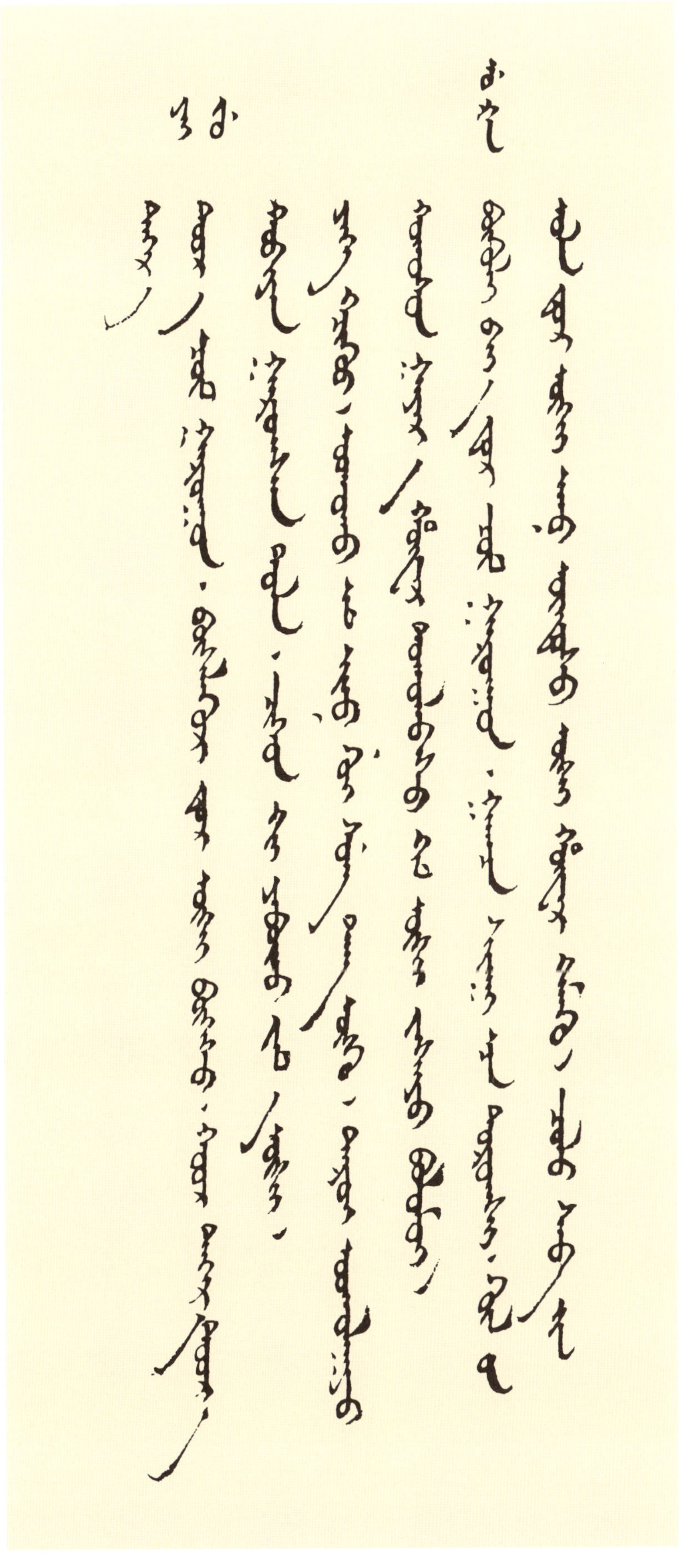

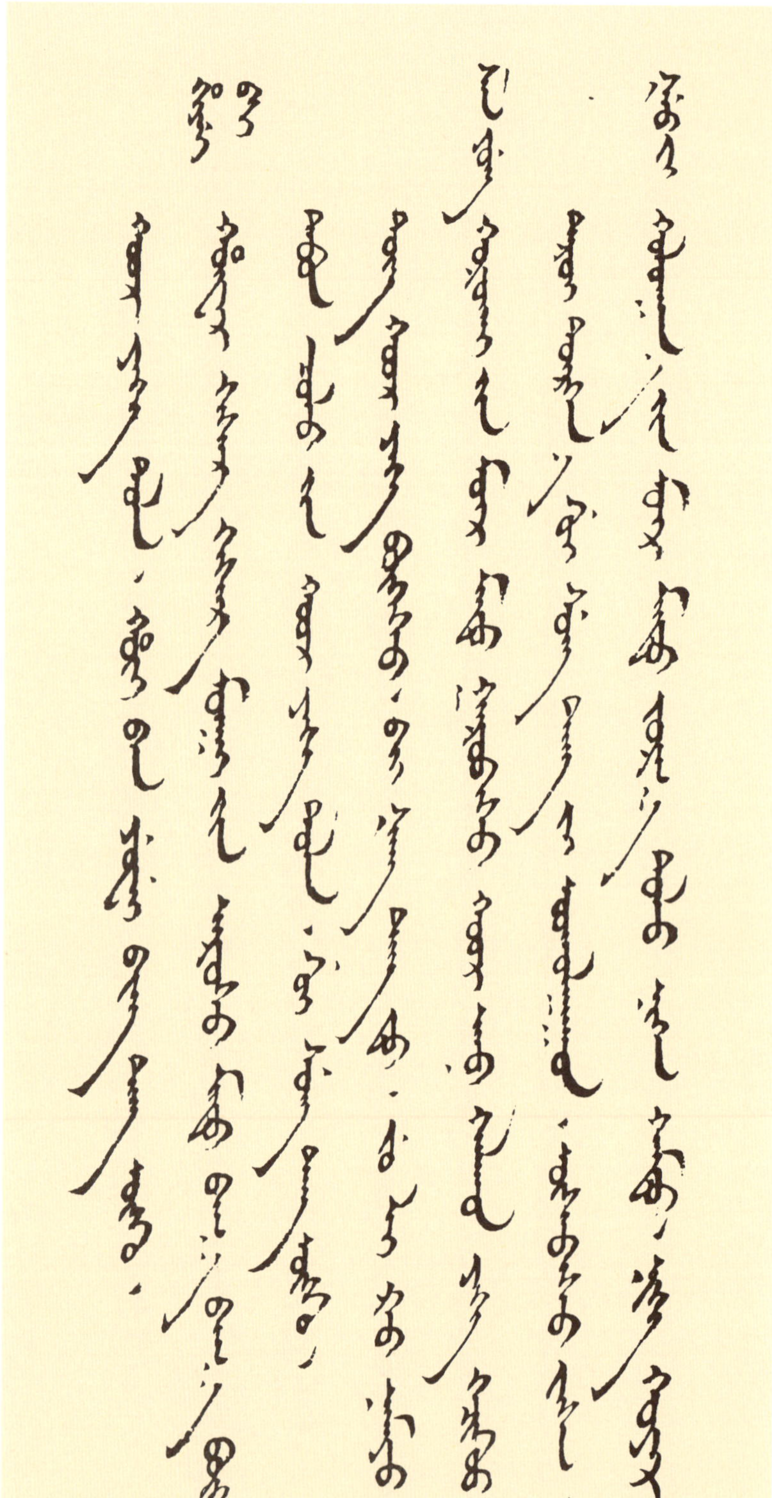

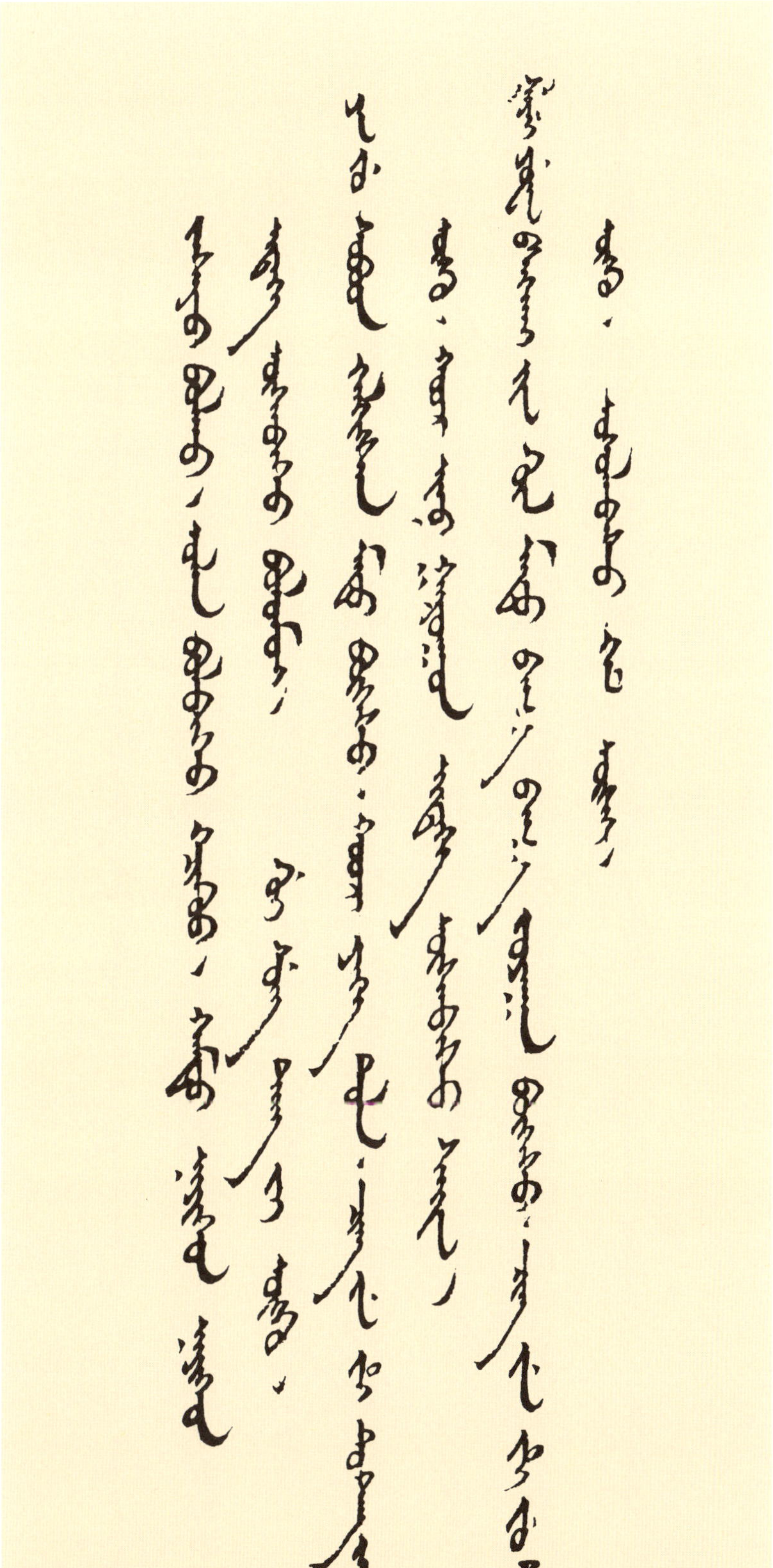

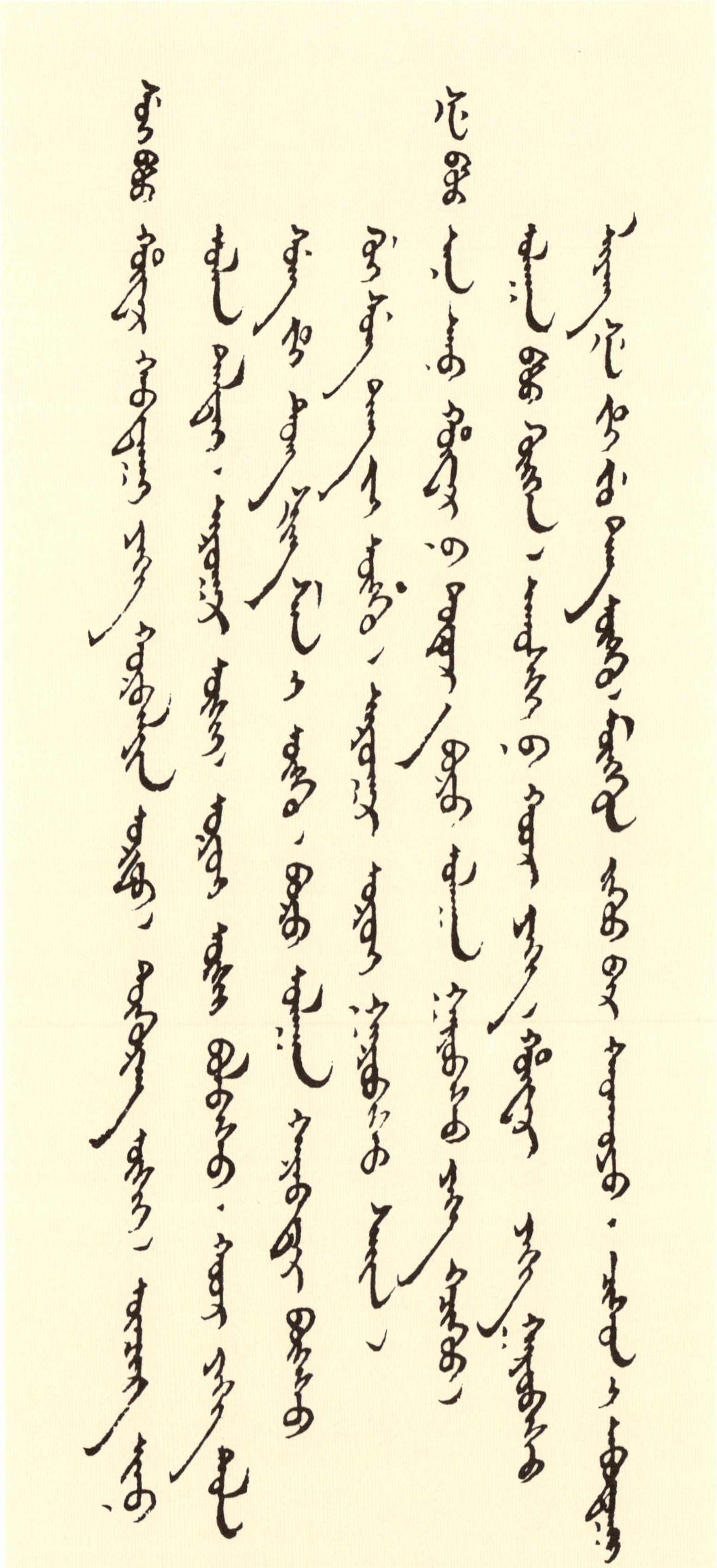

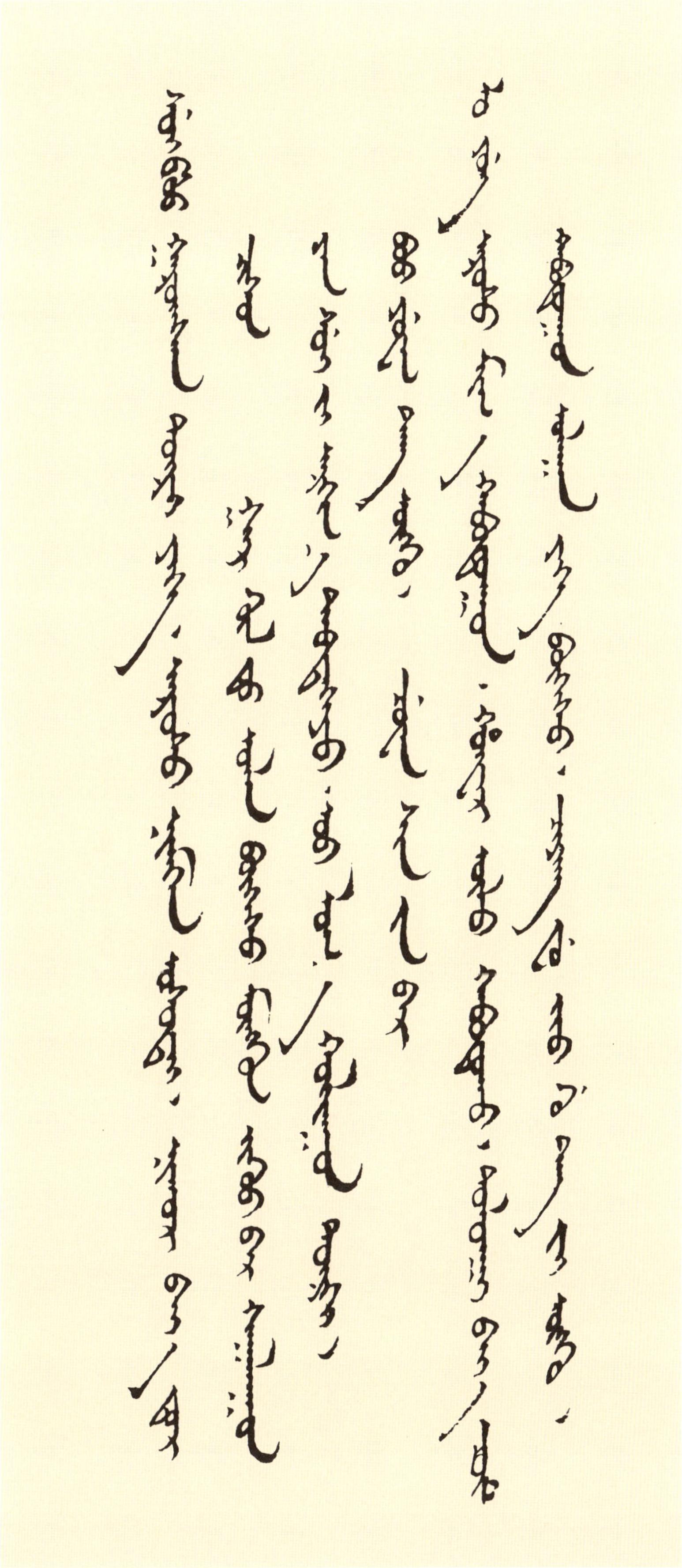

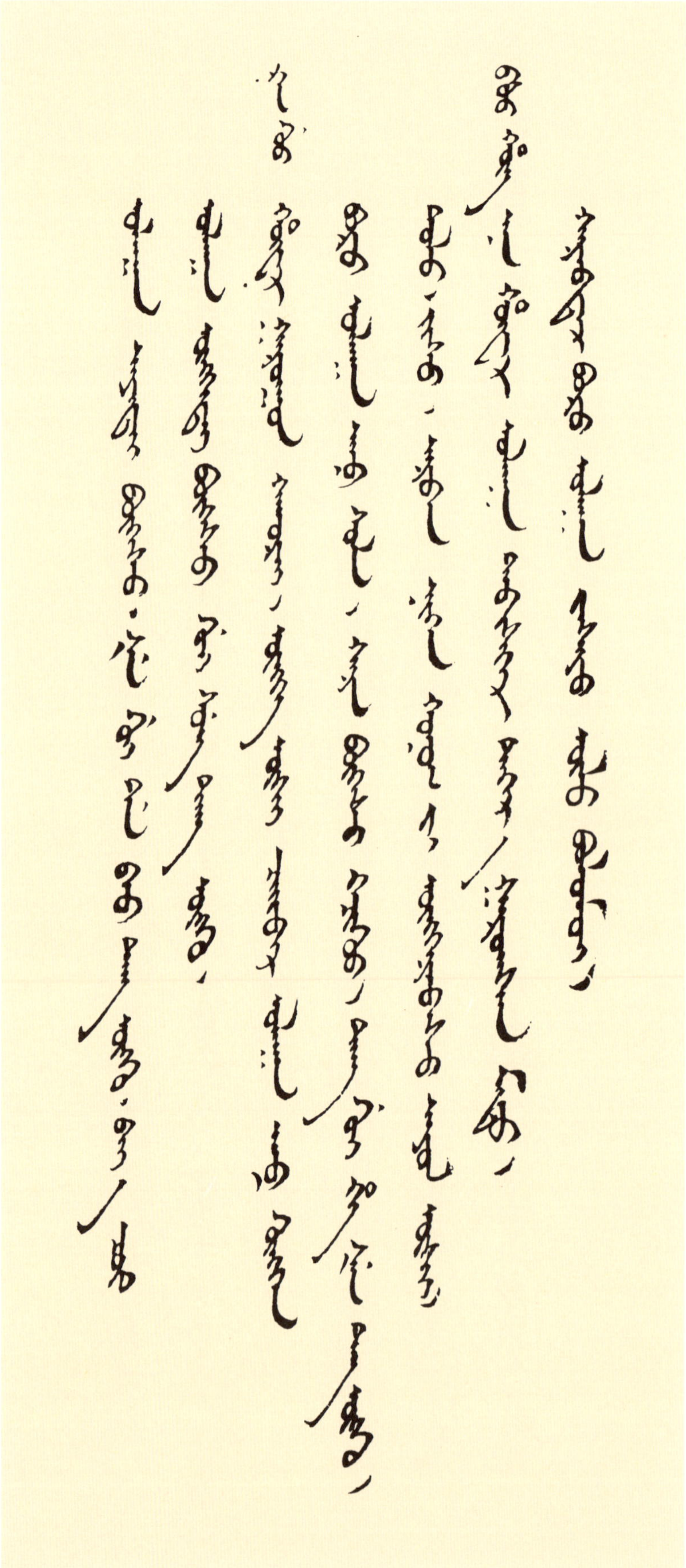

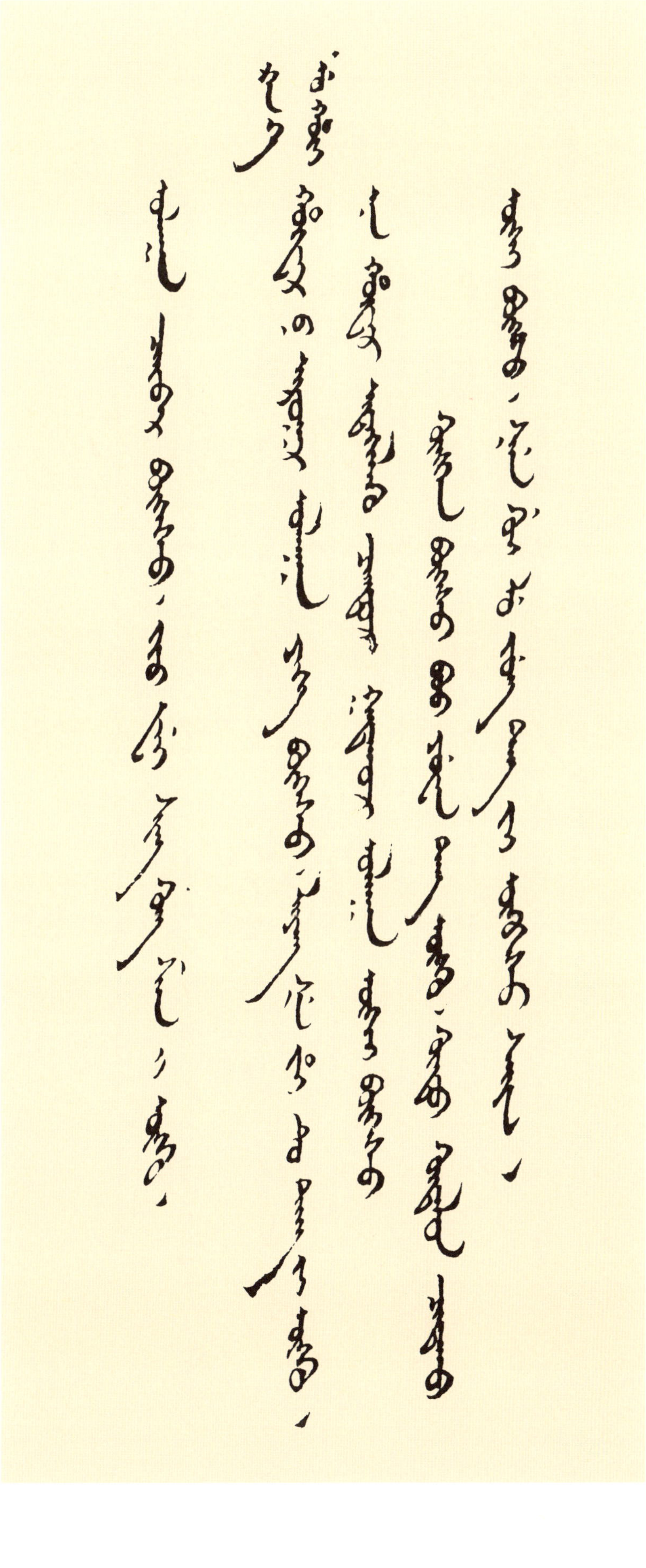

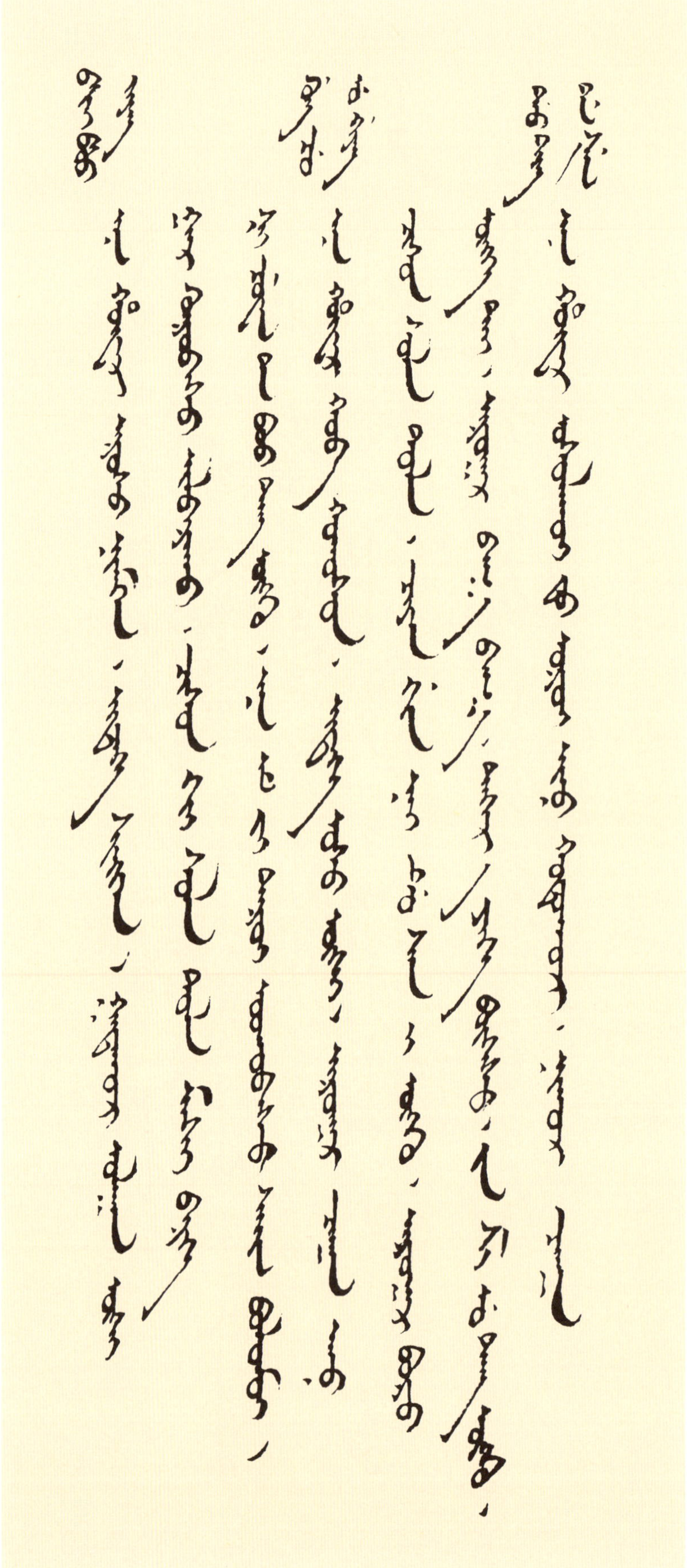

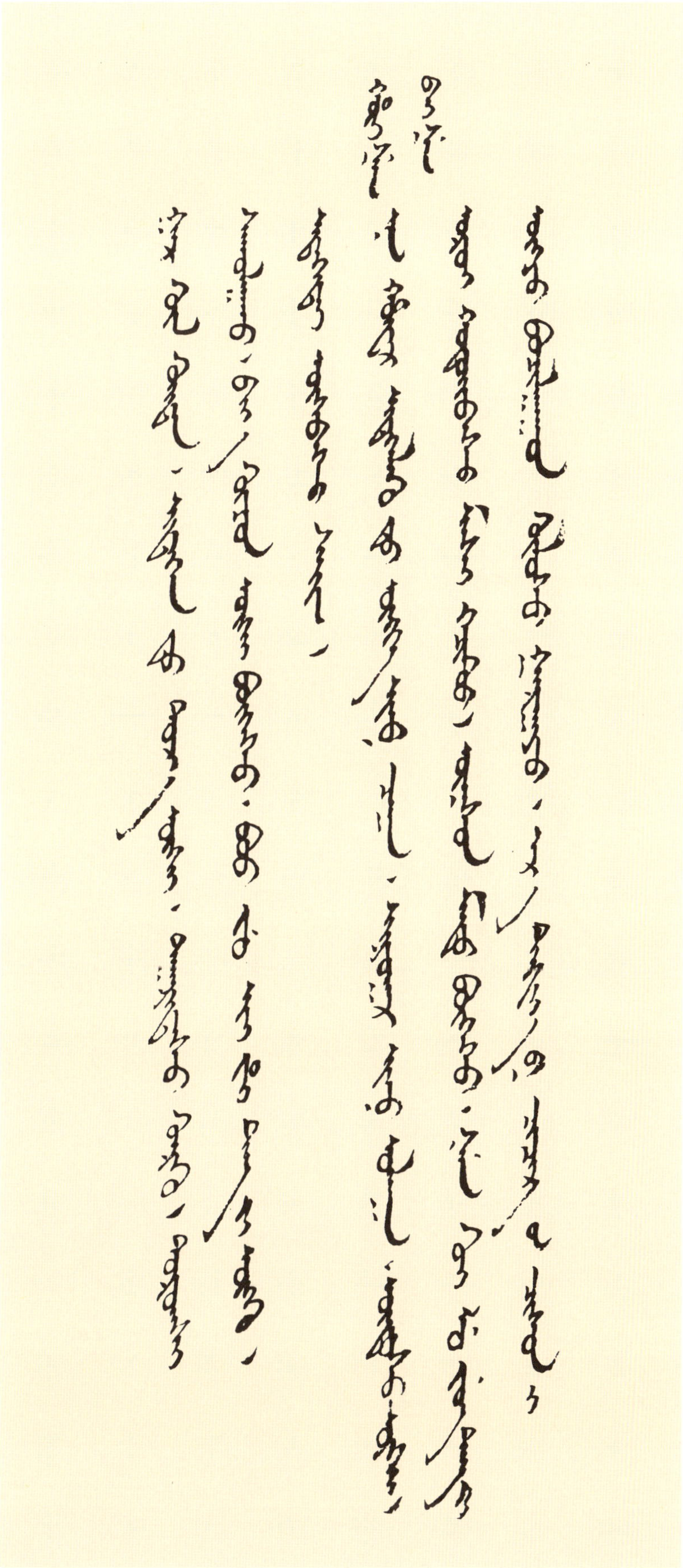

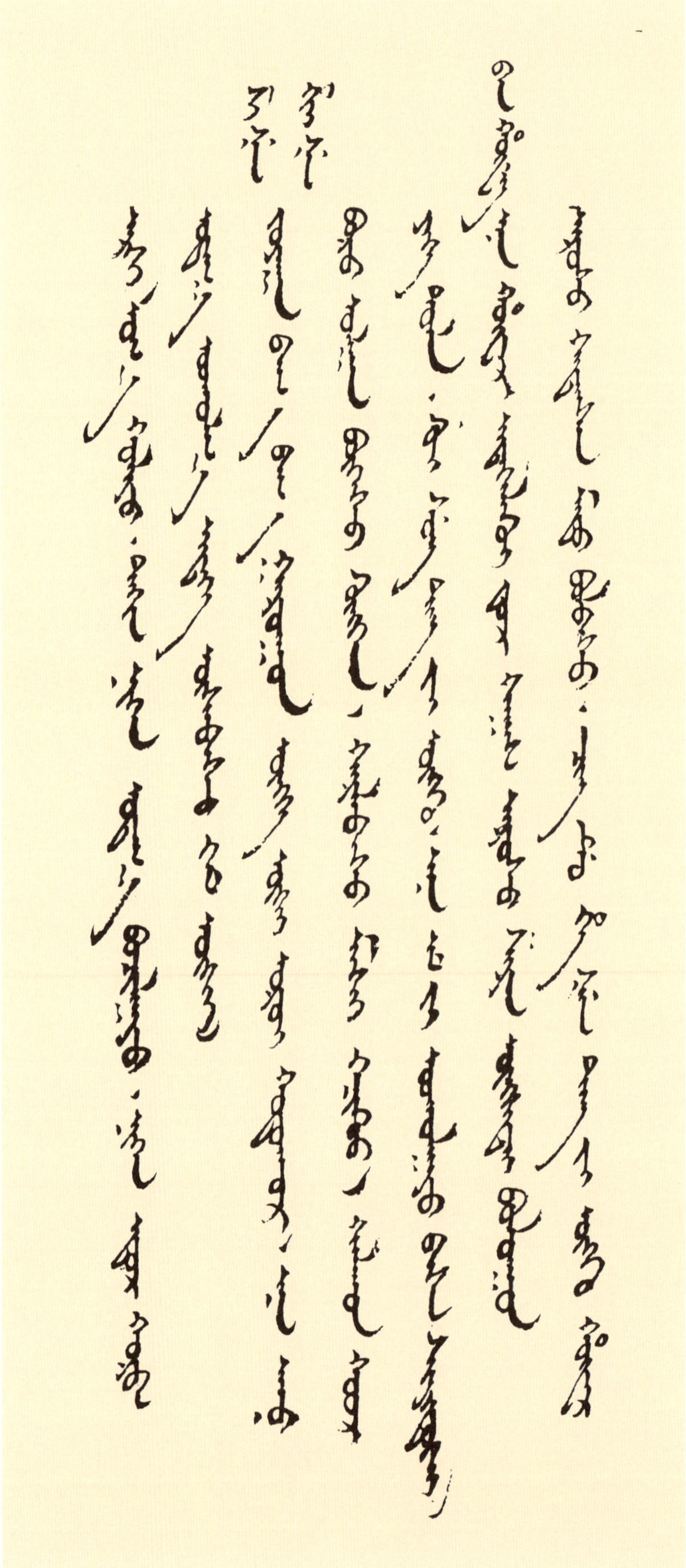

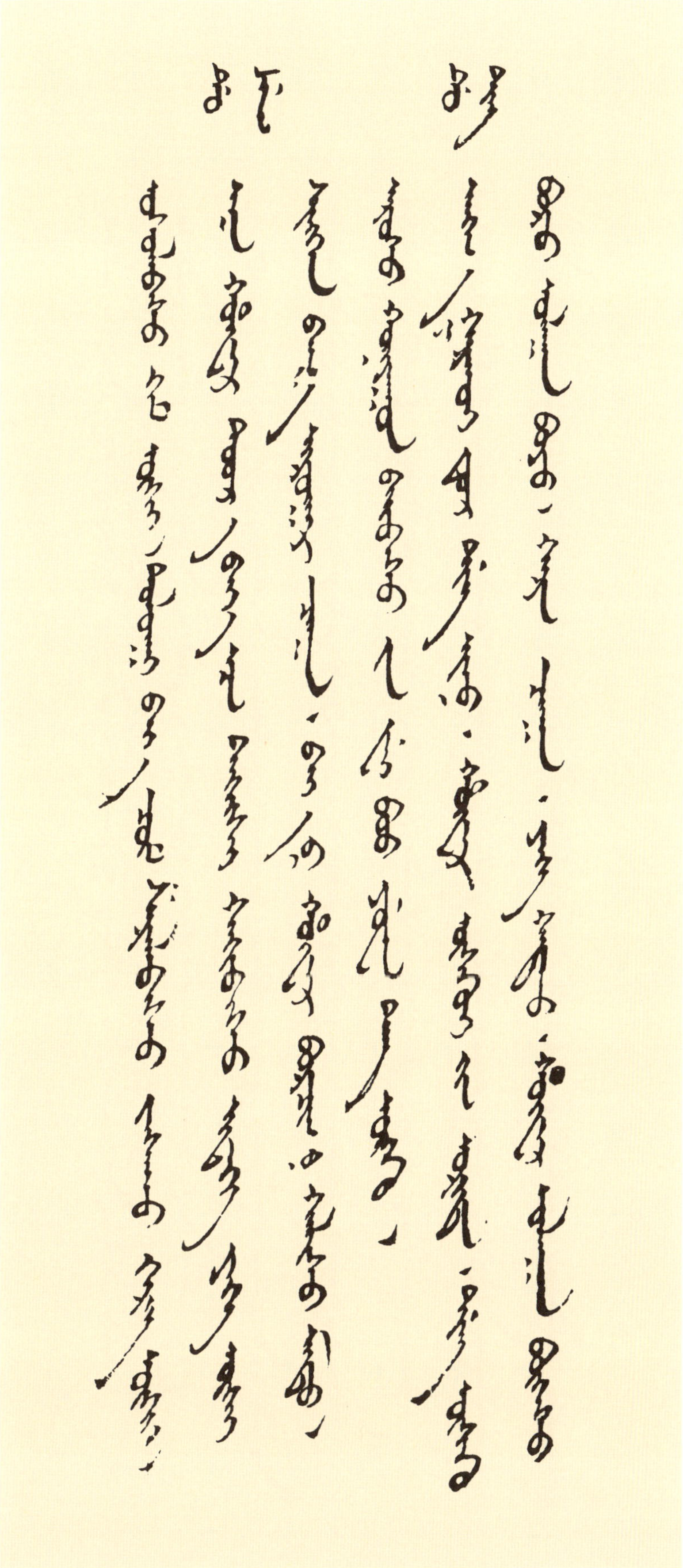

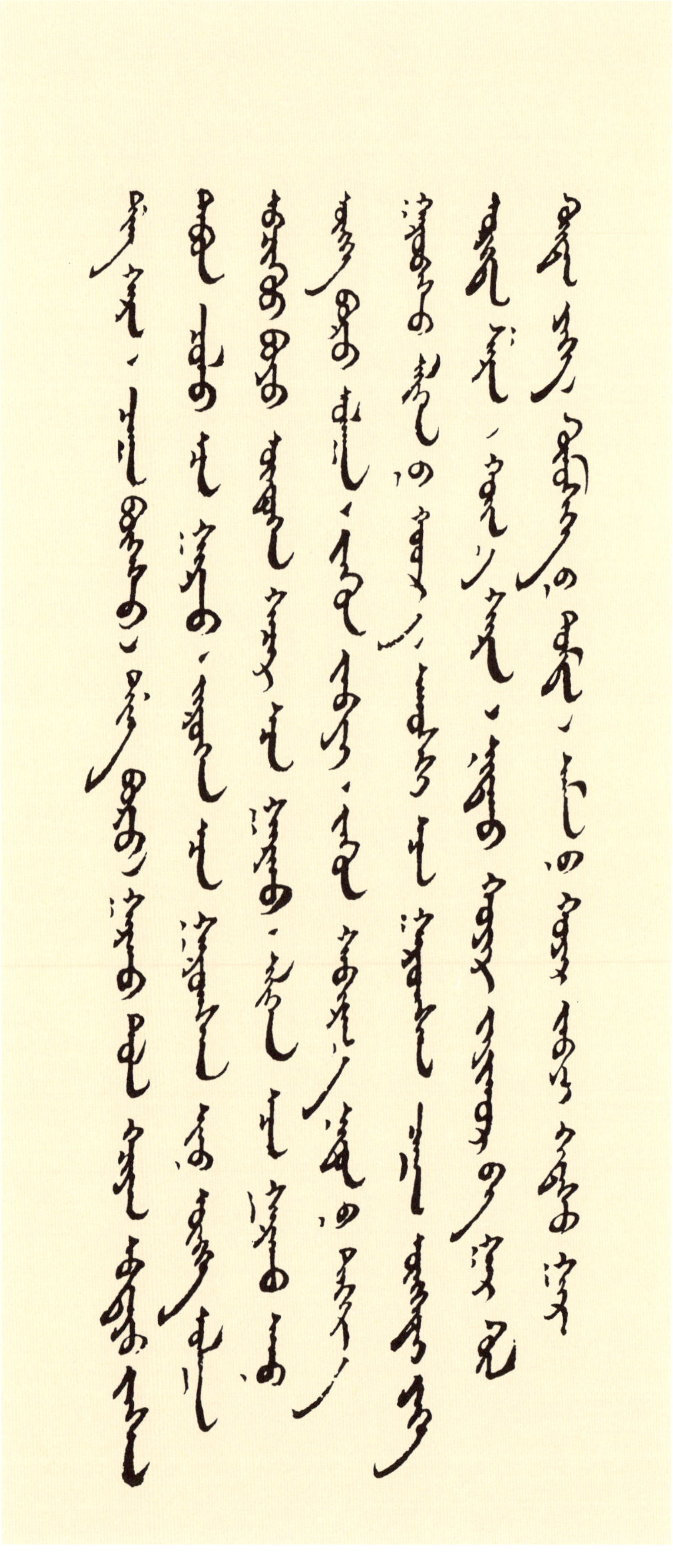

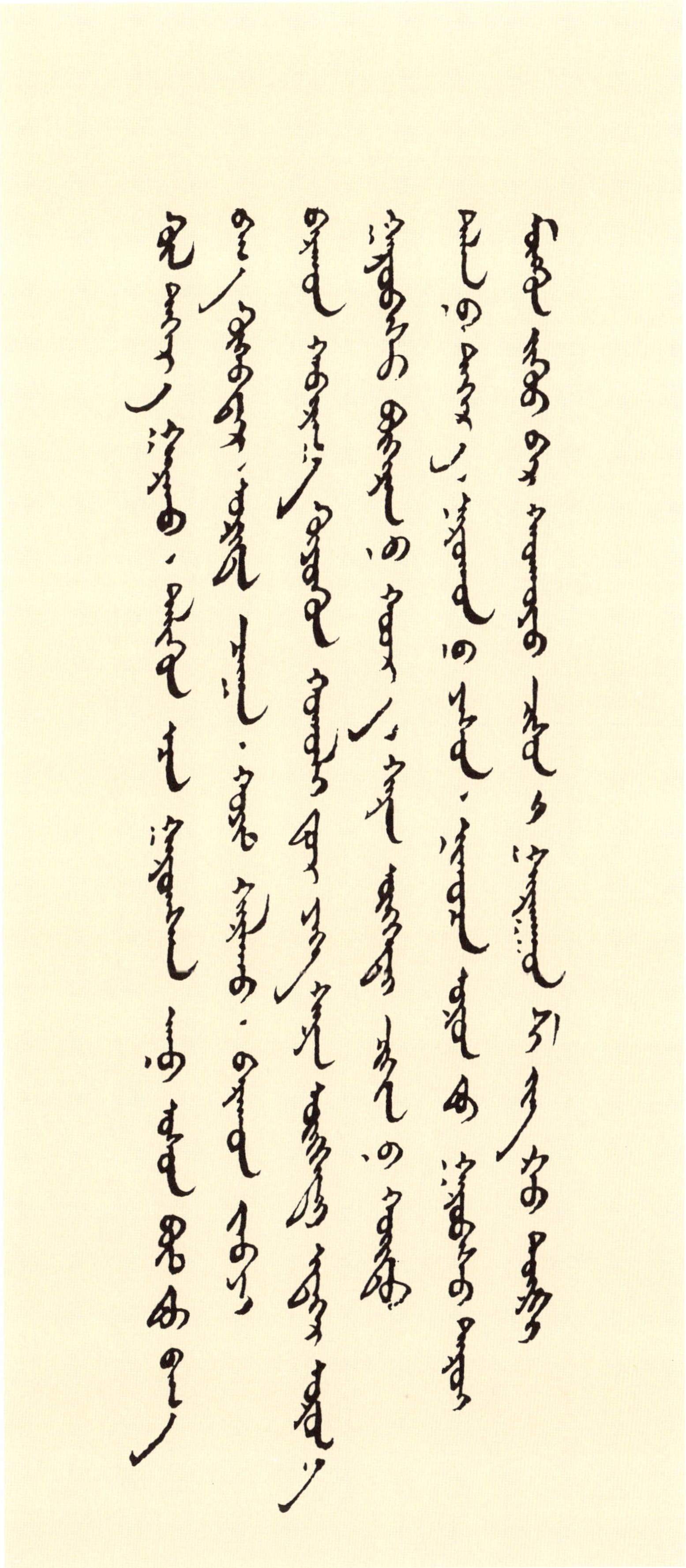

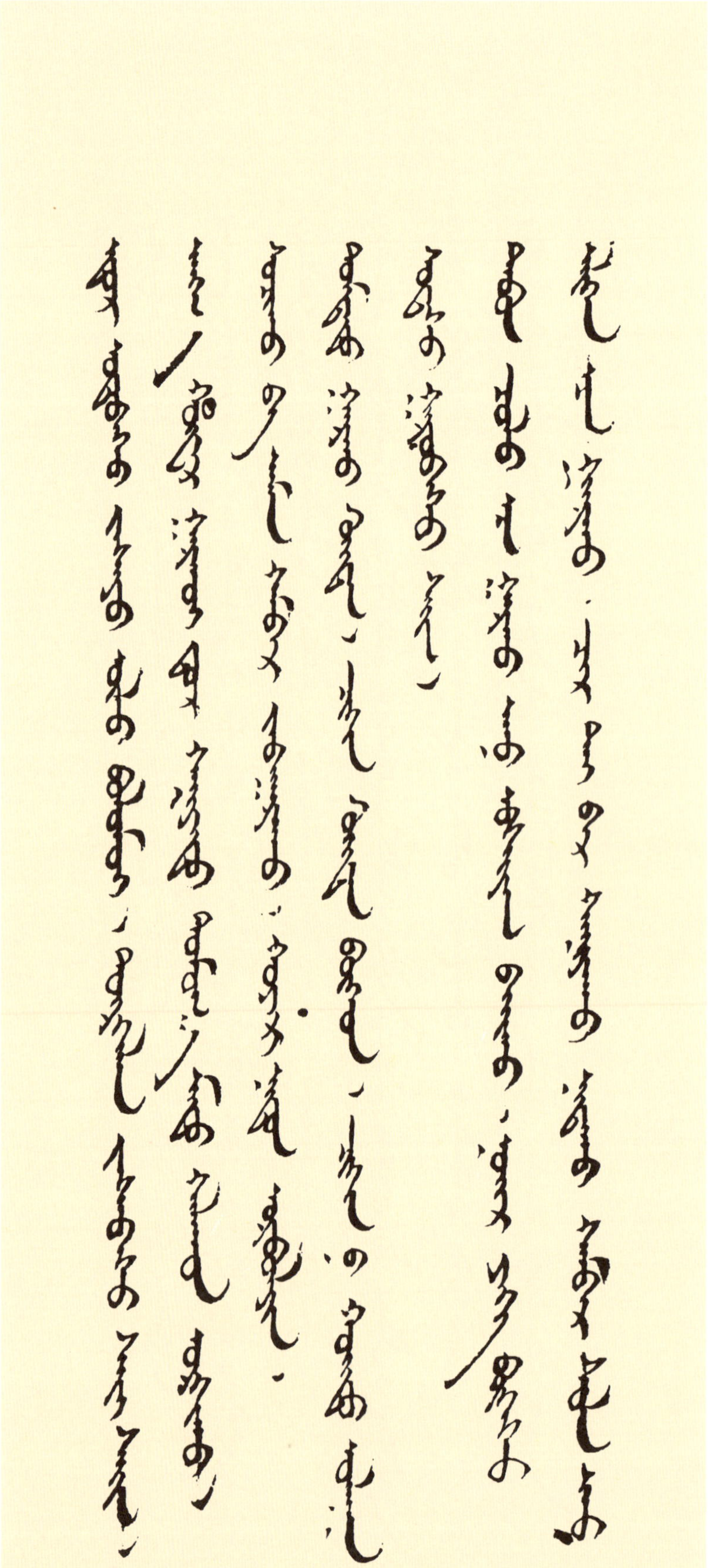

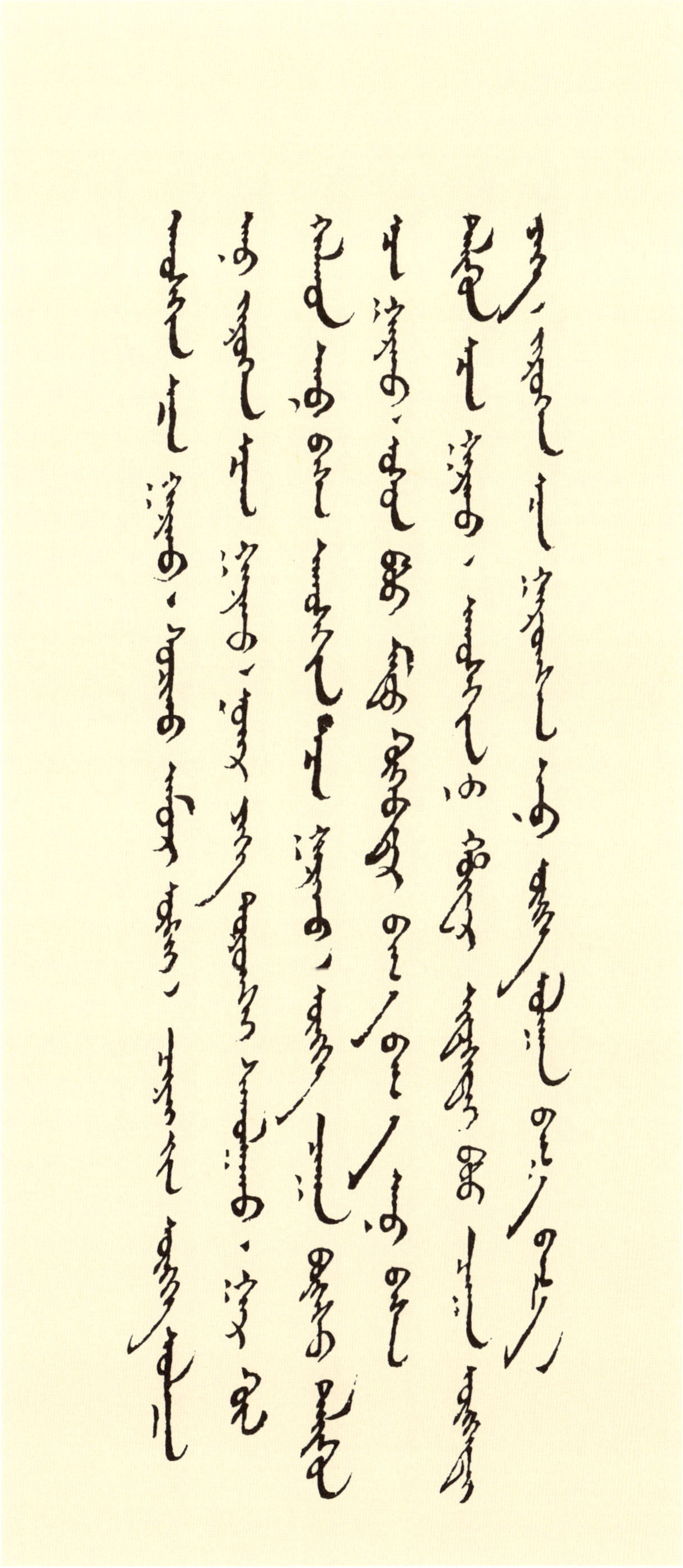

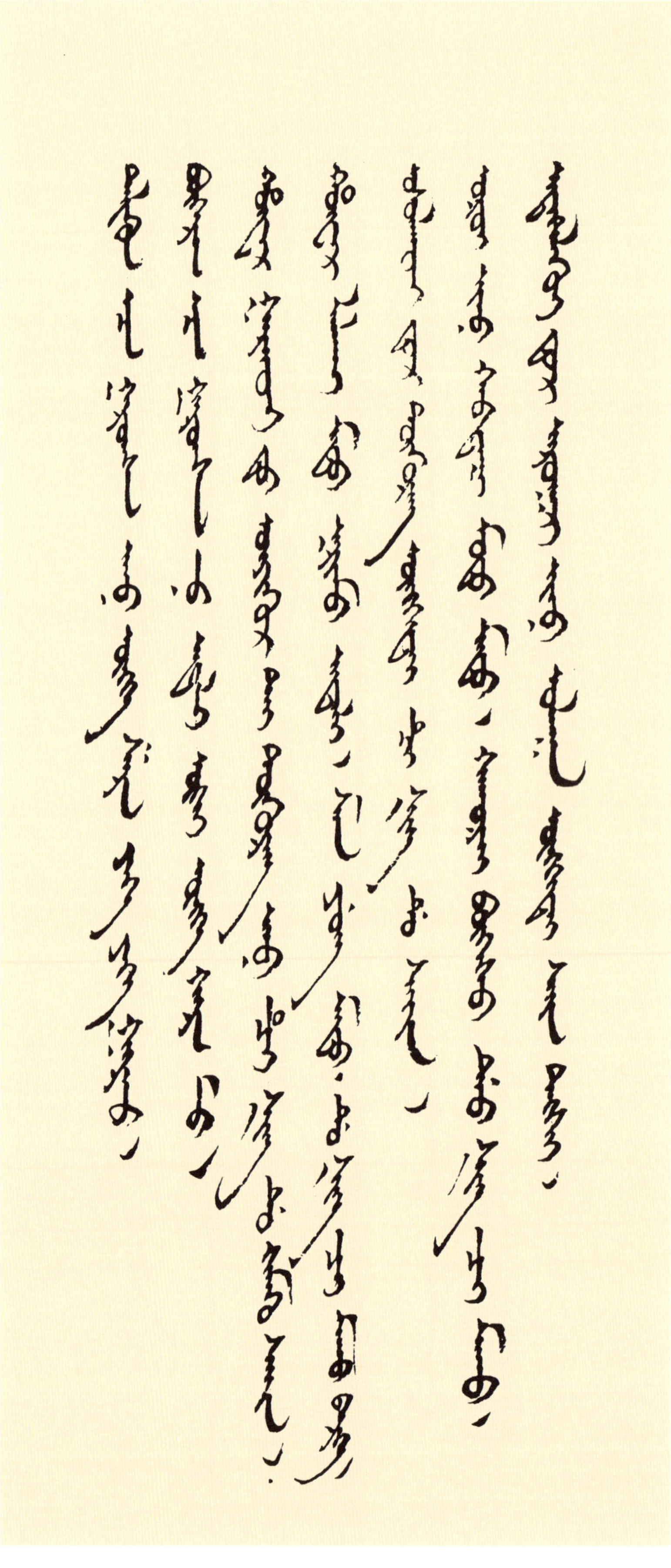

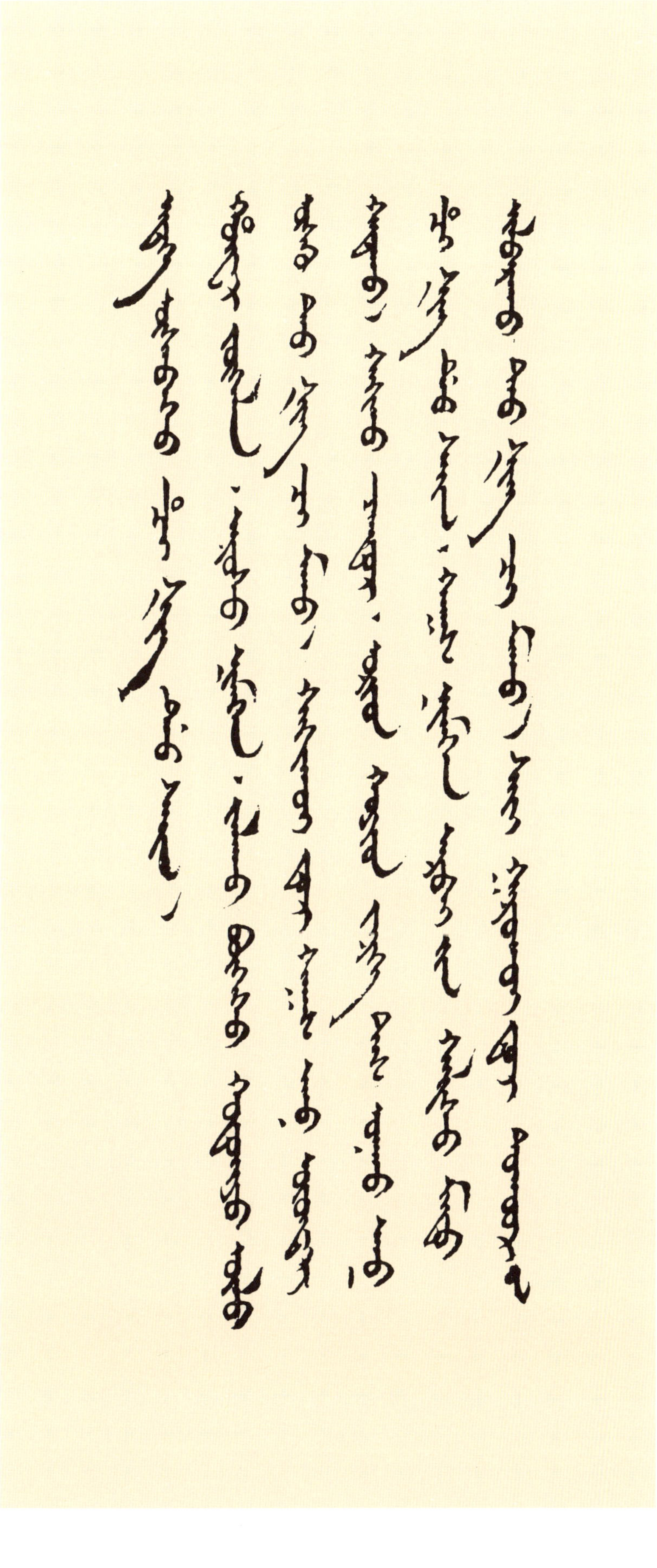

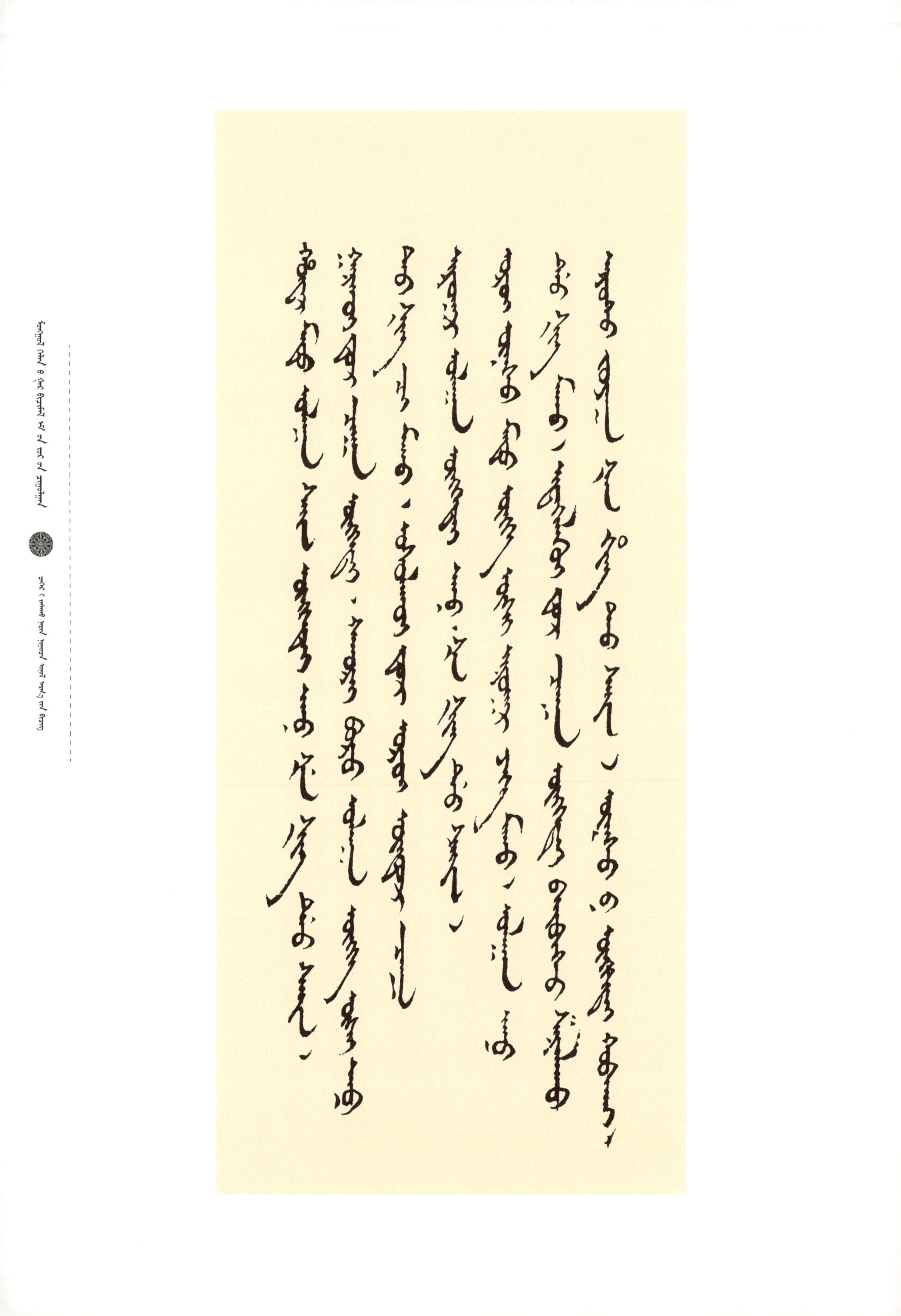

[illegible]

[illegible]

[illegible]

[illegible]

[illegible]

[illegible]

[illegible]

[illegible]

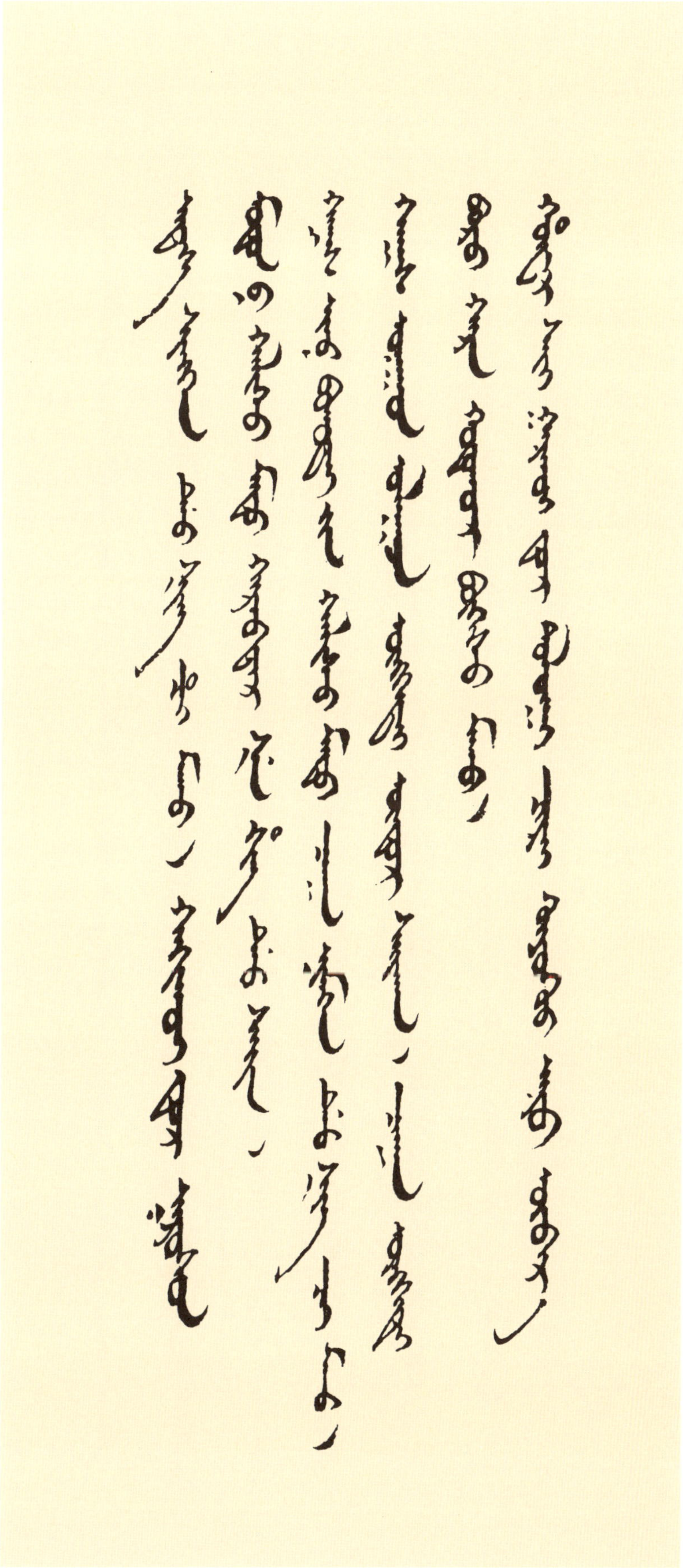

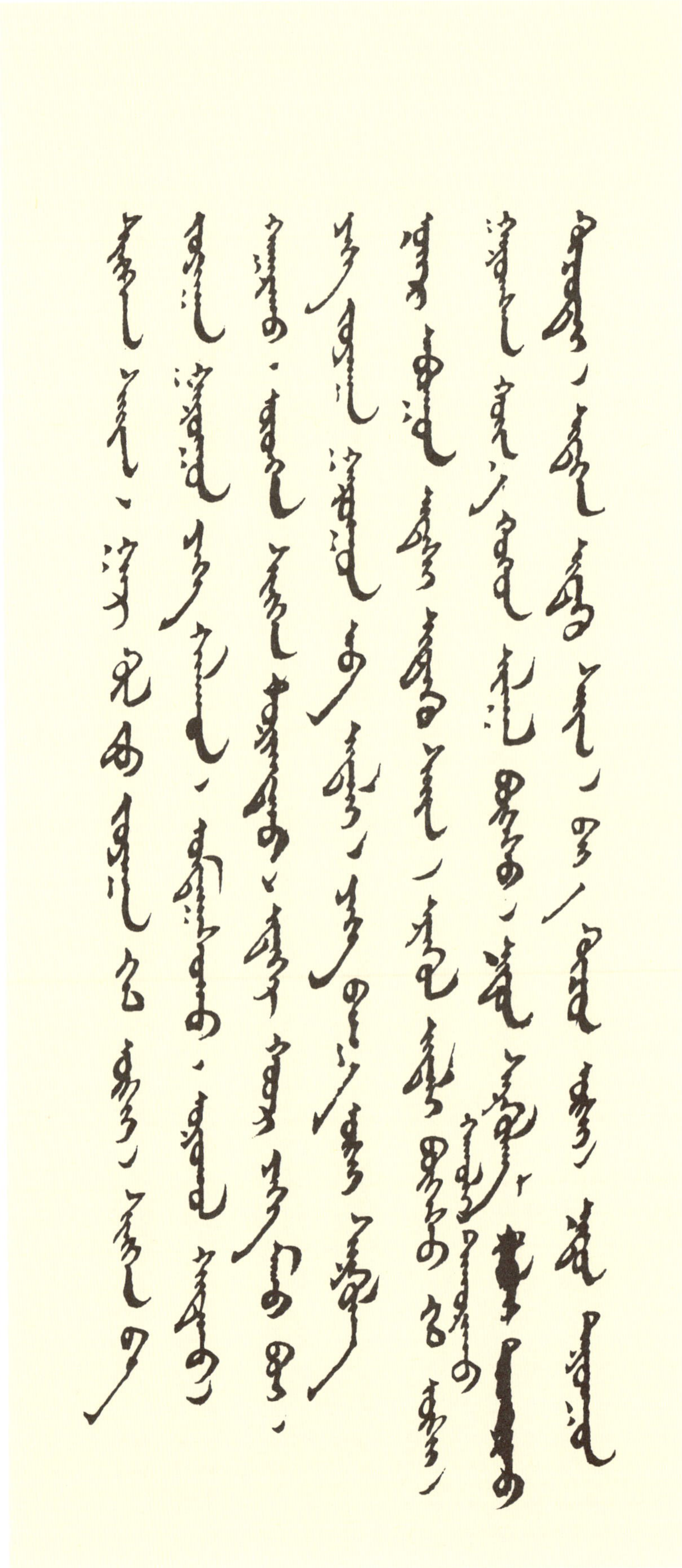

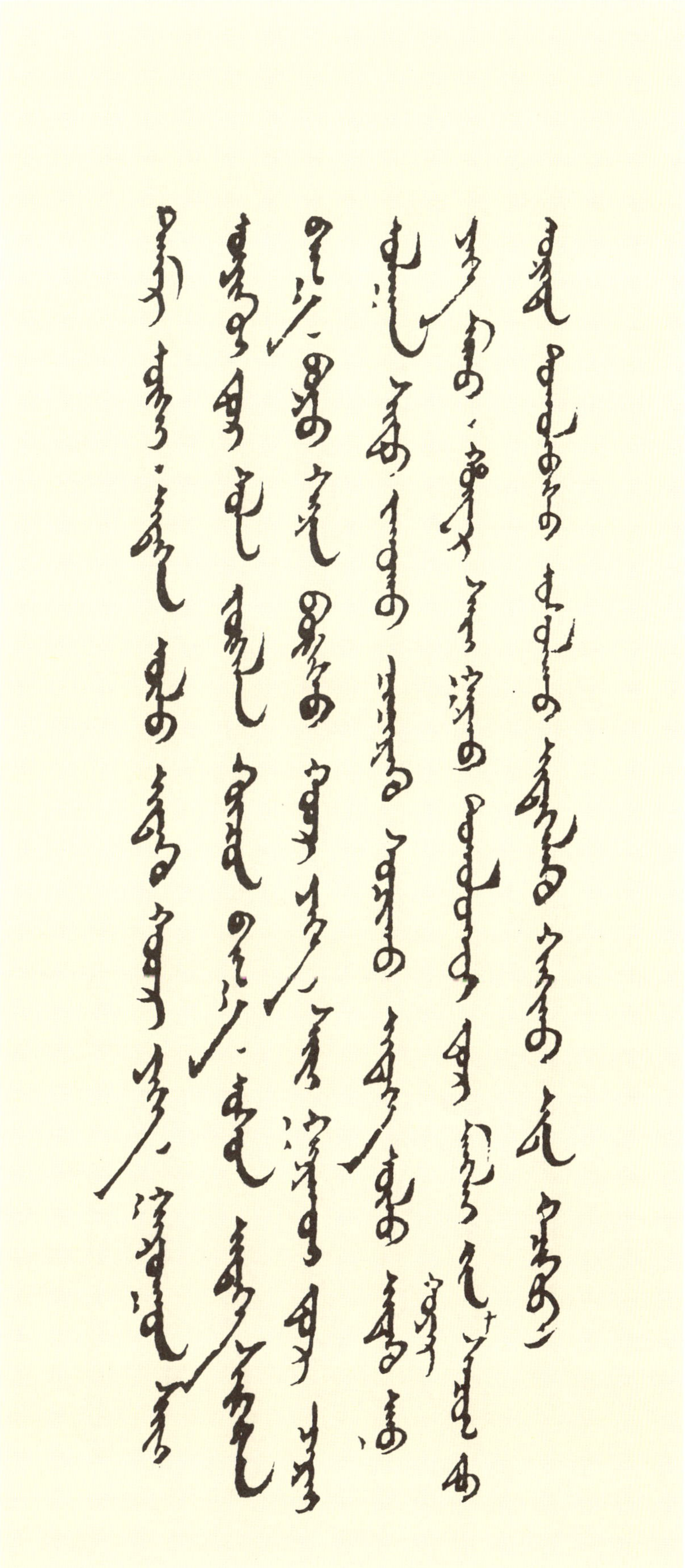

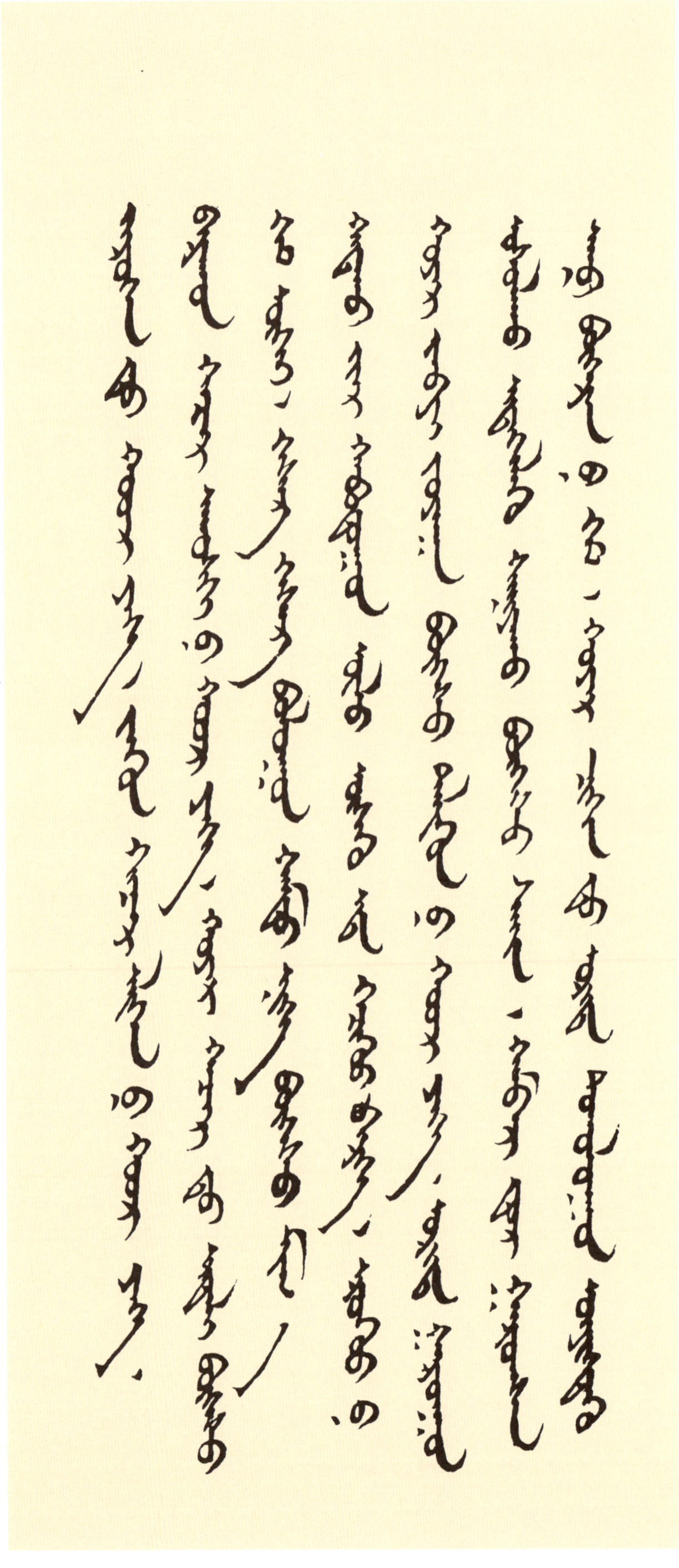

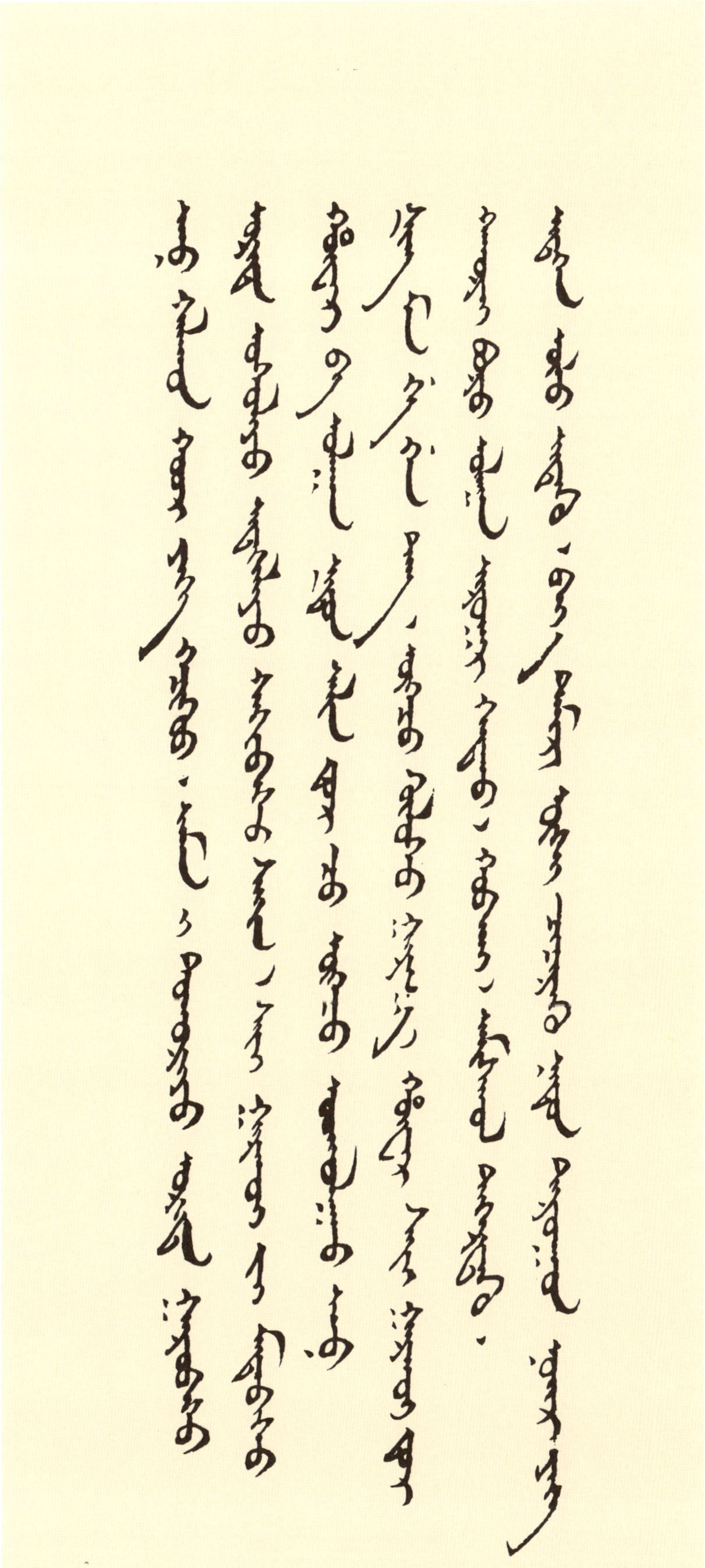

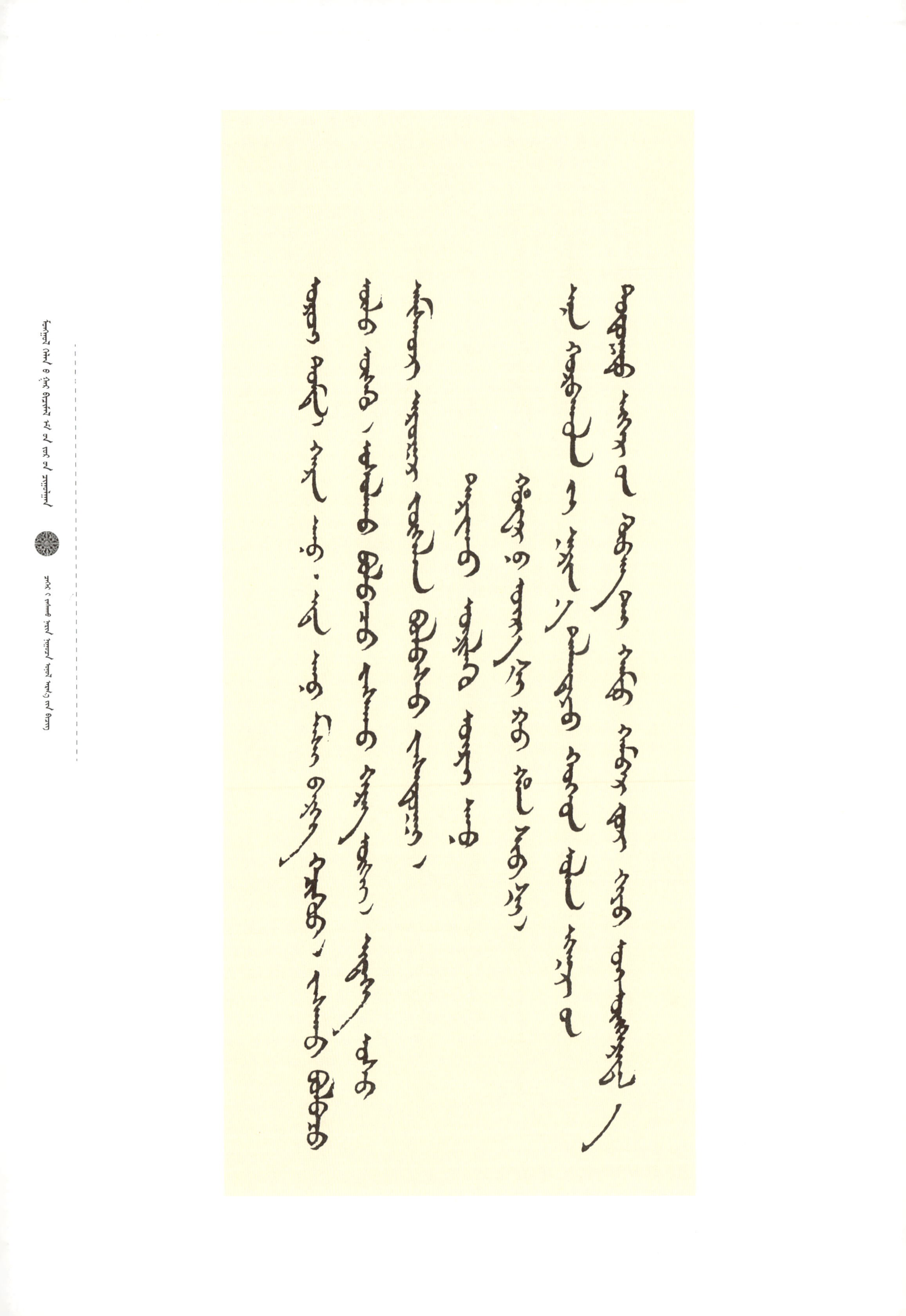

[illegible]

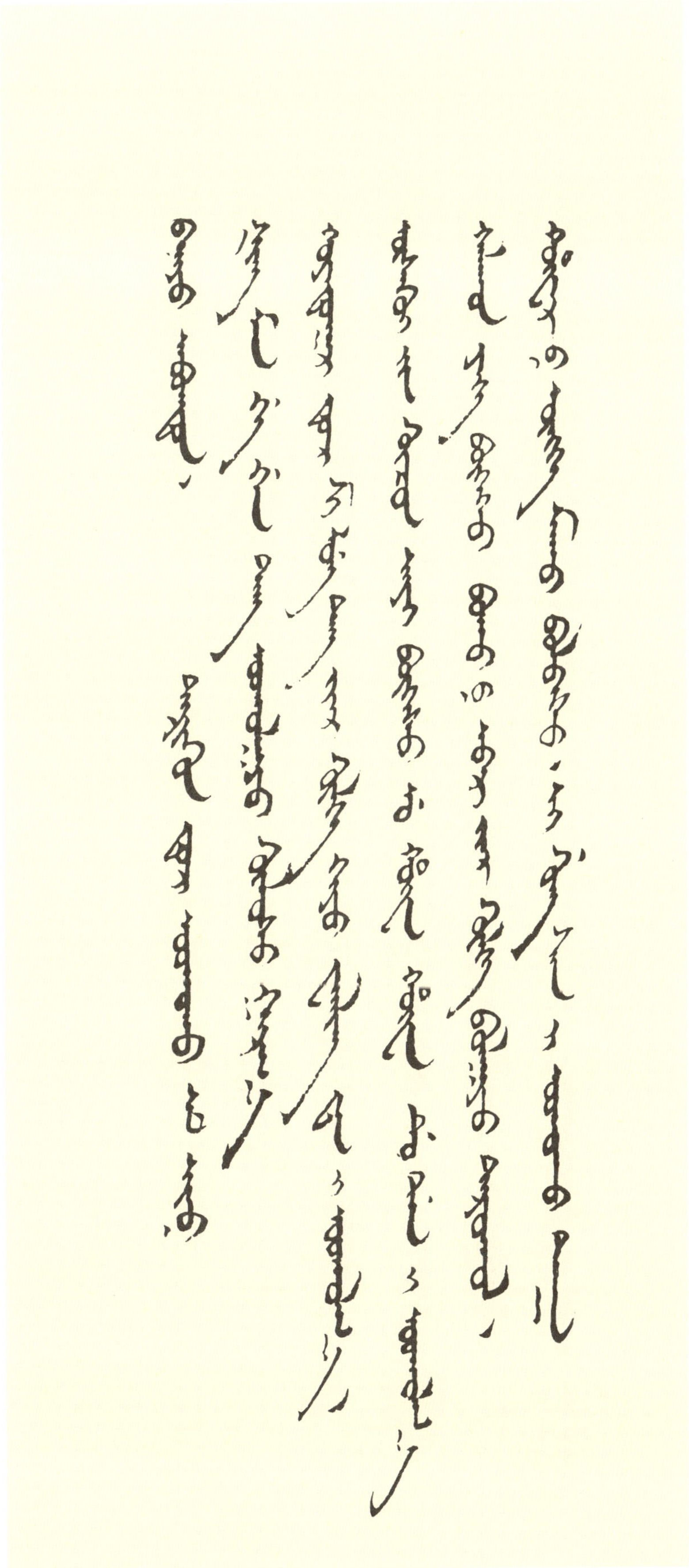

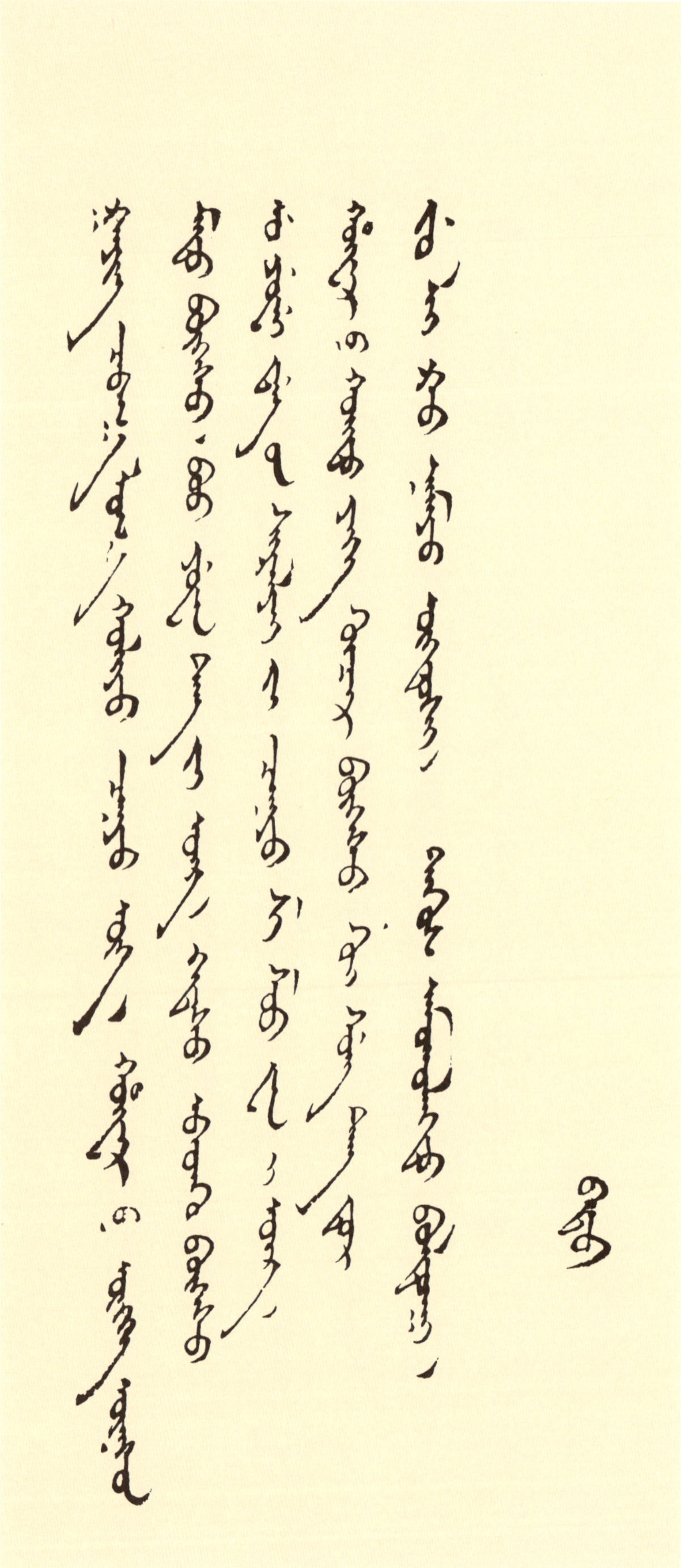

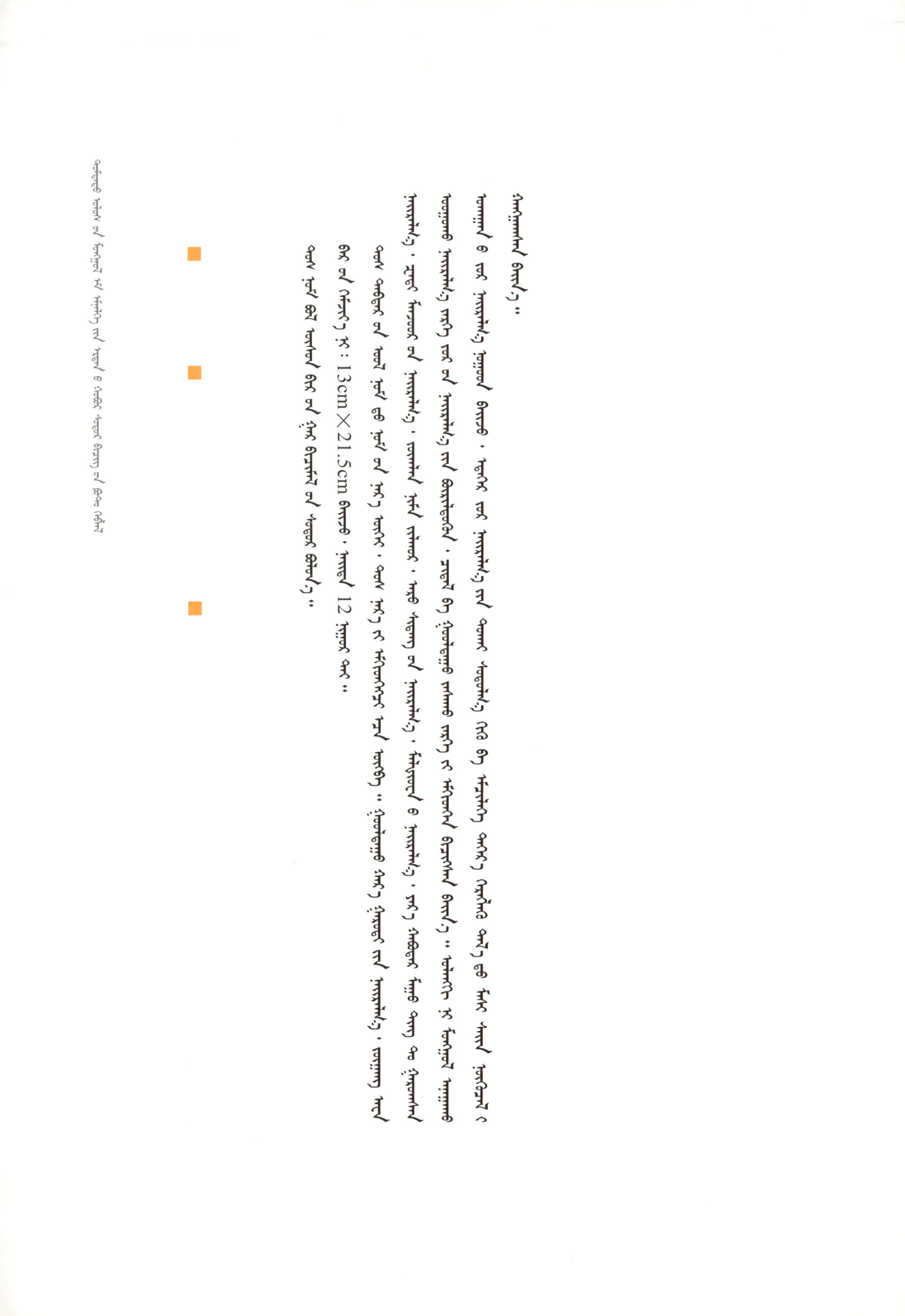

ᠮᠣᠩᠭᠣᠯ ᠬᠡᠯᠡ ᠪᠢᠴᠢᠭ ᠤᠨ ᠬᠡᠯᠪᠡᠷᠢ ᠶᠢᠨ ᠬᠡᠮᠵᠢᠶ᠎ᠡ ᠨᠢ᠄ 13cm×21.5cm ᠪᠣᠯᠤᠭᠰᠠᠨ᠂ ᠨᠡᠢᠲᠡ 12 ᠨᠢᠭᠤᠷ ᠲᠠᠢ᠃

■ ■ ■

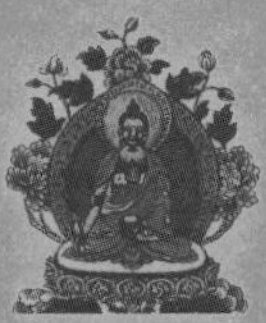

Prescriptions of Various Diseases

治疗各种疾病的药方

6

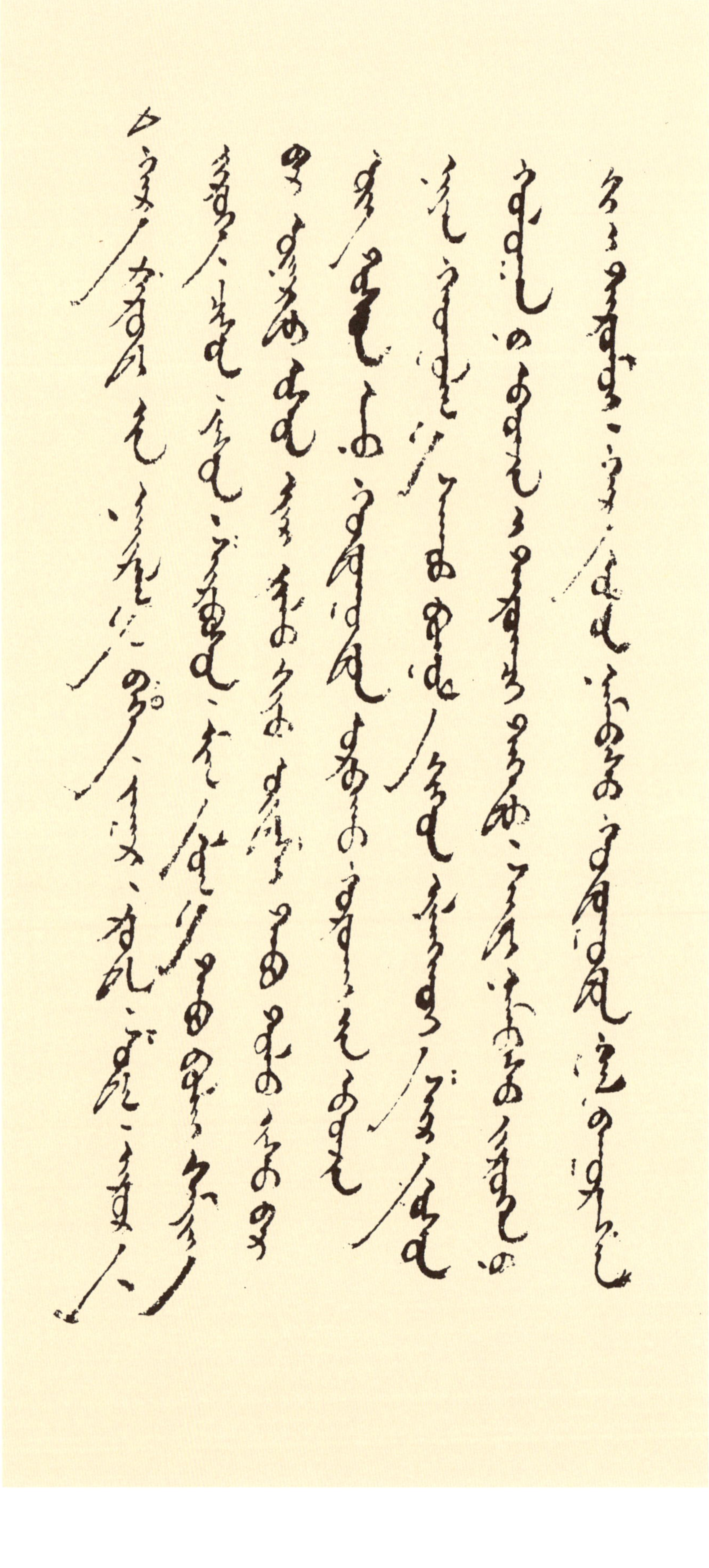

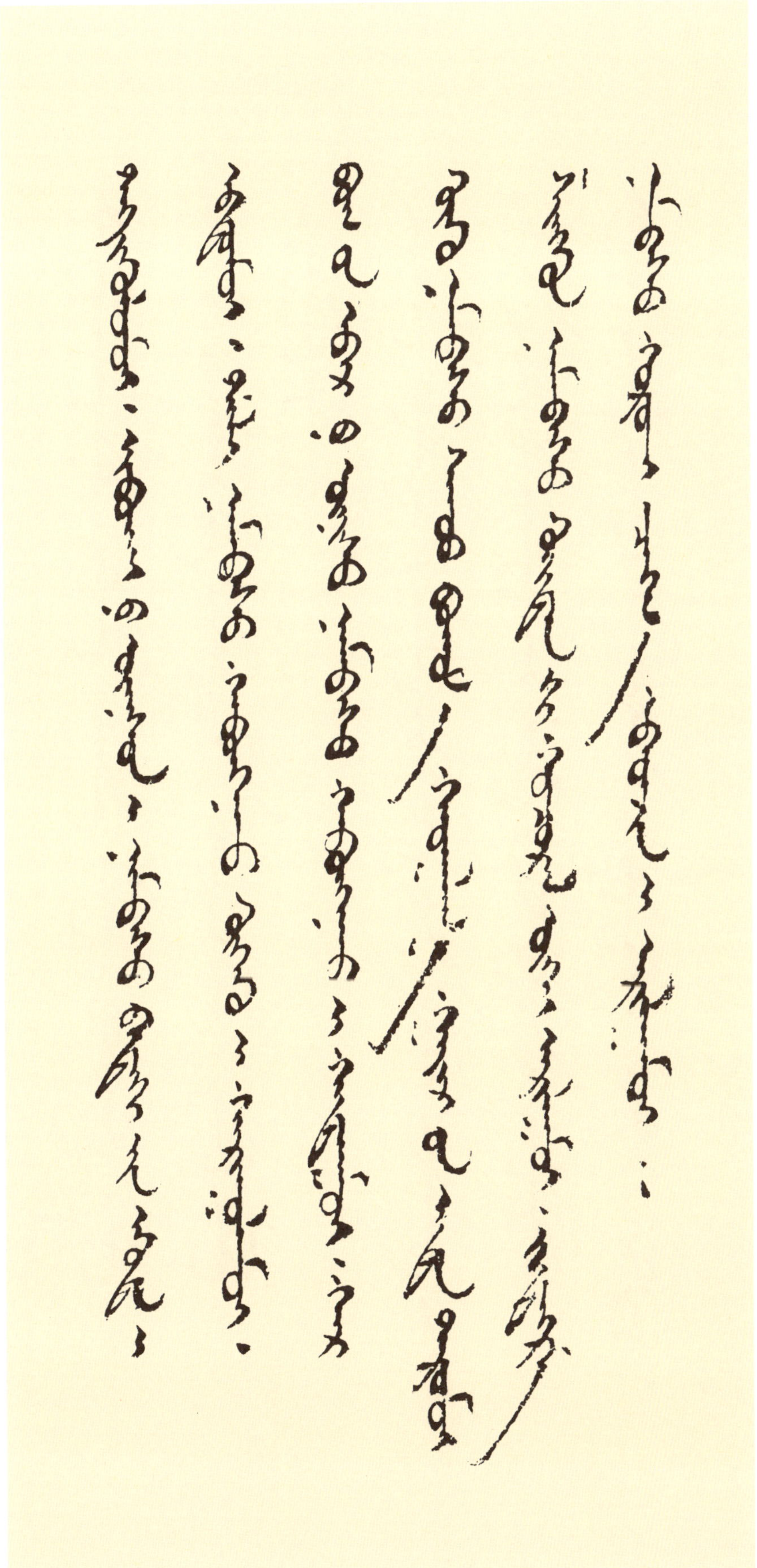

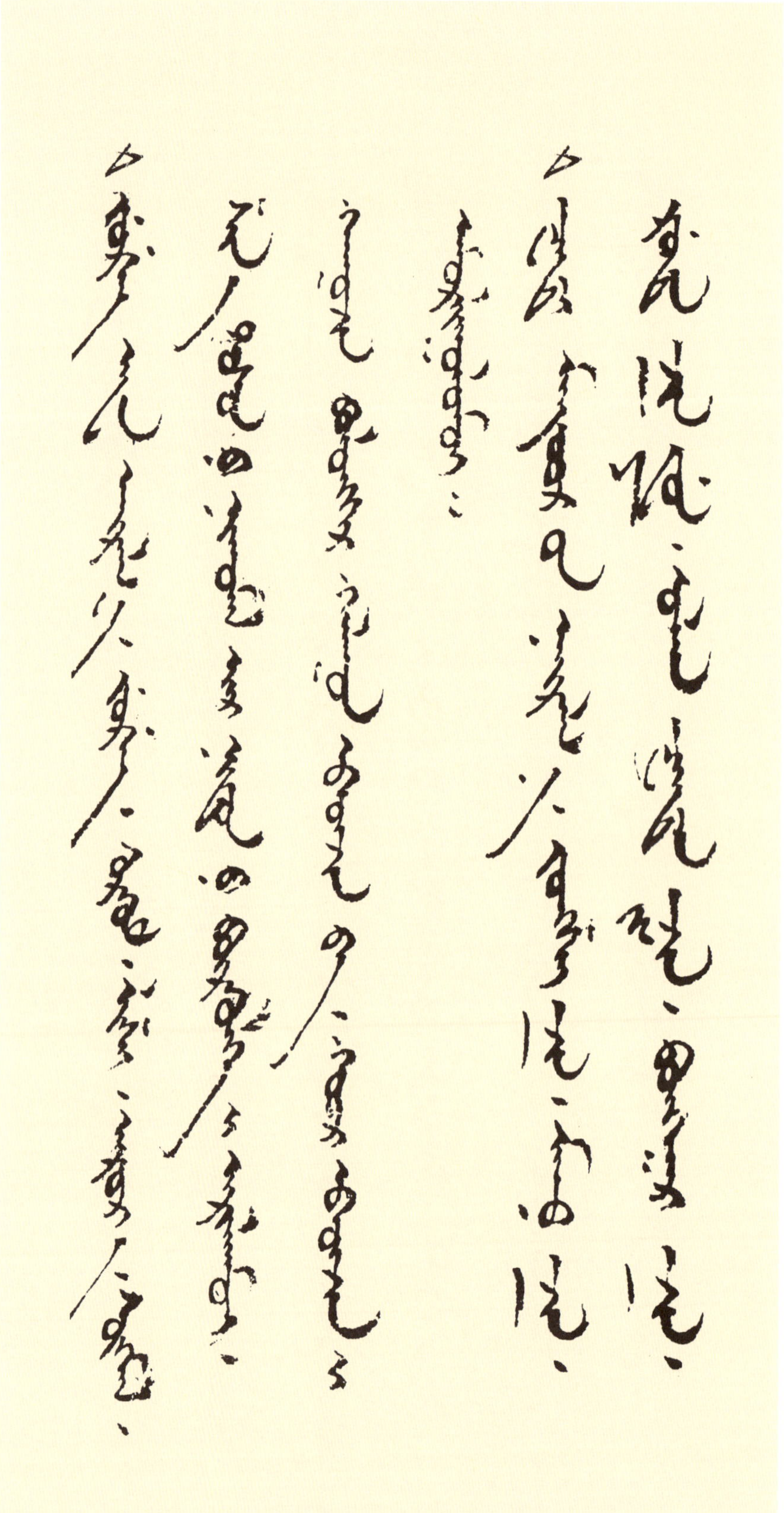

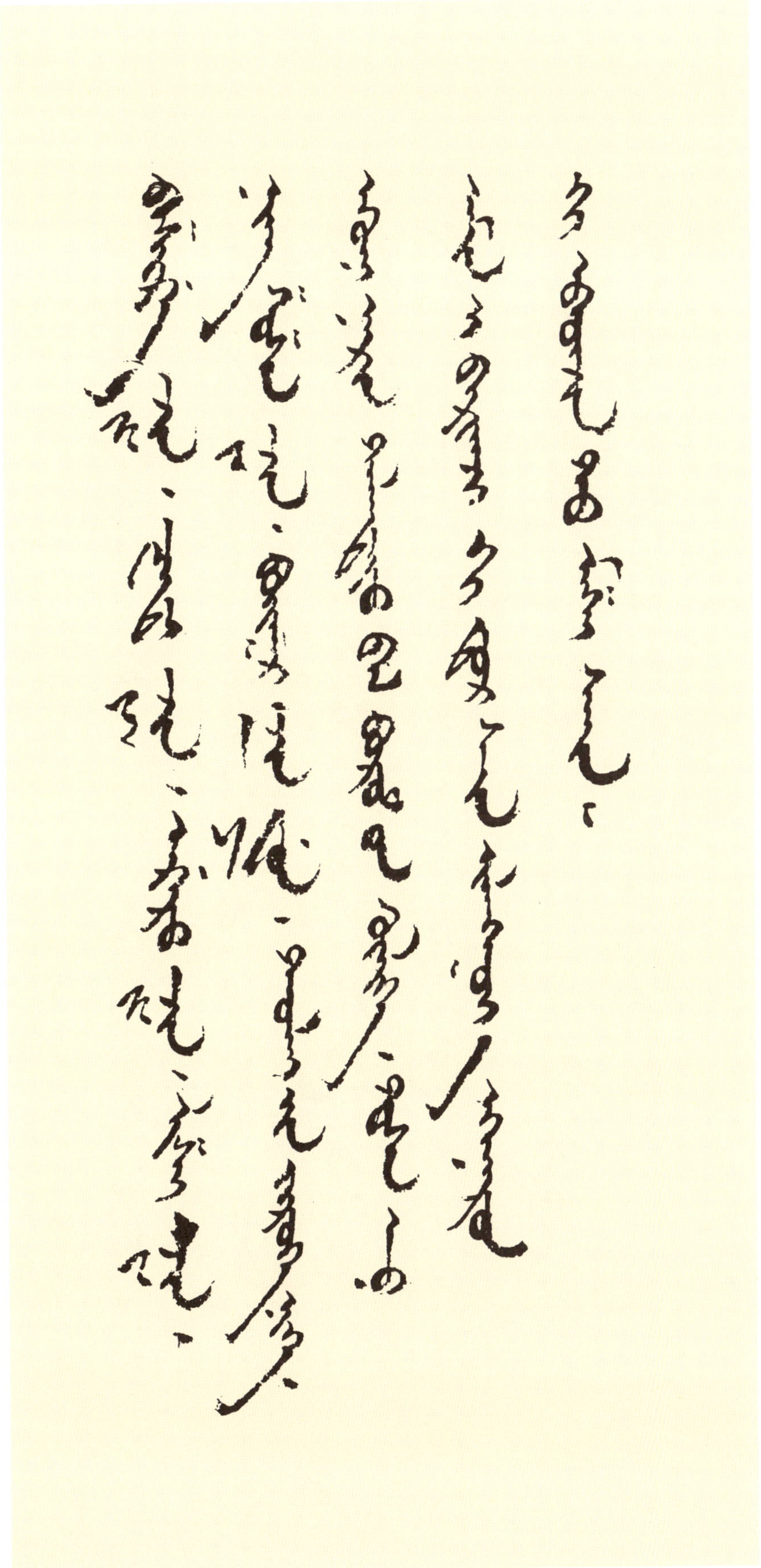

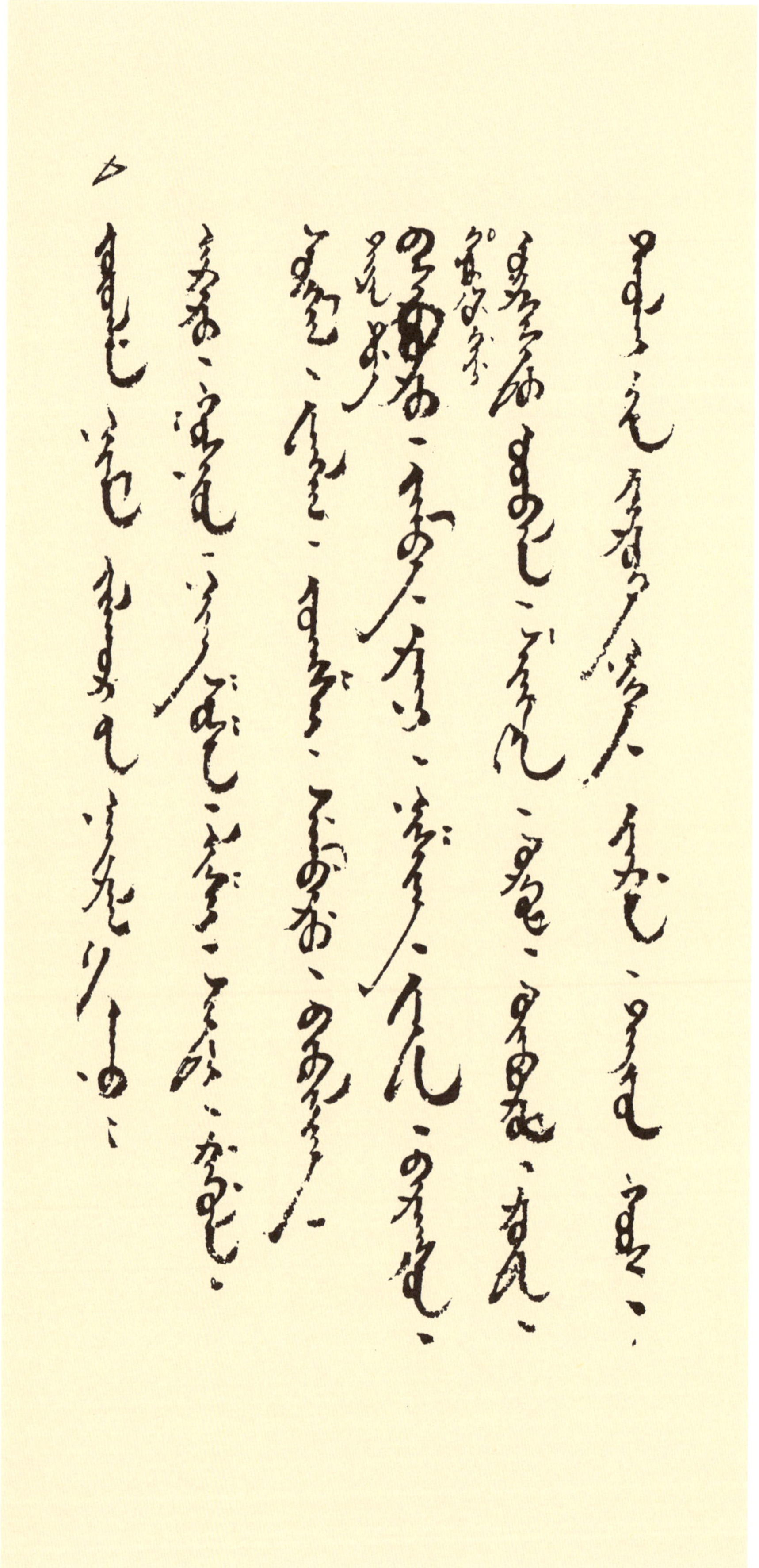

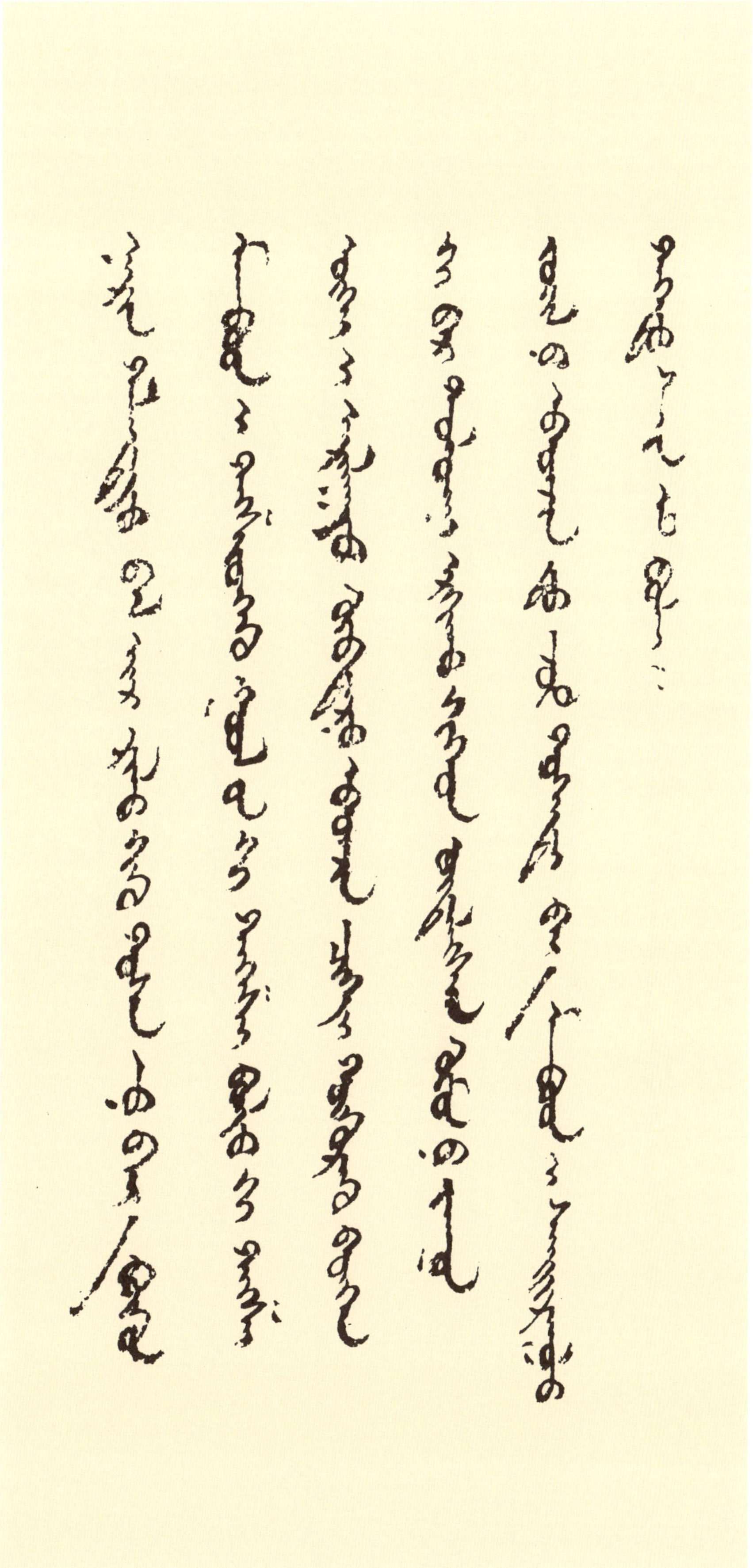

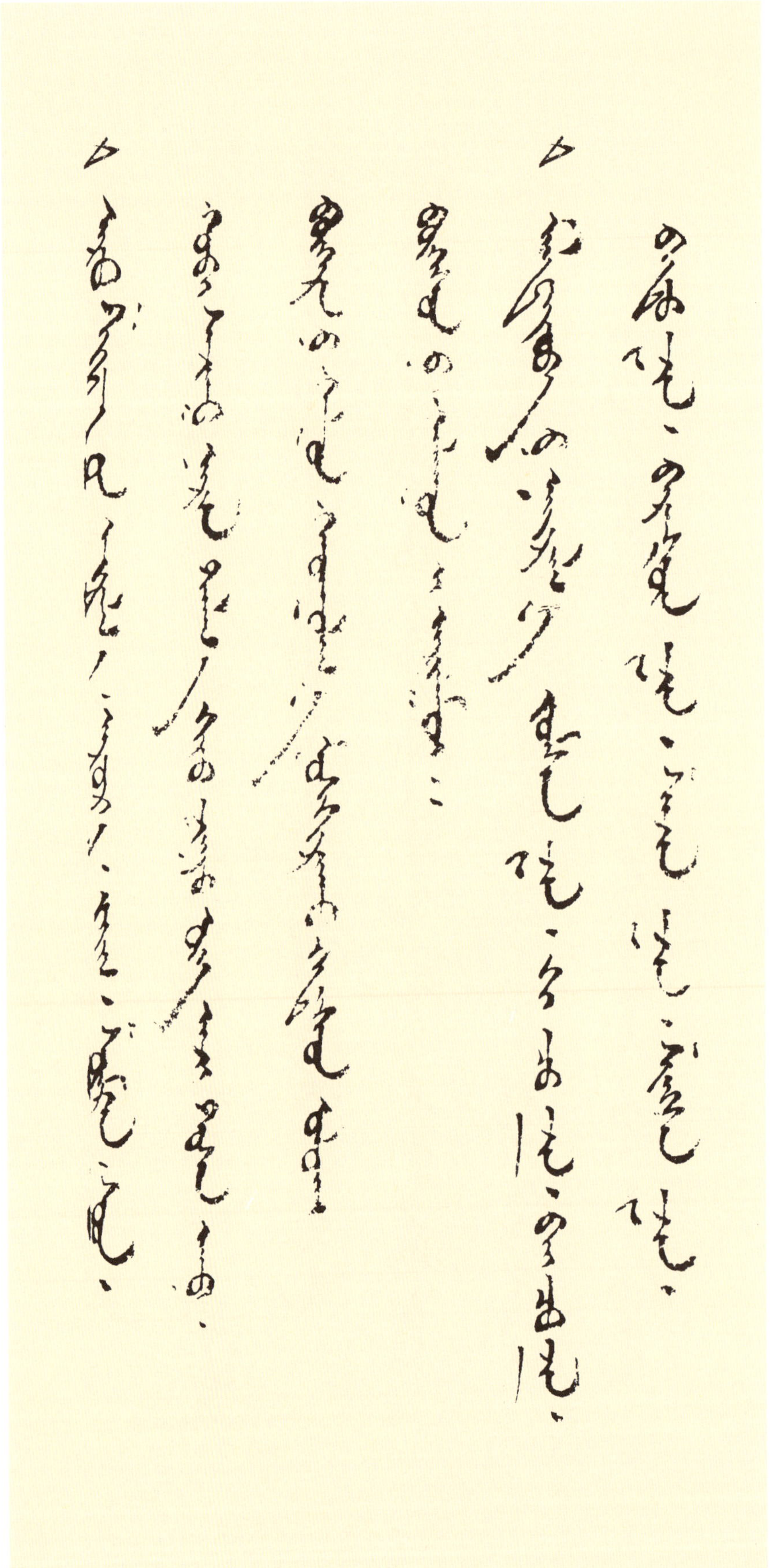

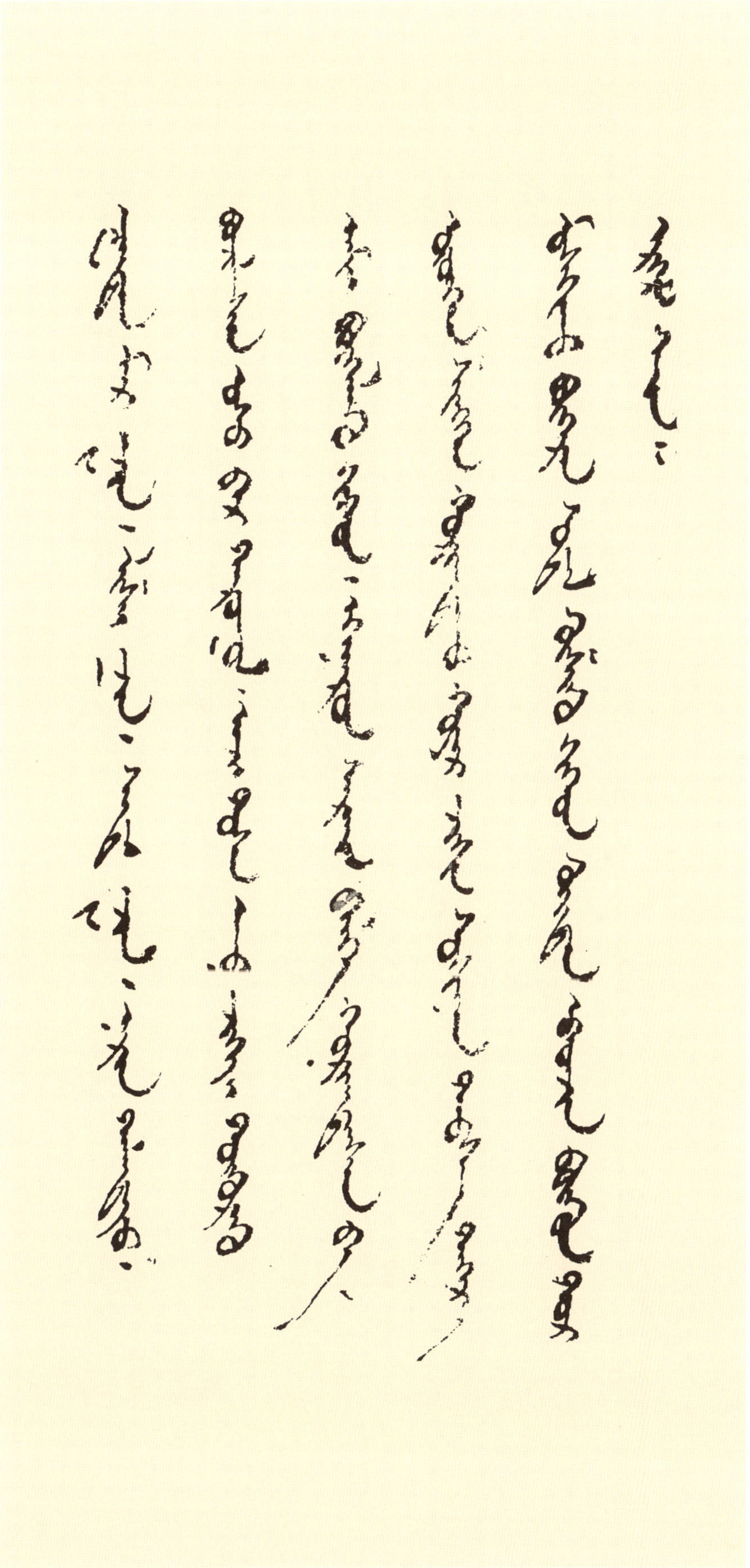

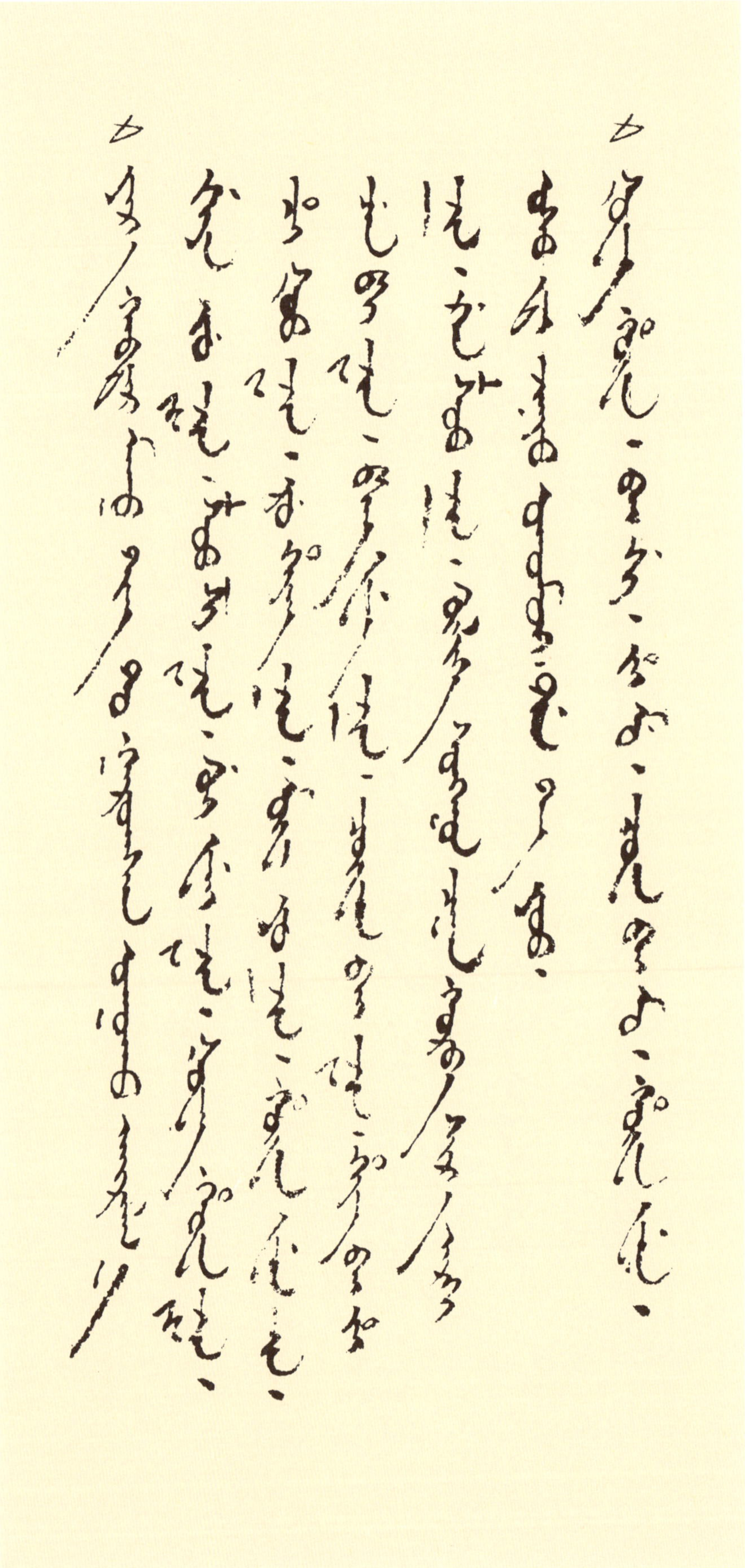

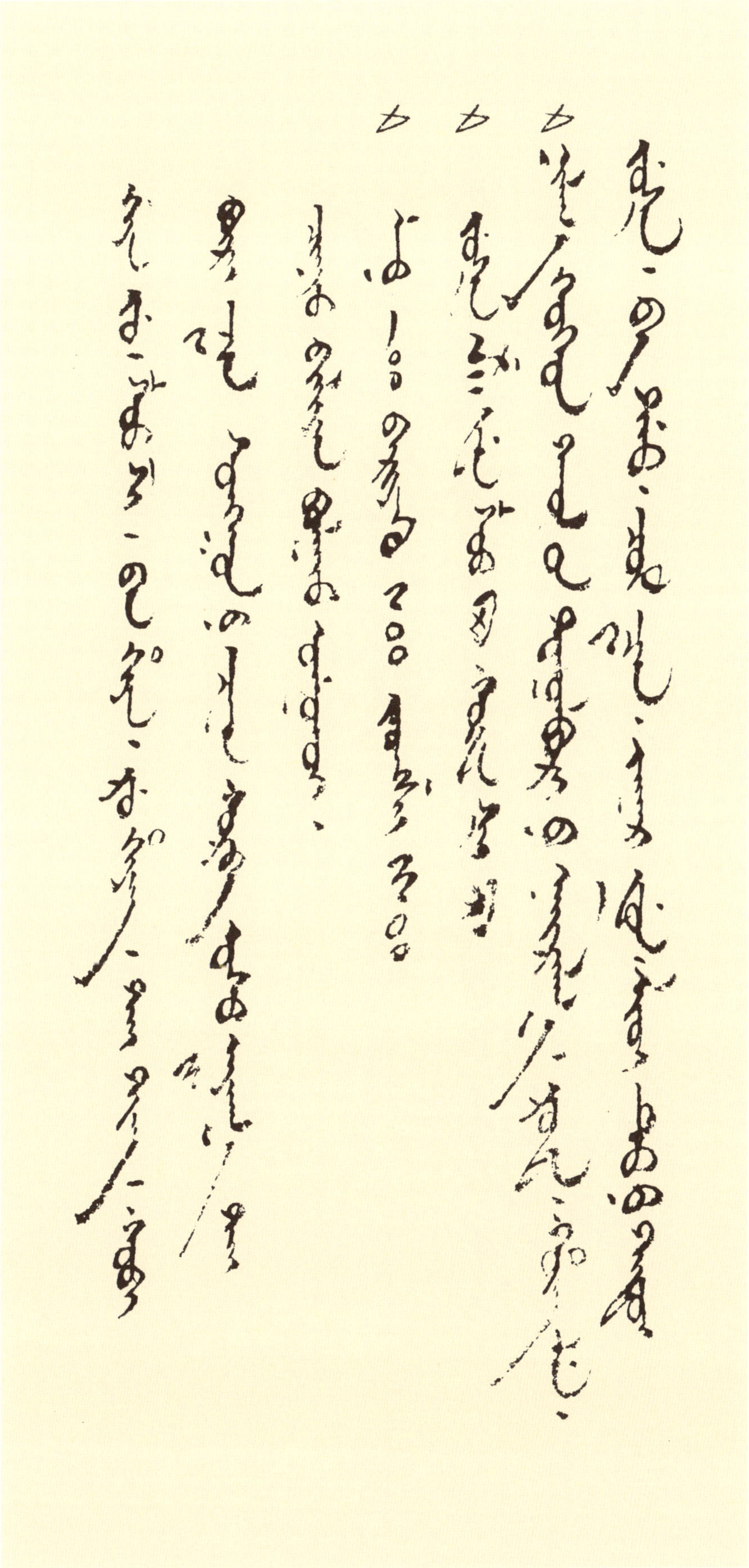

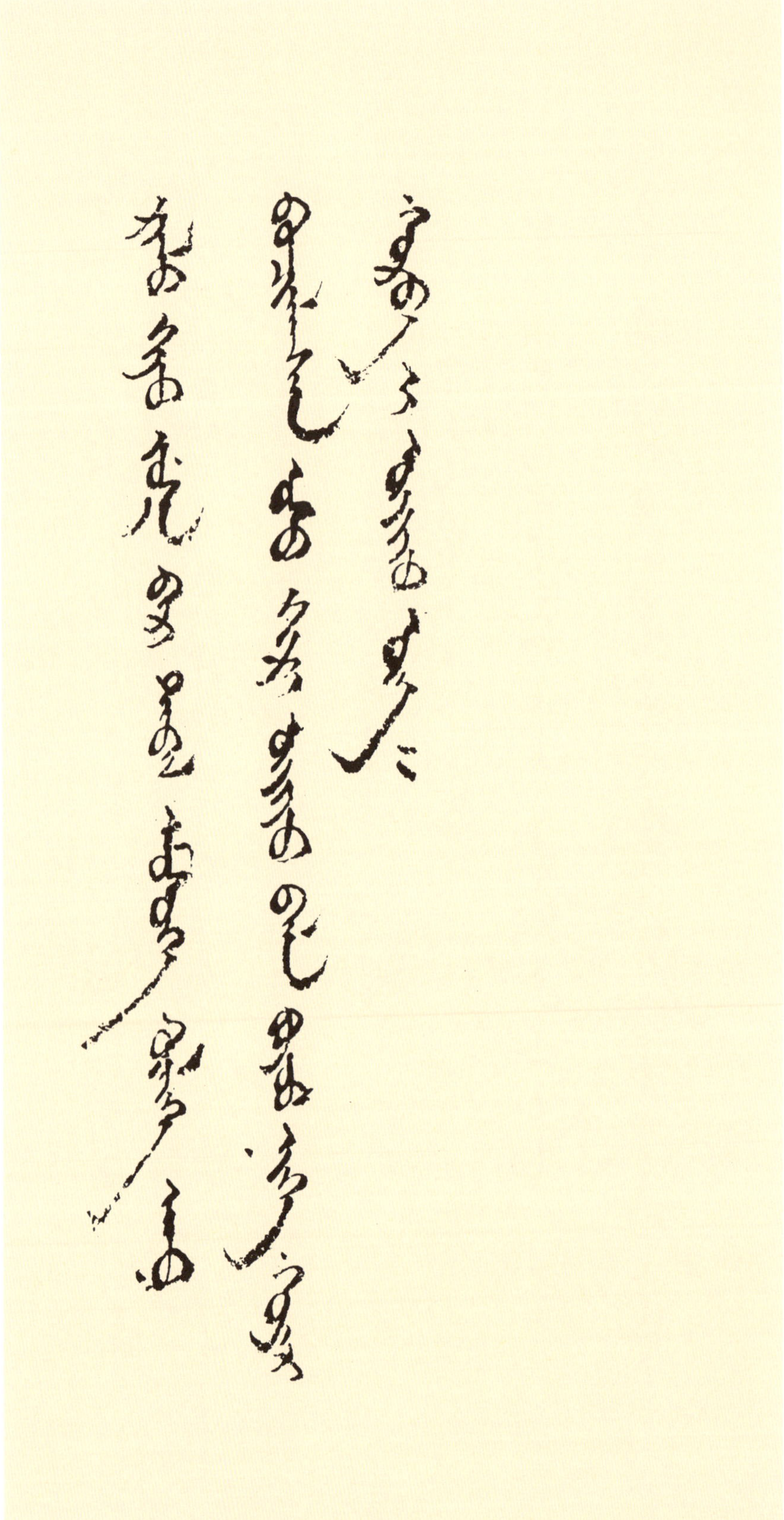

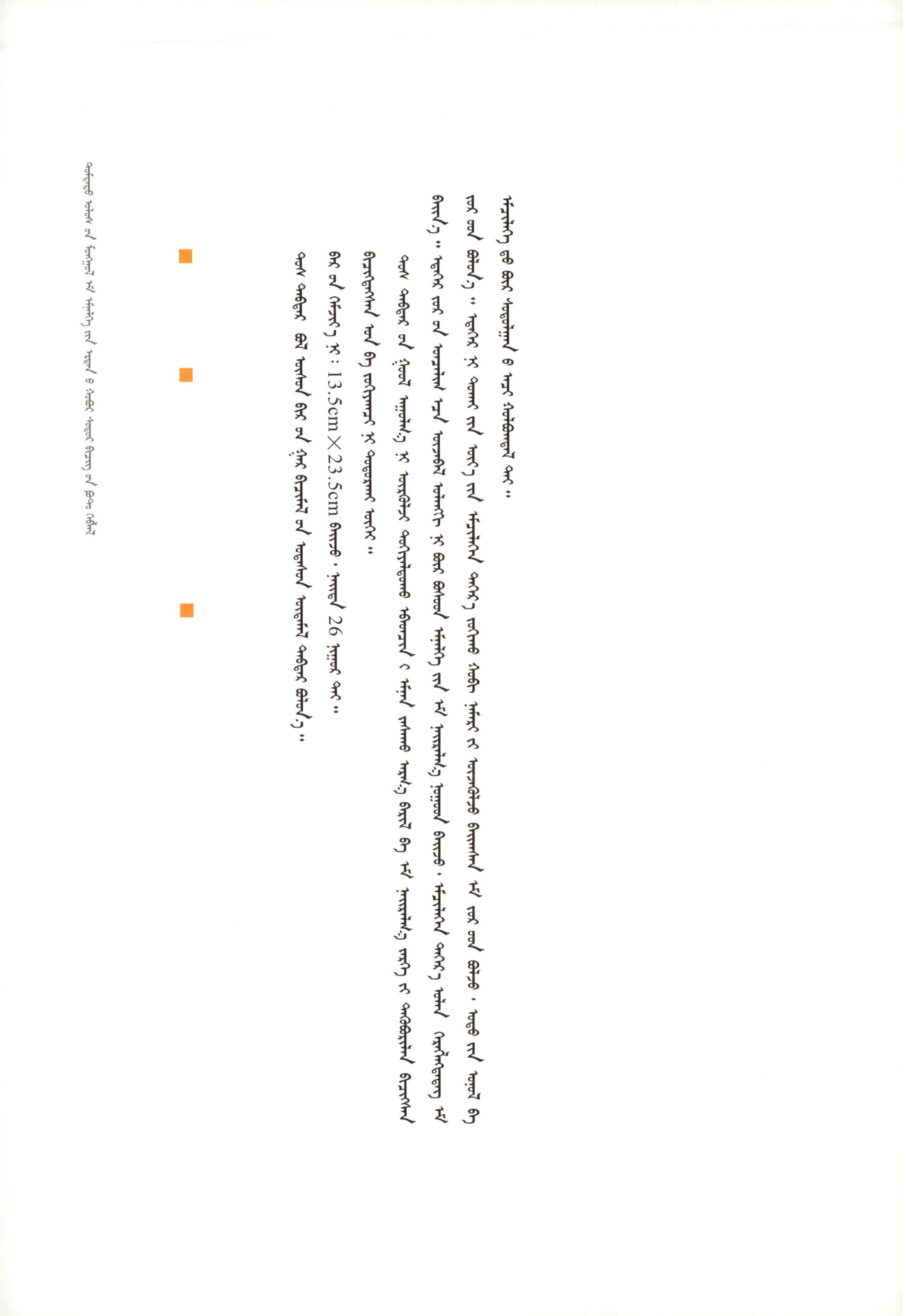

ᠨᠣᠮ ᠤᠨ ᠬᠡᠮᠵᠢᠶ᠎ᠡ ᠨᠢ : 13.5cm × 23.5cm ᠪᠣᠯᠤᠭᠠᠳ · ᠨᠢᠭᠤᠷ 26 ᠨᠢᠭᠤᠷ ᠲᠠᠢ ::

7

太医院七十二症奇方（一）

72 Prescriptions of Imperial Academy of Medicine (1)

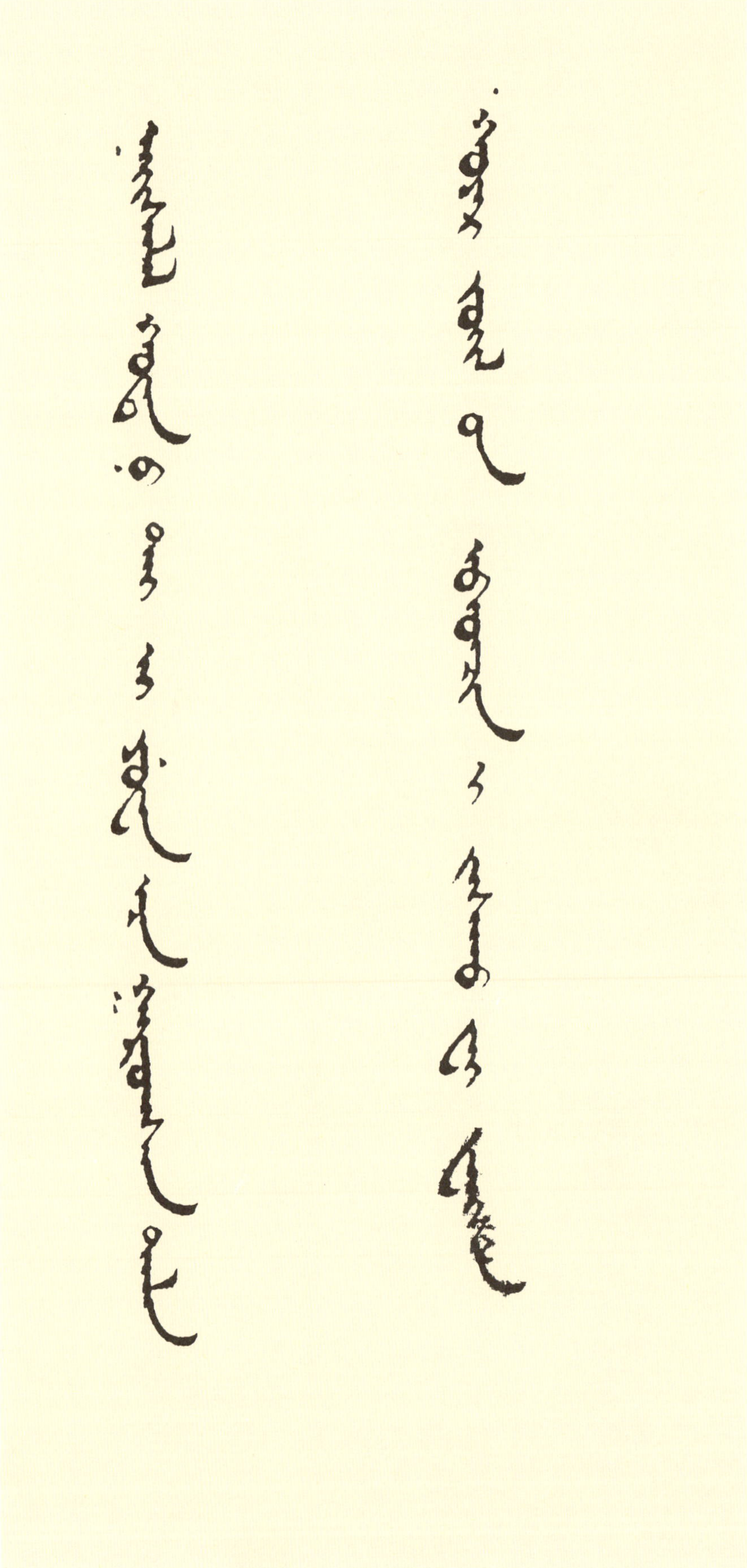

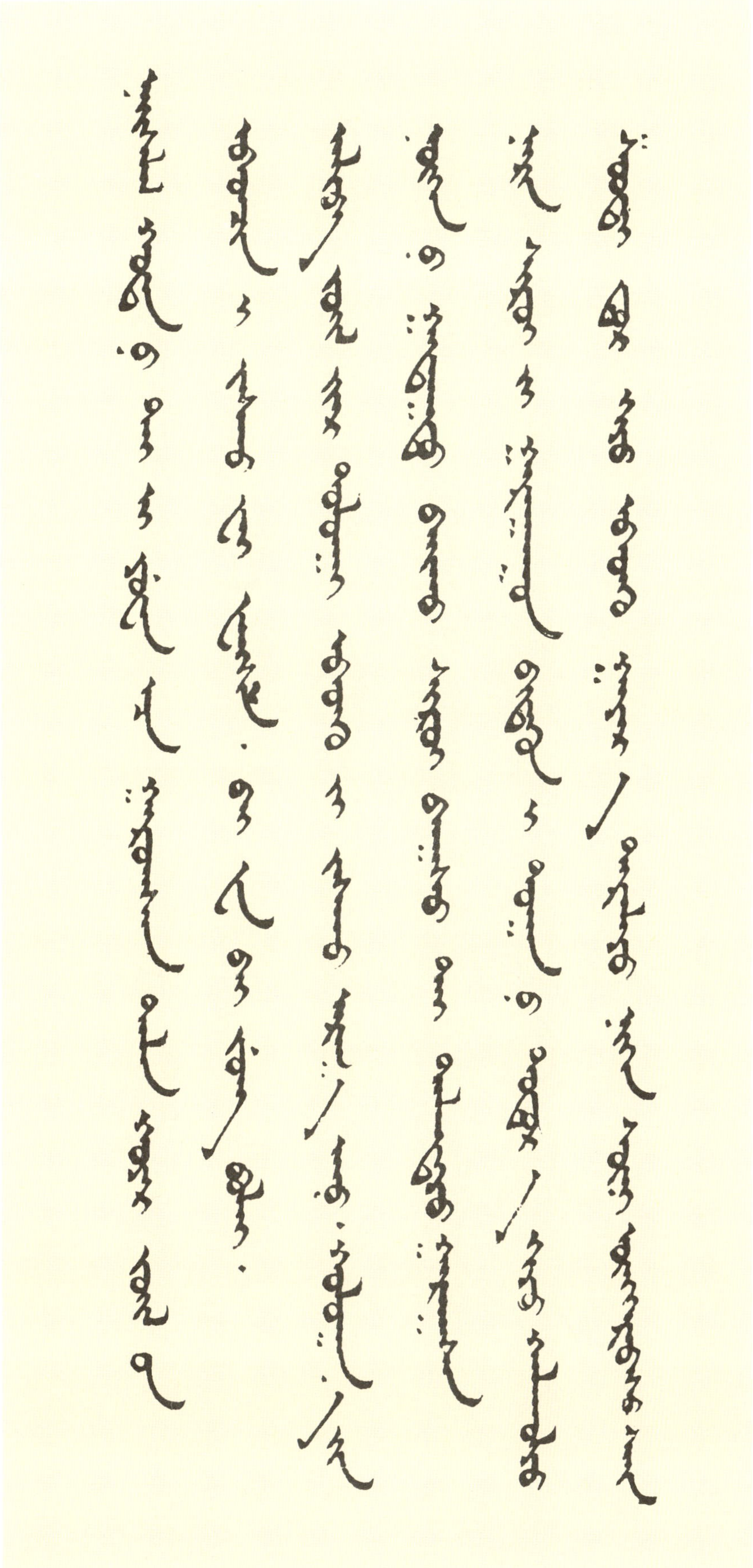

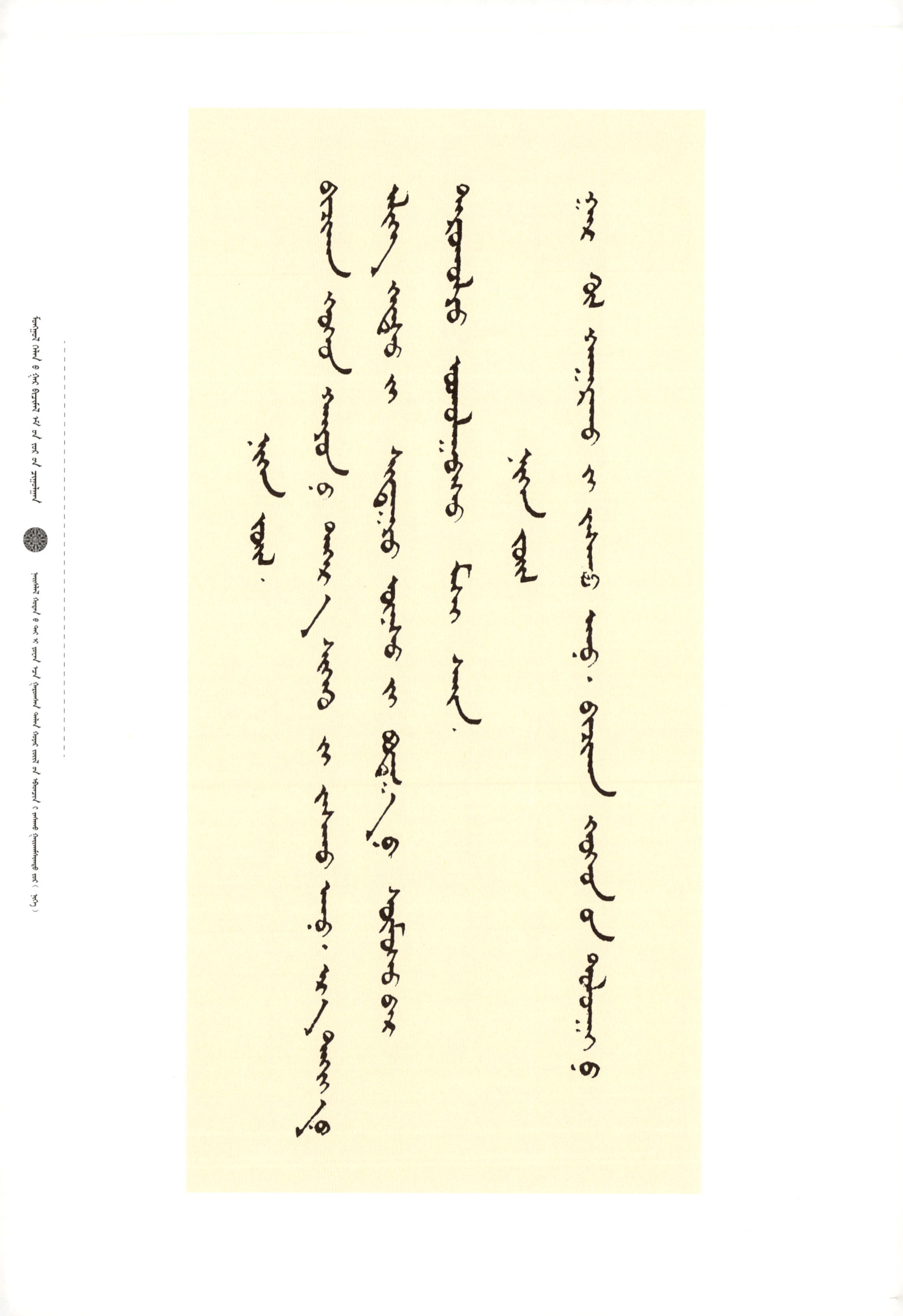

[illegible]

[illegible]

[illegible]

[illegible]

[illegible]

[illegible]

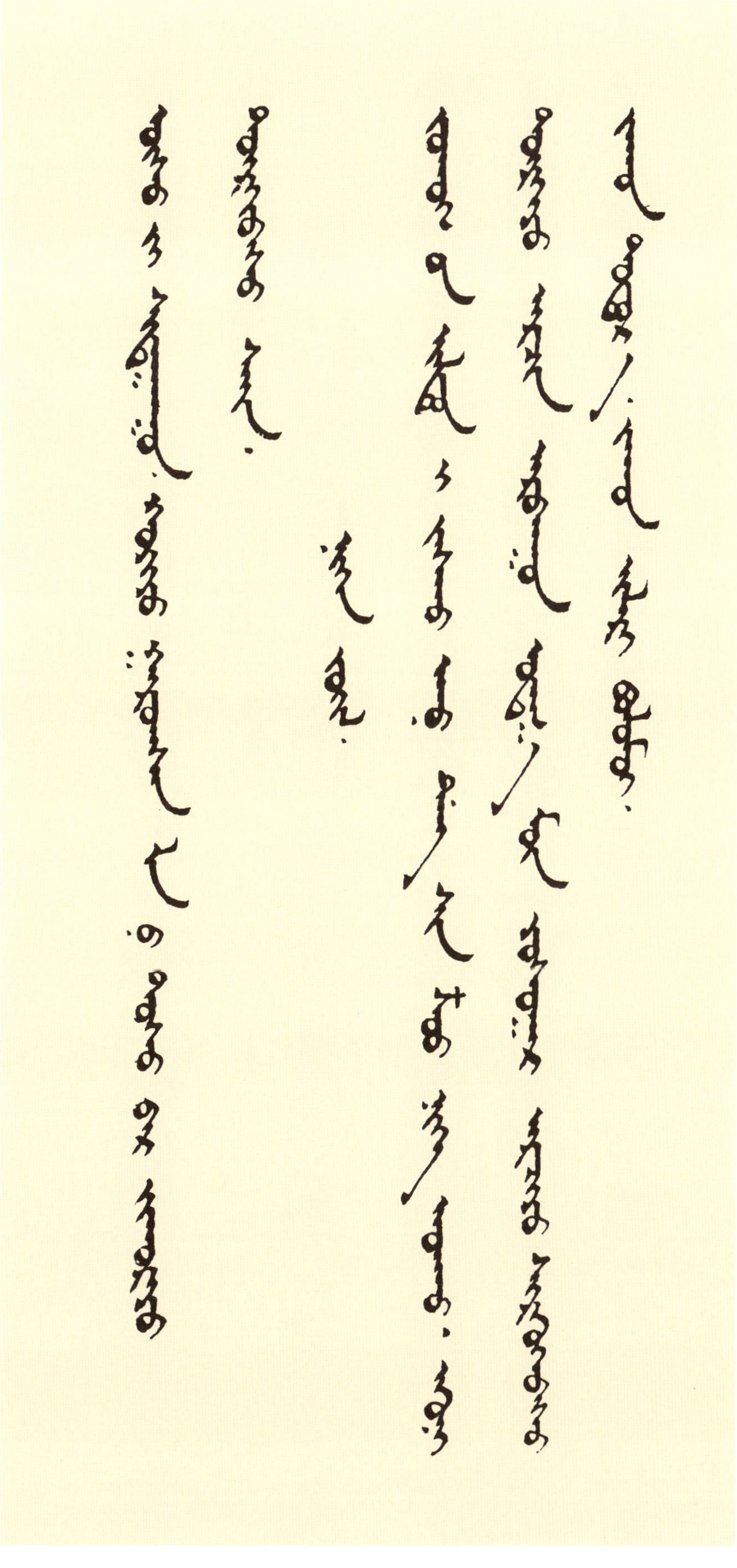

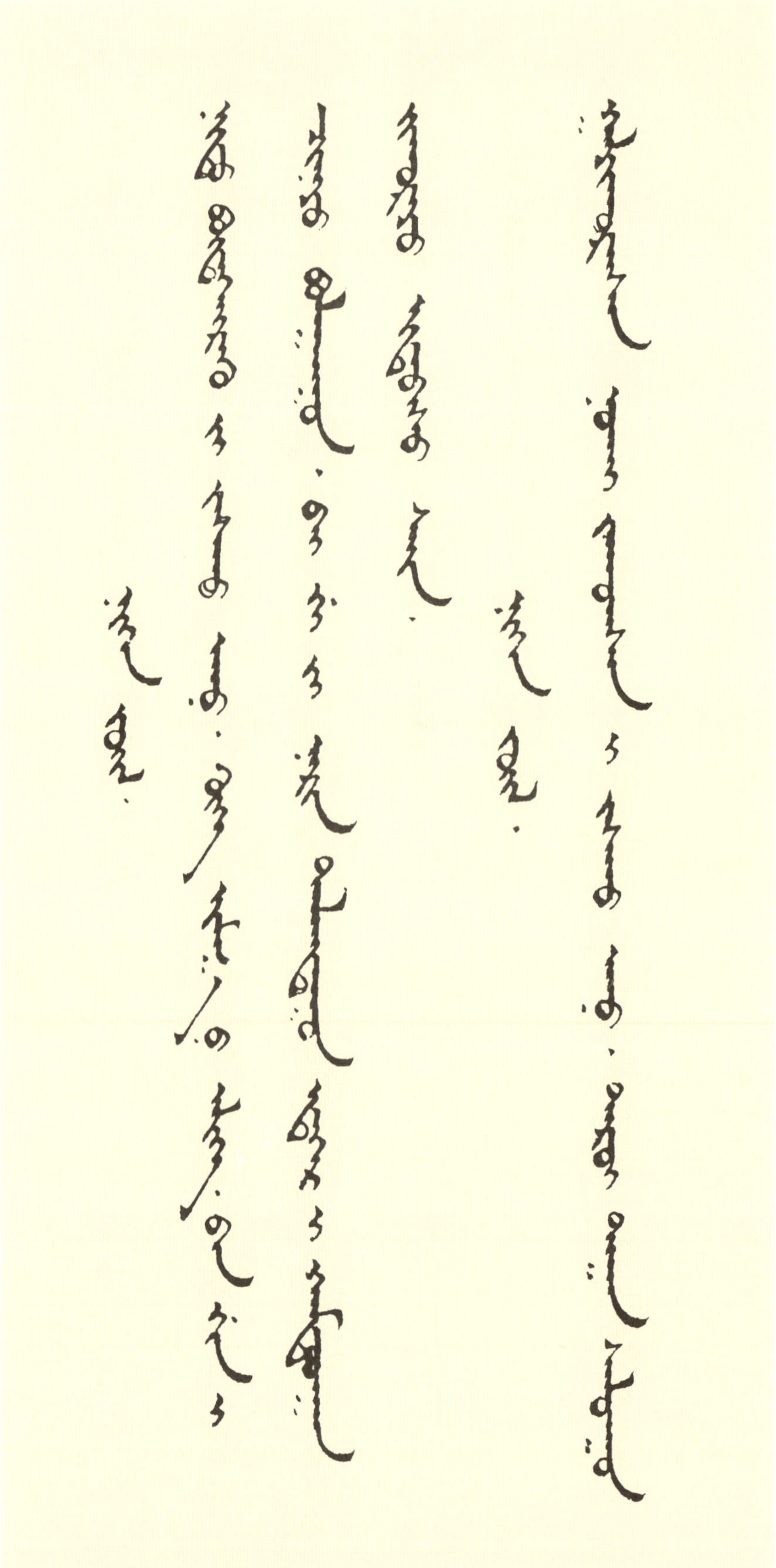

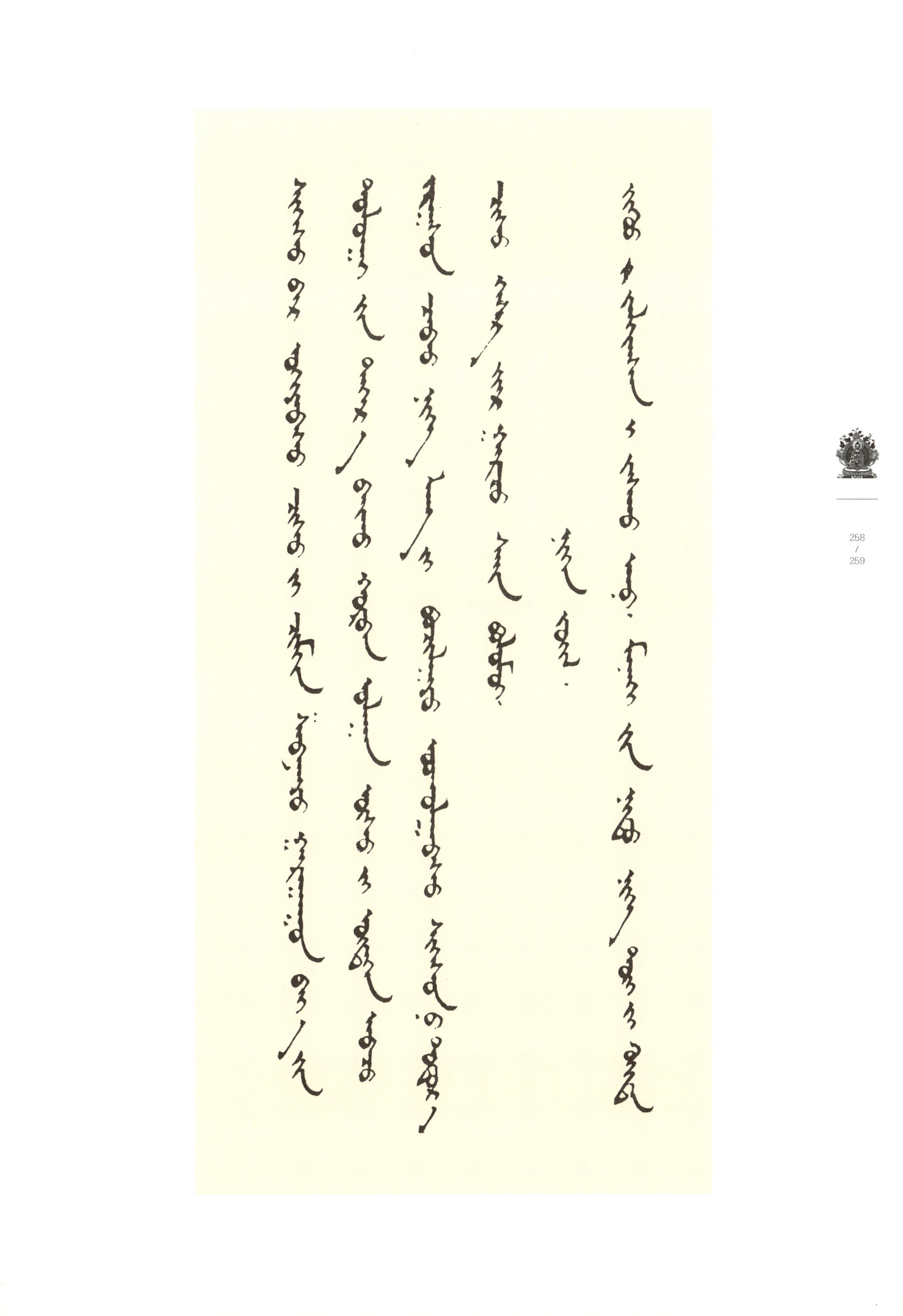

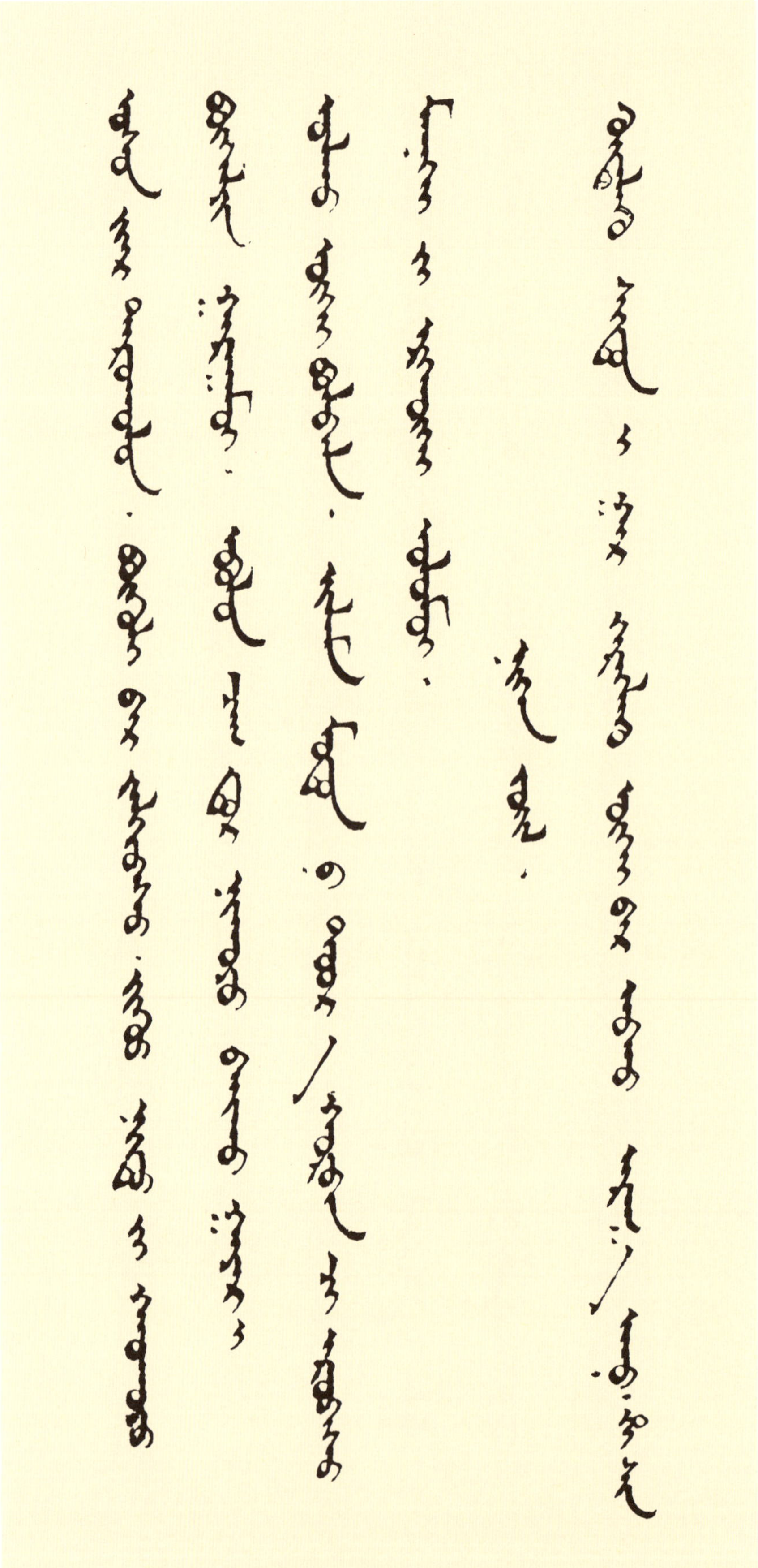

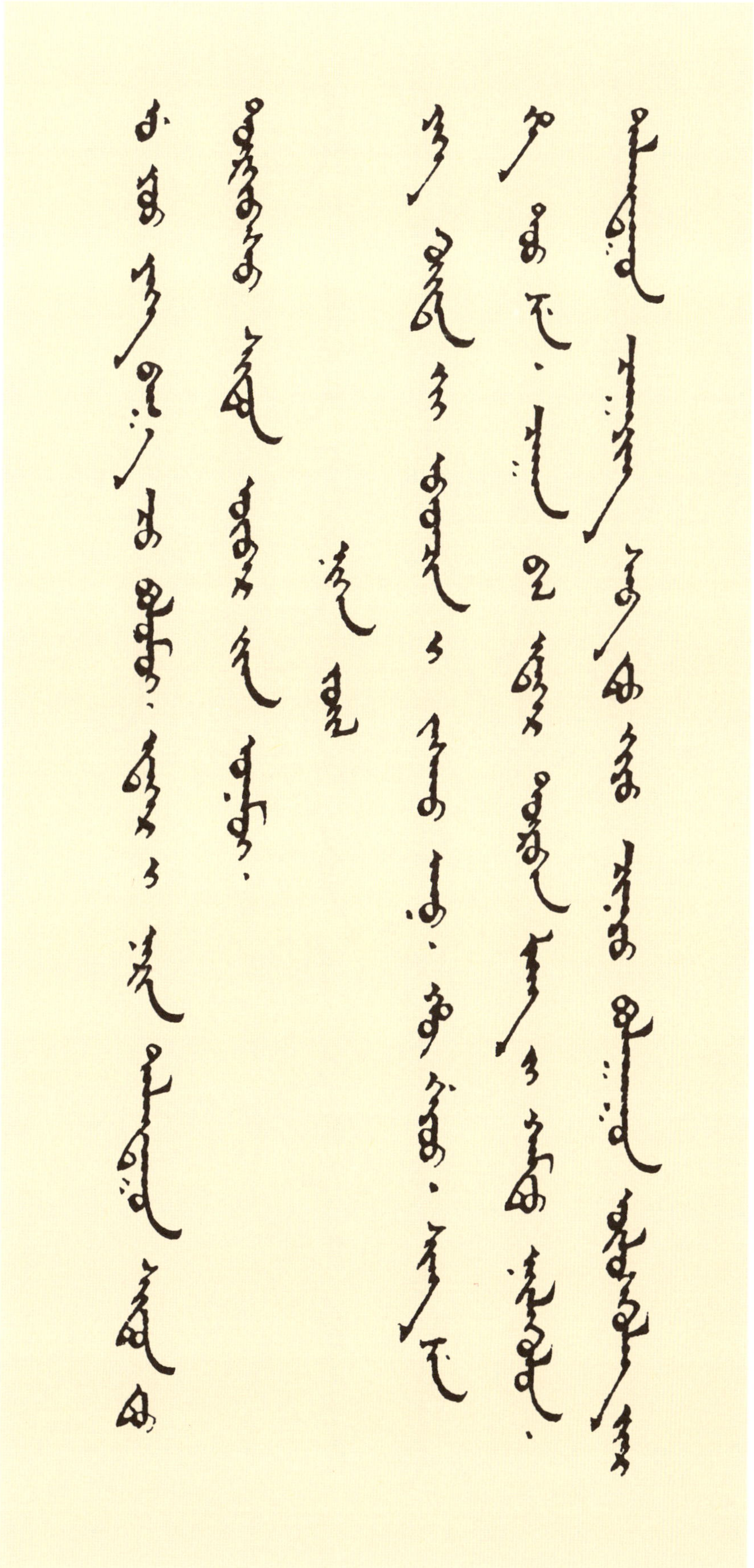

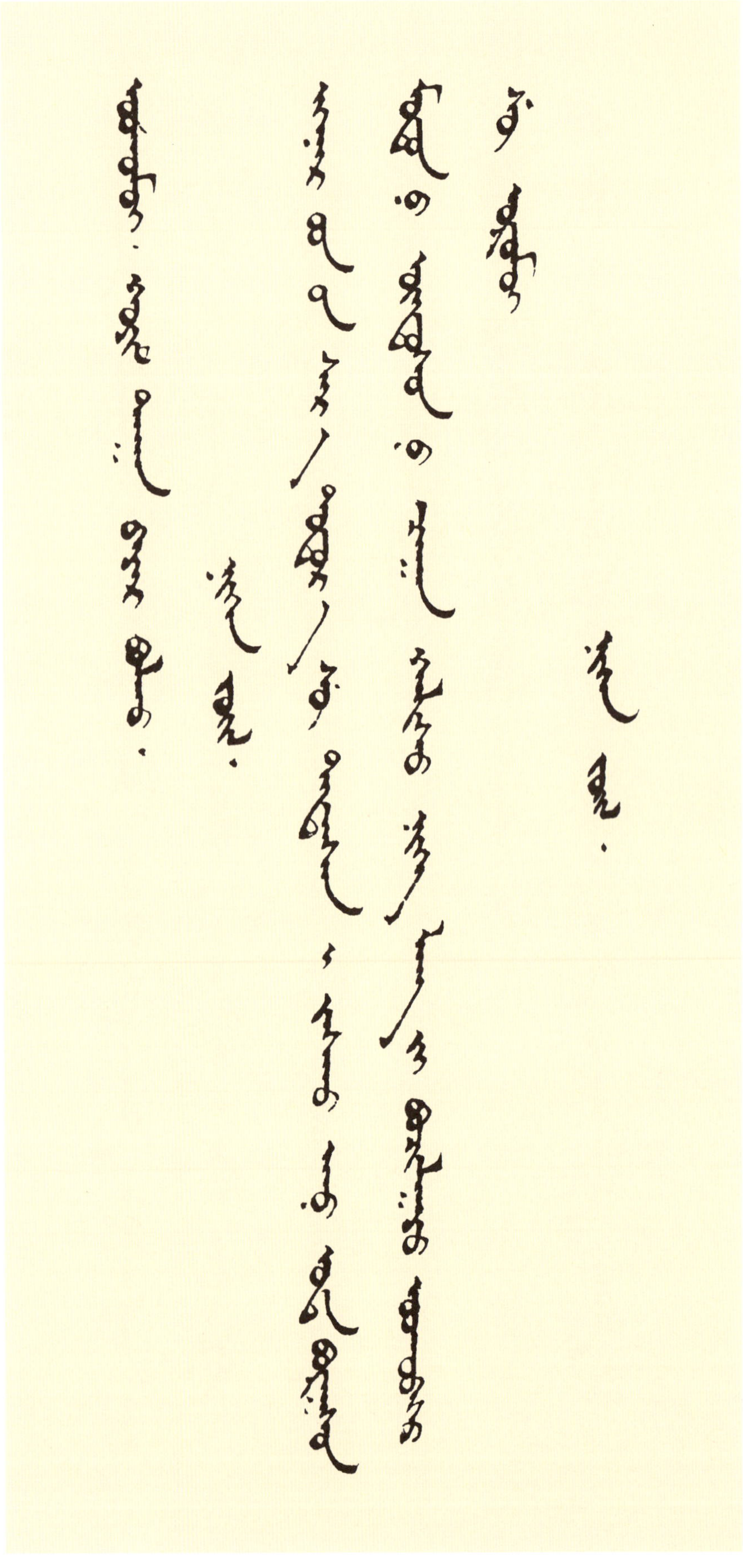

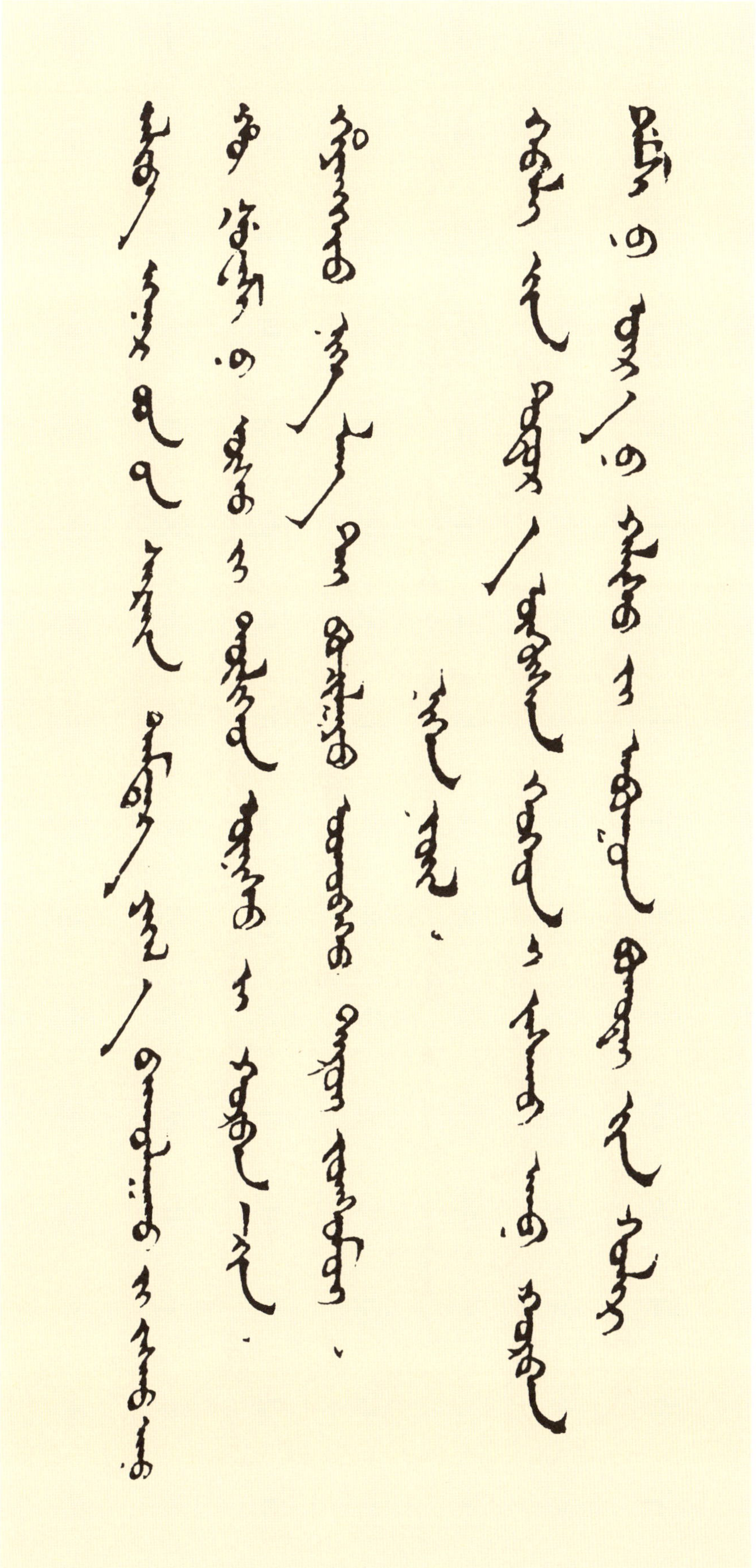

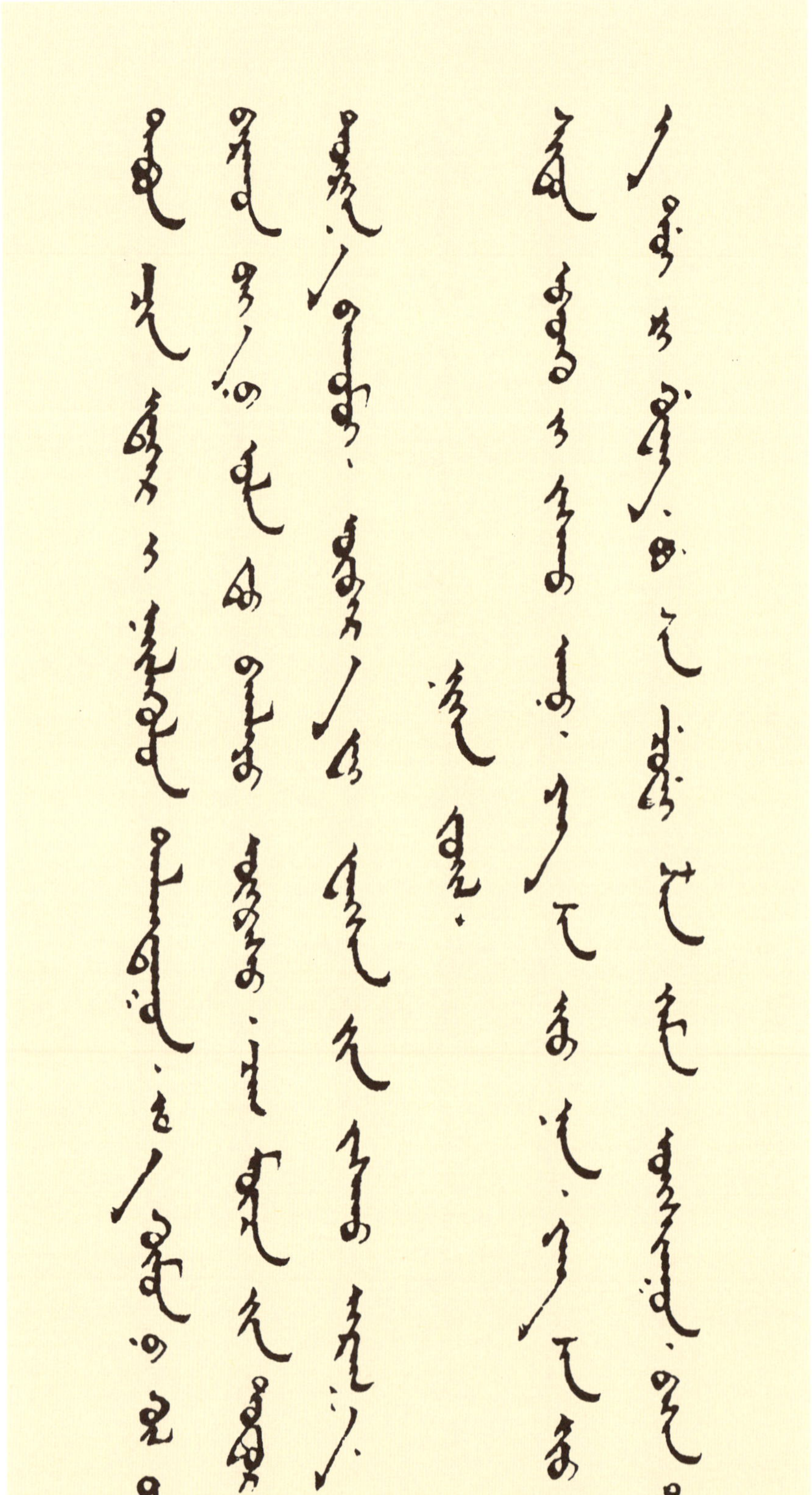

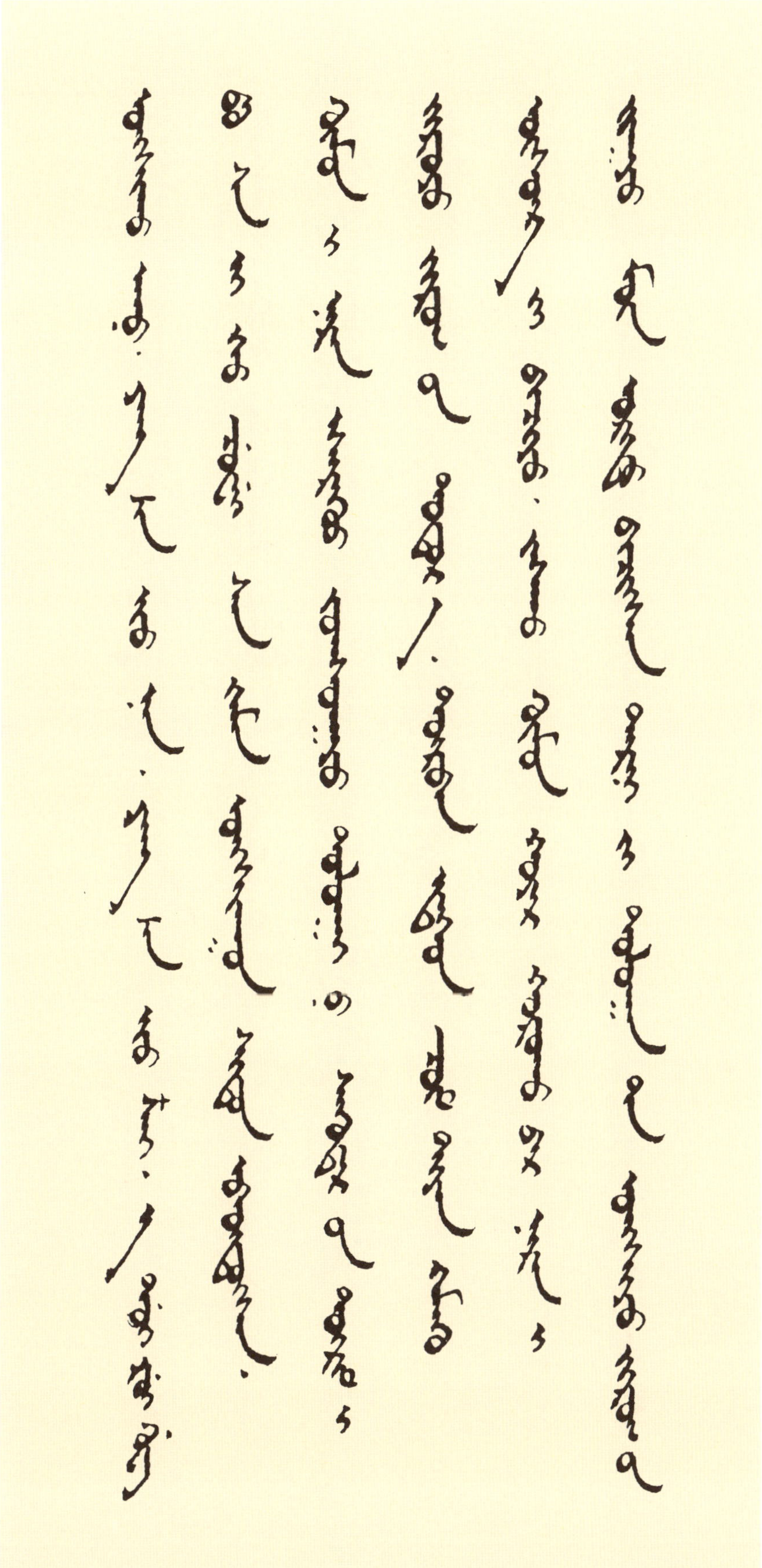

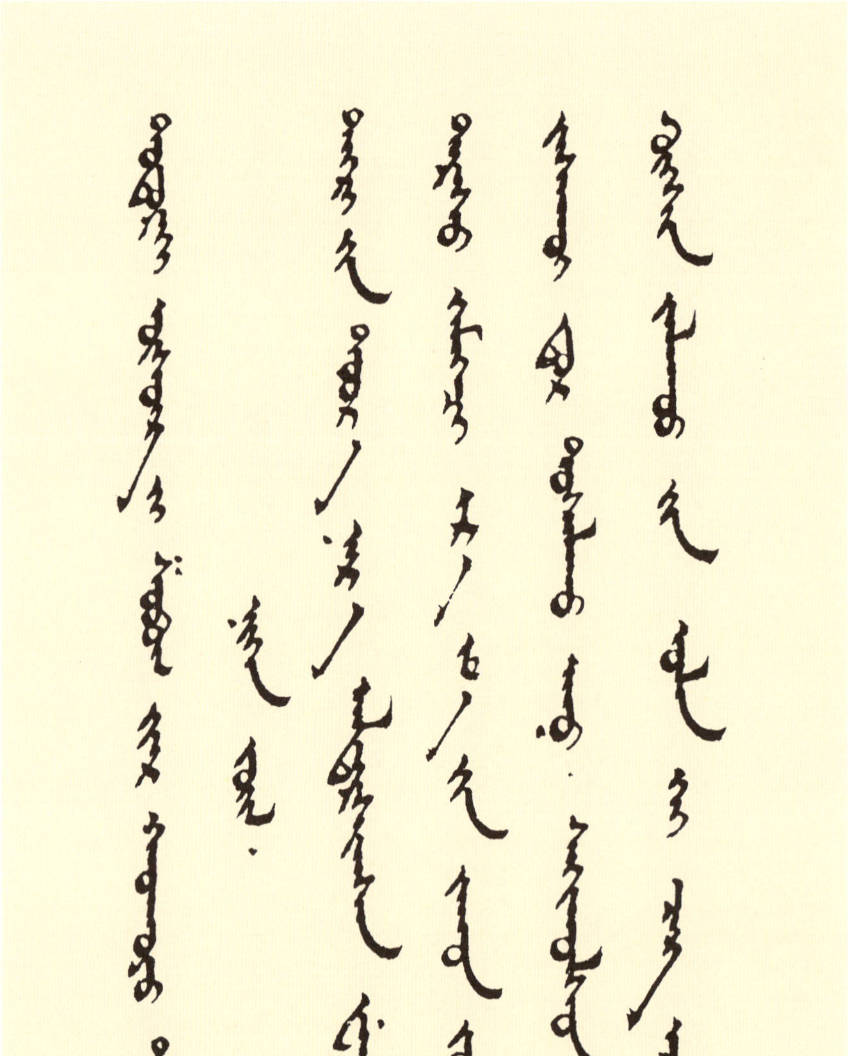

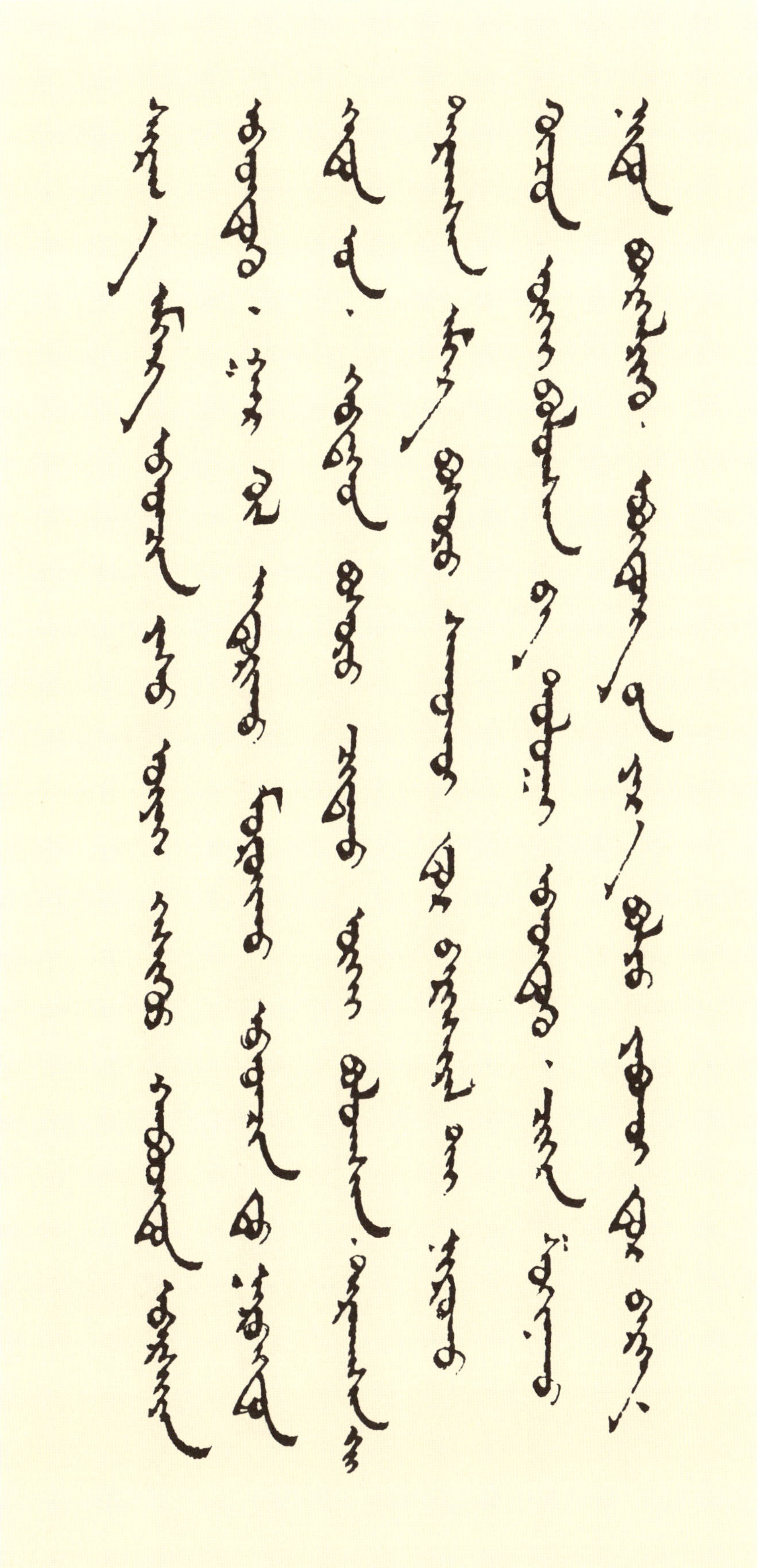

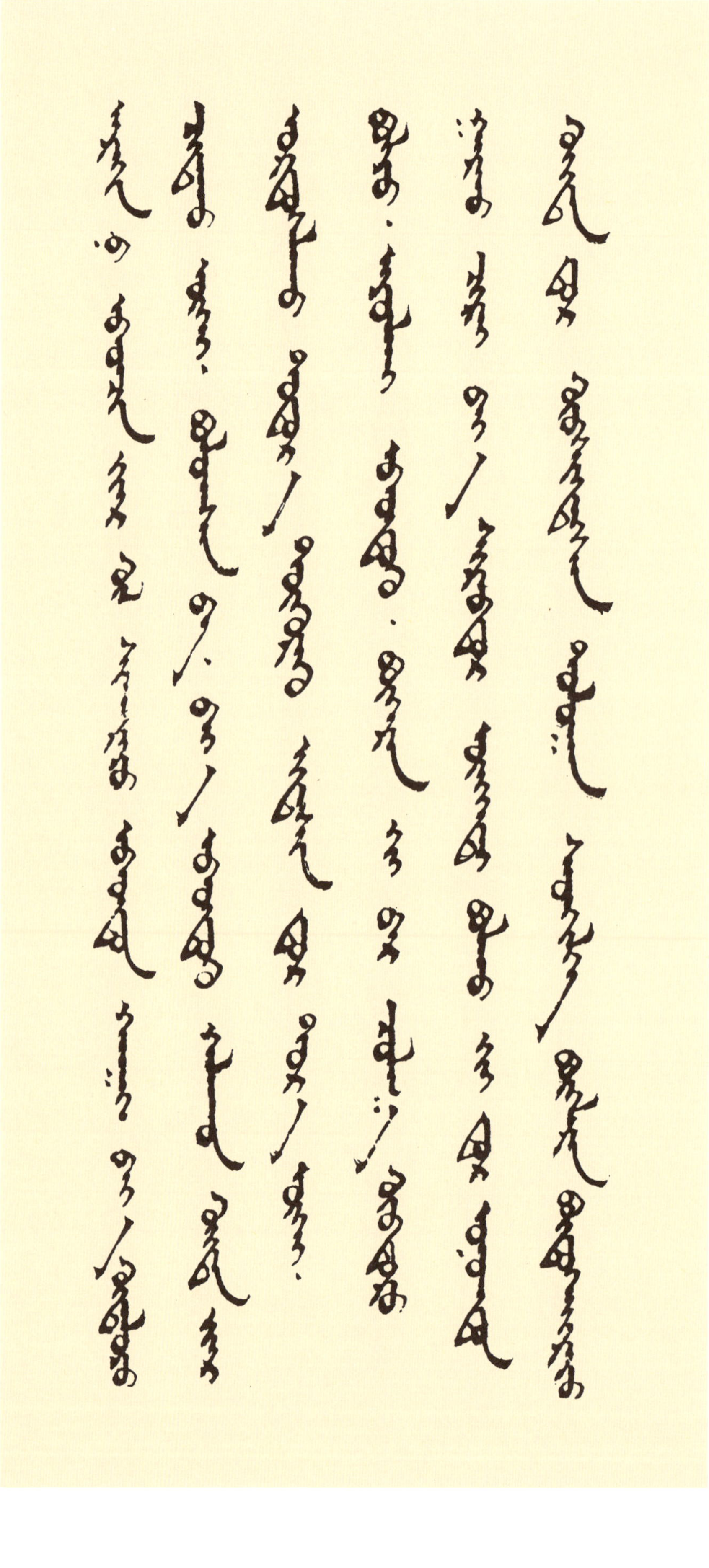

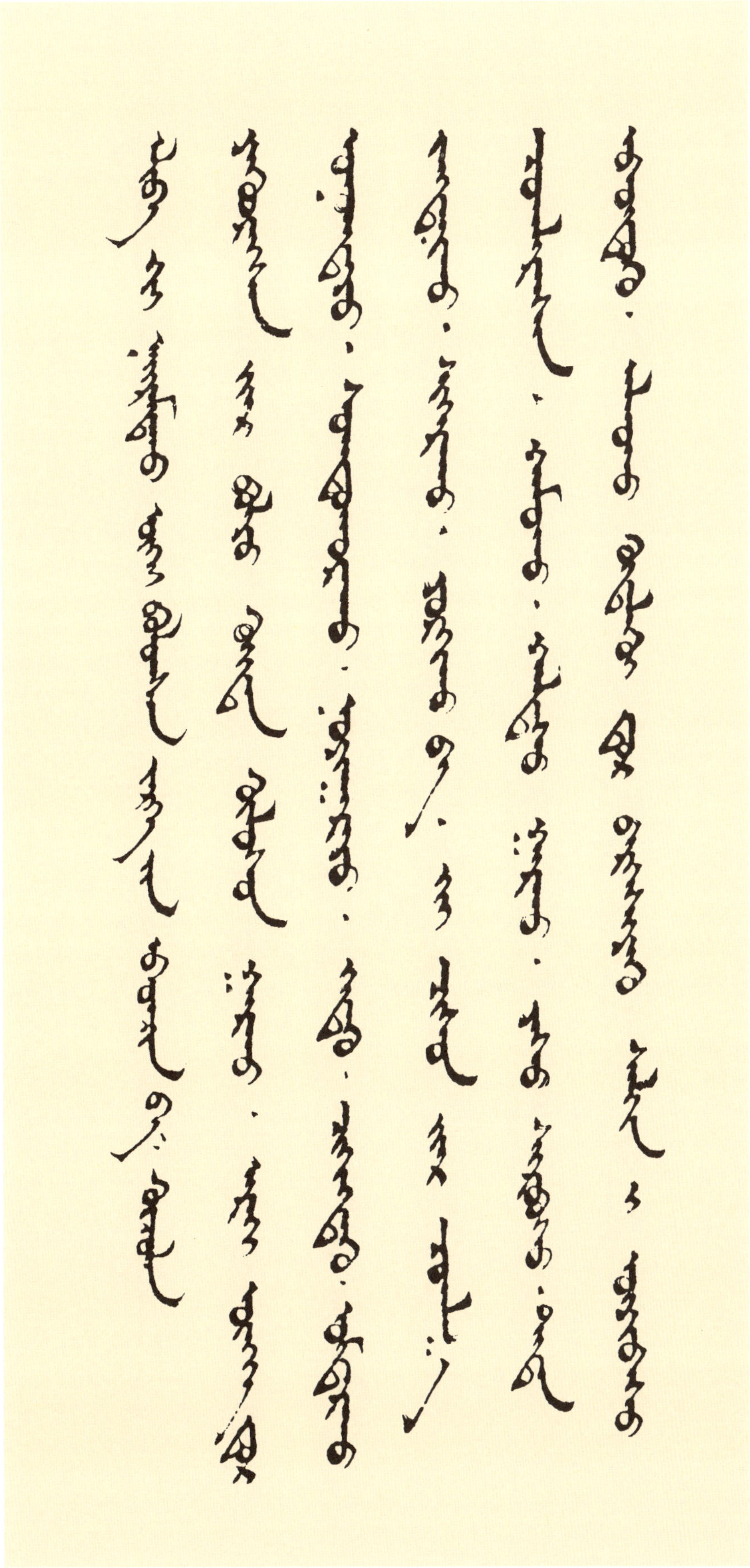

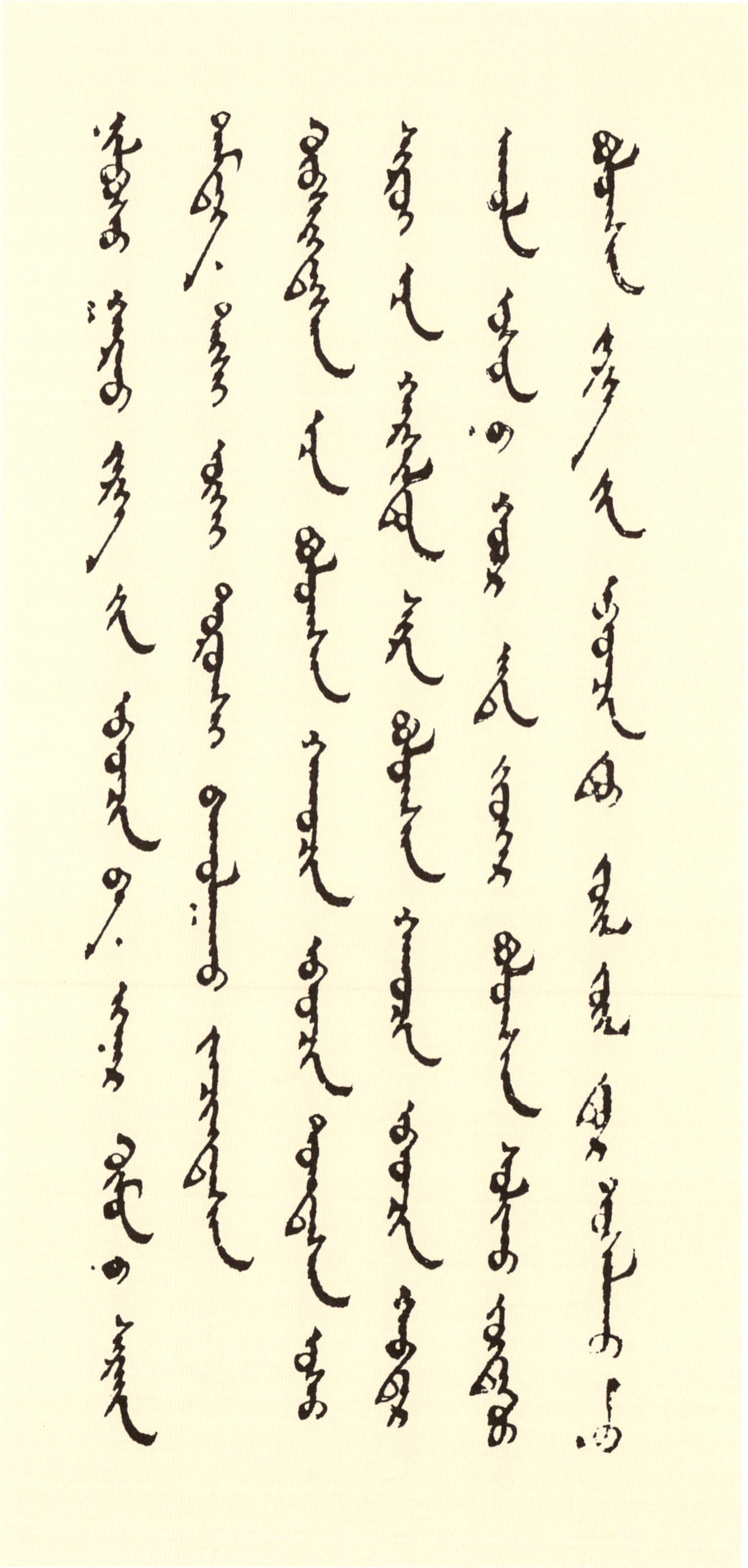

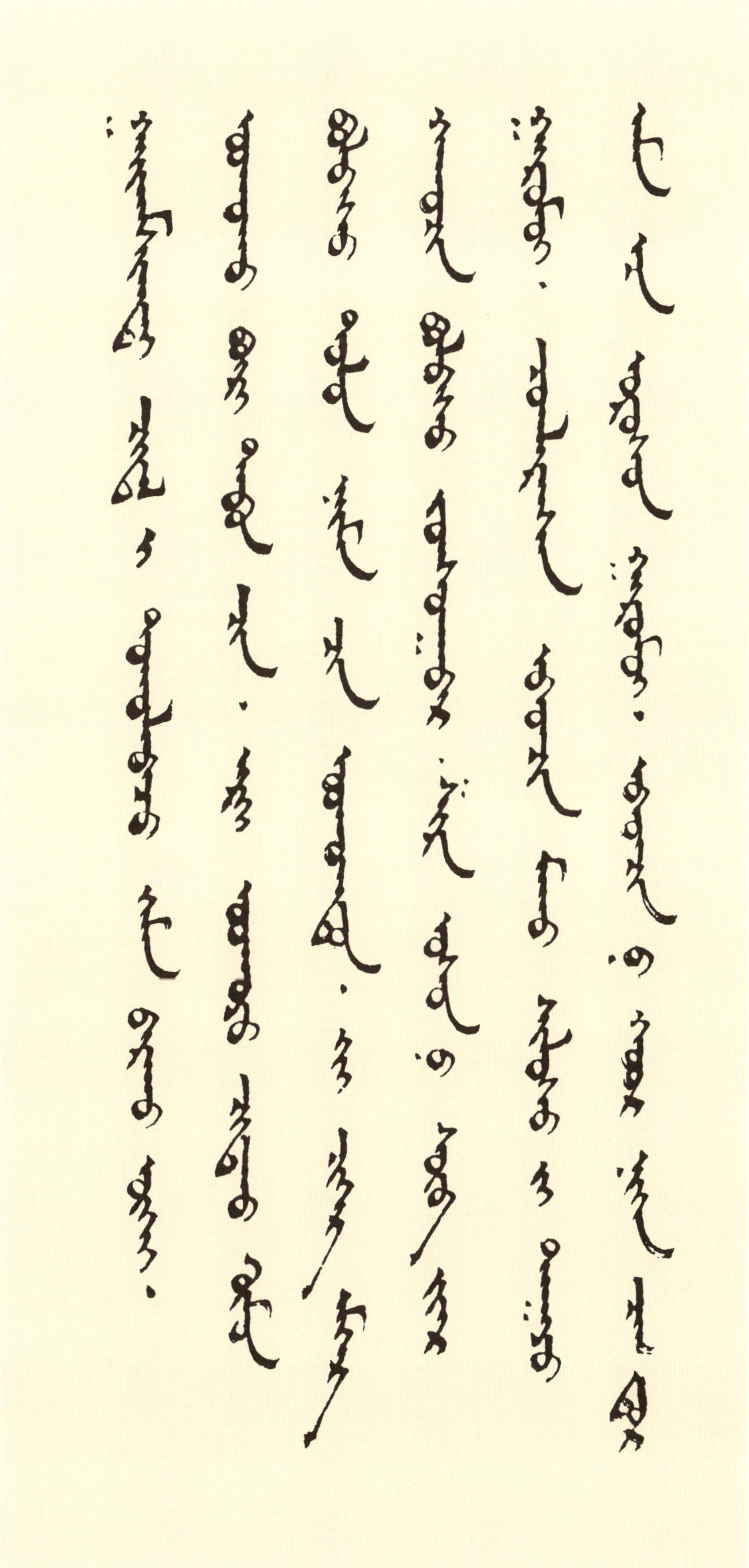

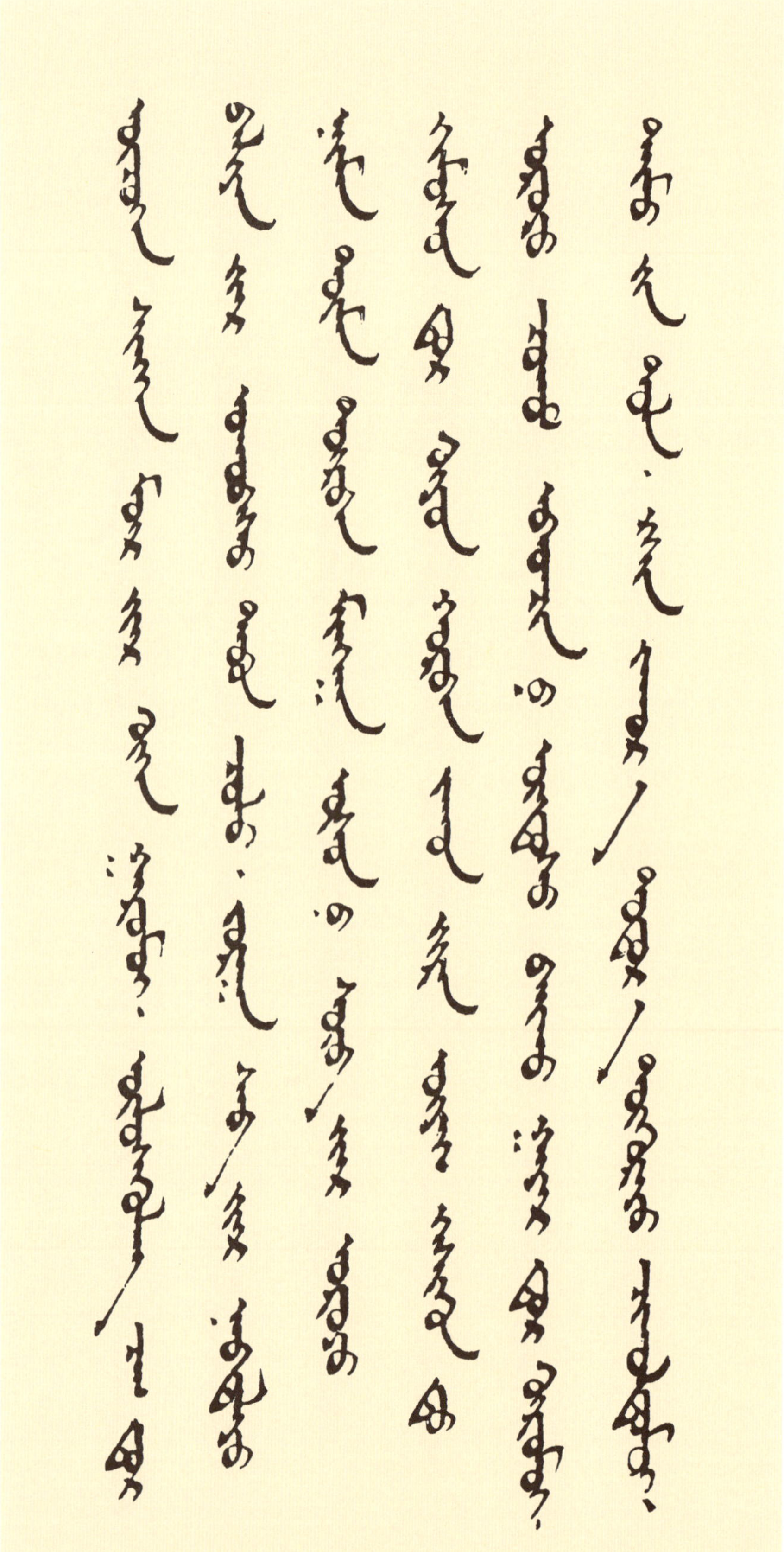

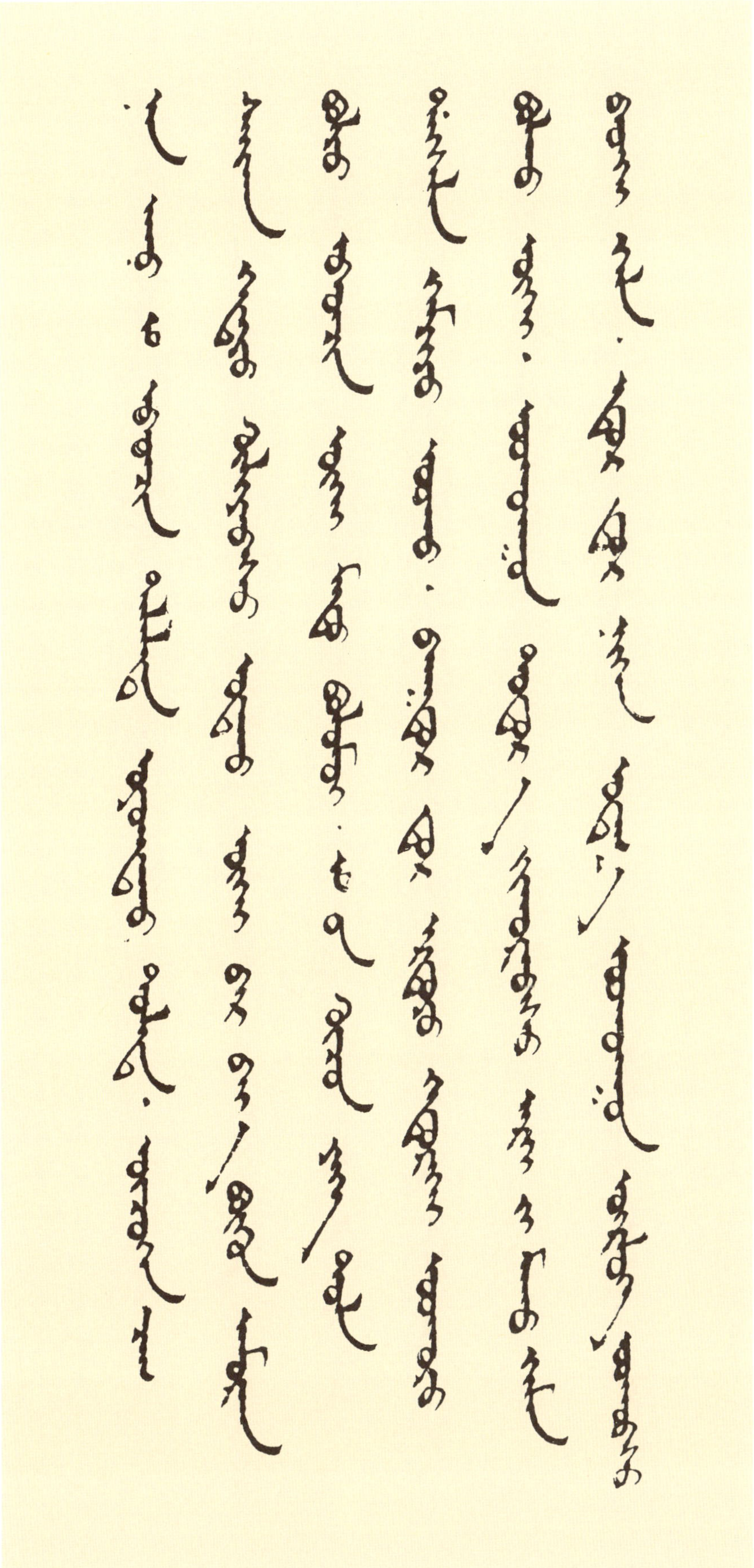

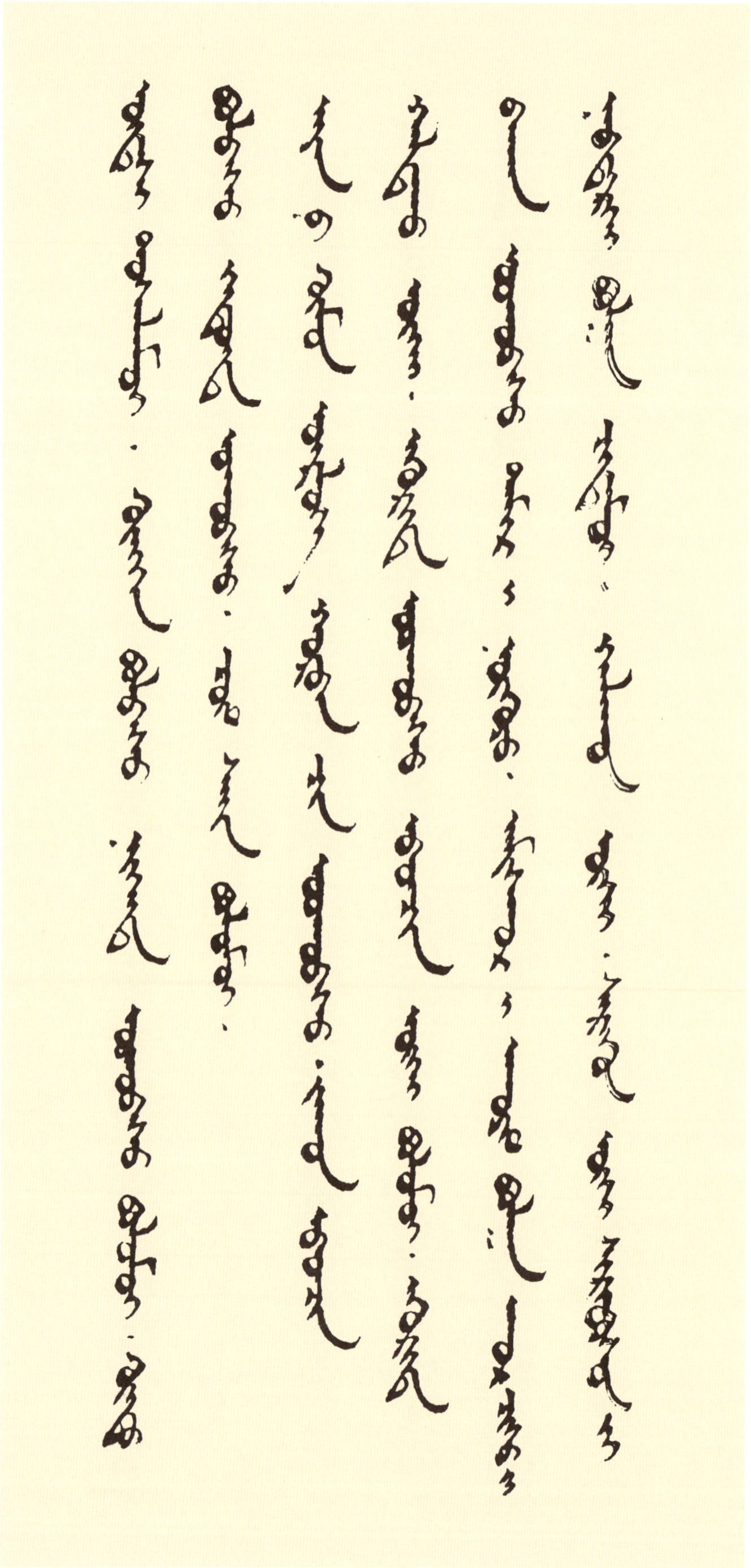

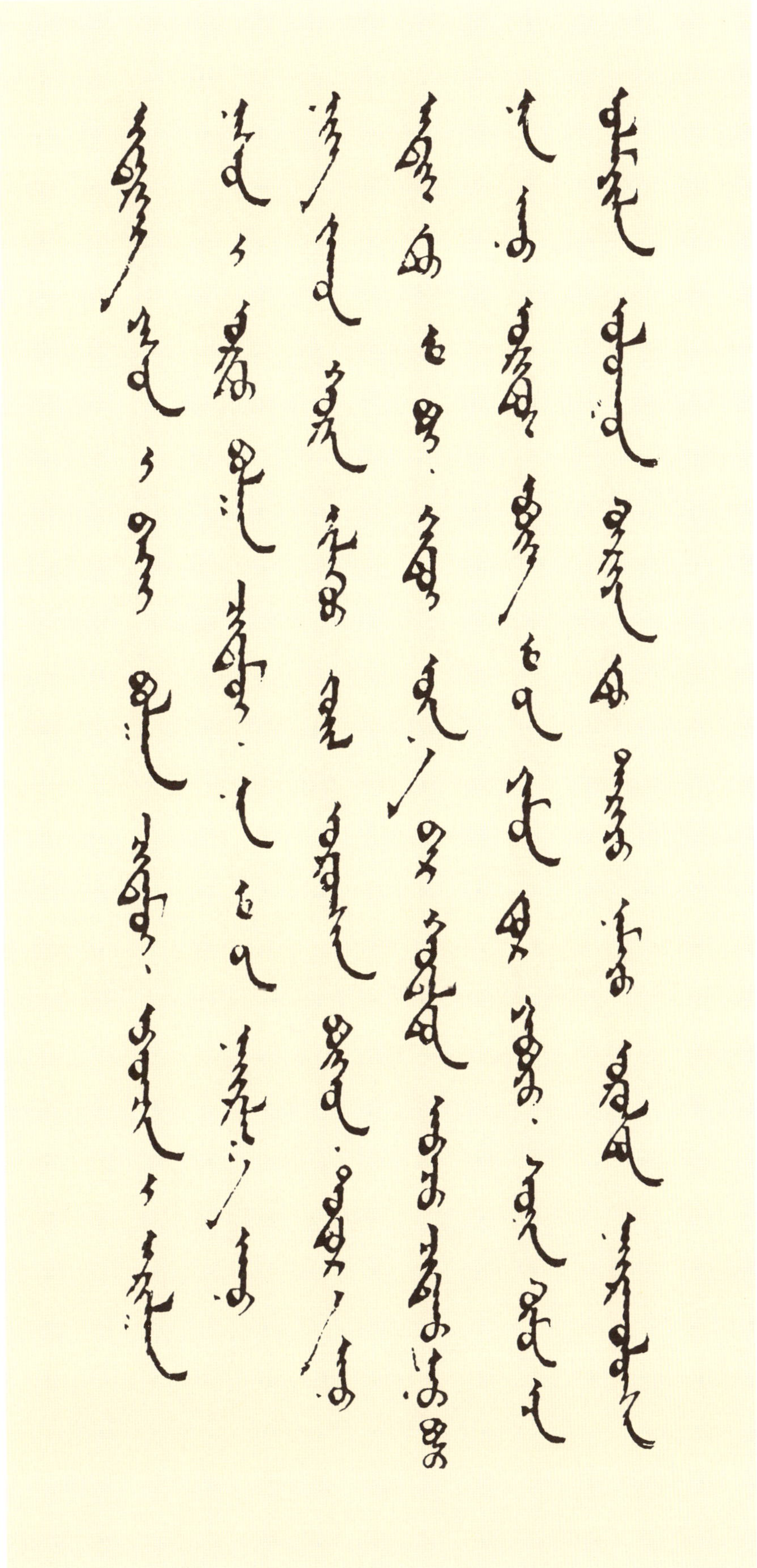

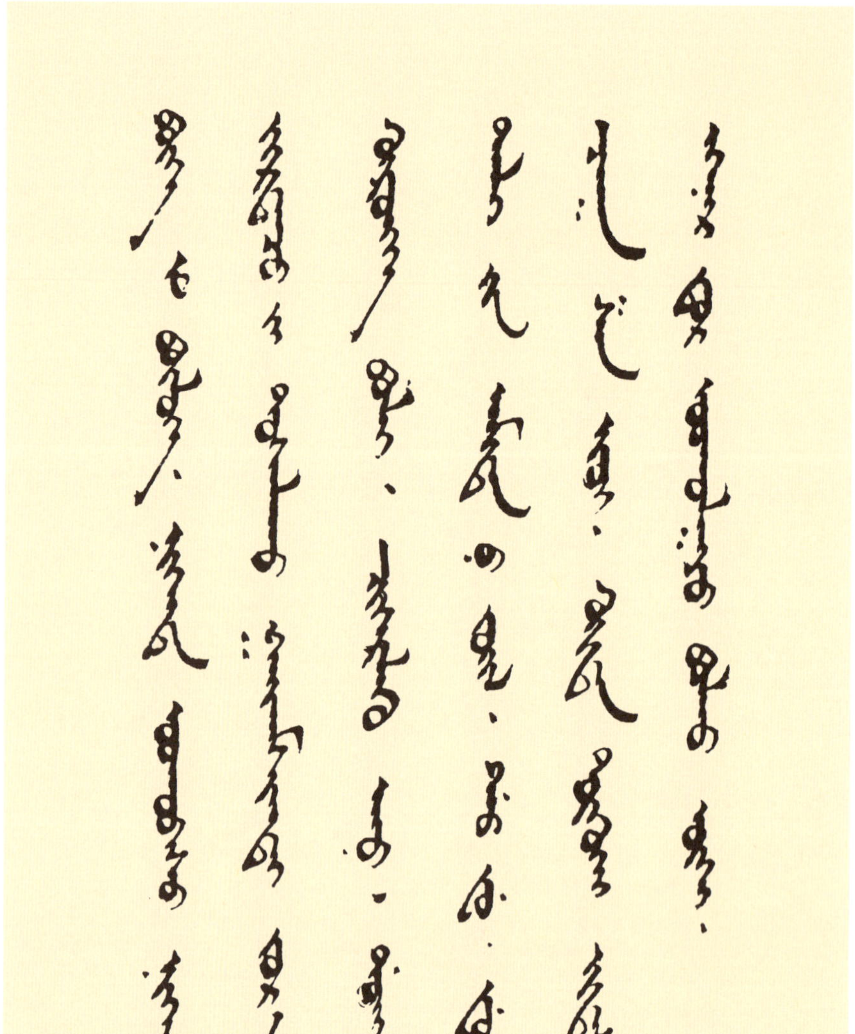

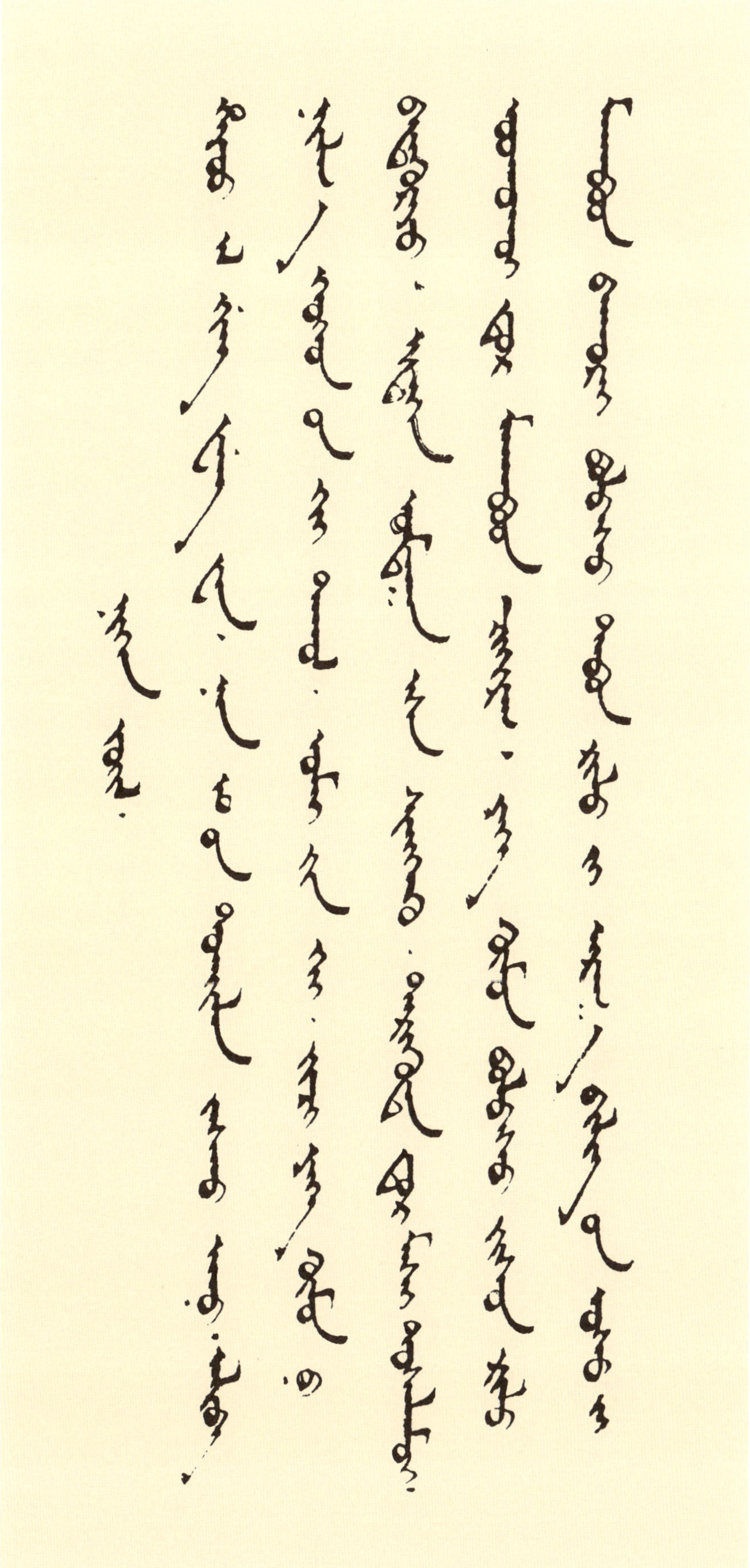

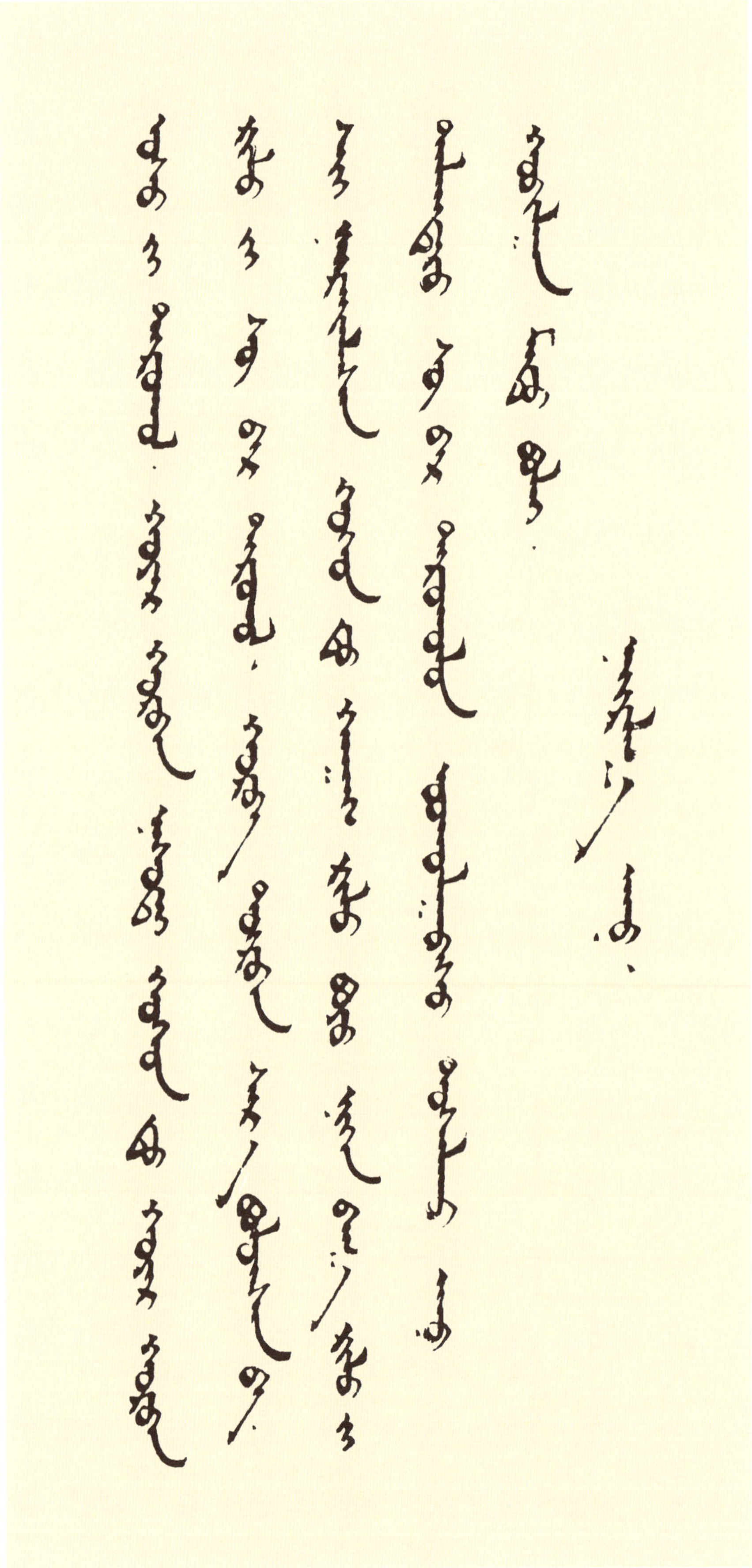

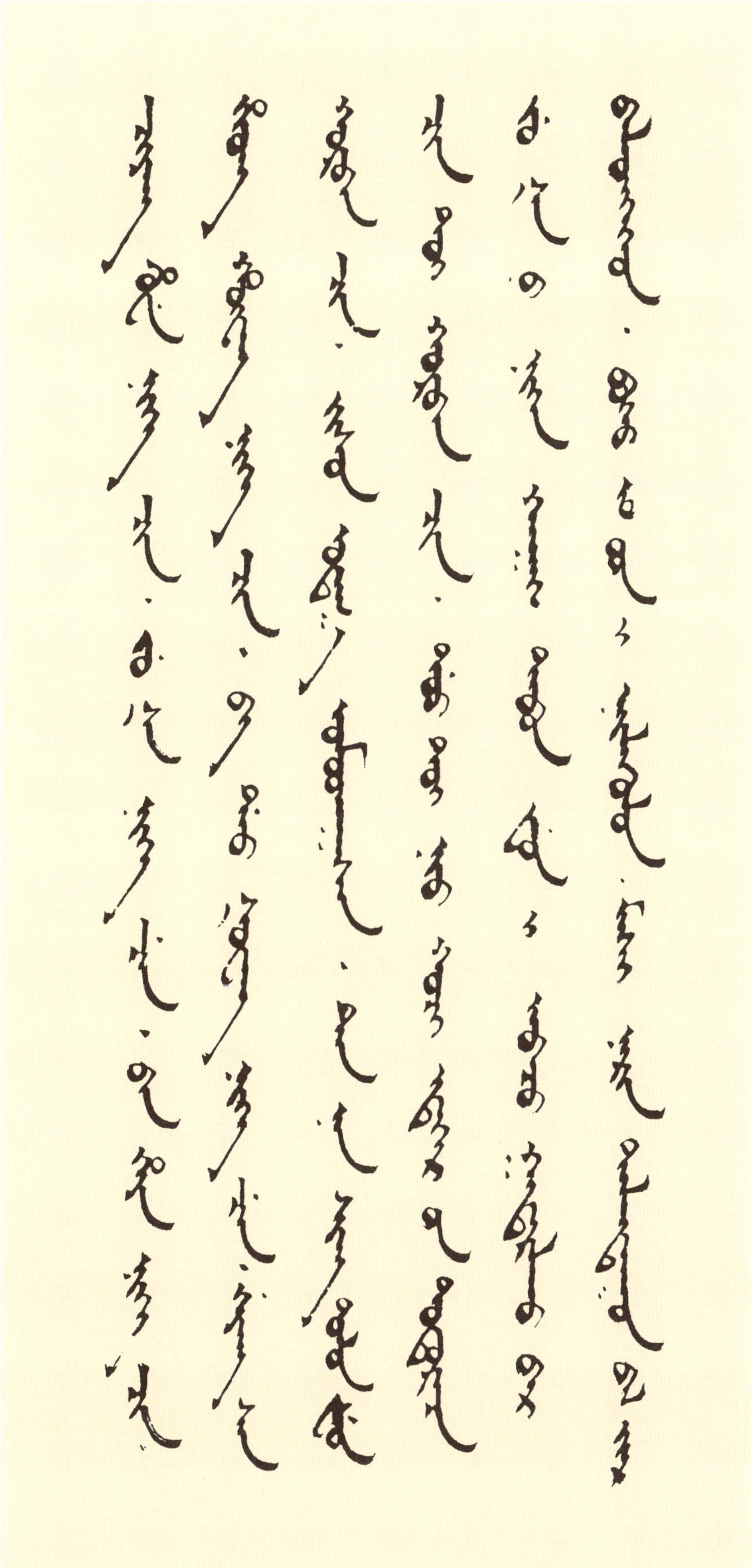

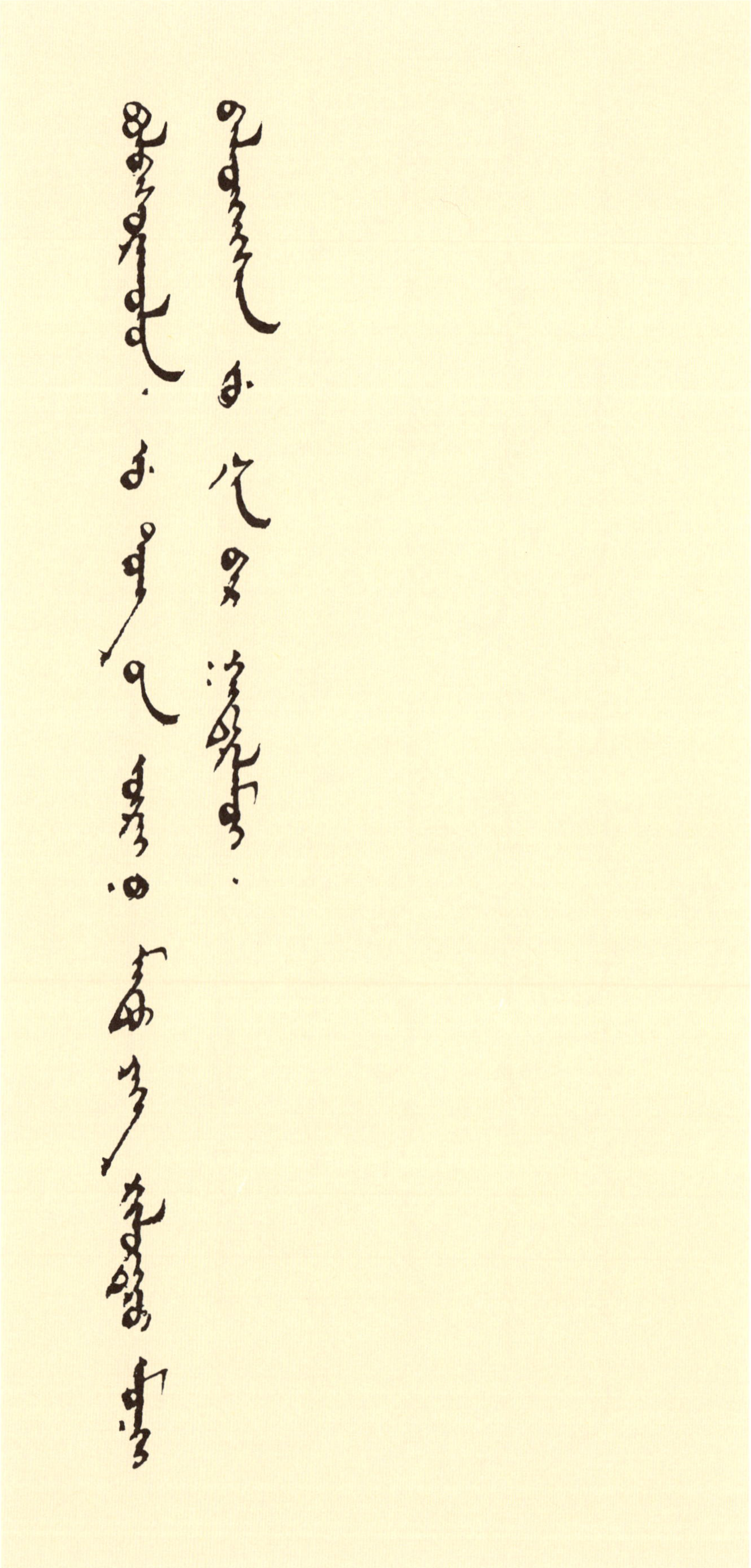

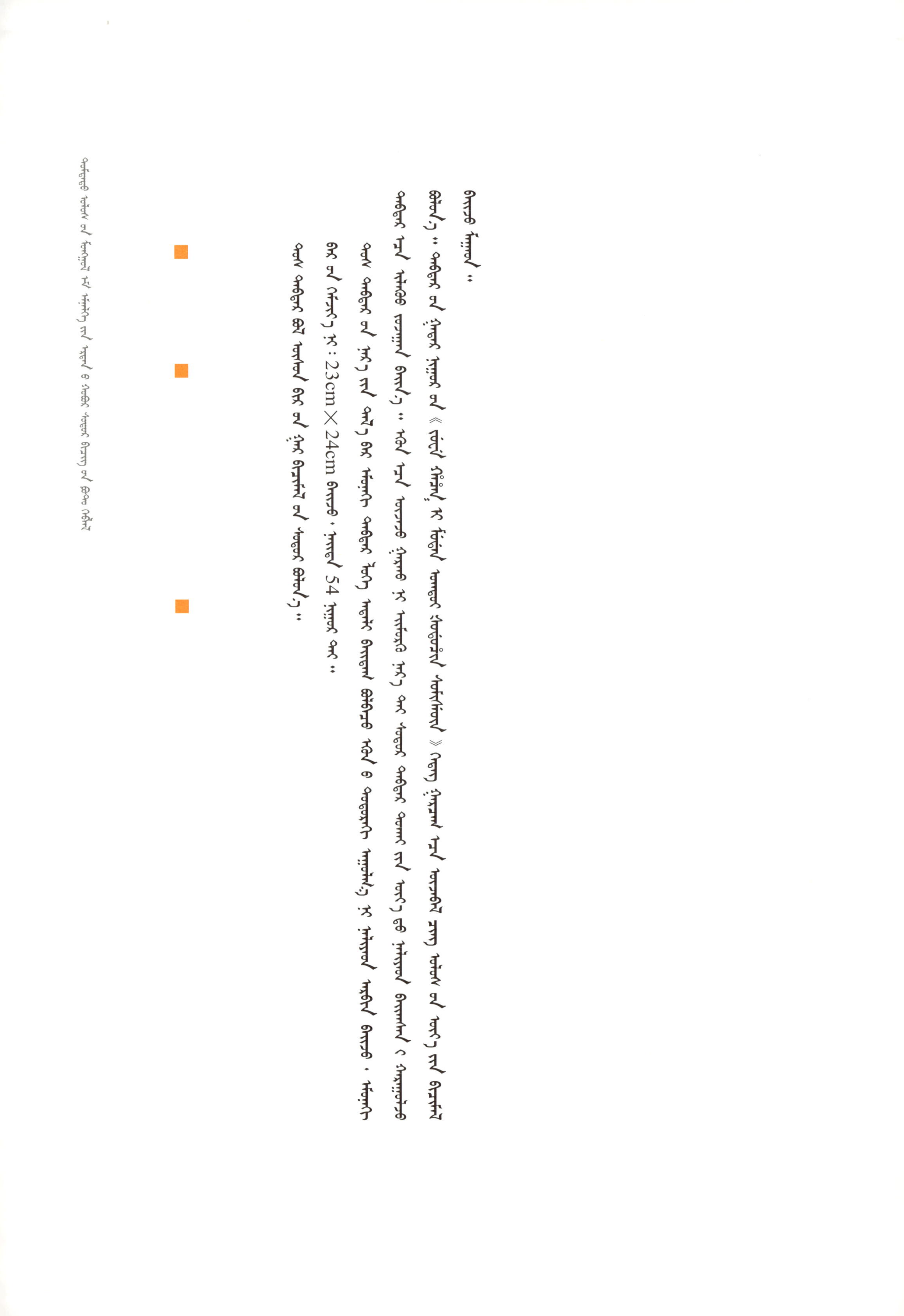

ᠬᠡᠪ ᠦᠨ ᠬᠡᠮᠵᠢᠶ᠎ᠡ ᠨᠢ : 23cm × 24cm ᠪᠣᠯᠤᠨ᠎ᠠ ᠂ ᠨᠡᠶᠢᠲᠡ 54 ᠨᠢᠭᠤᠷ ᠲᠠᠢ ::

太医院七十二症奇方（二）

72 Prescriptions of Imperial Academy of Medicine (2)

8

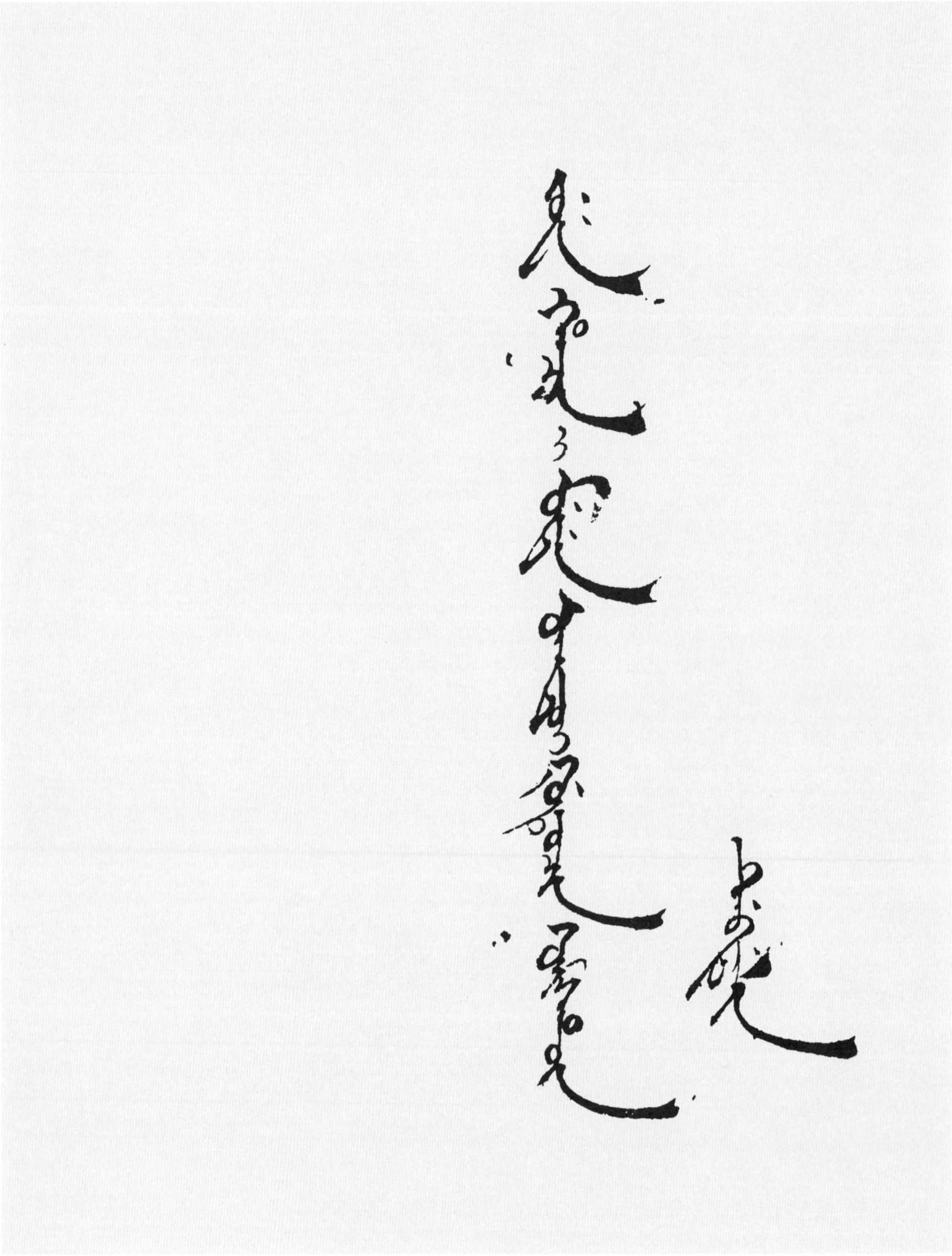

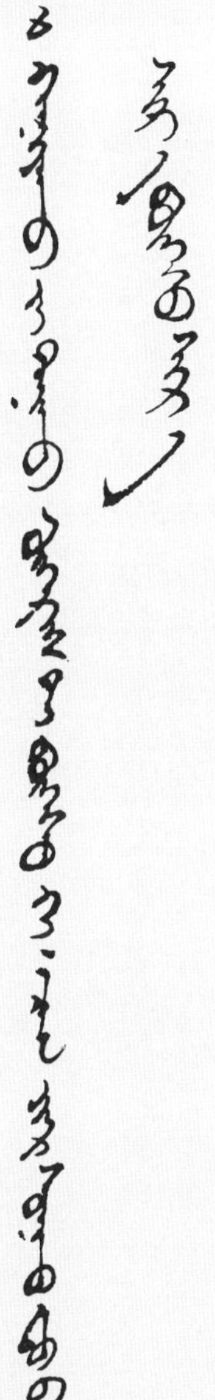

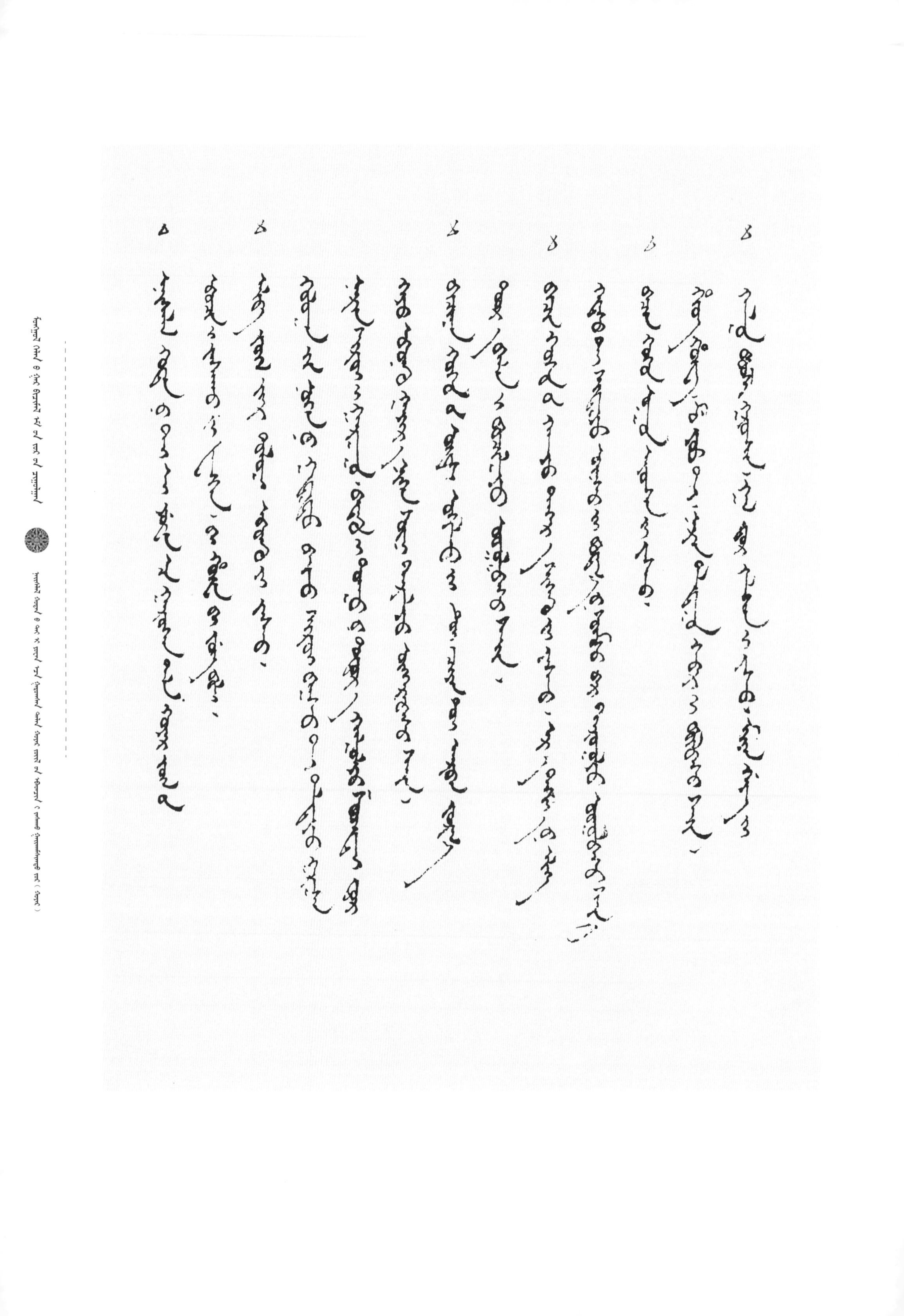

[illegible]

[illegible]

[illegible]

[illegible]

[illegible]

[illegible]

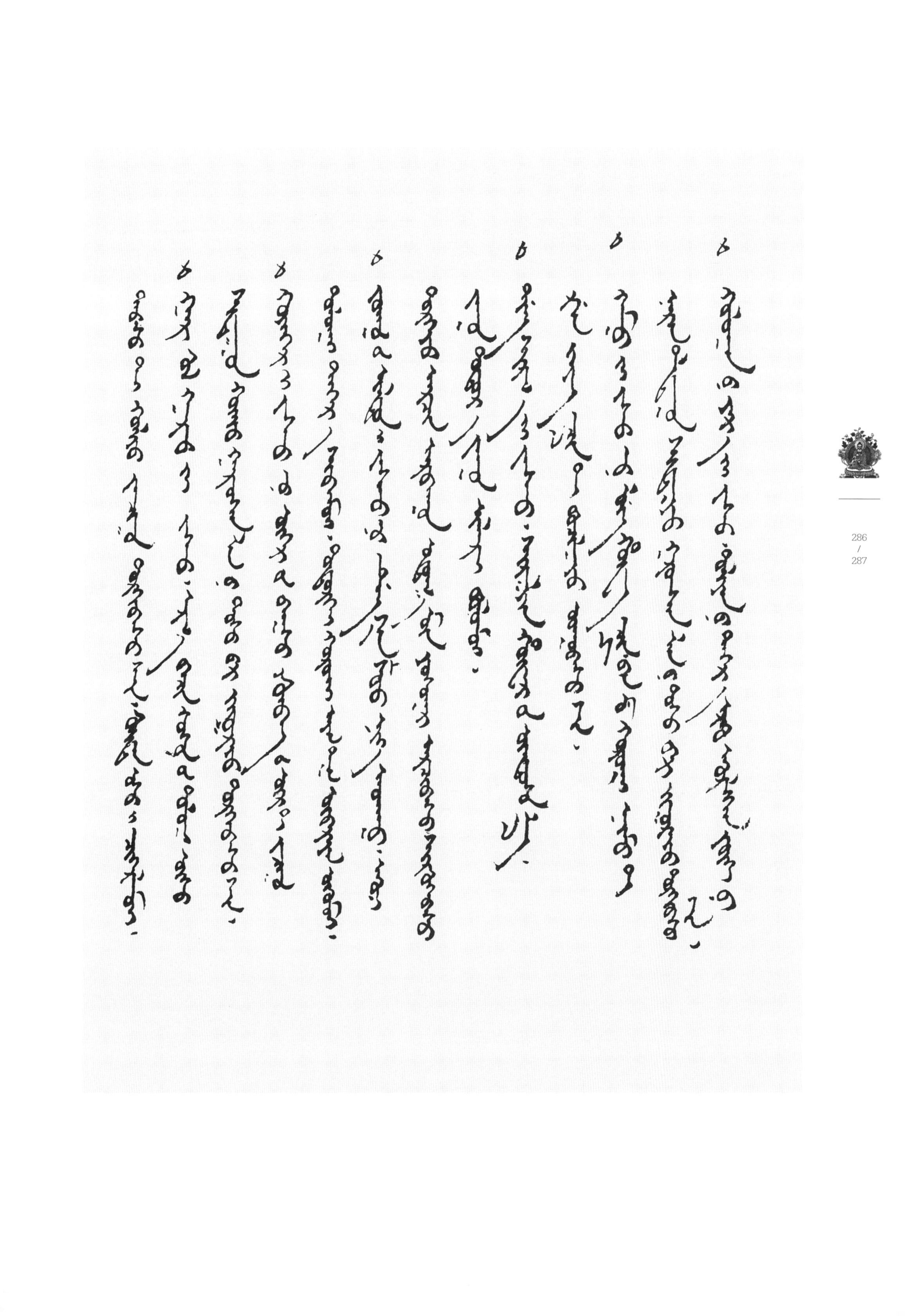

[illegible]

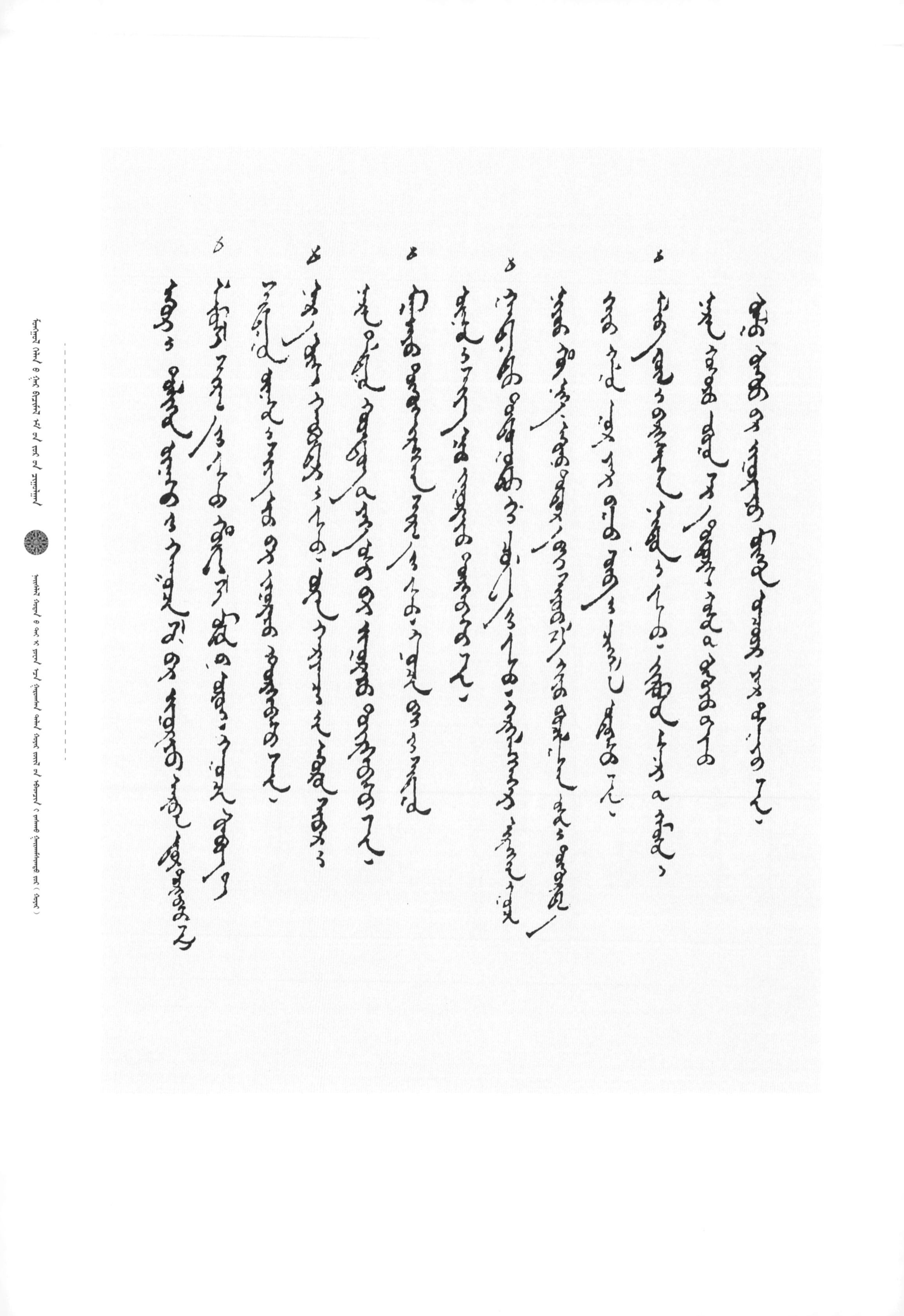

[illegible]

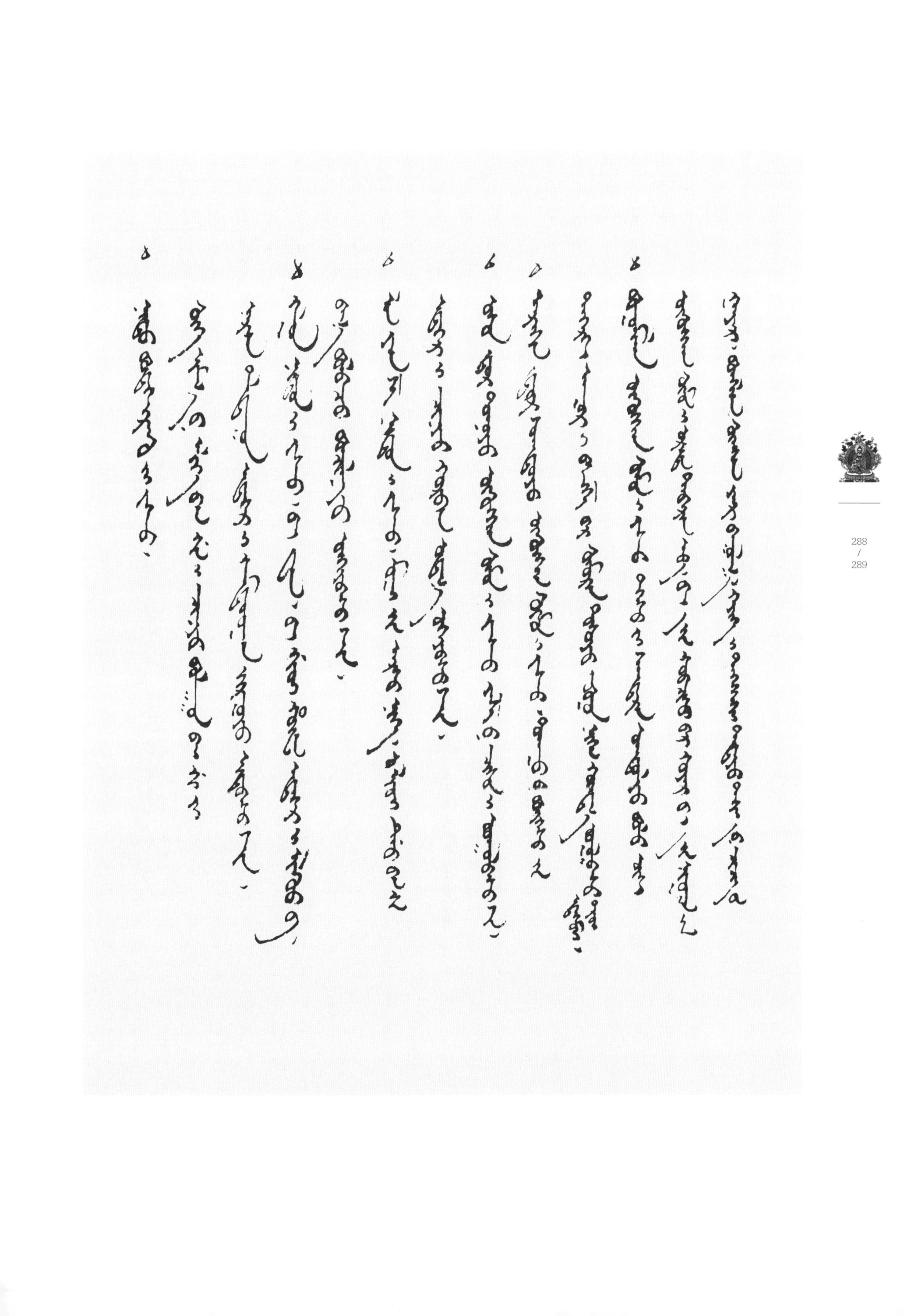

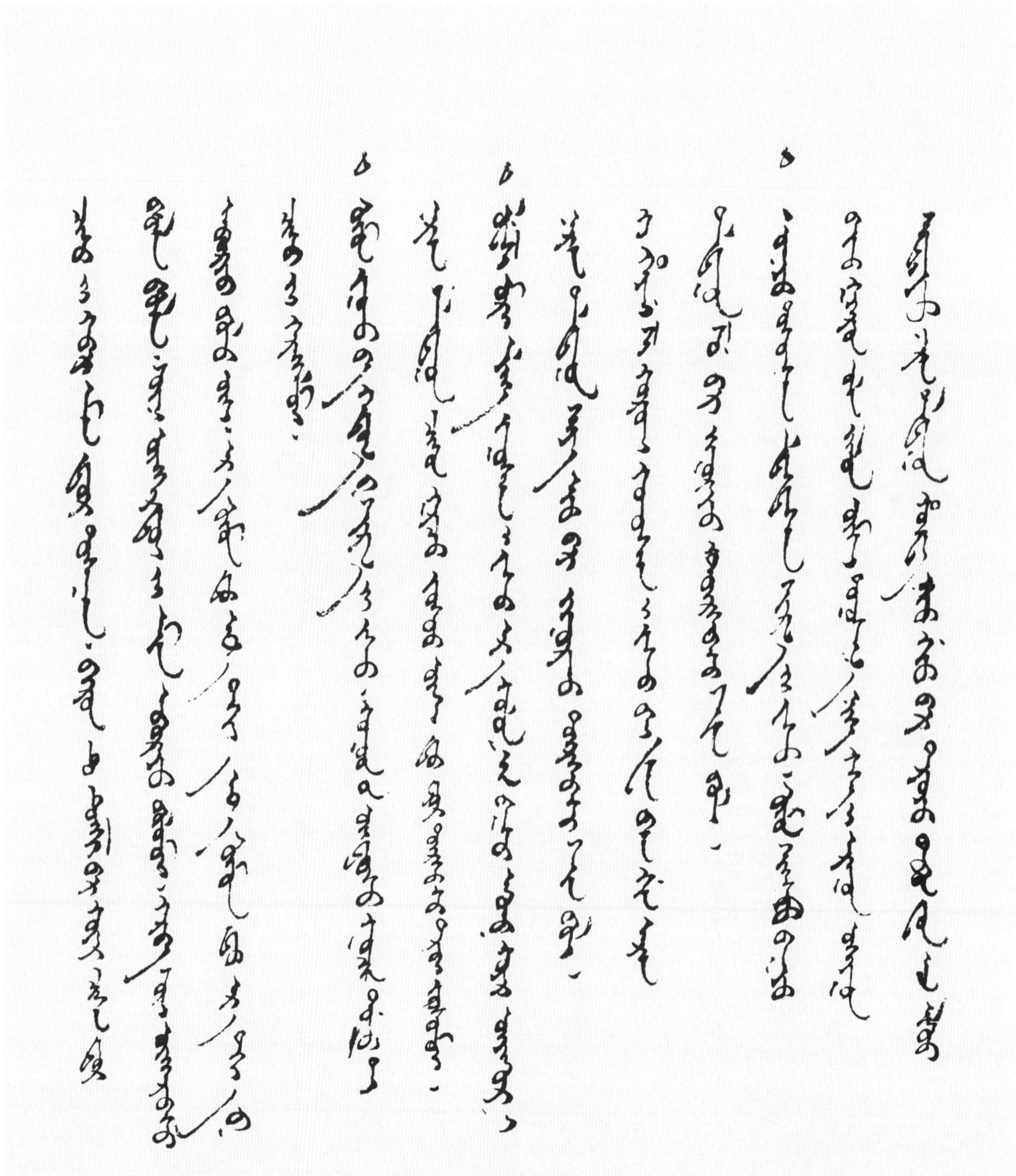

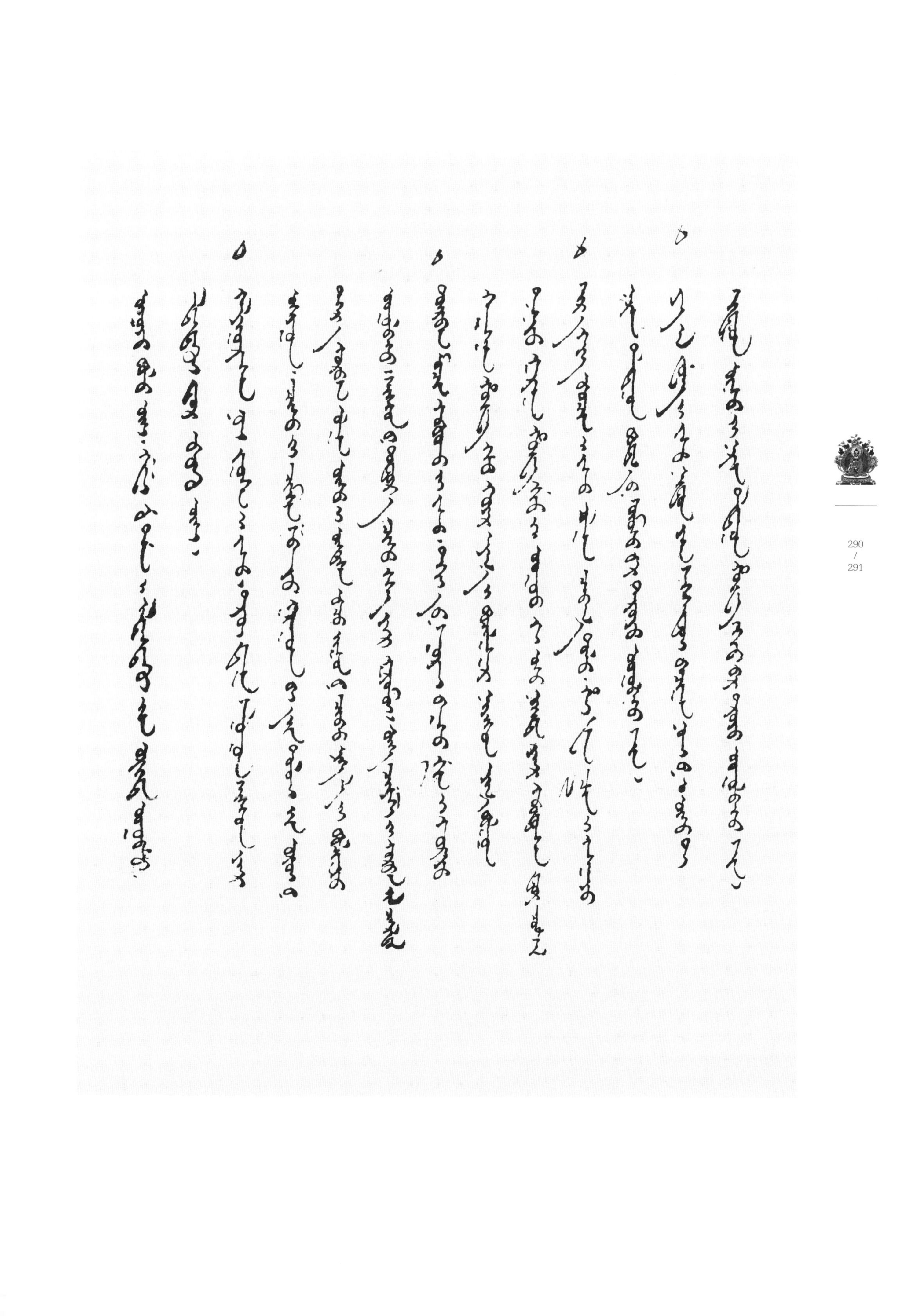

[illegible]

[illegible]

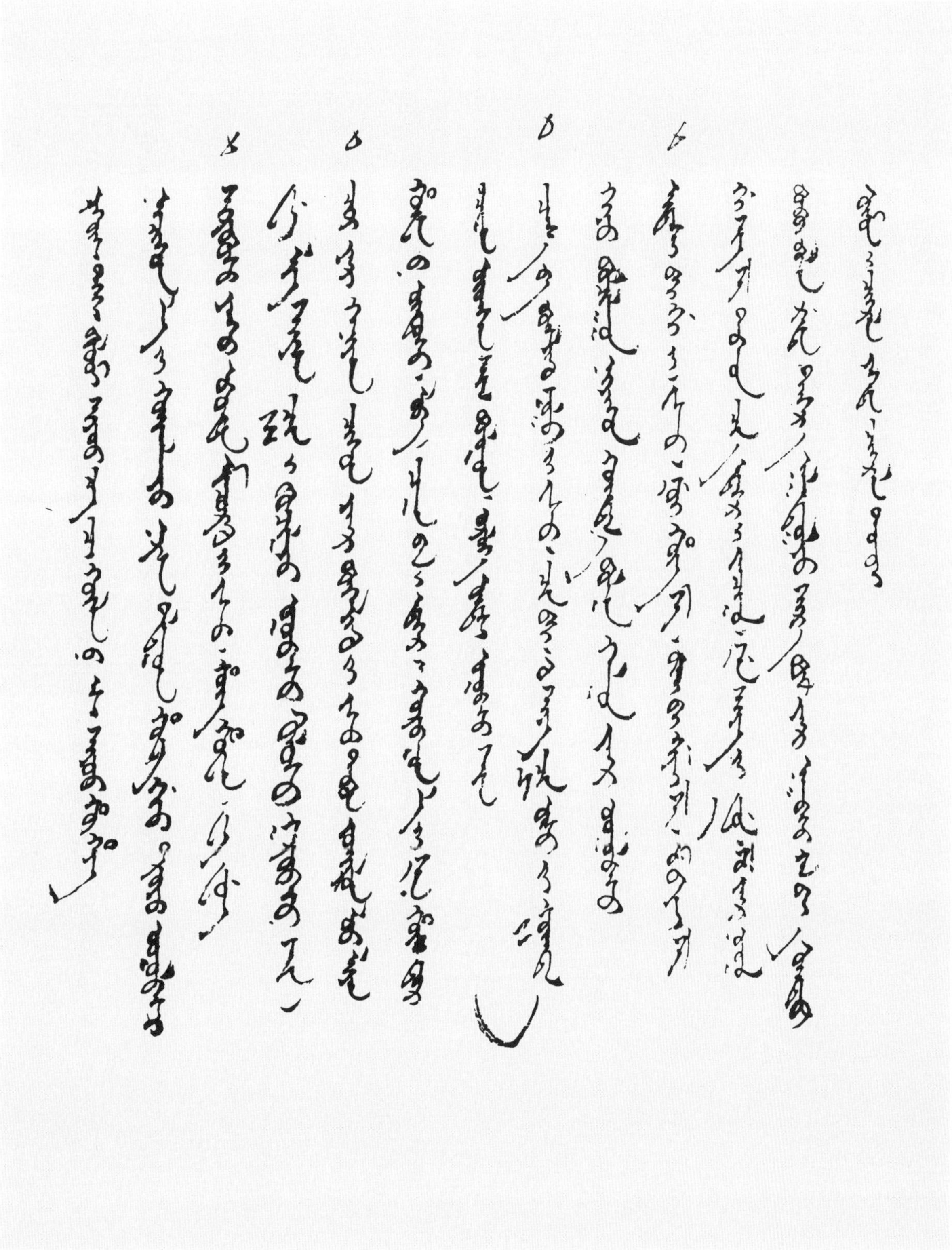

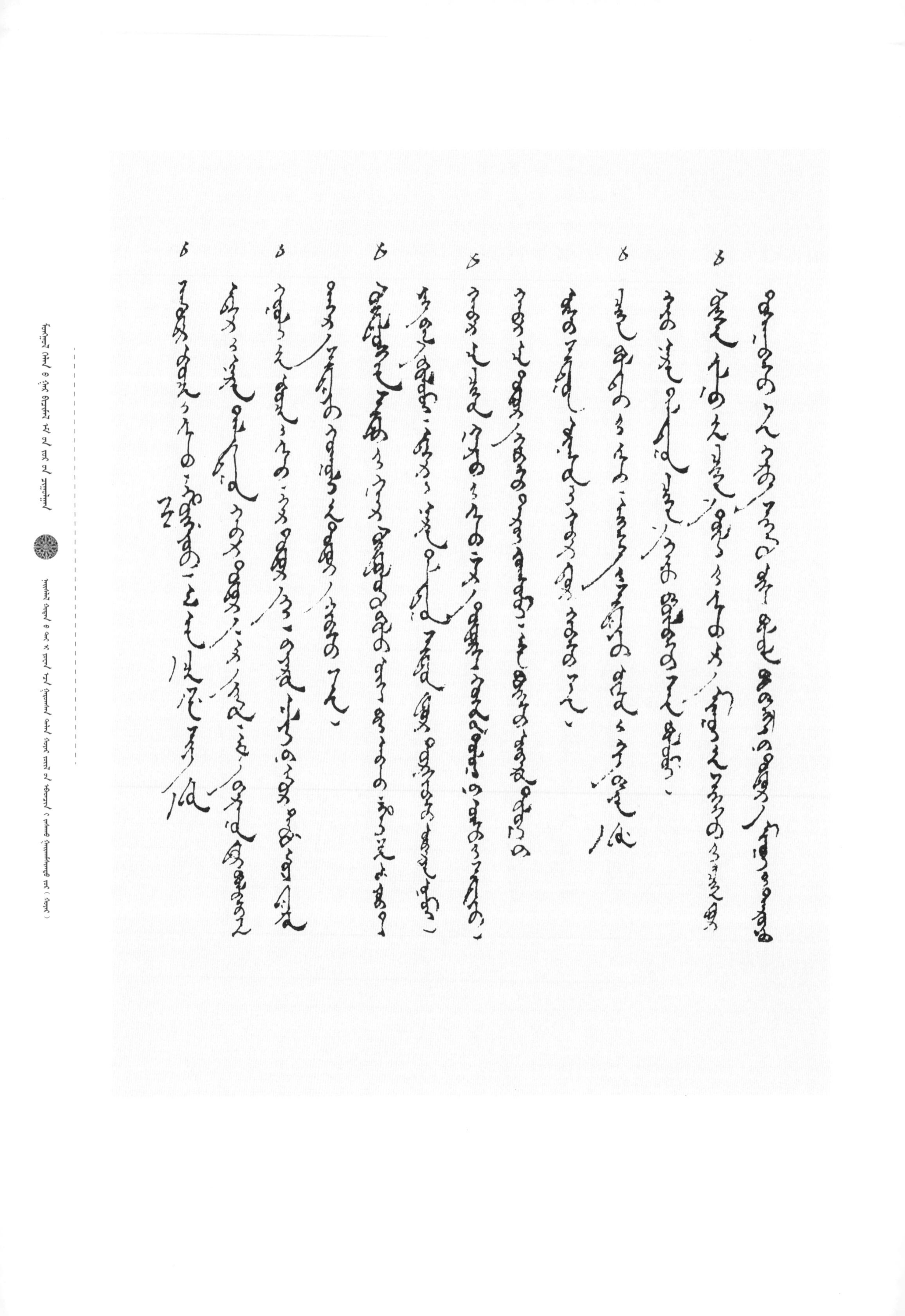

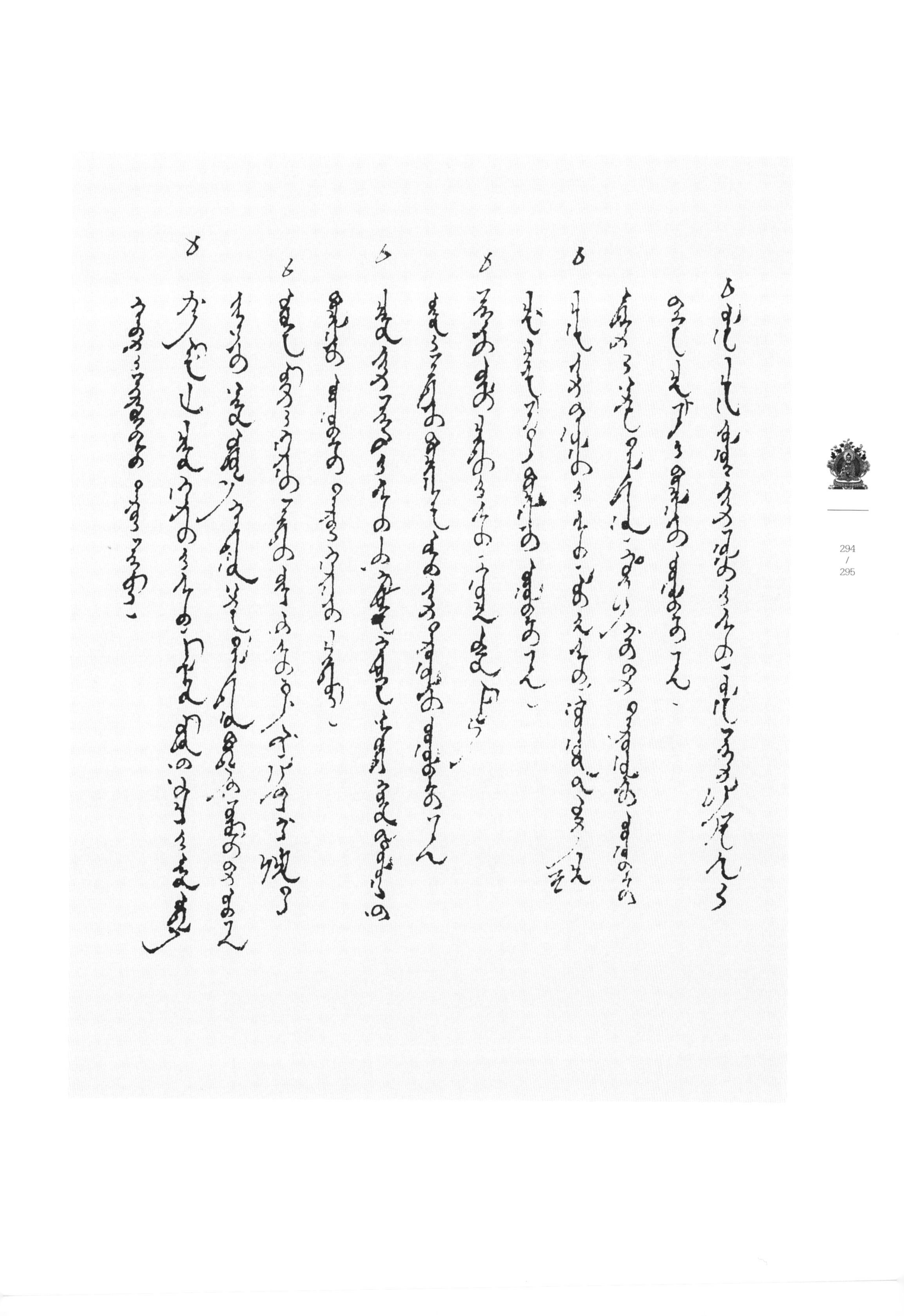

[illegible]

[illegible]

[illegible]

[illegible]

[illegible]

[illegible]

[illegible]

[illegible]

[illegible]

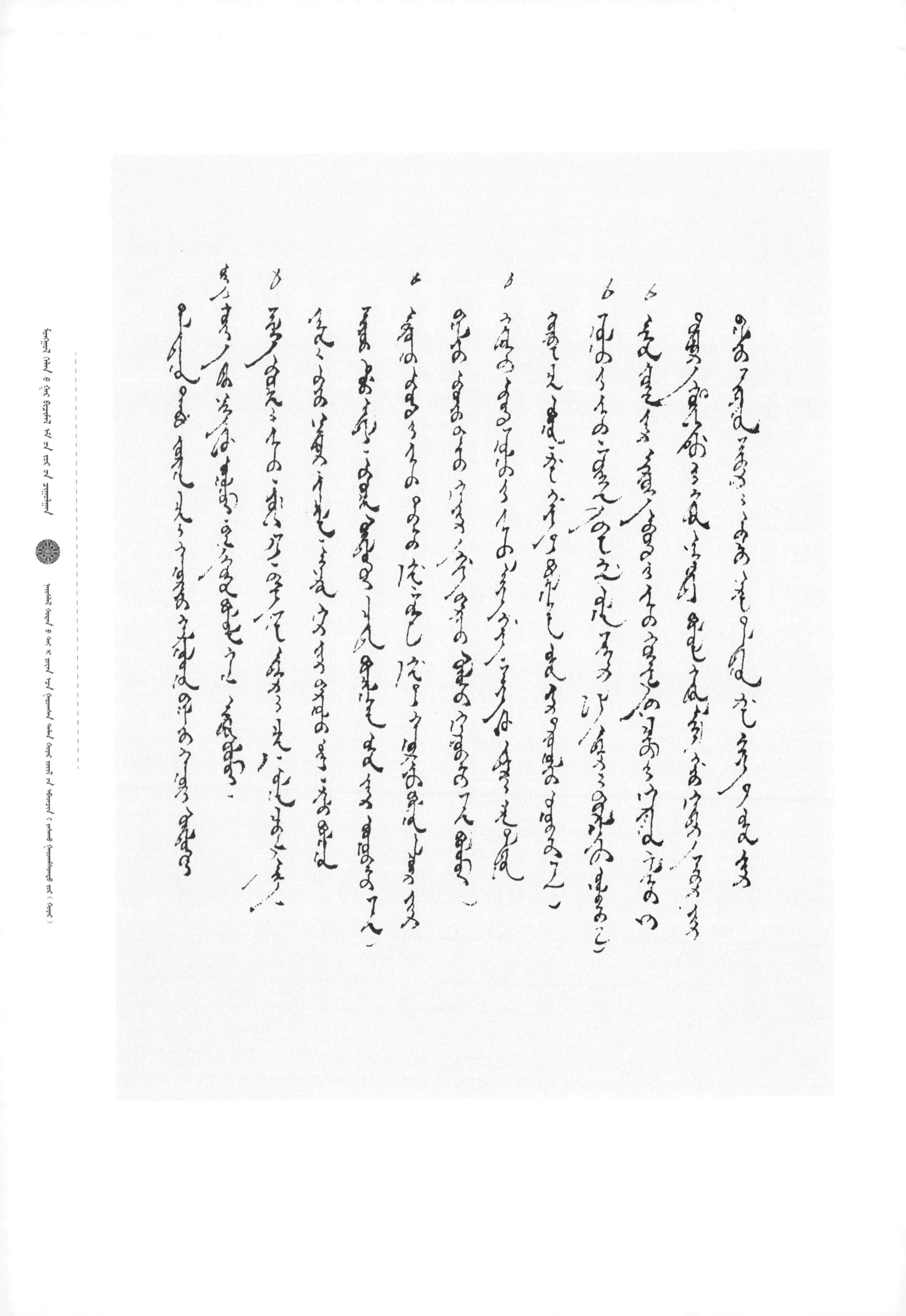

[illegible]
[illegible]
[illegible]
[illegible]
[illegible]
[illegible]
[illegible]
[illegible]
[illegible]
[illegible]
[illegible]
[illegible]
[illegible]

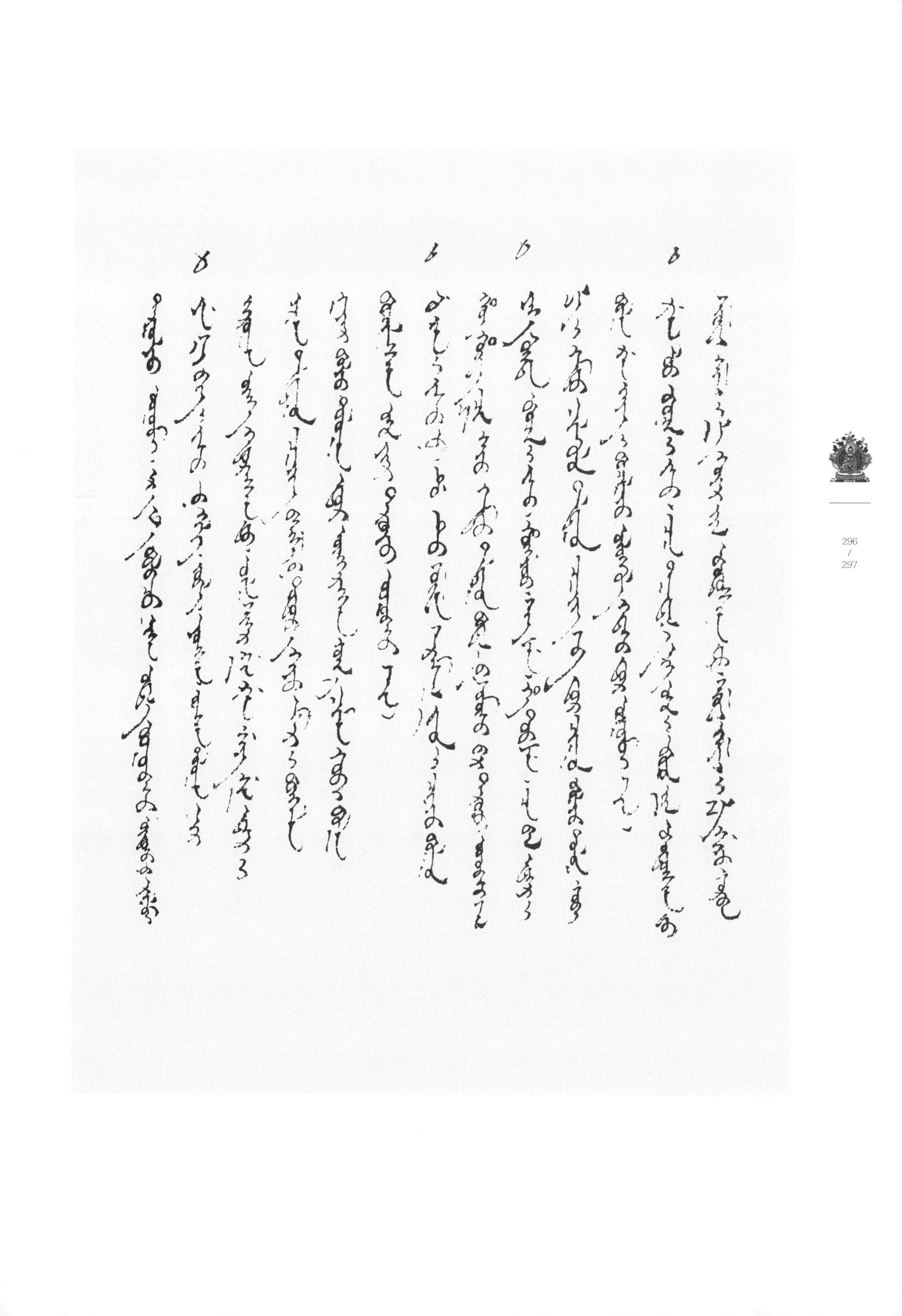

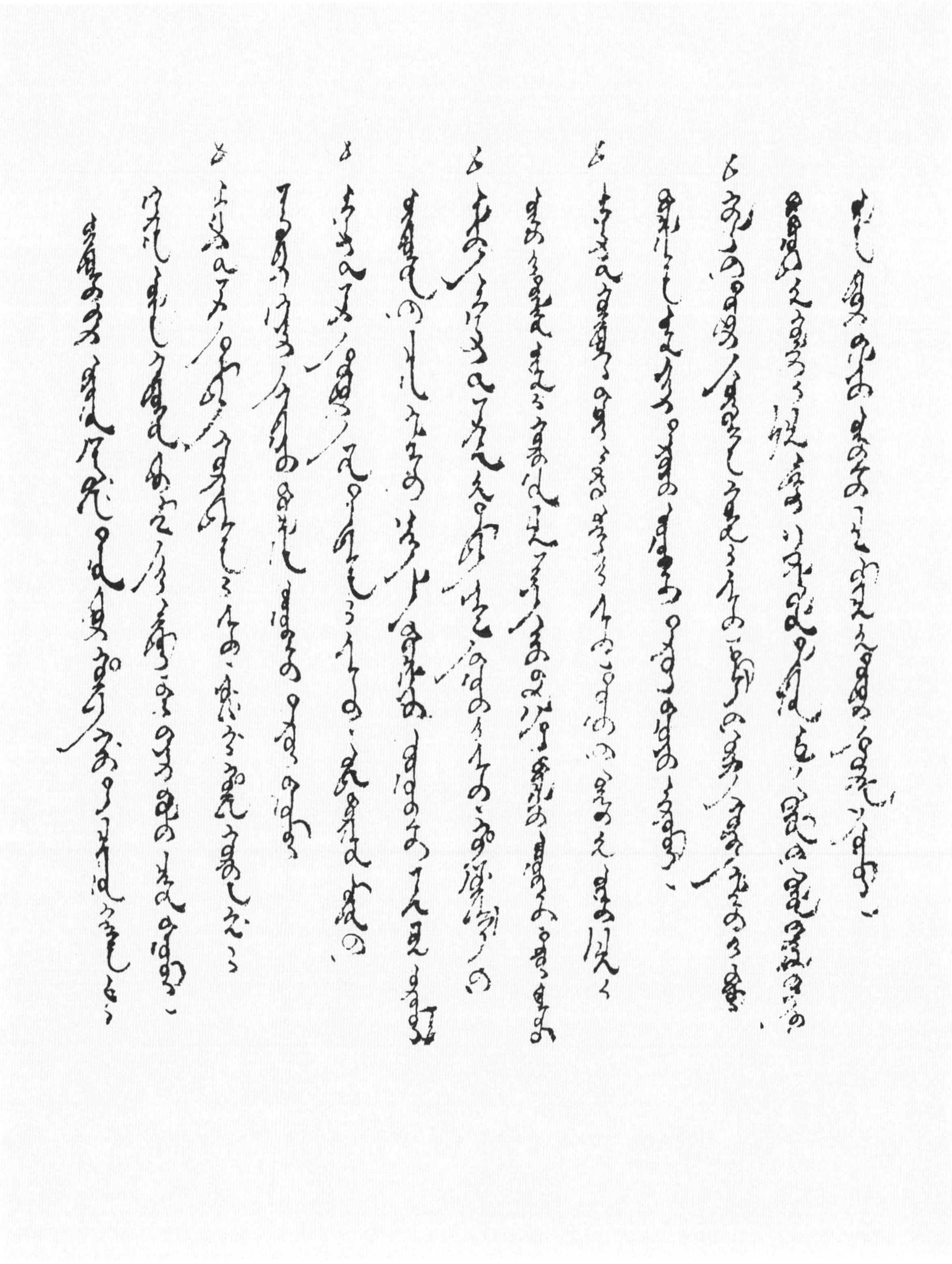

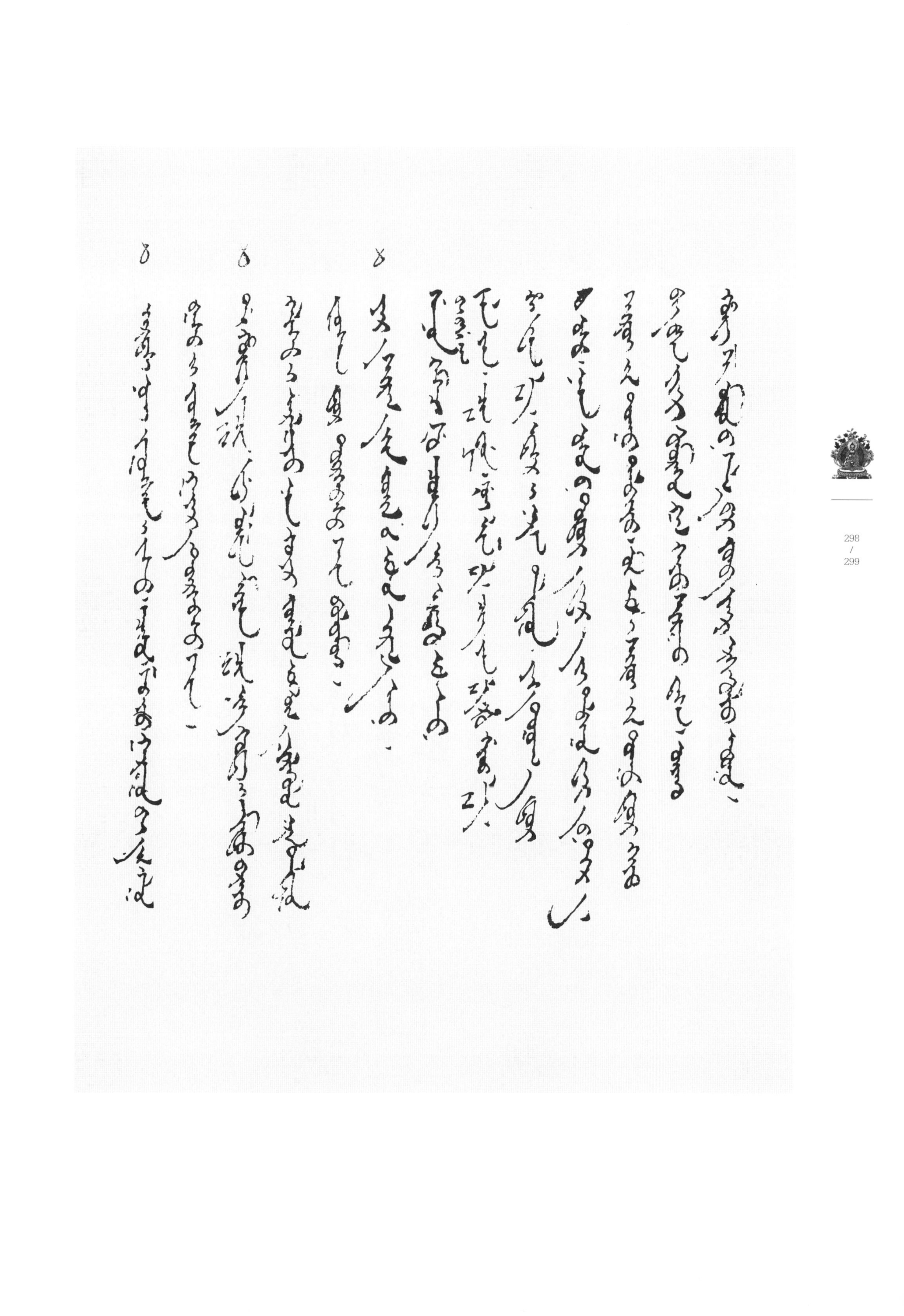

[illegible]

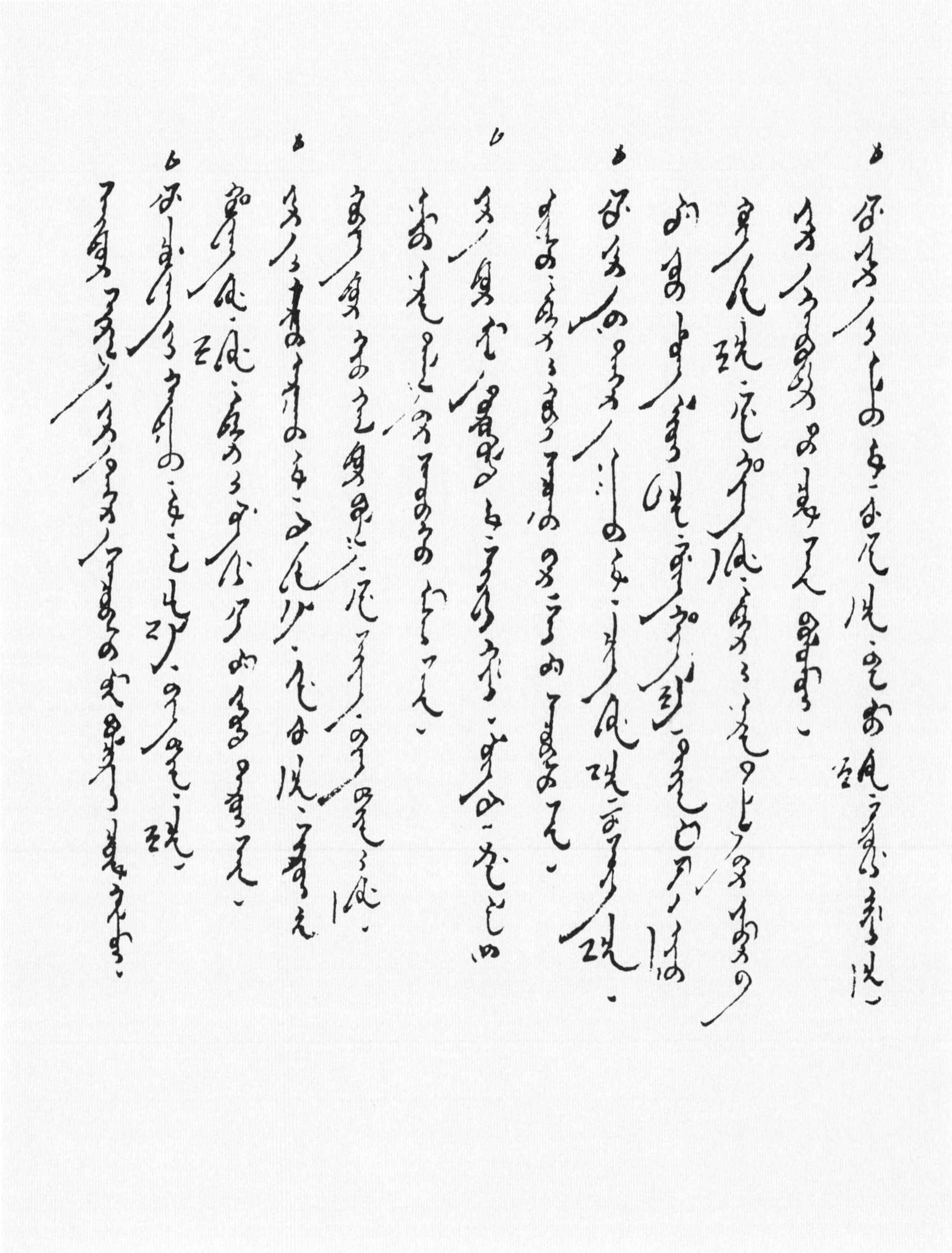

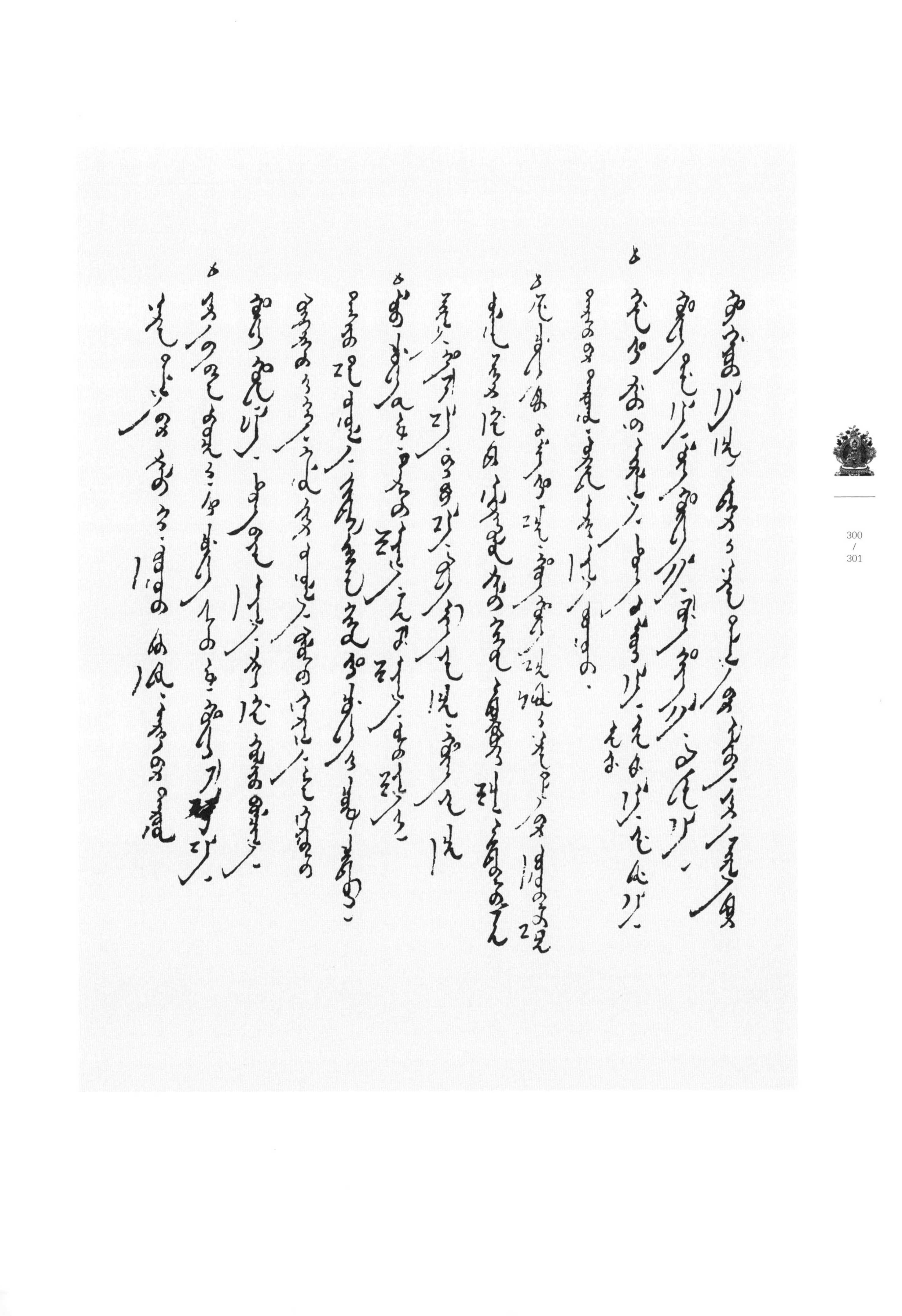

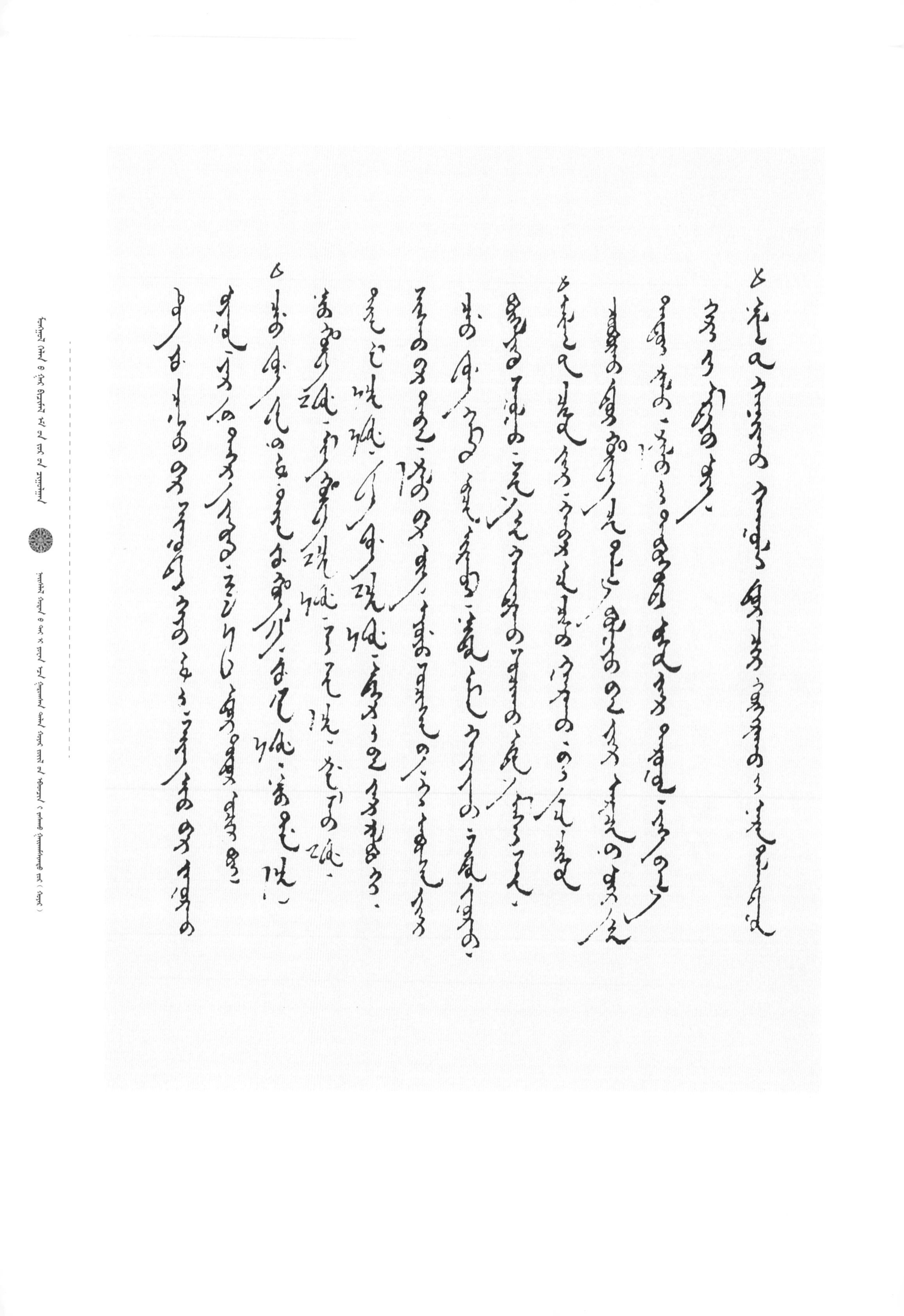

[illegible]
[illegible]
[illegible]
[illegible]
[illegible]
[illegible]
[illegible]
[illegible]
[illegible]
[illegible]
[illegible]
[illegible]
[illegible]
[illegible]

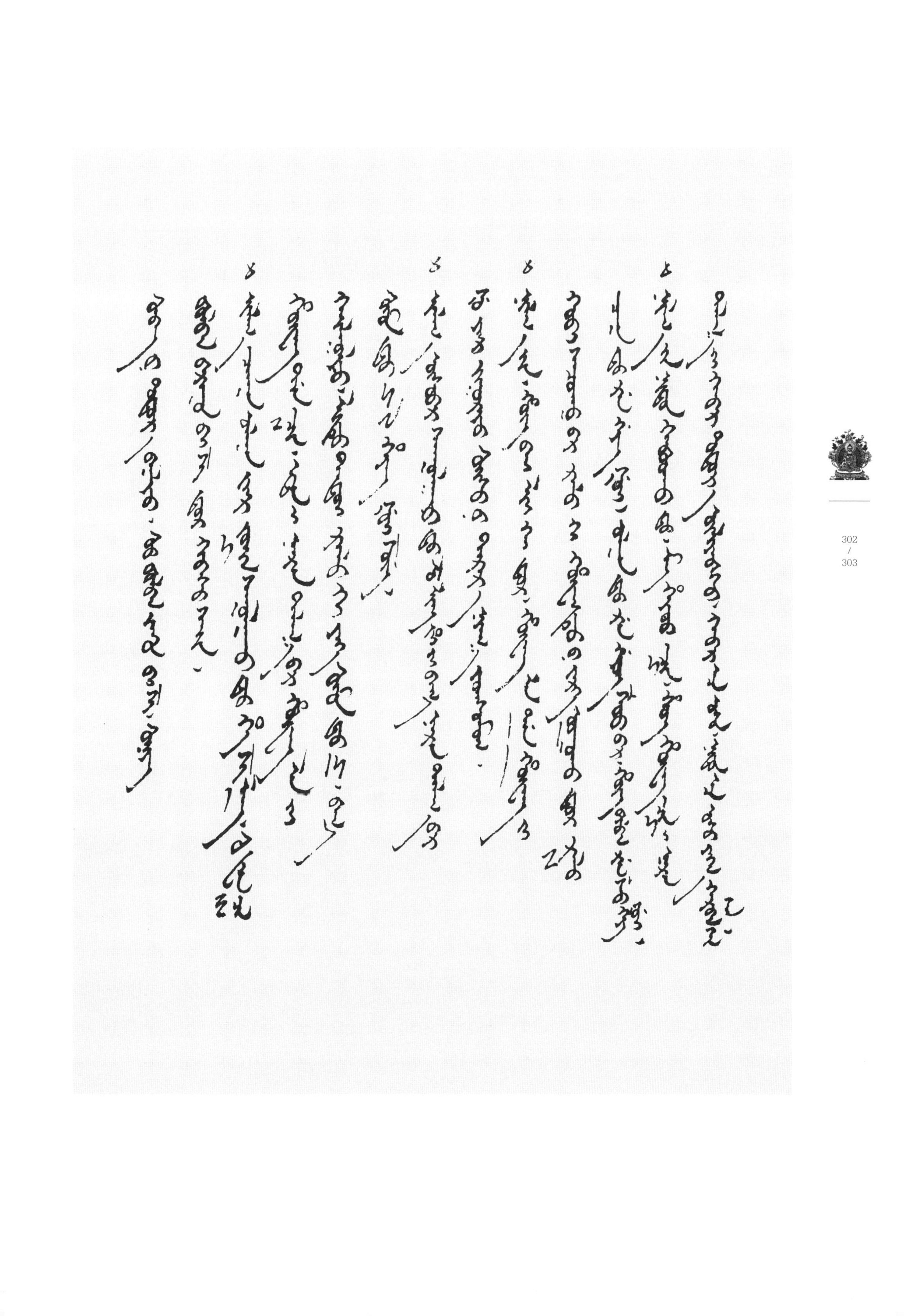

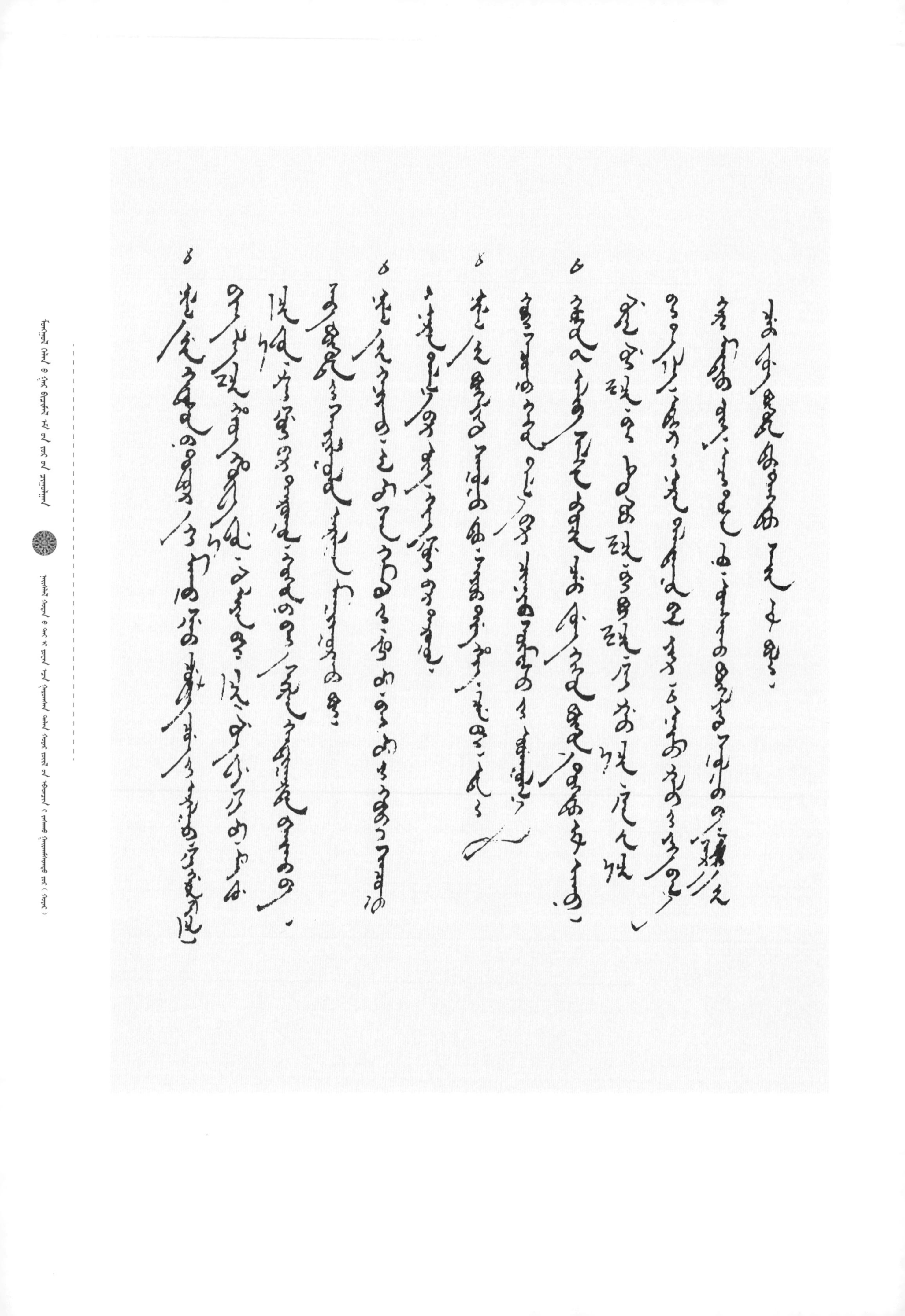

[illegible]

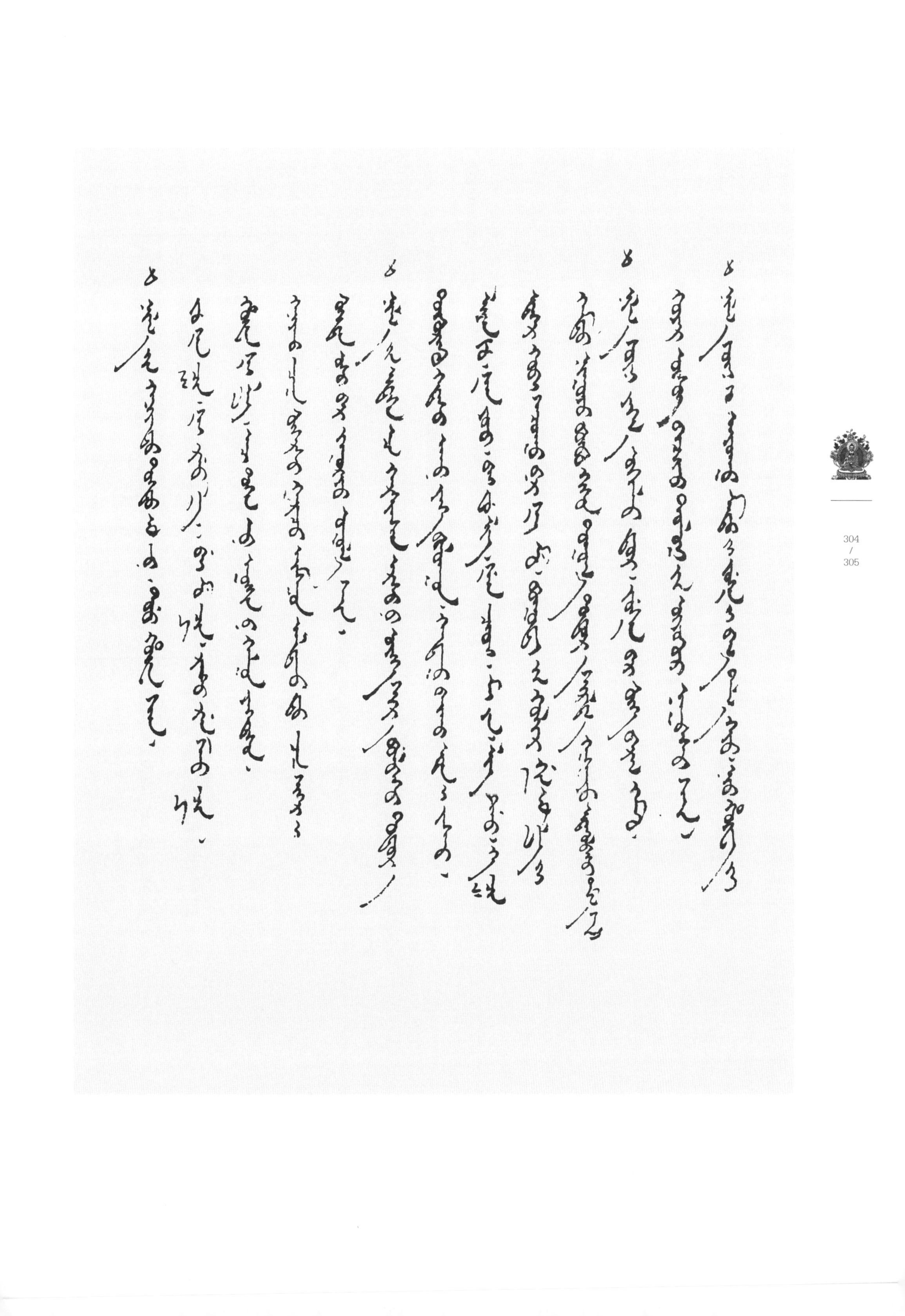

[illegible]

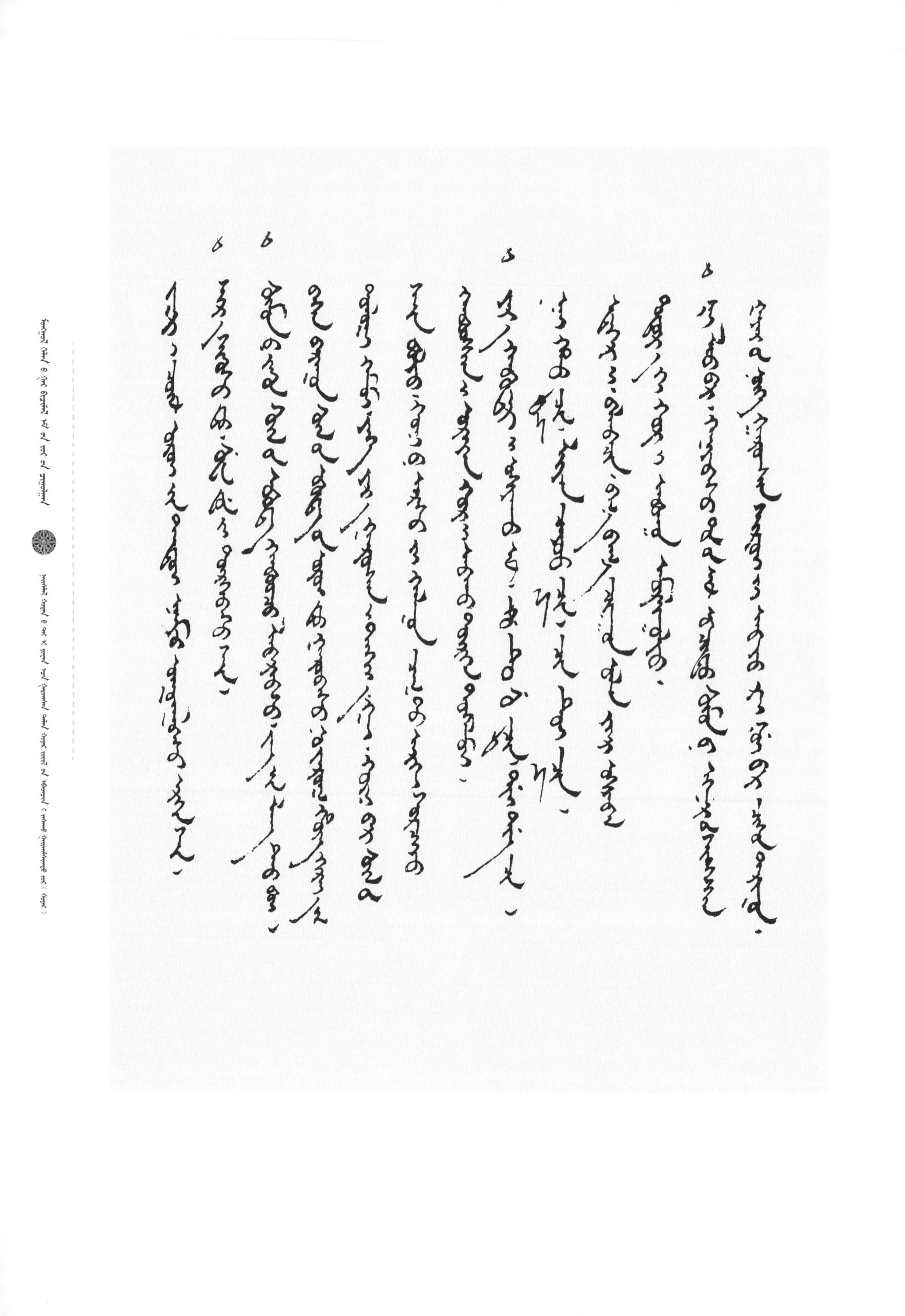

[illegible]
[illegible]
[illegible]
[illegible]
[illegible]
[illegible]
[illegible]
[illegible]
[illegible]
[illegible]
[illegible]
[illegible]
[illegible]

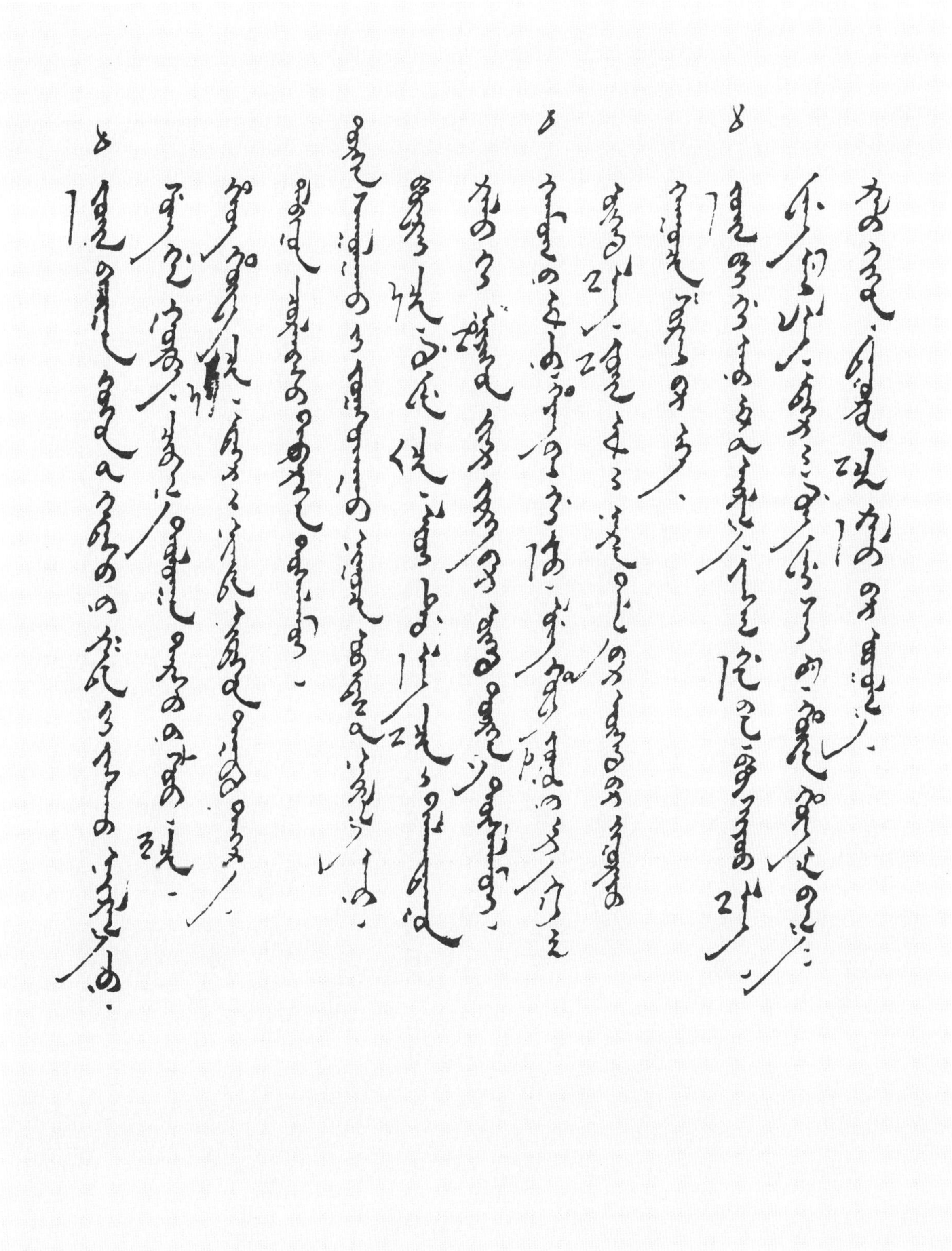

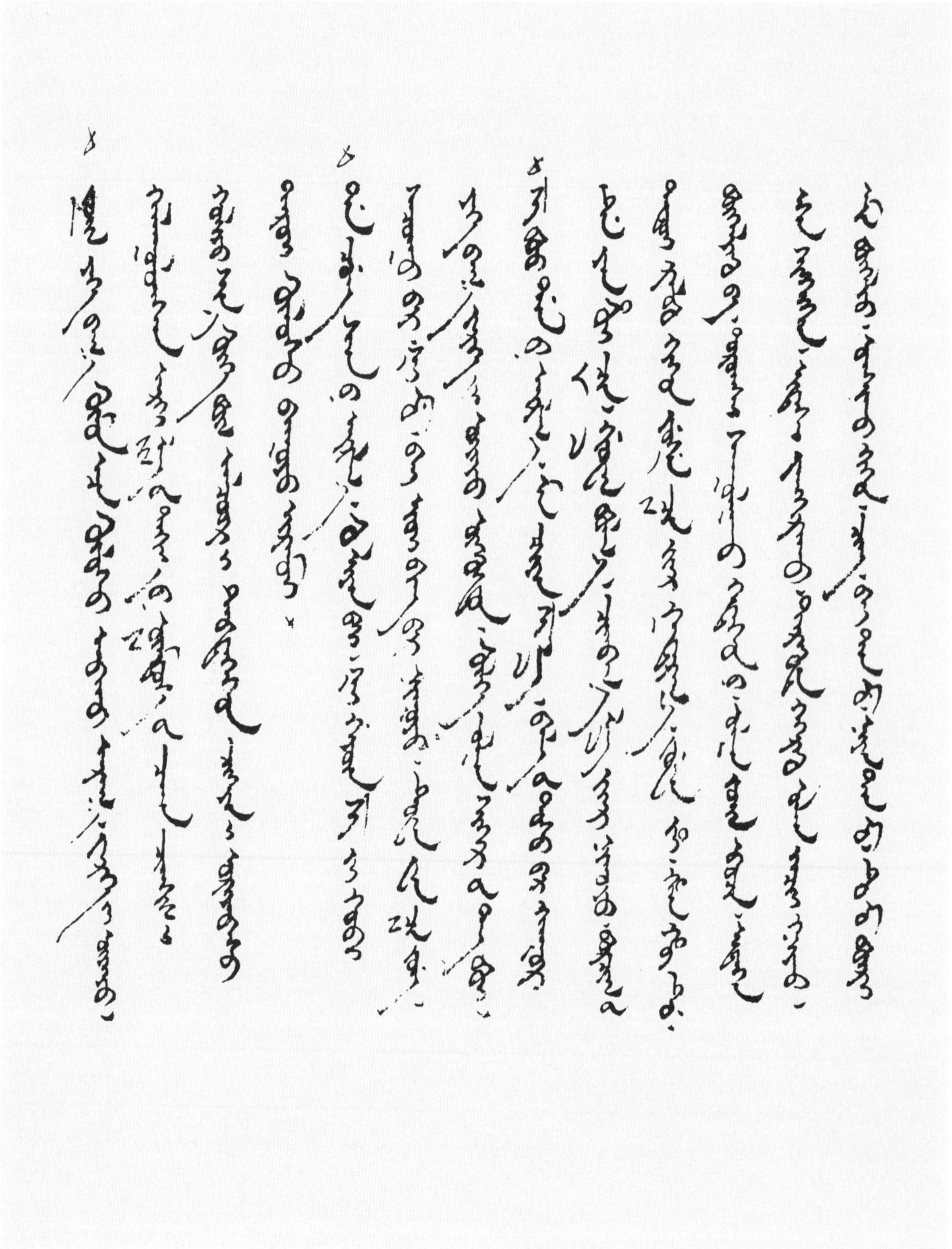

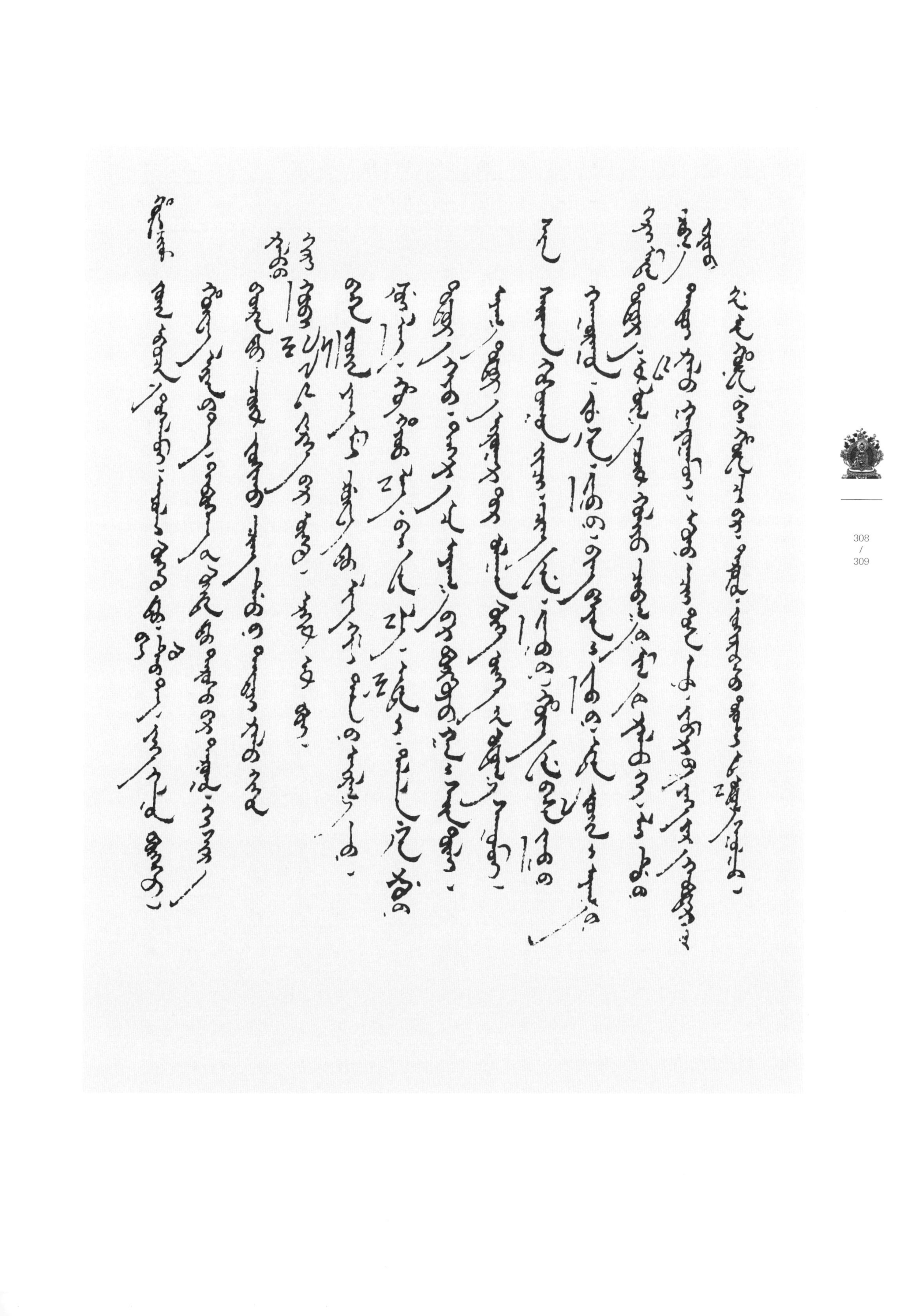

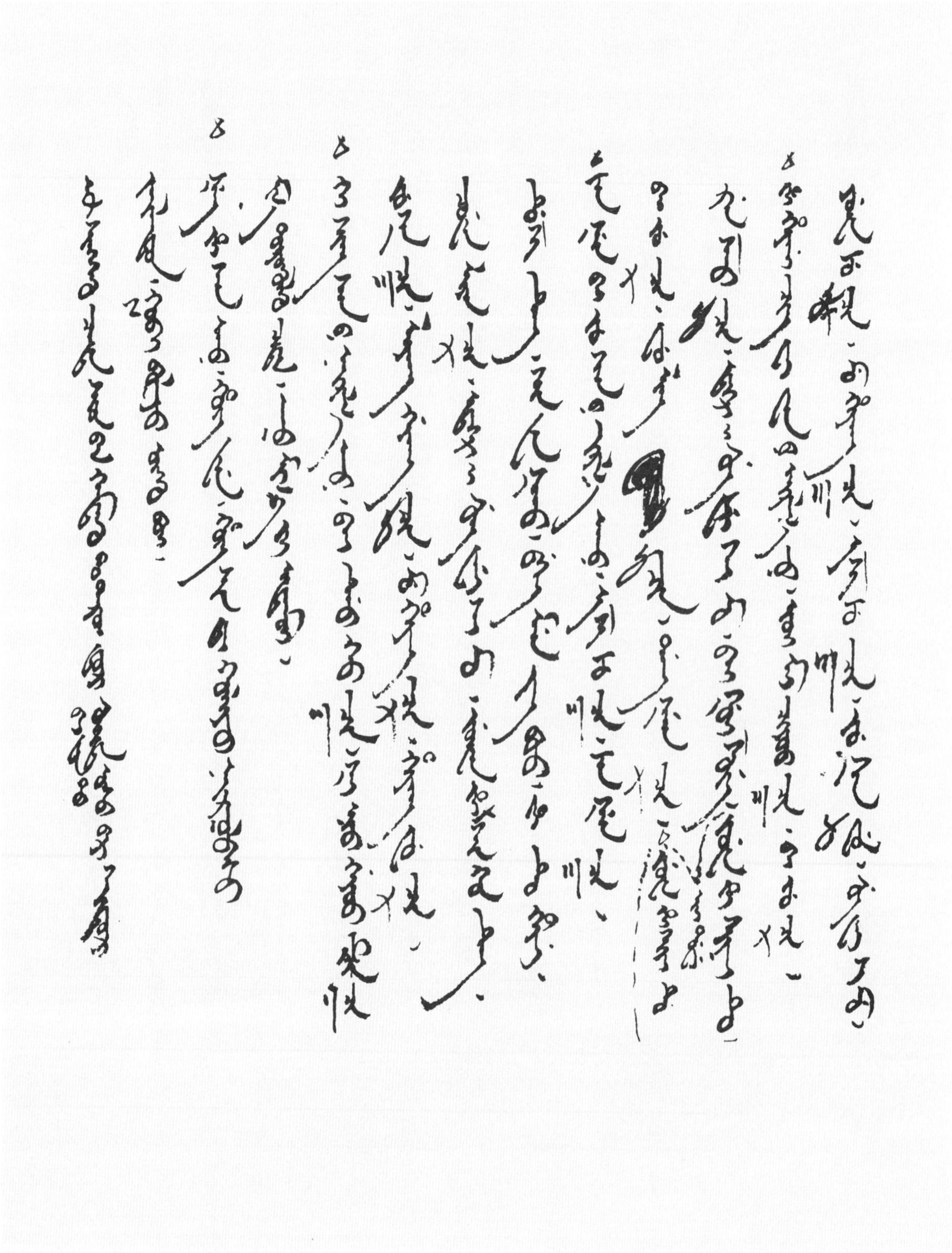

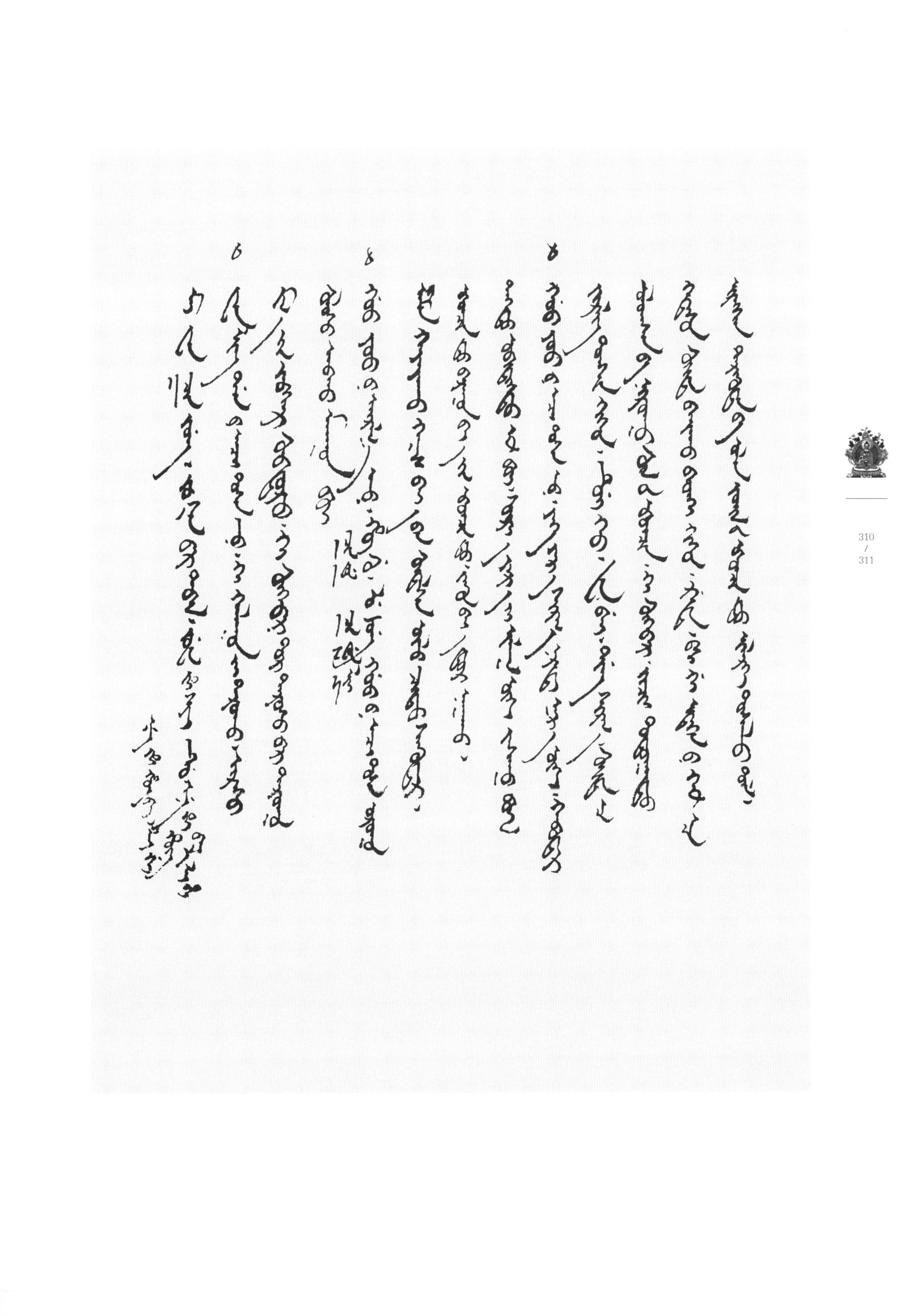

[illegible]

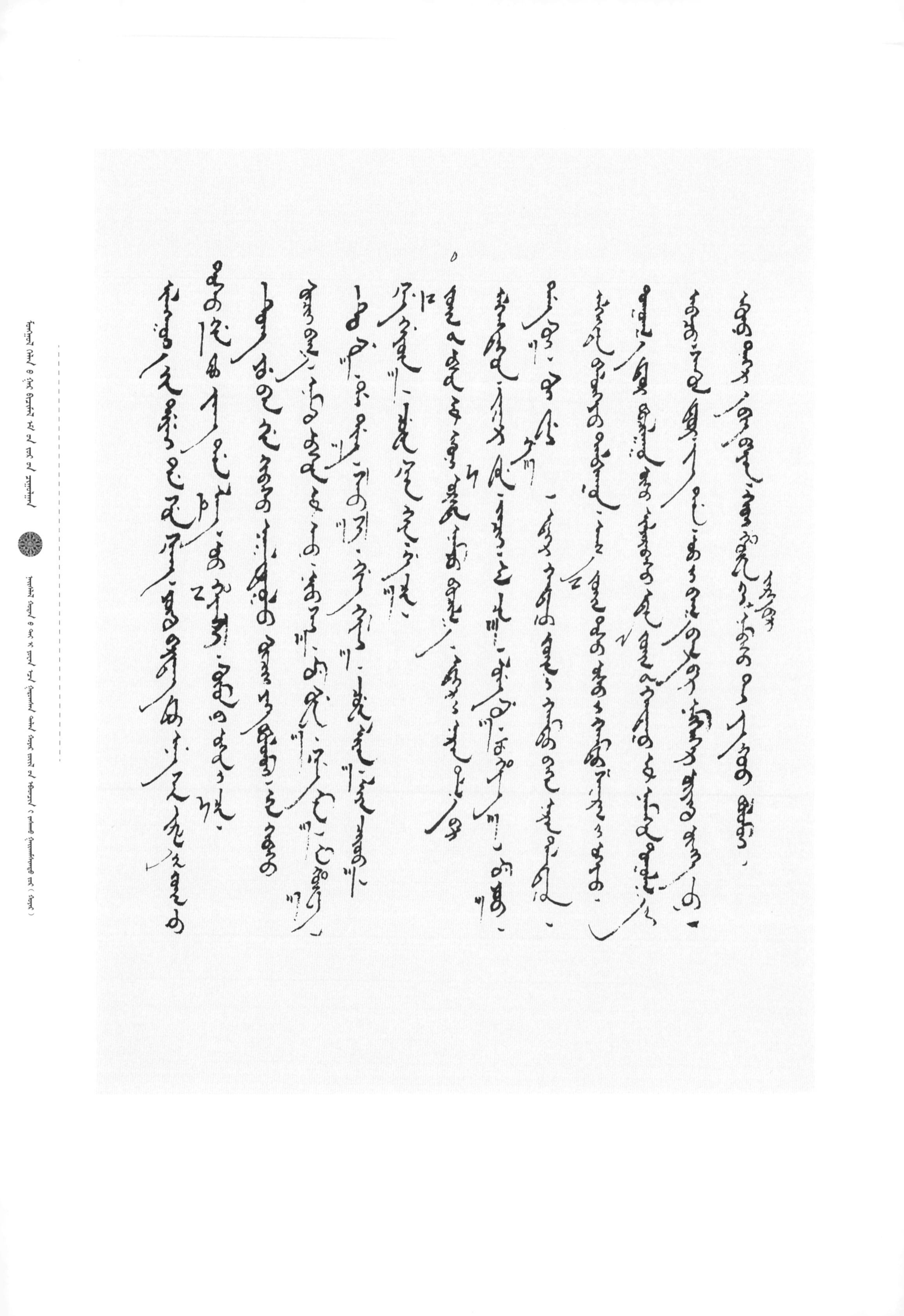

[illegible]

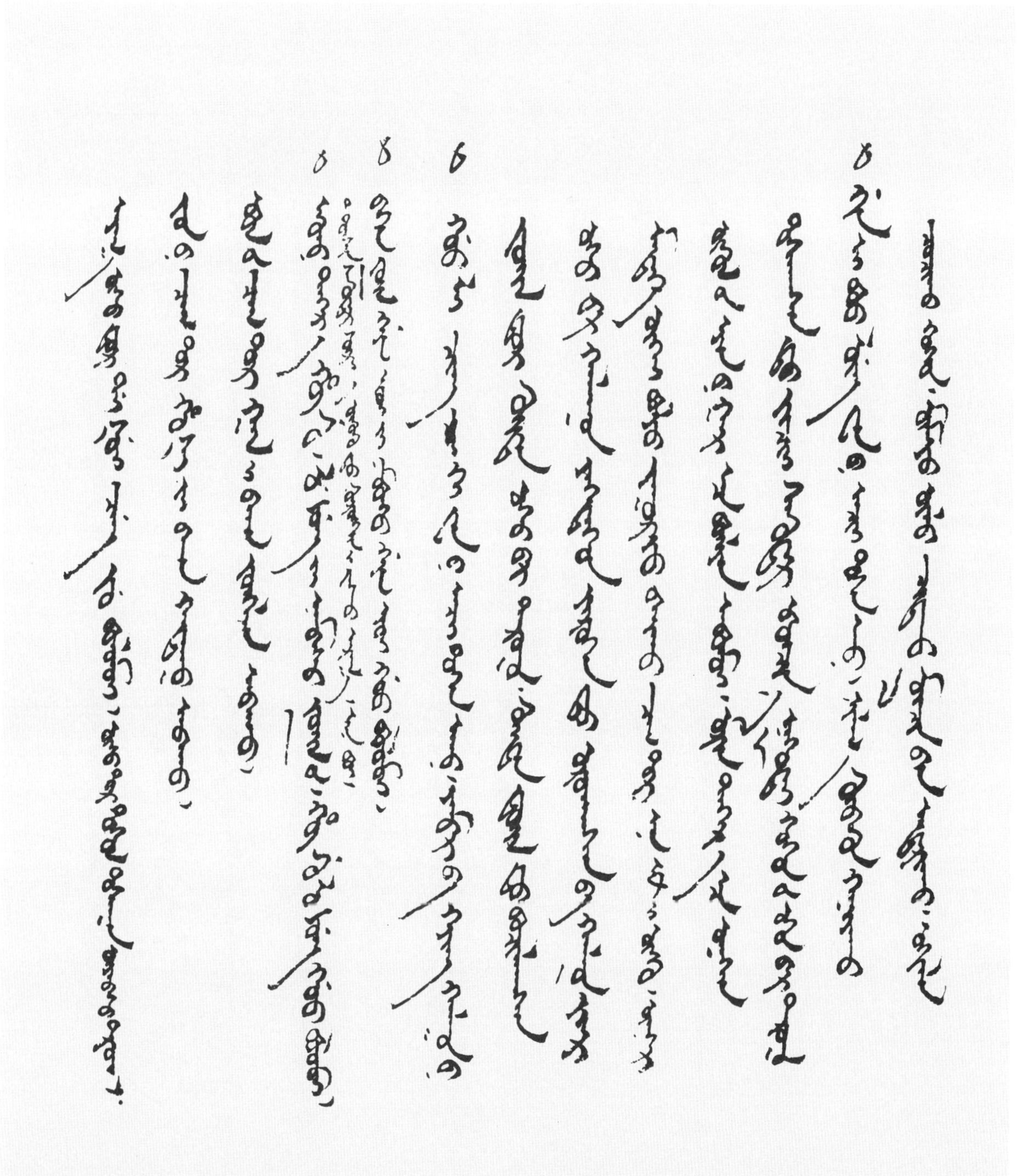

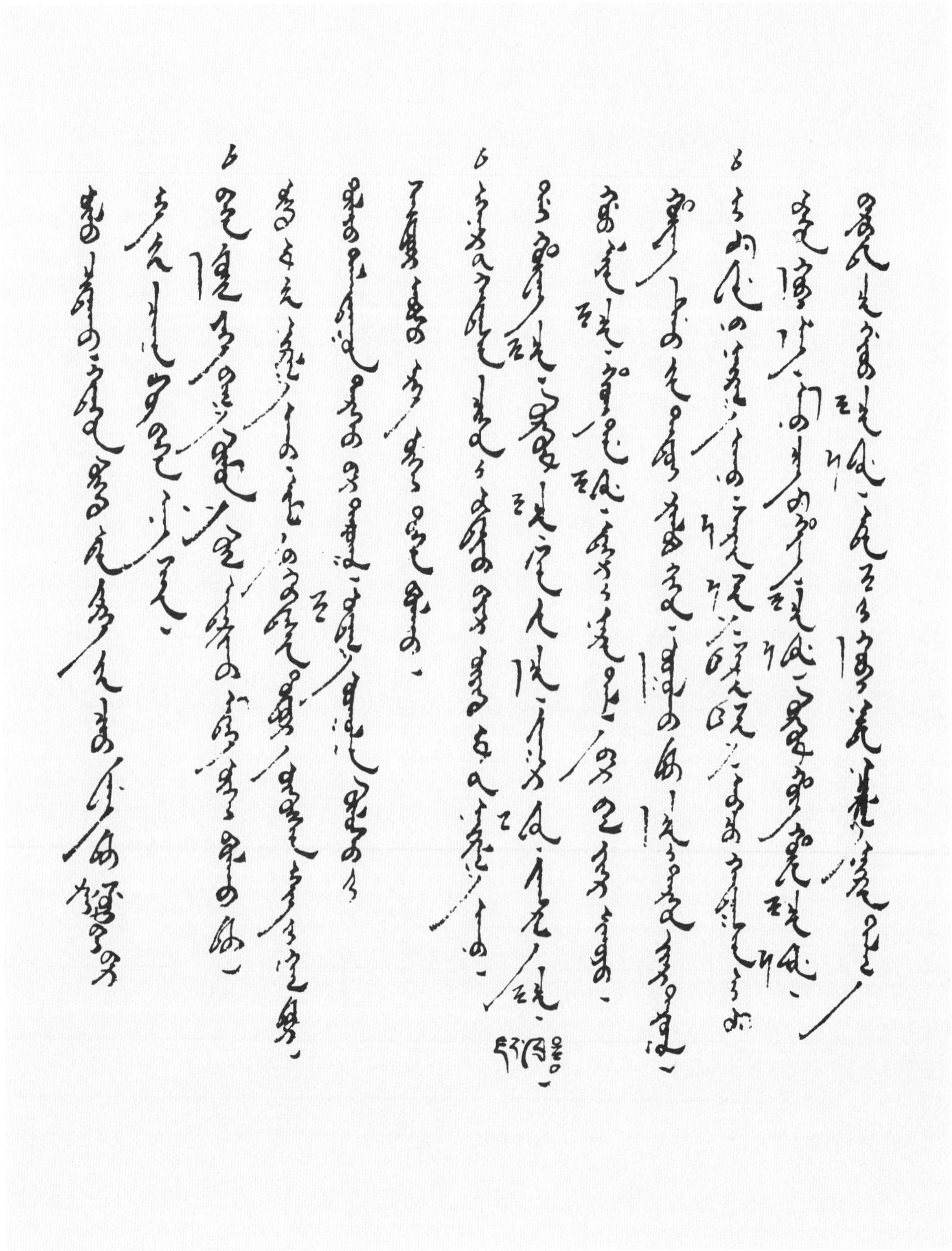

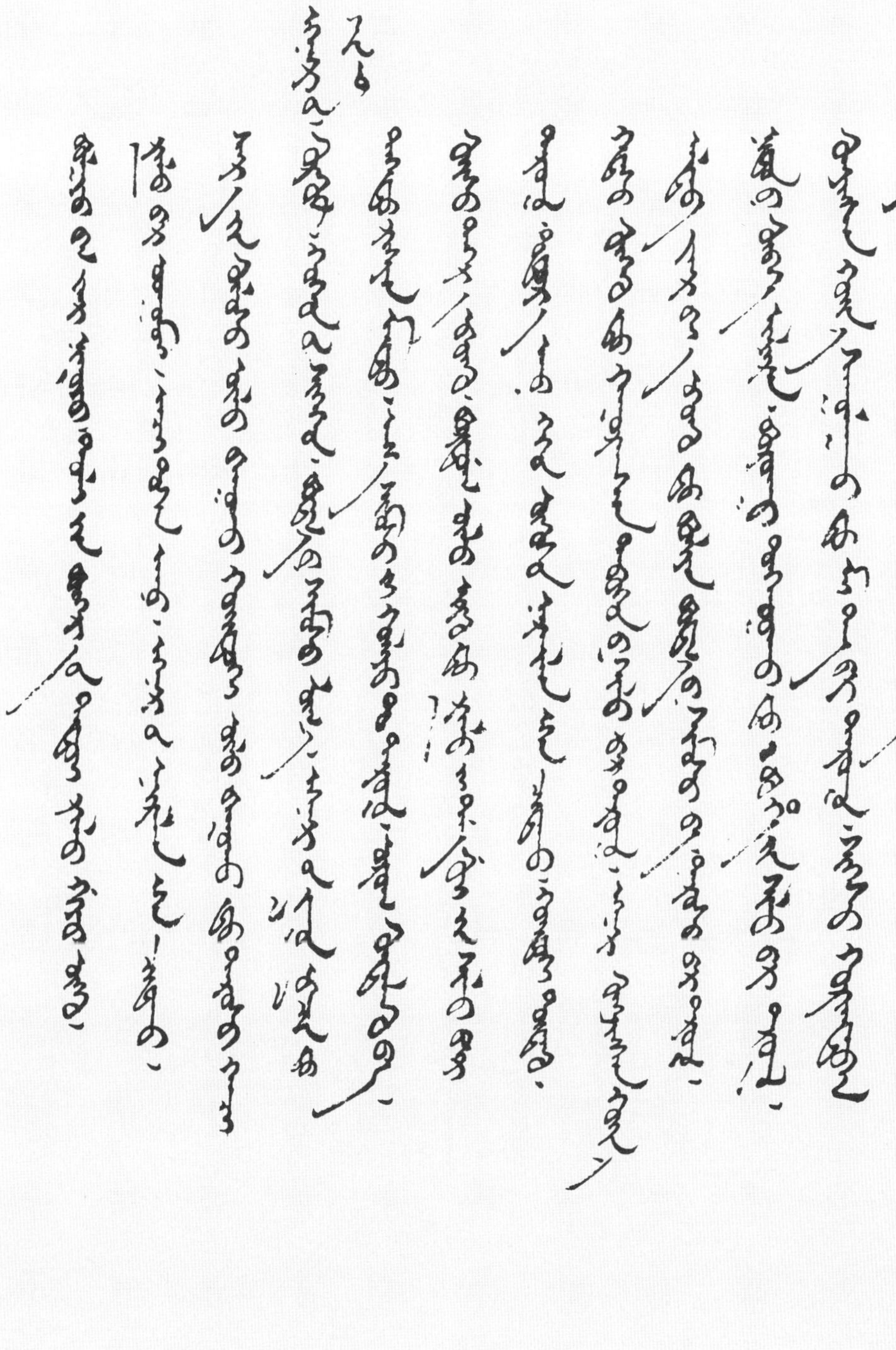

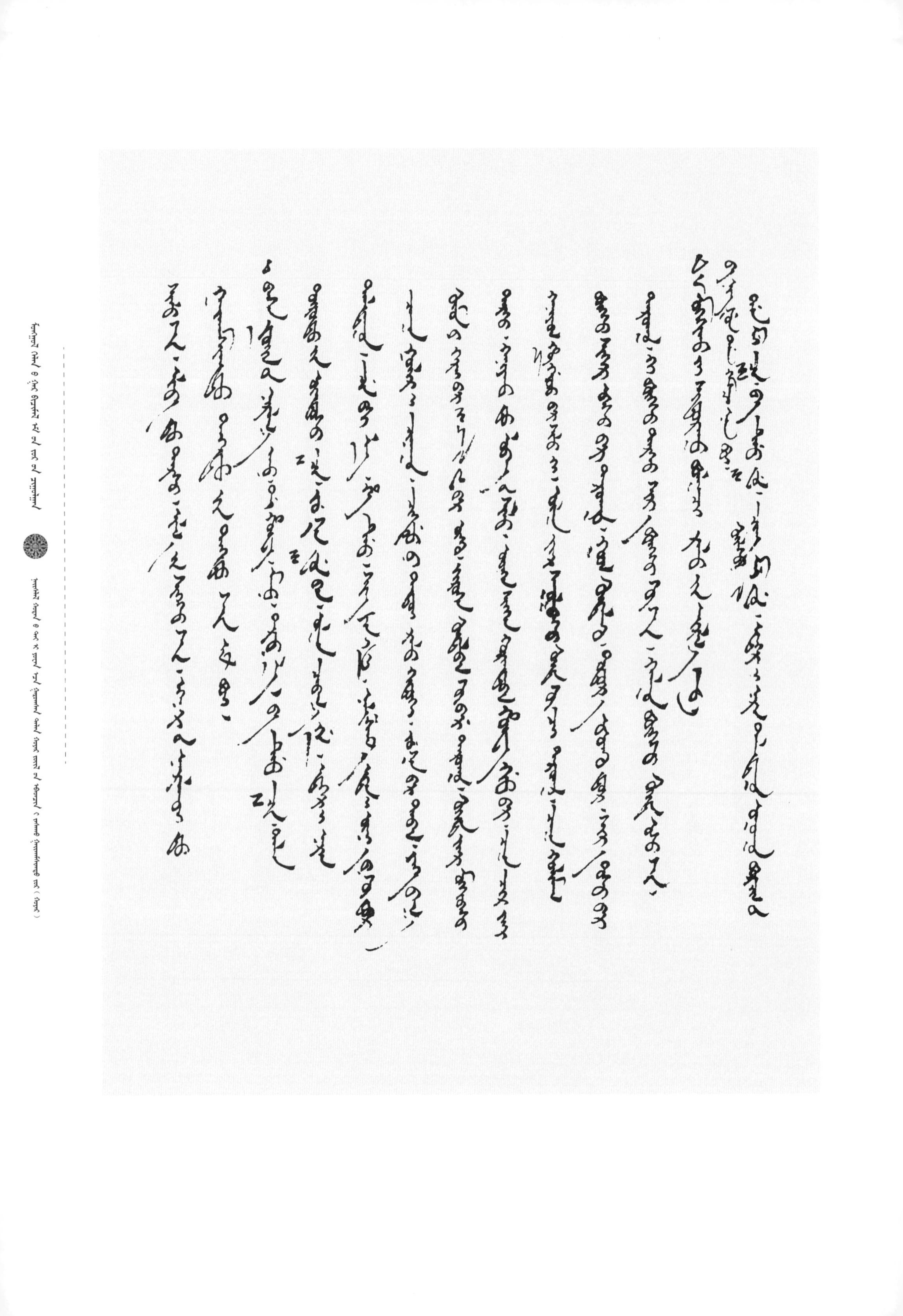

[illegible]

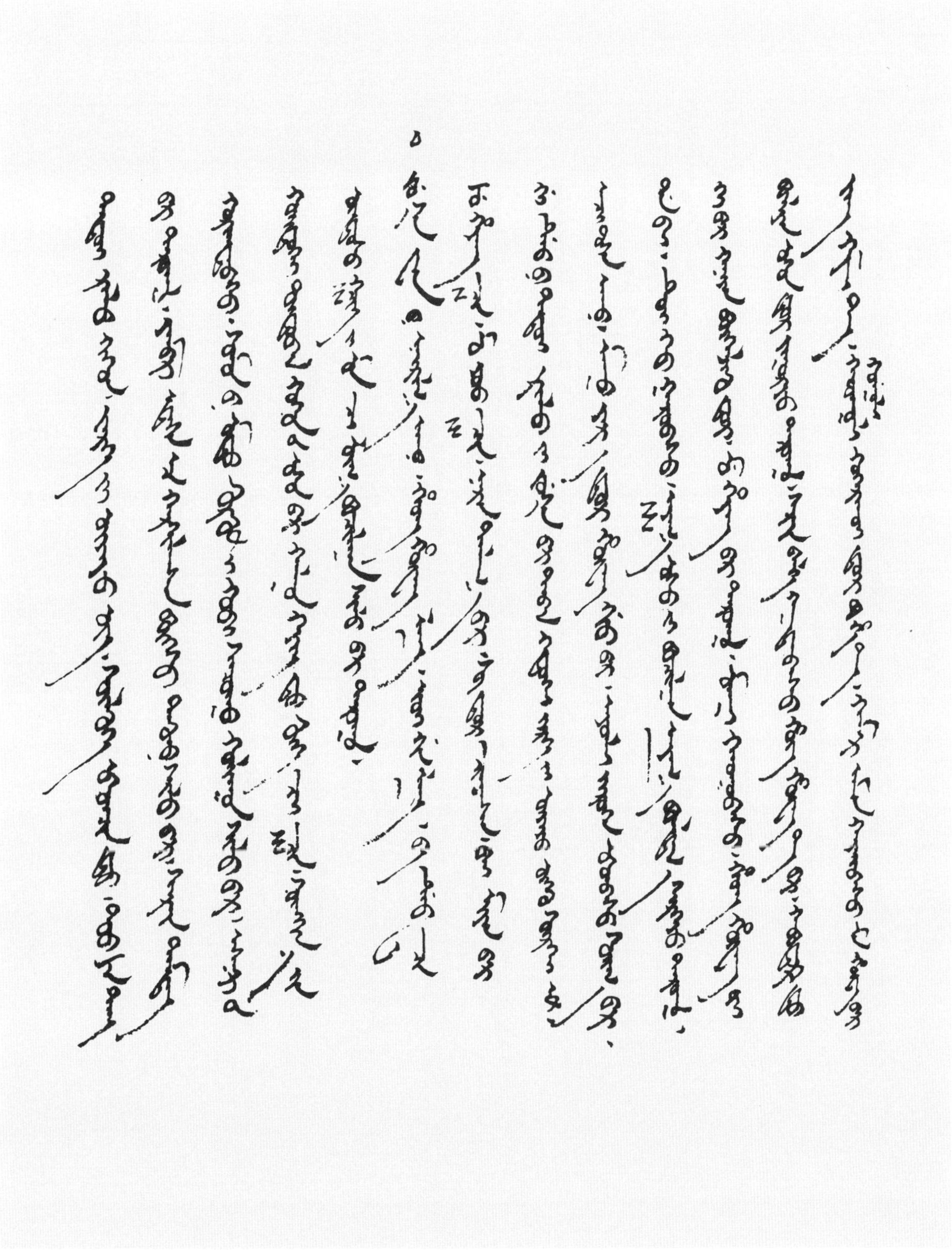

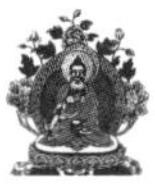

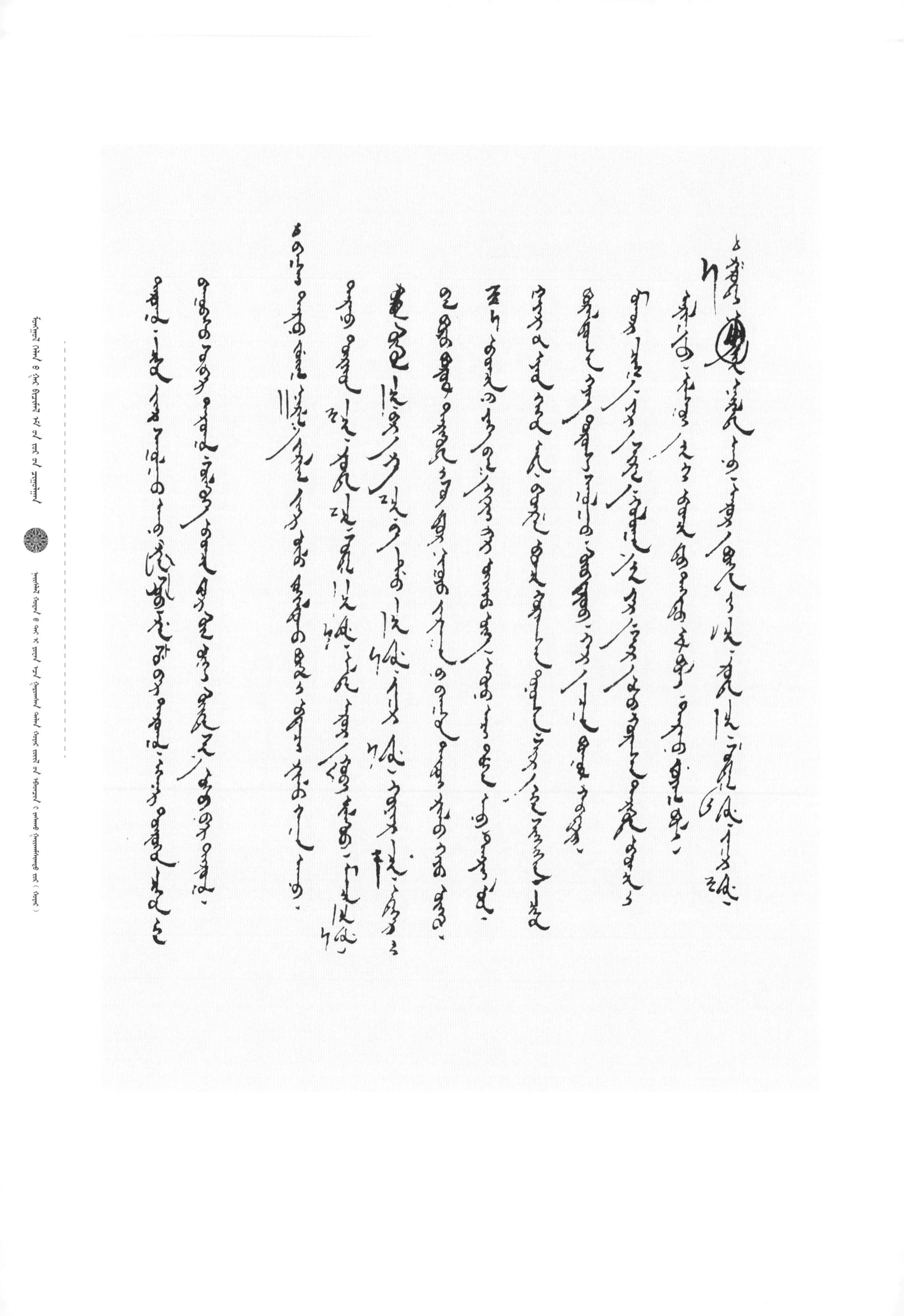

[illegible]

[illegible]

[illegible]

[illegible]

[illegible]

[illegible]

[illegible]

[illegible]

[illegible]

[illegible]

[illegible]

[illegible]

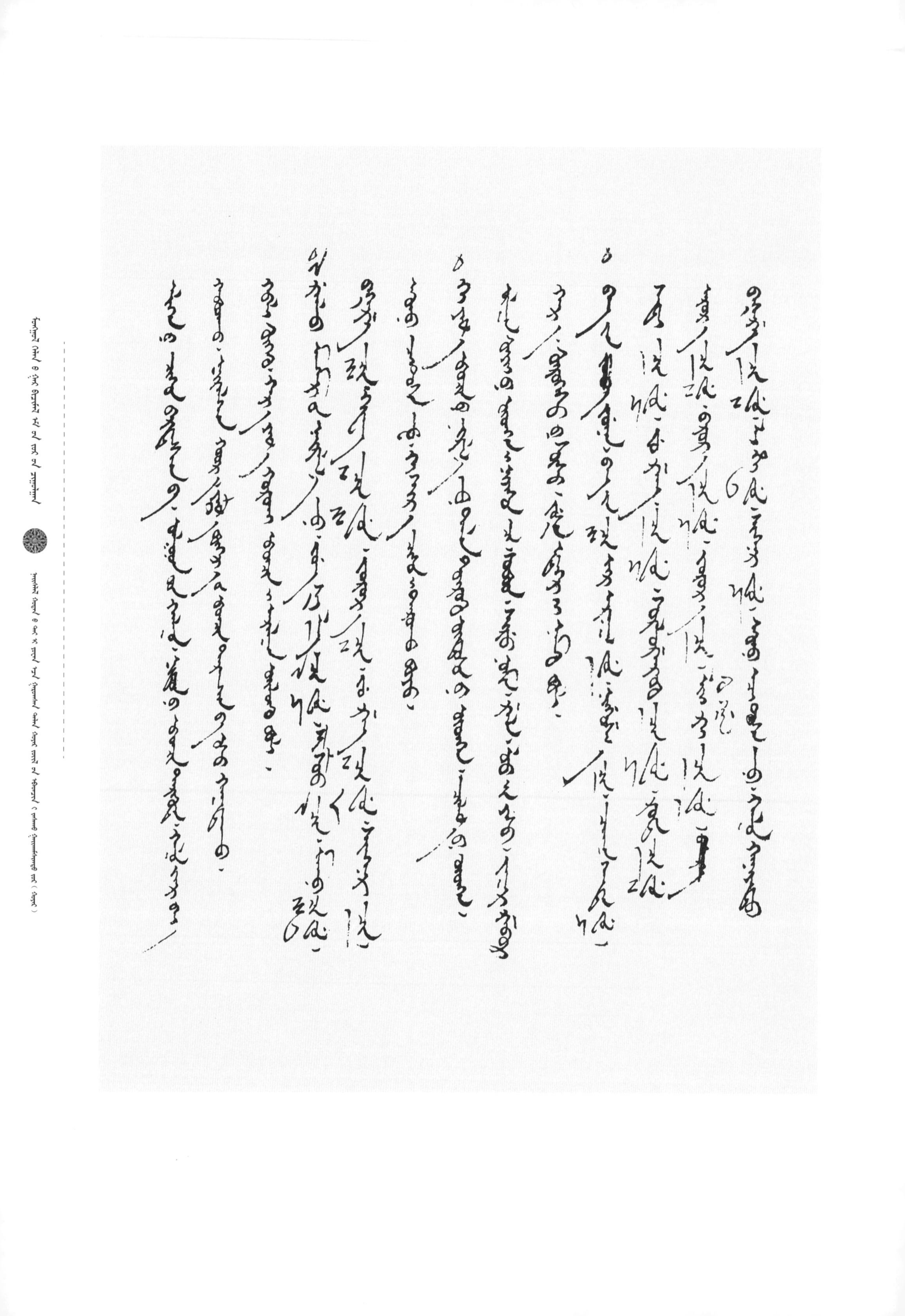

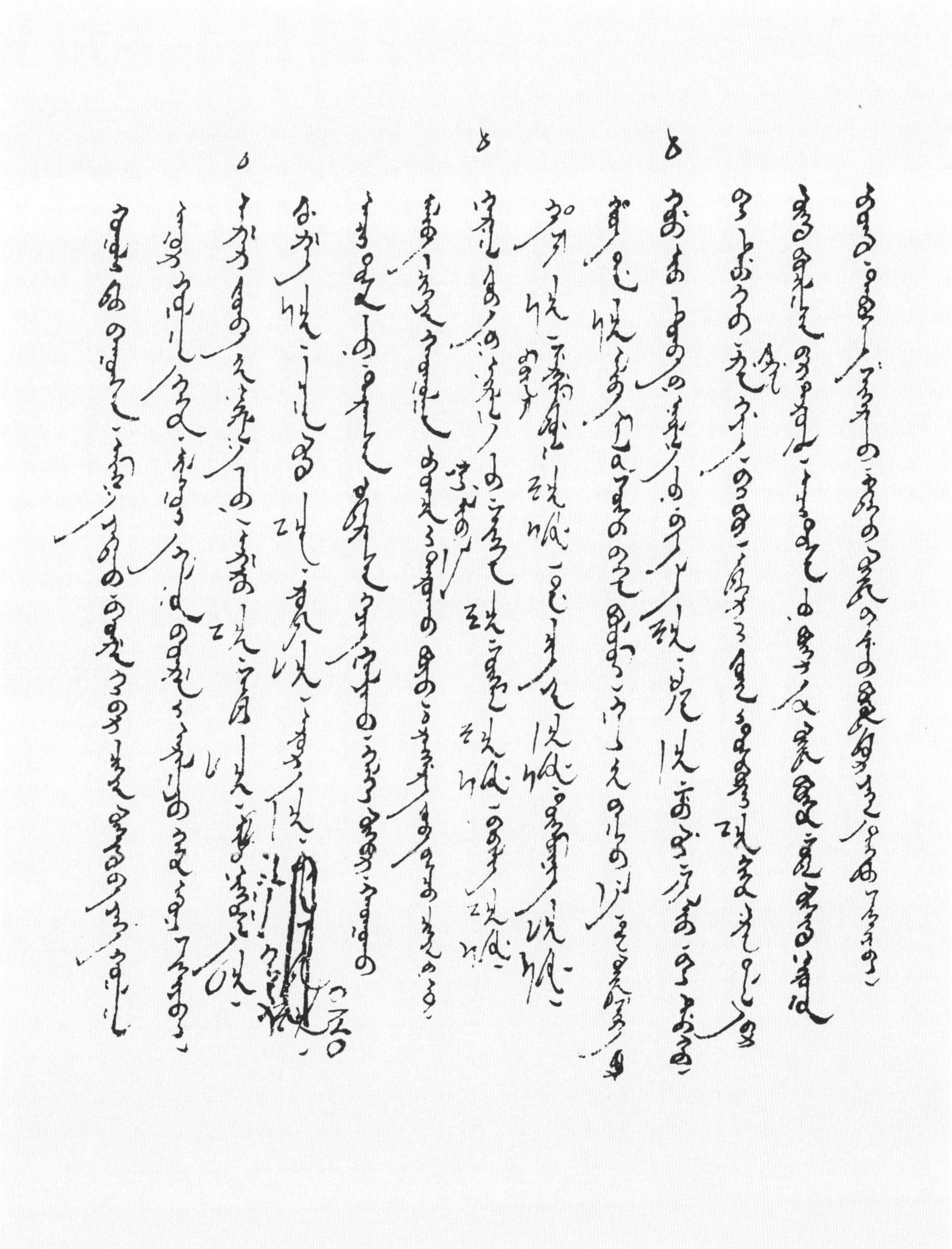

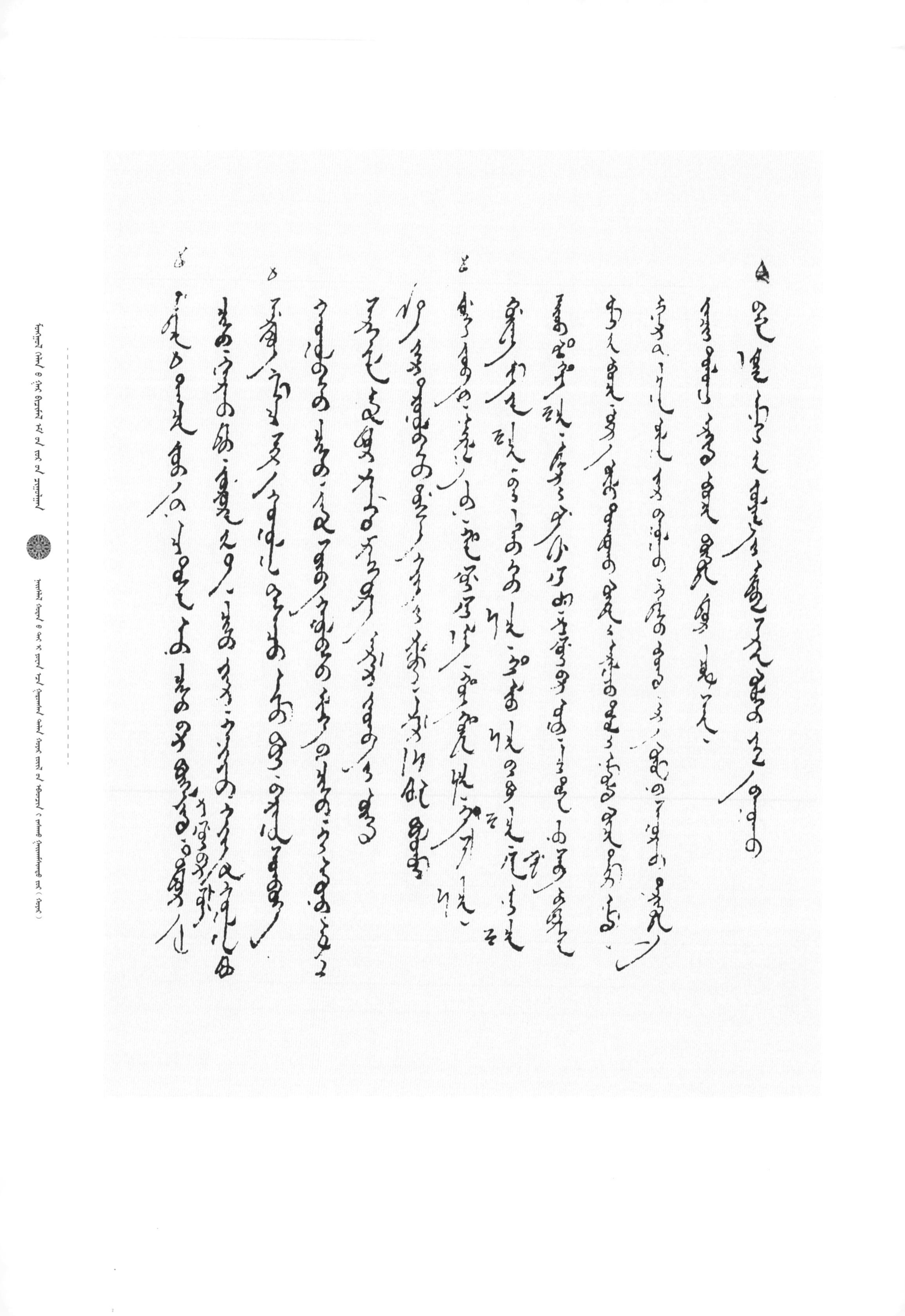

[illegible]

[illegible]

[illegible]

[illegible]

[illegible]

[illegible]

[illegible]

[illegible]

[illegible]

[illegible]

[illegible]

[illegible]

[illegible]

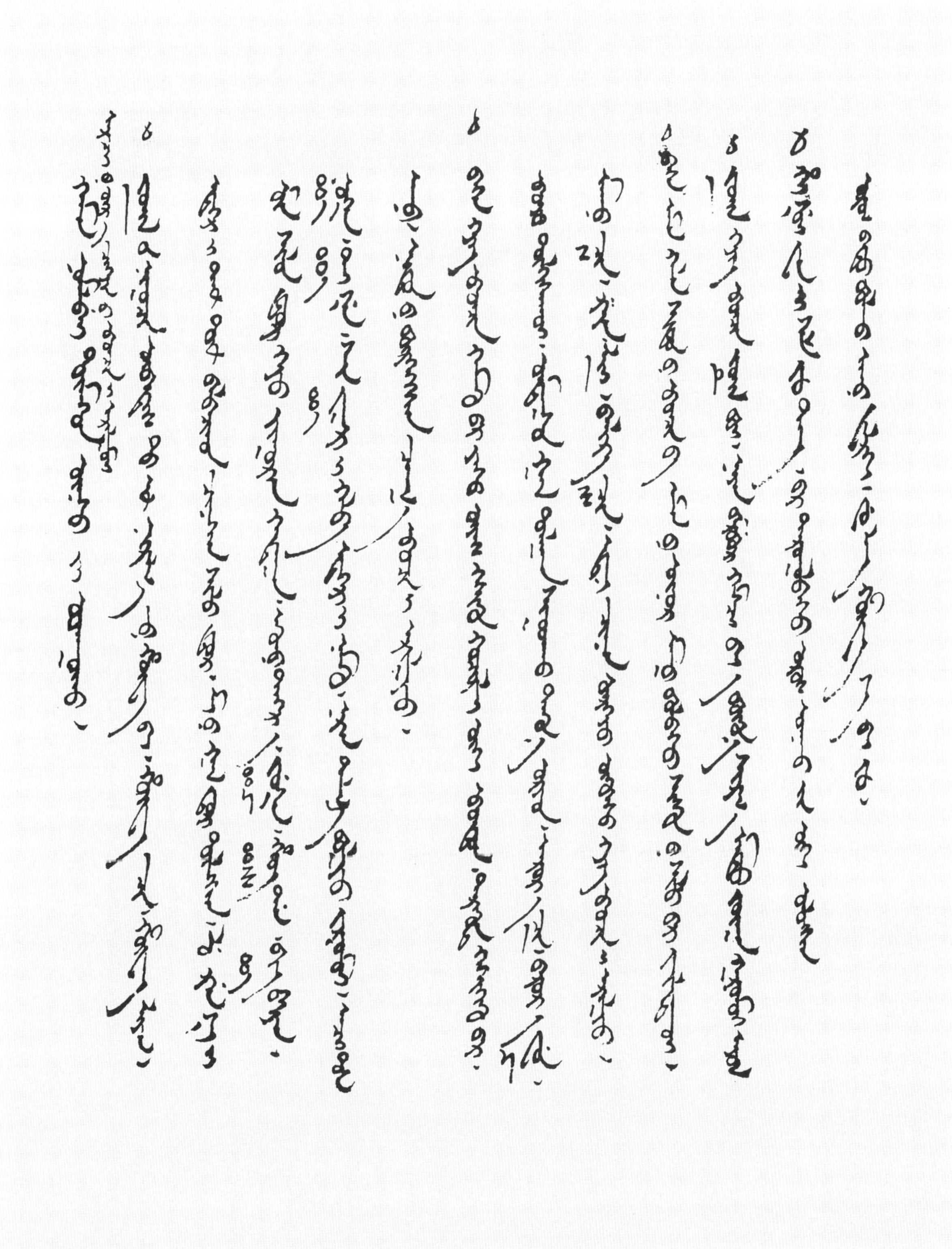

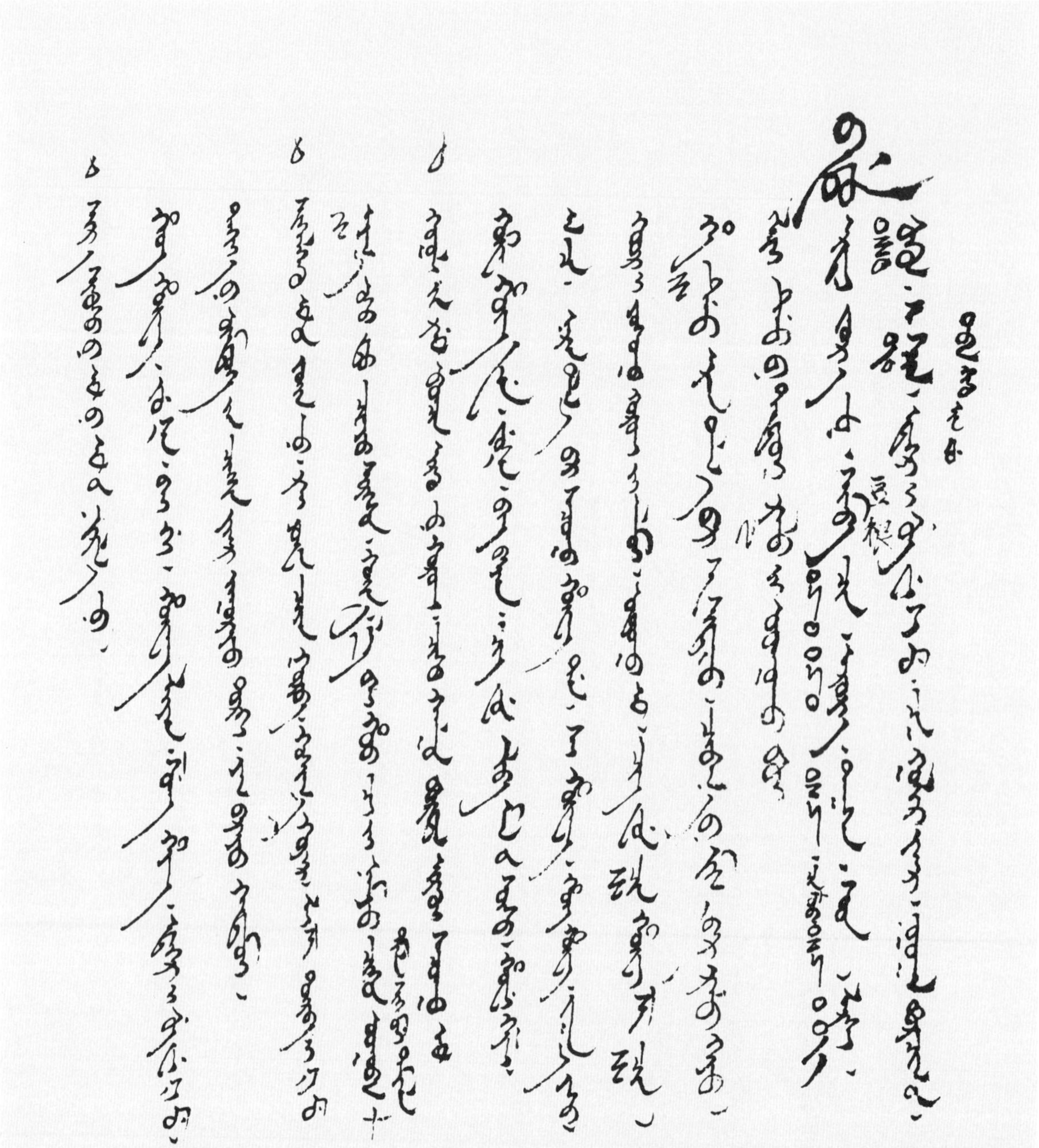

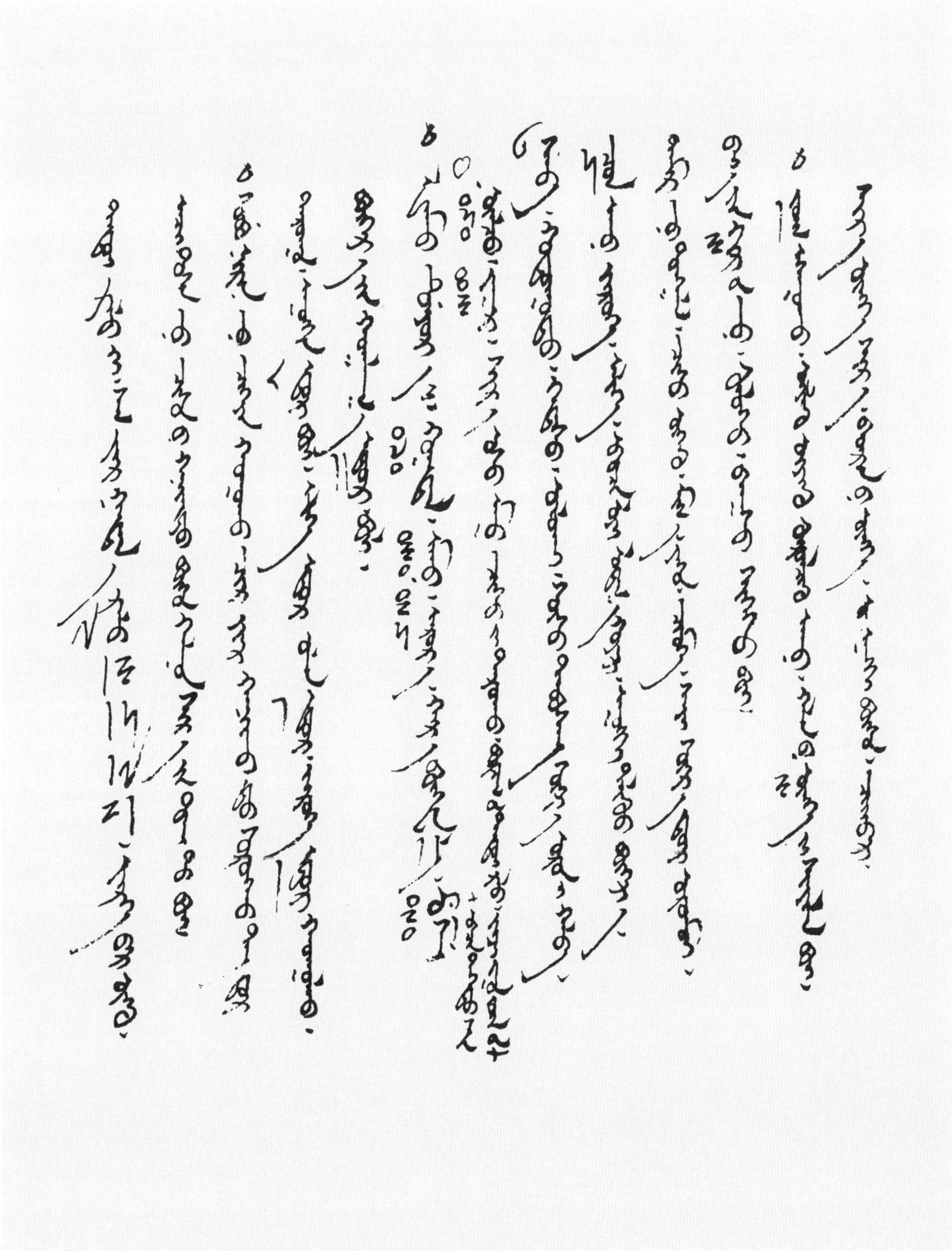

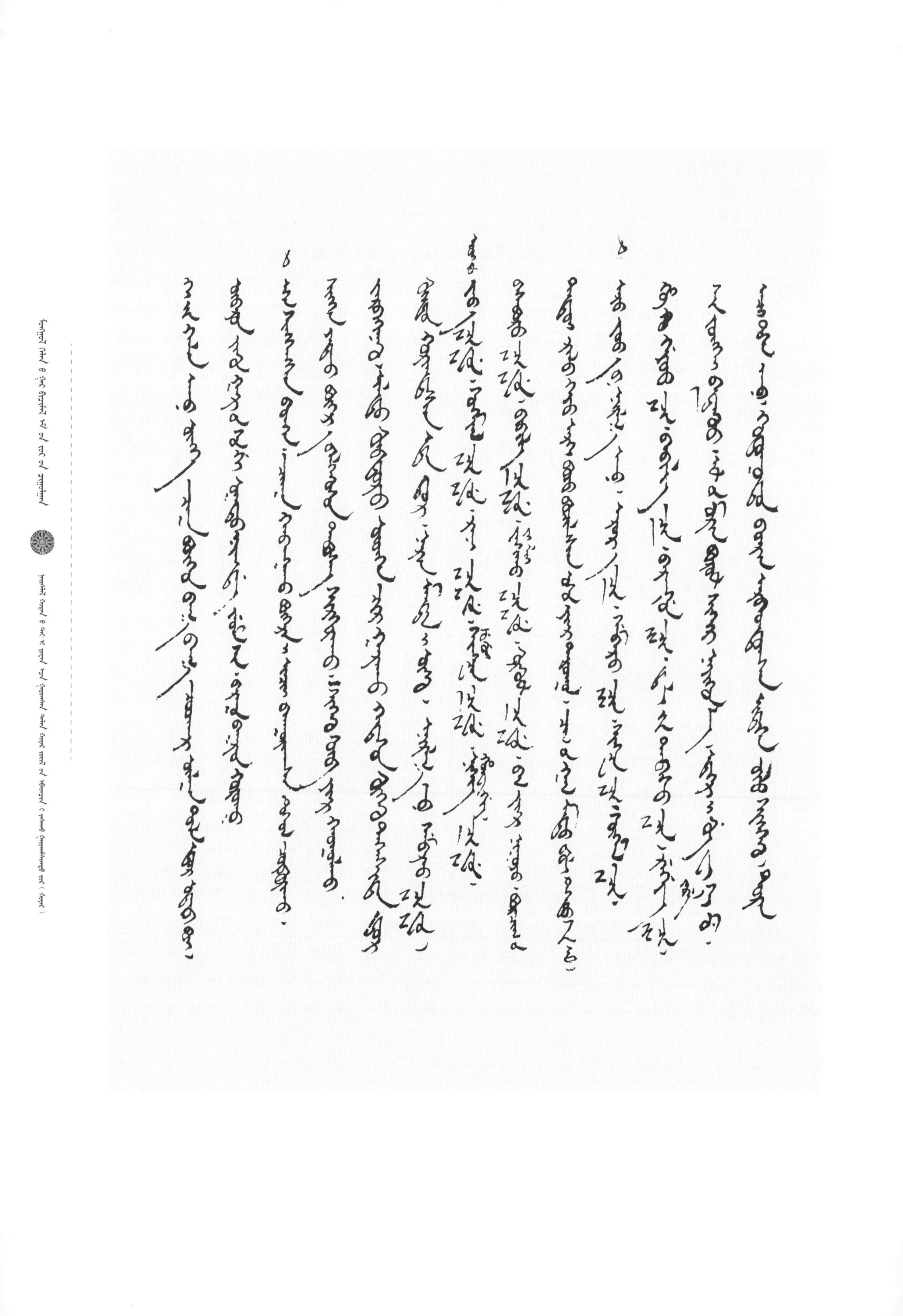

[illegible]

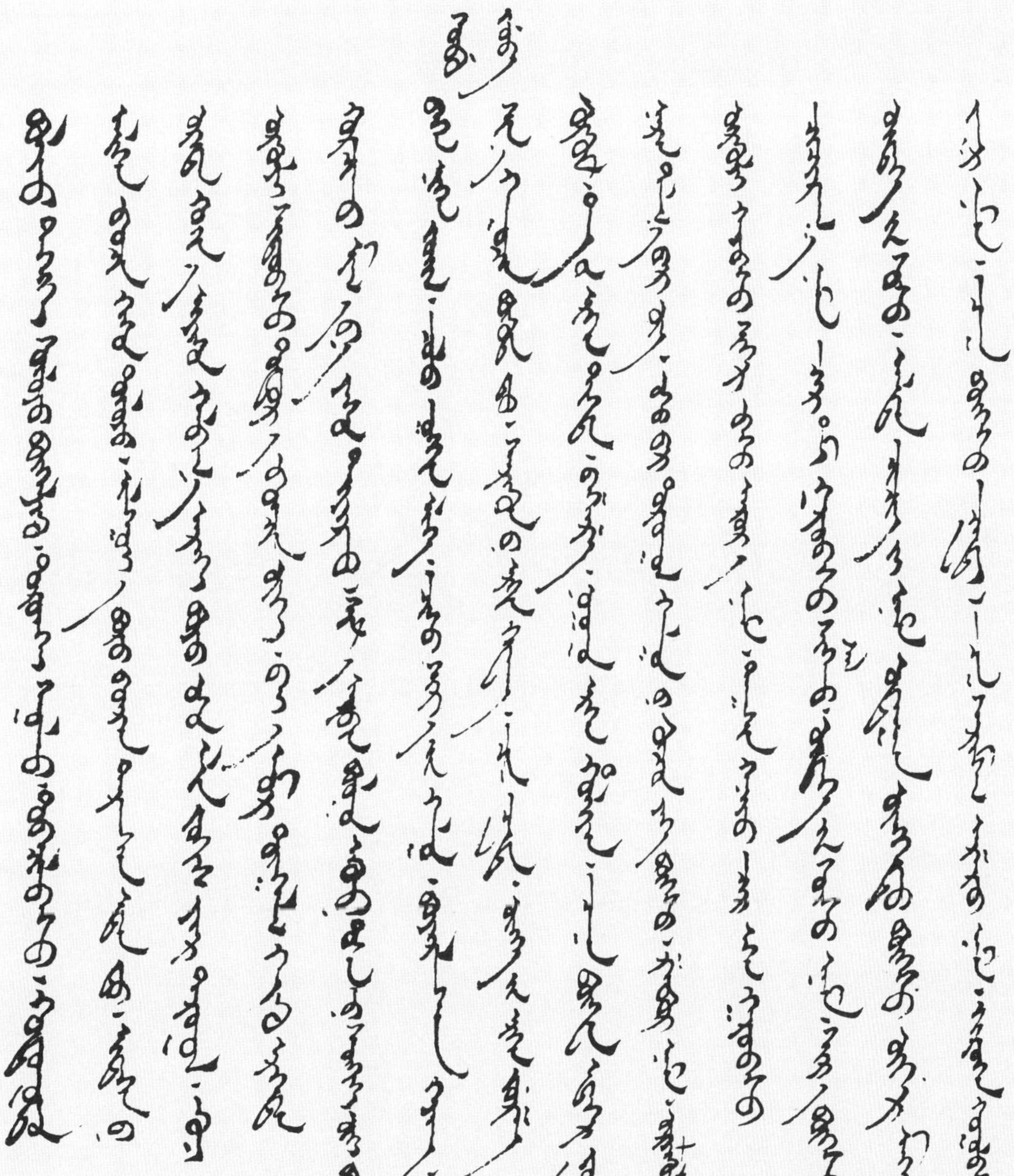

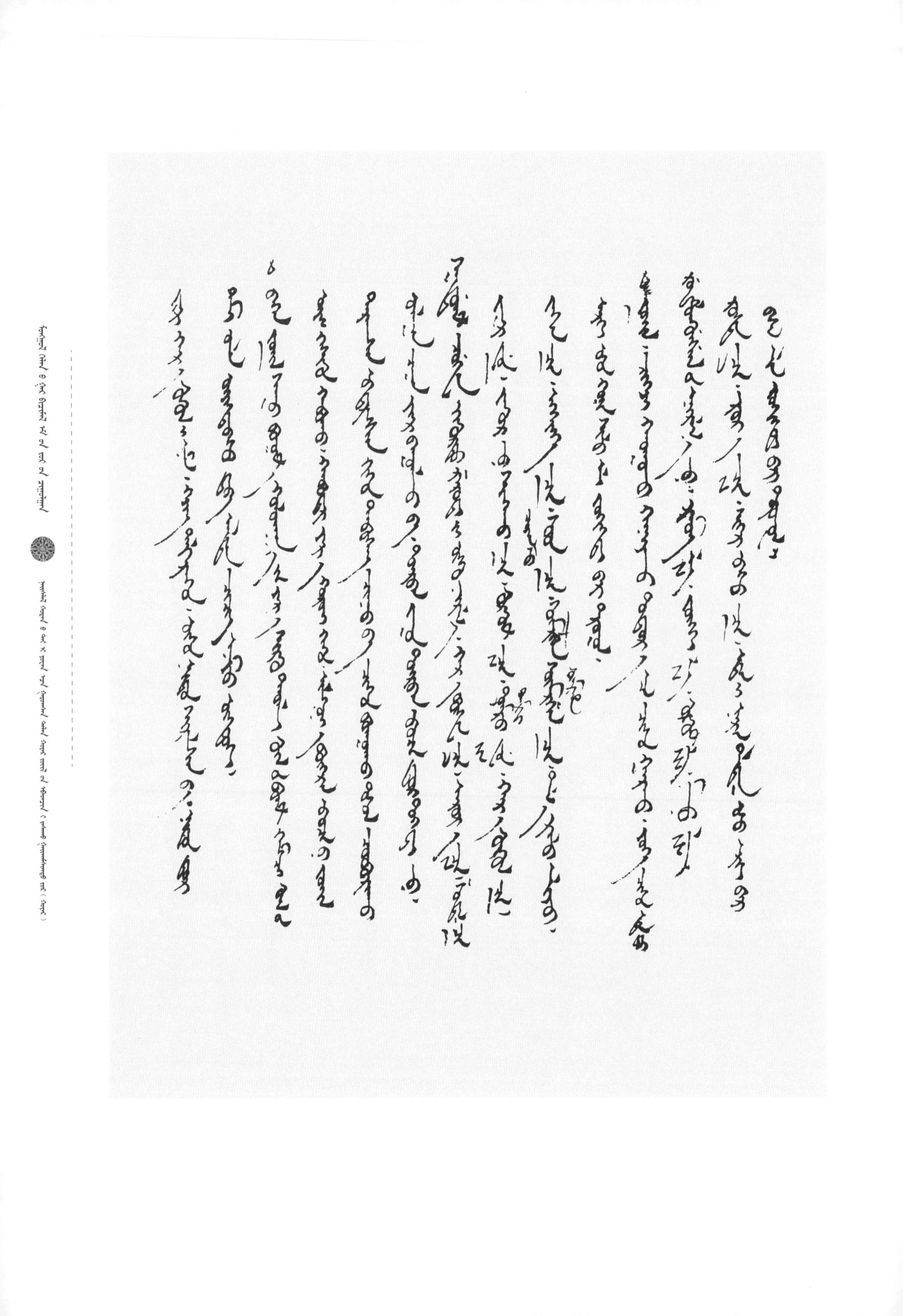

[illegible]

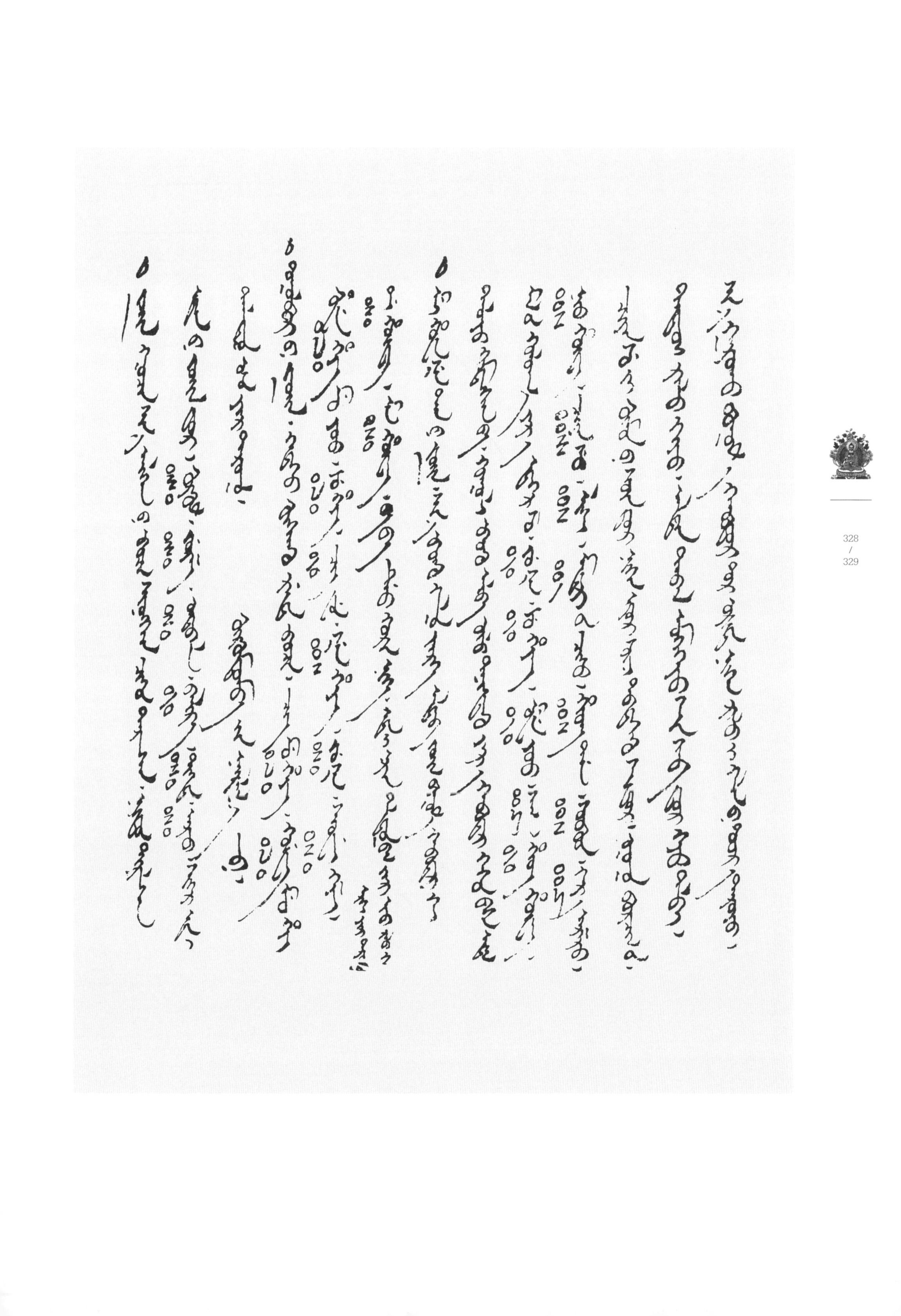

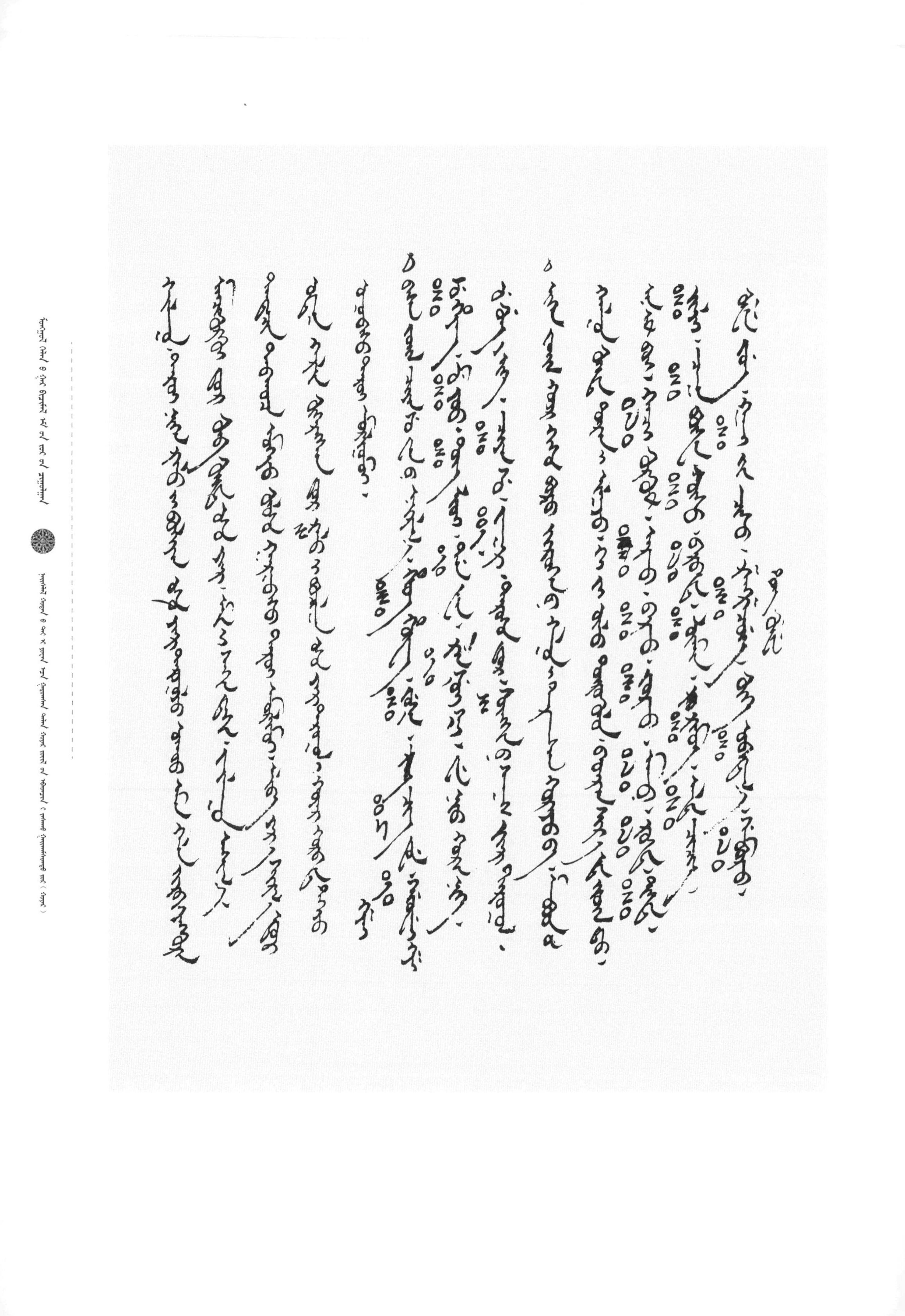

[illegible]

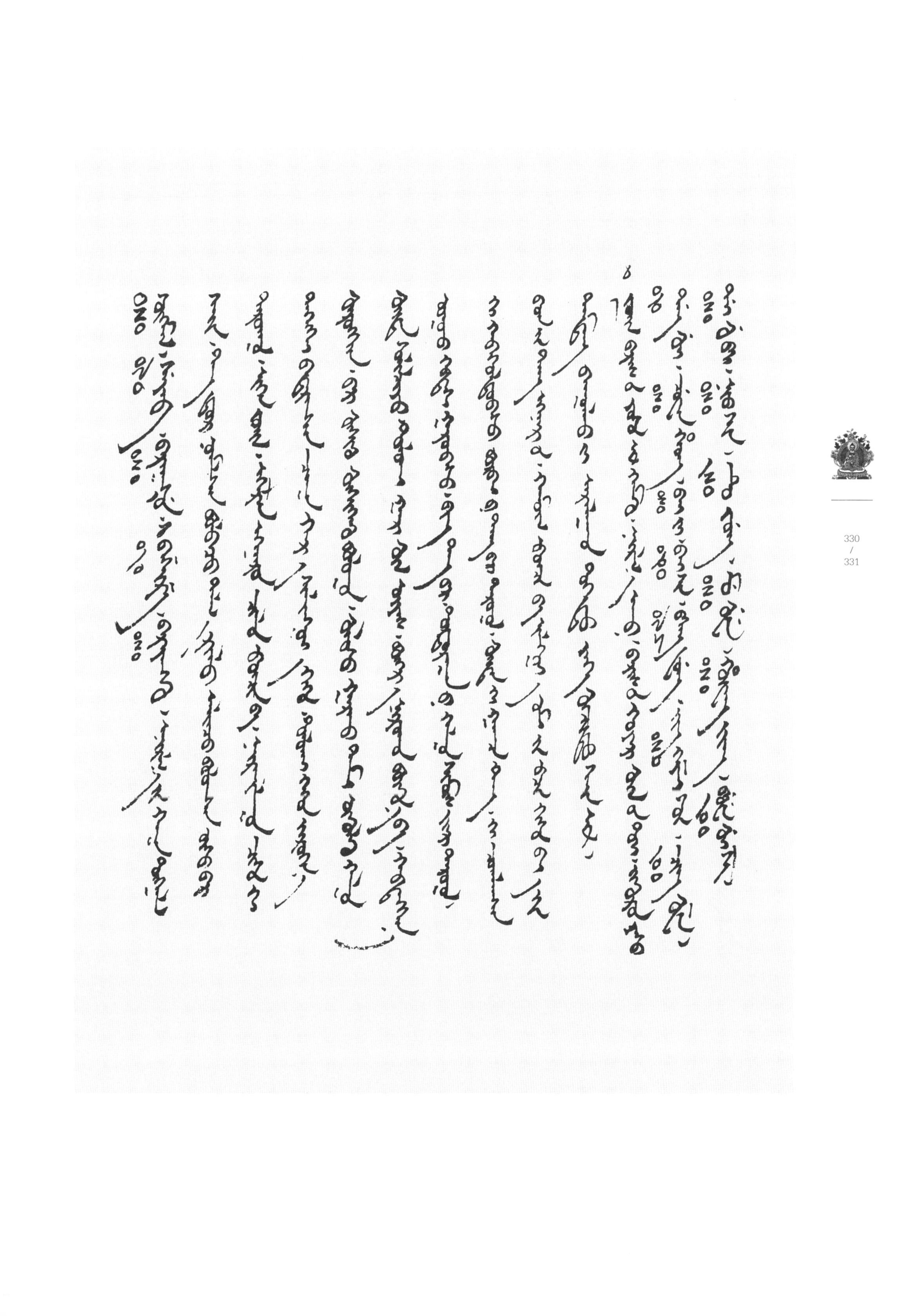

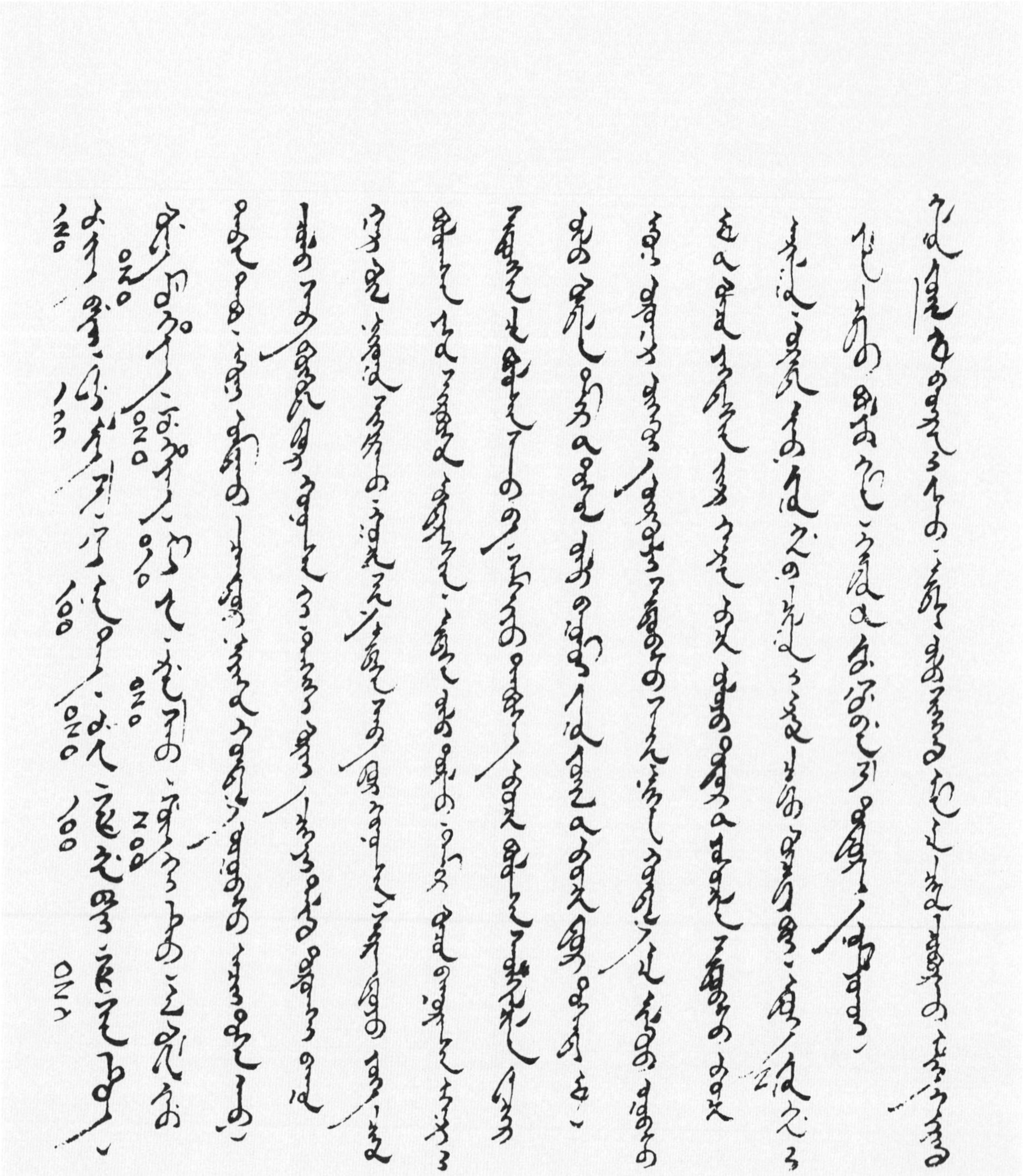

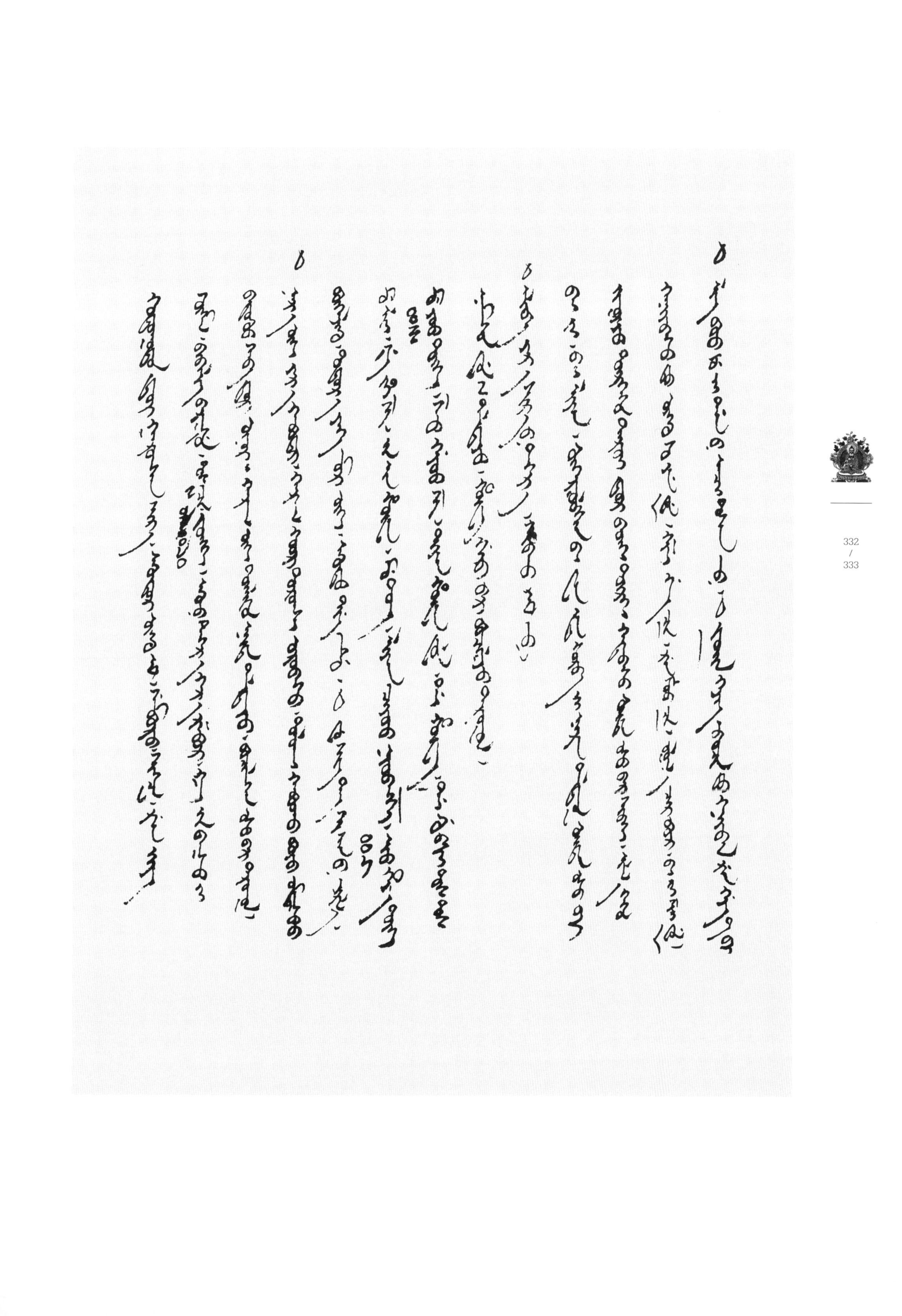

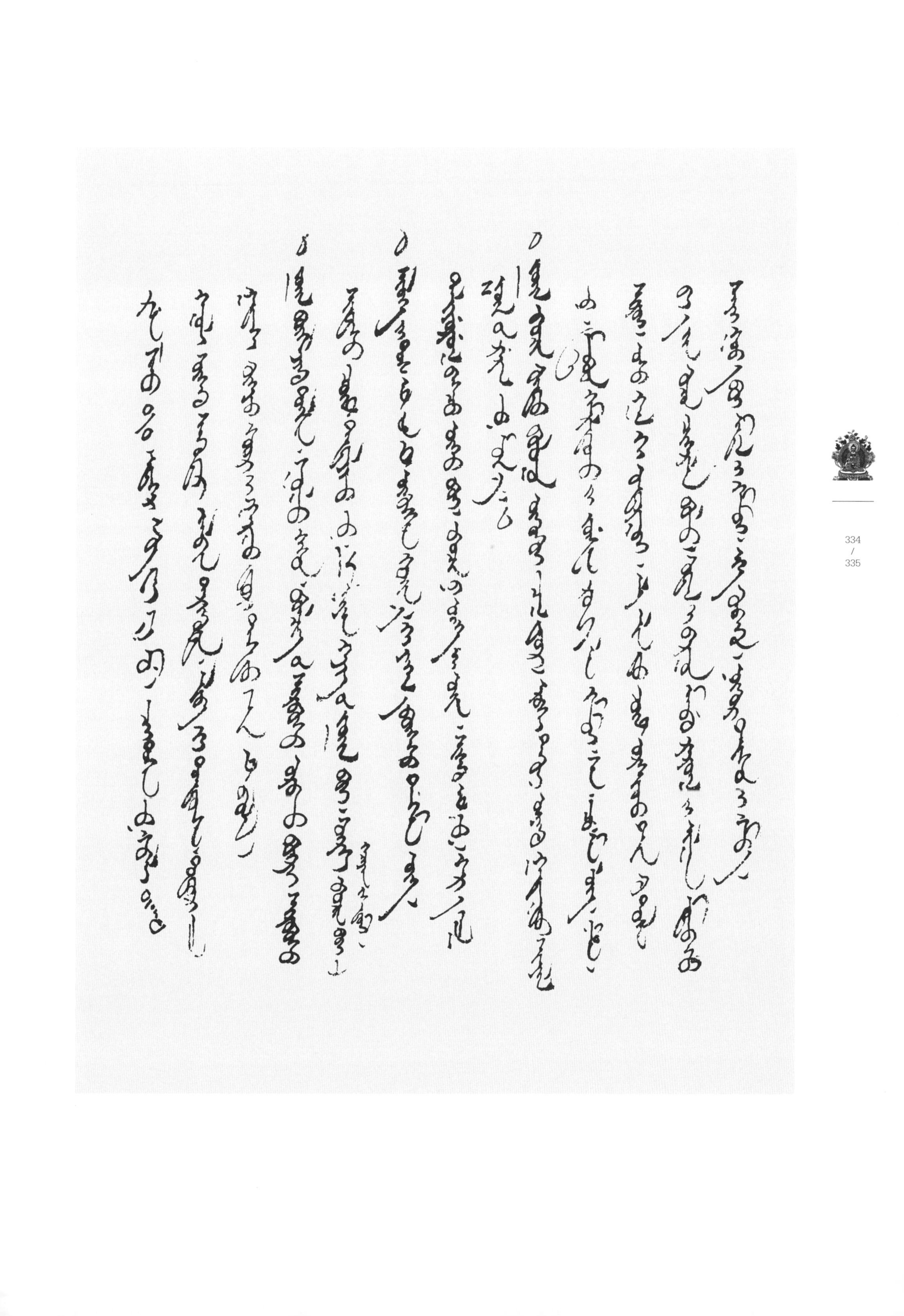

[illegible]

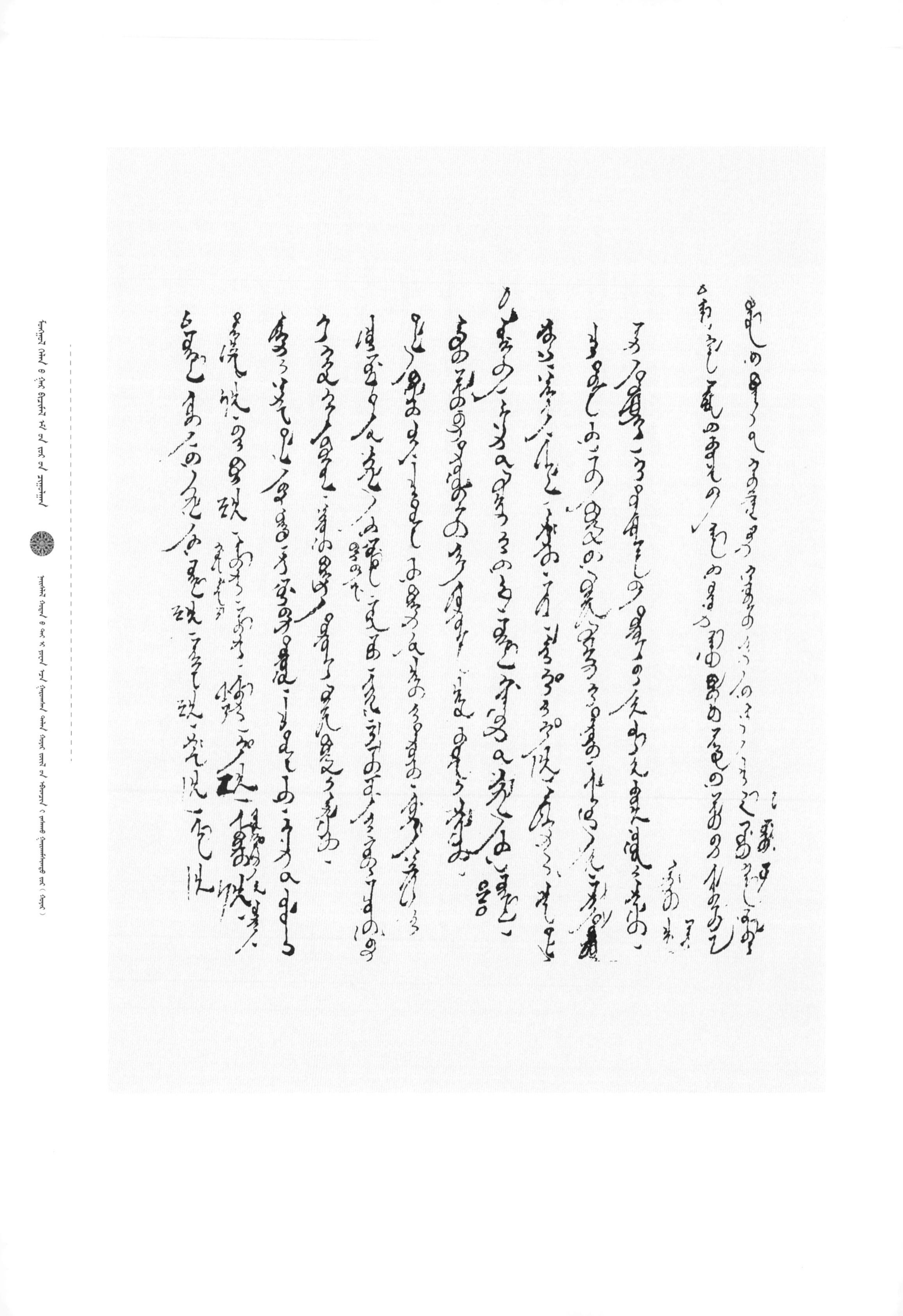

[illegible]

ᠳᠠᠭᠤ ᠰᠣᠩᠰᠣᠭᠠᠳ ᠬᠣᠪᠢ ᠵᠢᠷᠤᠭᠲᠤ ᠮᠣᠩᠭᠣᠯ ᠤᠨ ᠪᠡᠶᠡᠵᠢᠭᠦᠯᠦᠭᠰᠡᠨ ᠳᠣᠬᠢᠶ᠎ᠠ（1893）ᠣᠨ ᠮᠣᠩᠭᠣᠯ ᠣᠨ ᠪᠦᠷᠢᠨ ᠪᠠᠢᠳᠠᠯ ᠤᠨ ᠬᠡᠪᠯᠡᠯ ᠪᠣᠯᠤᠨ᠎ᠠ ᠃ ᠲᠡᠪᠰᠢᠭᠦᠯᠦᠨ ᠣᠨ ᠰᠢᠨ᠎ᠡ ᠪᠡᠷ ᠪᠡᠶᠡᠵᠢᠭᠦᠯᠦᠨ ᠬᠡᠪ ᠦᠨ ᠬᠡᠮᠵᠢᠶ᠎ᠡ ᠨᠢ : 19.5cm×18.5cm ᠪᠣᠯᠤᠨ᠎ᠠ ᠂ ᠨᠢᠭᠤᠷ 34 ᠨᠢᠭᠤᠷ ᠲᠠᠢ ᠃

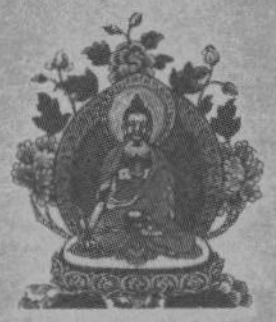

Books on the Treatment of Wounds, Abscesses and Other Diseases

治疗各种创伤、脓包以及疾病书

9

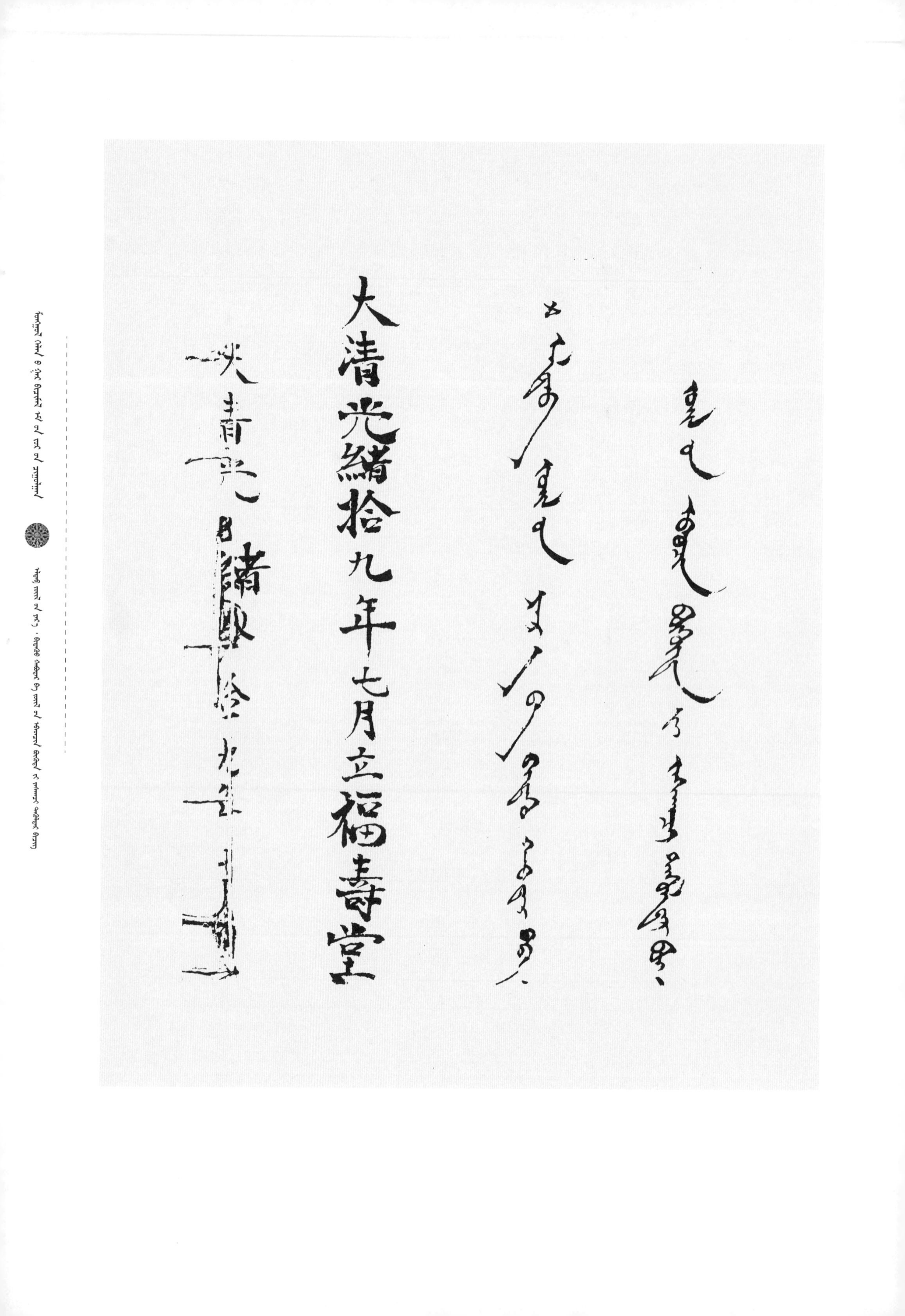

大清光緒拾九年七月立福壽堂

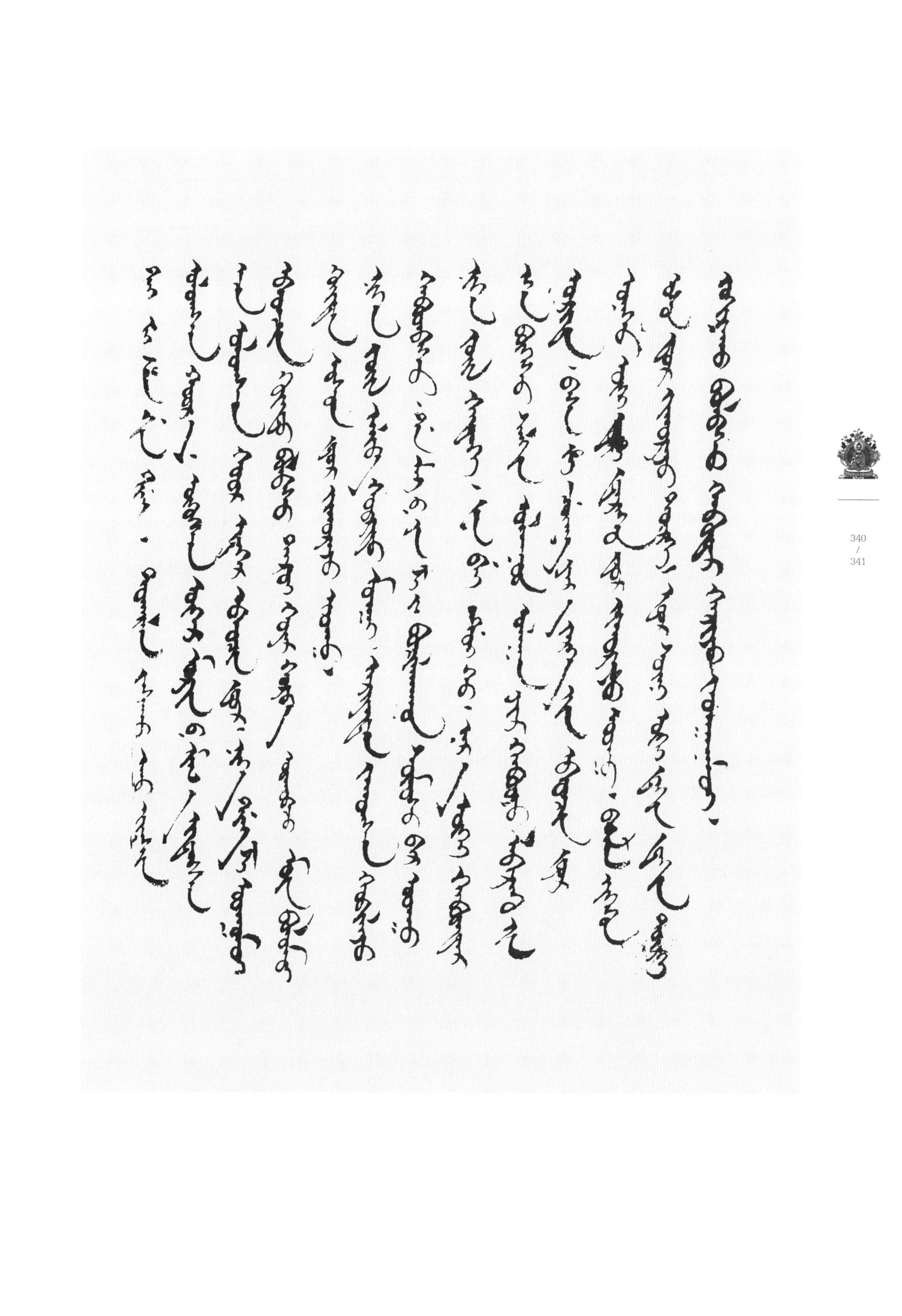

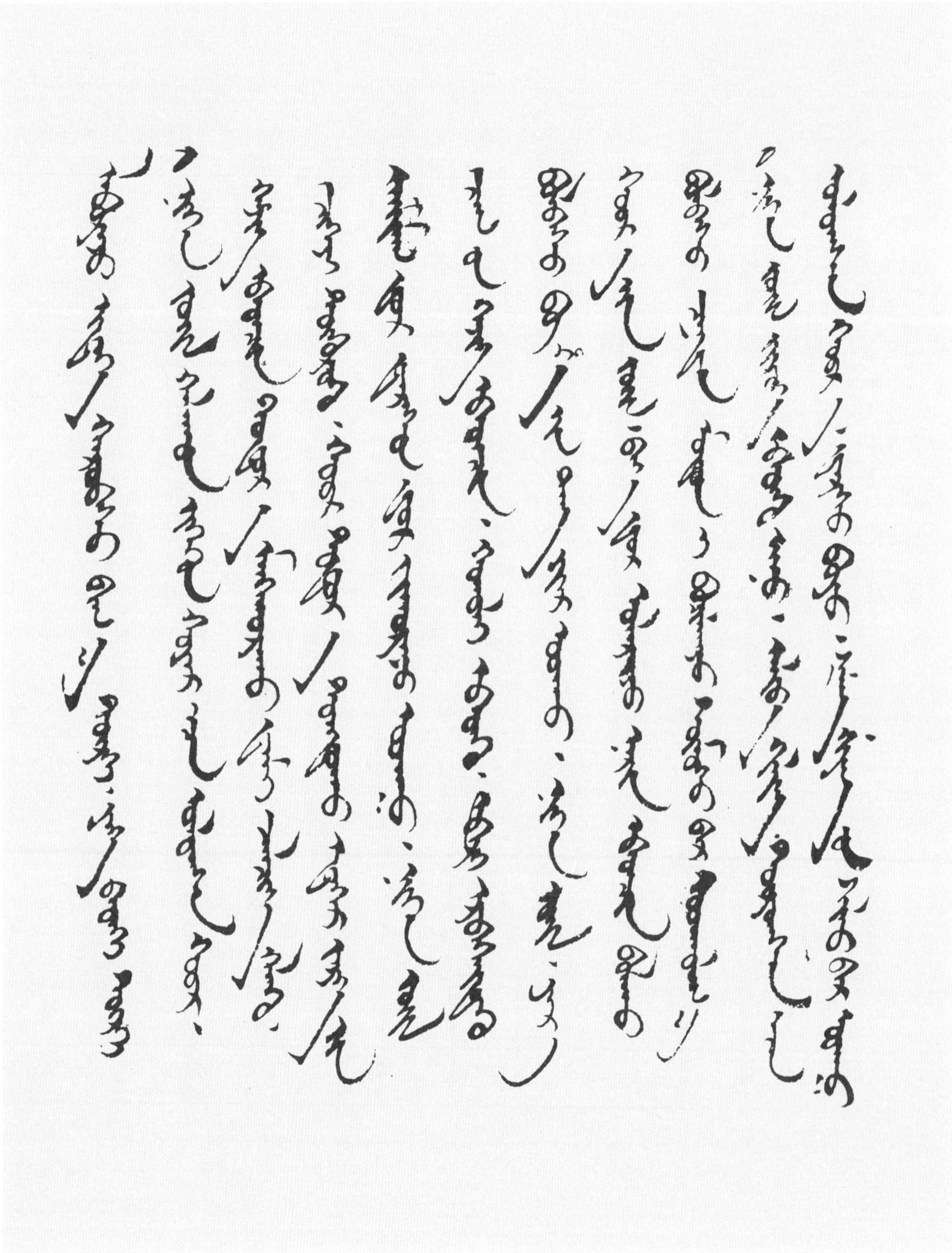

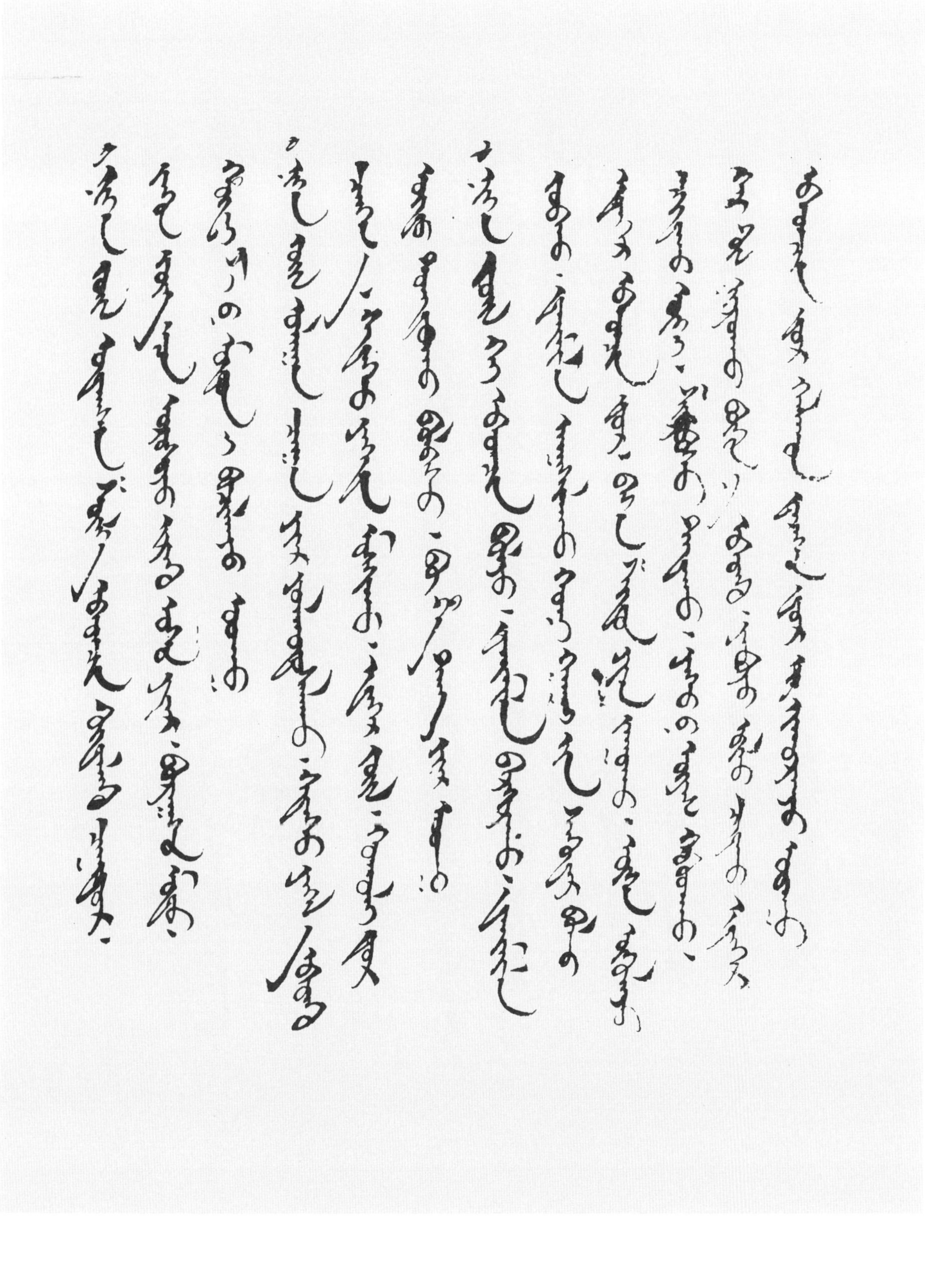

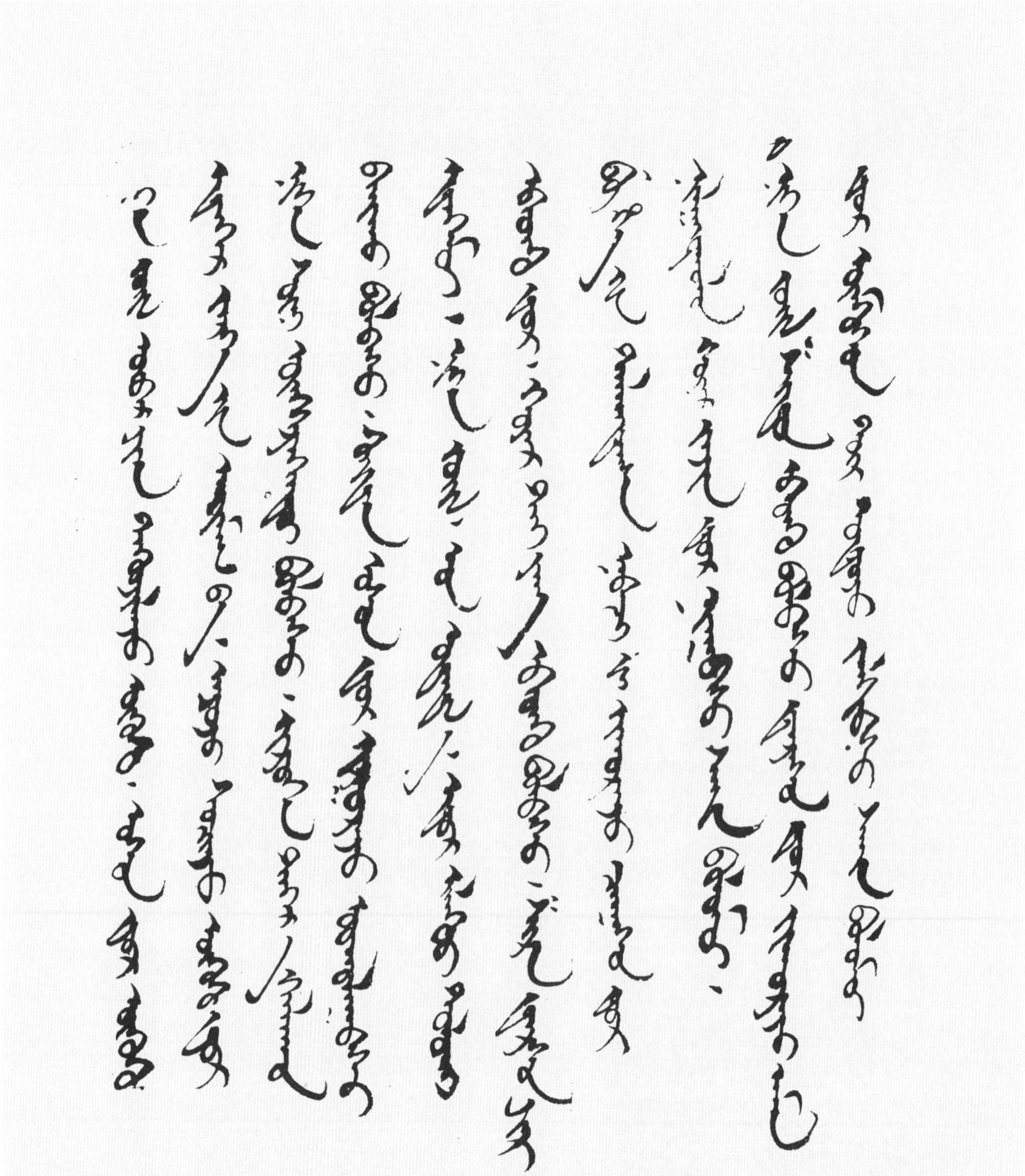

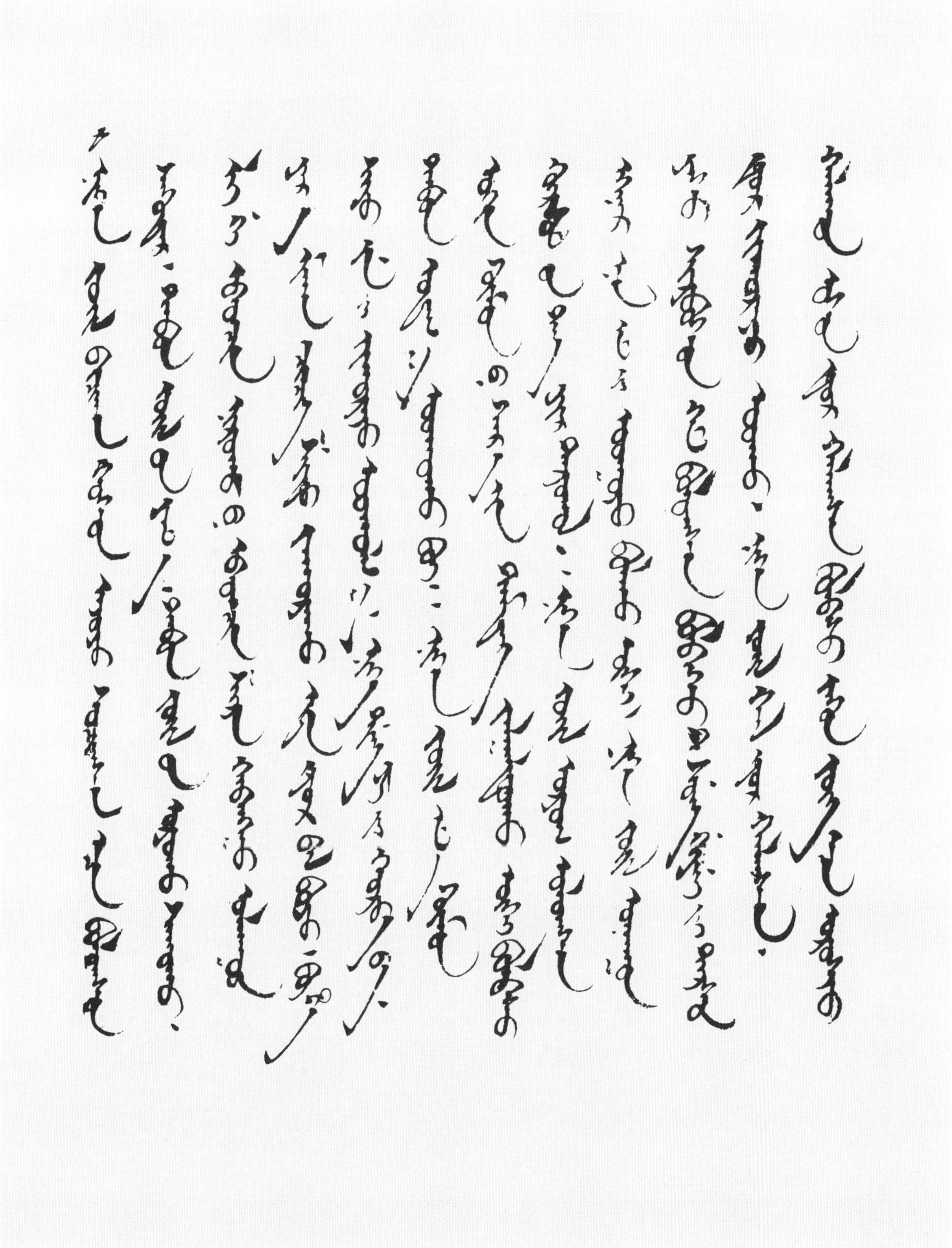

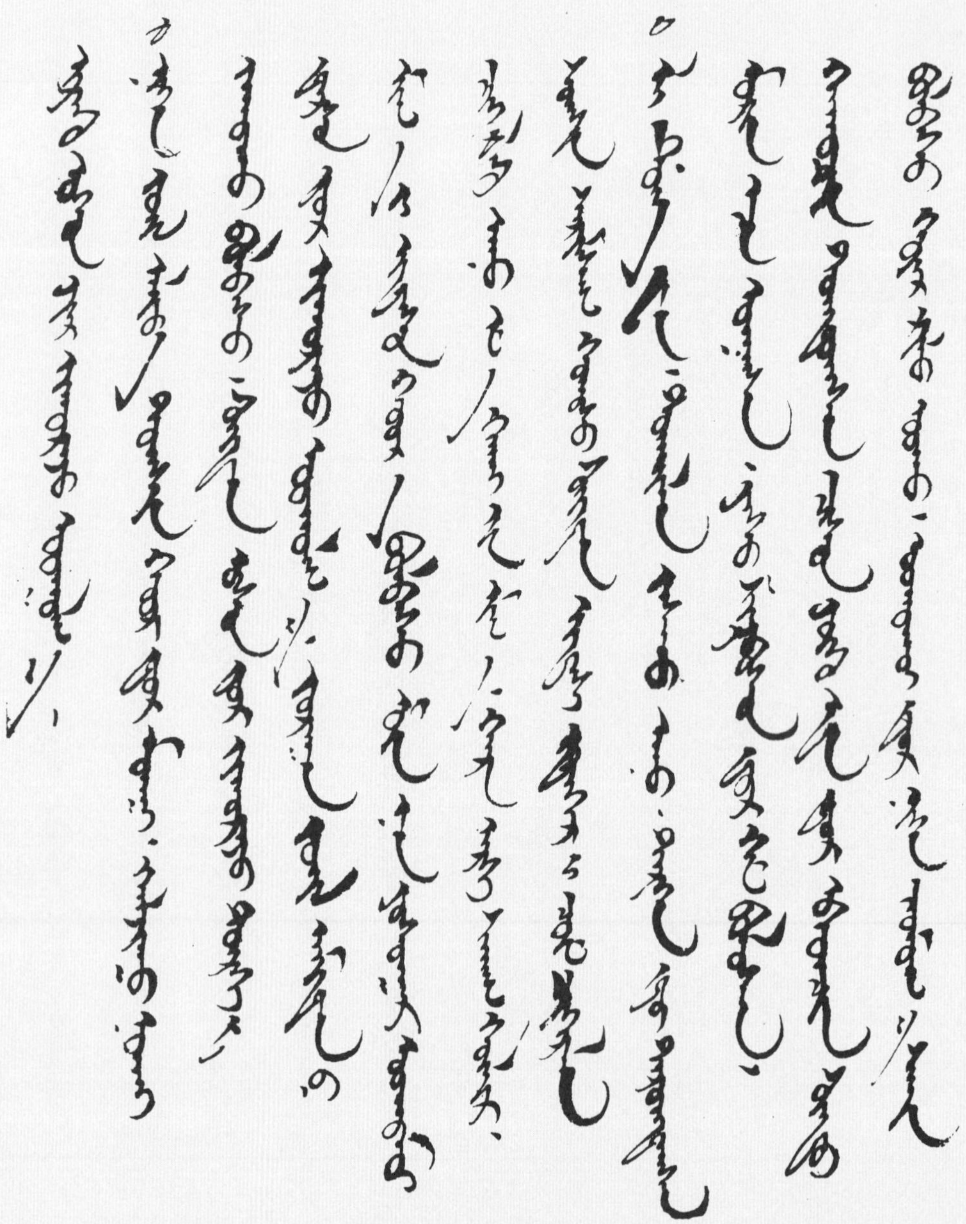

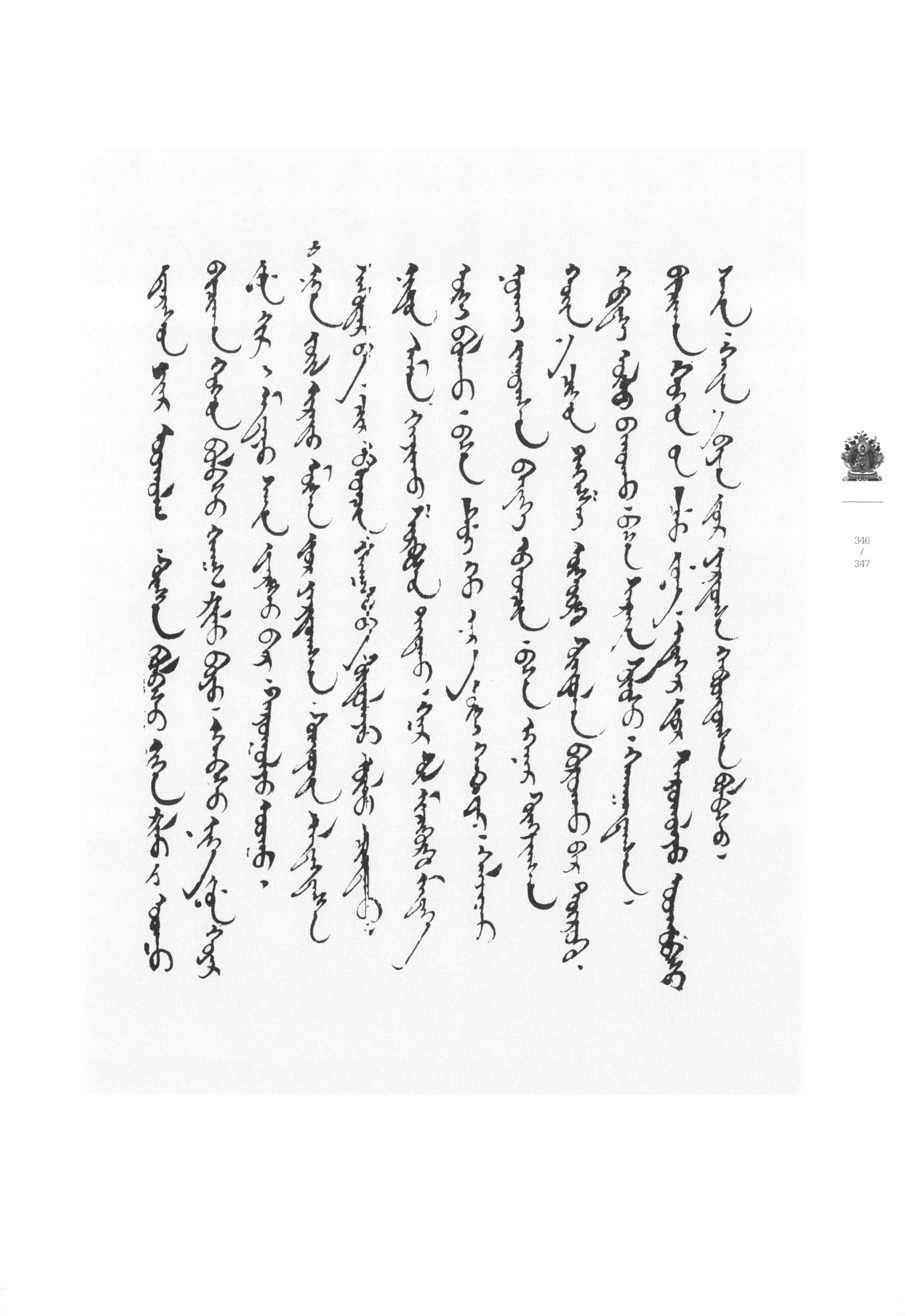

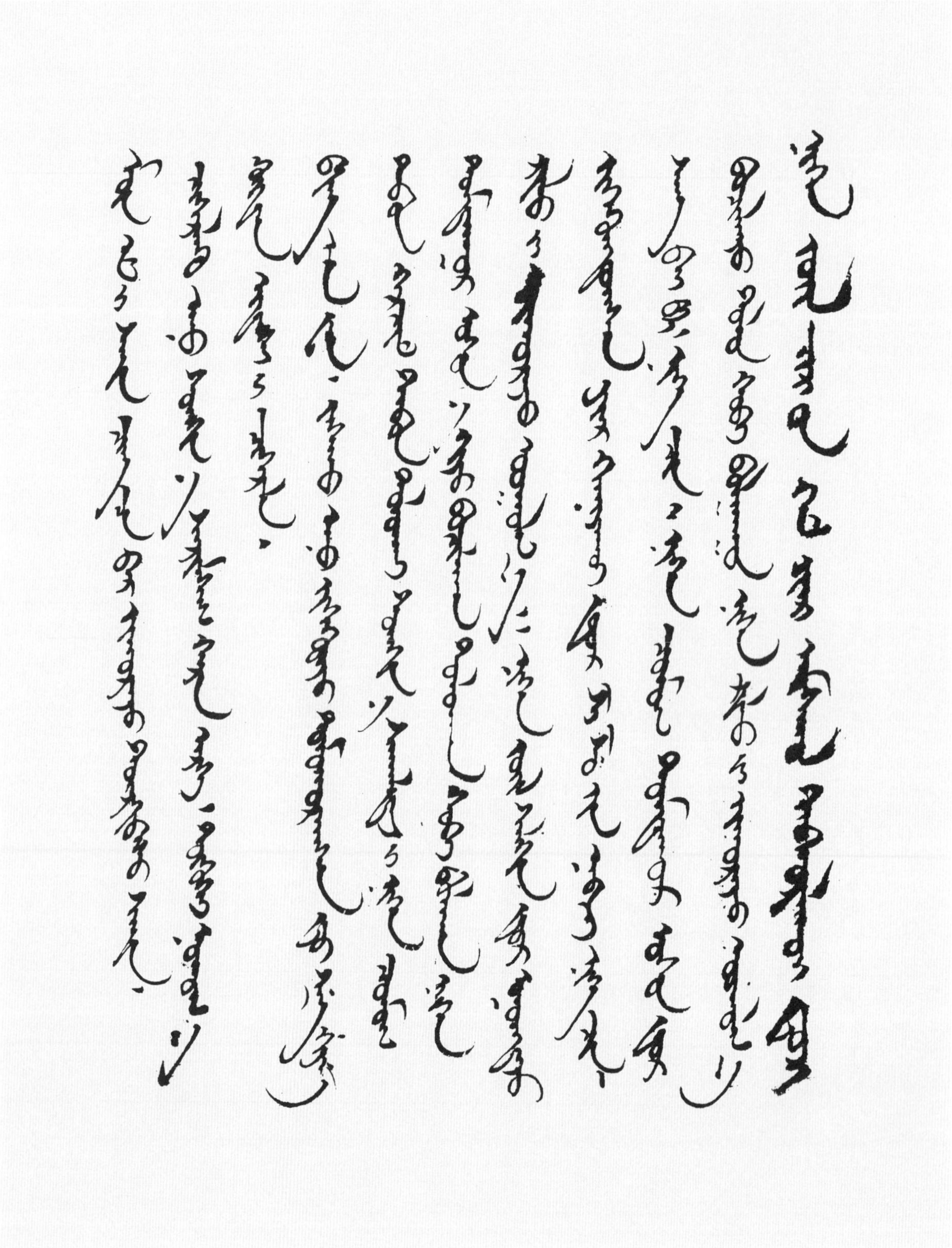

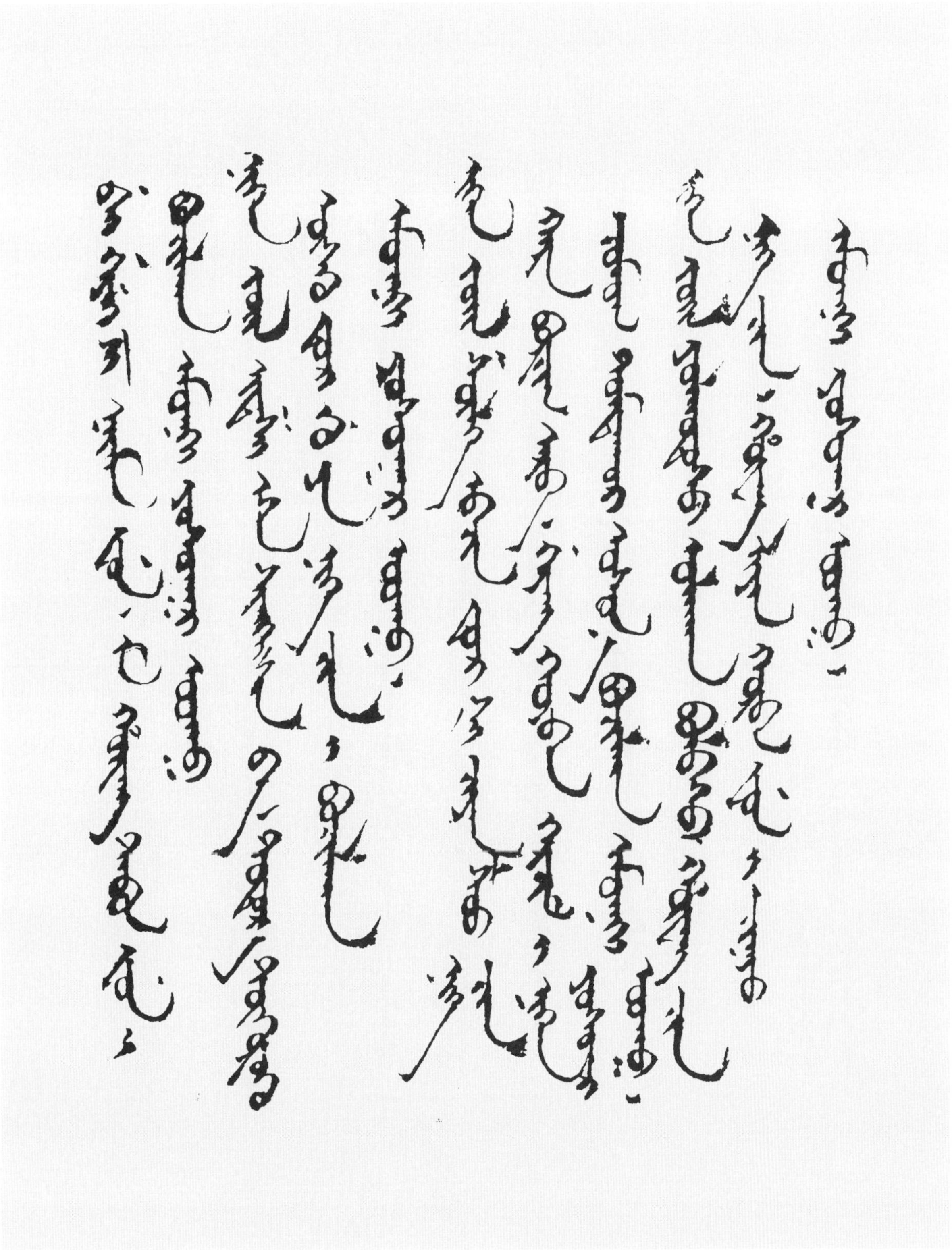

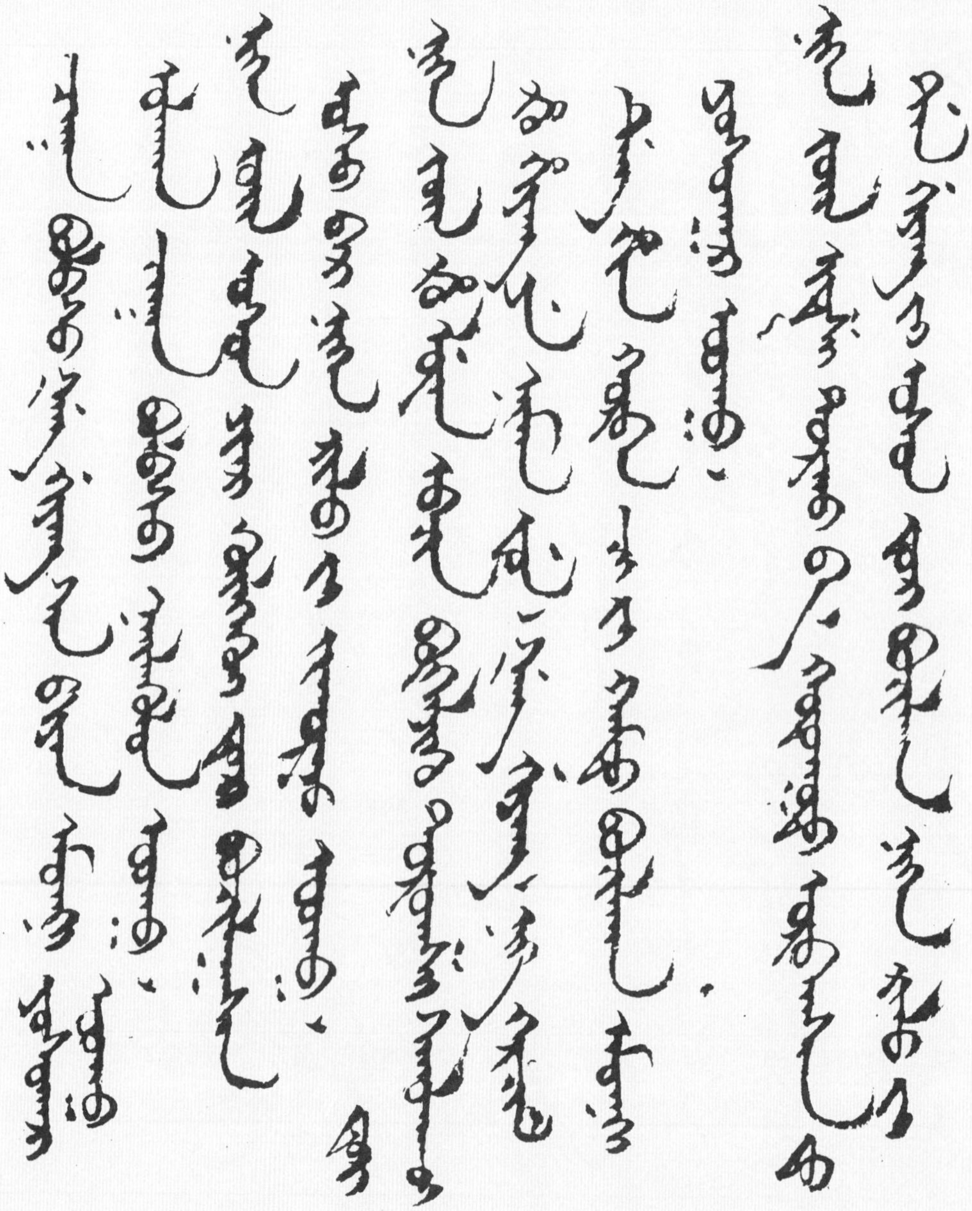

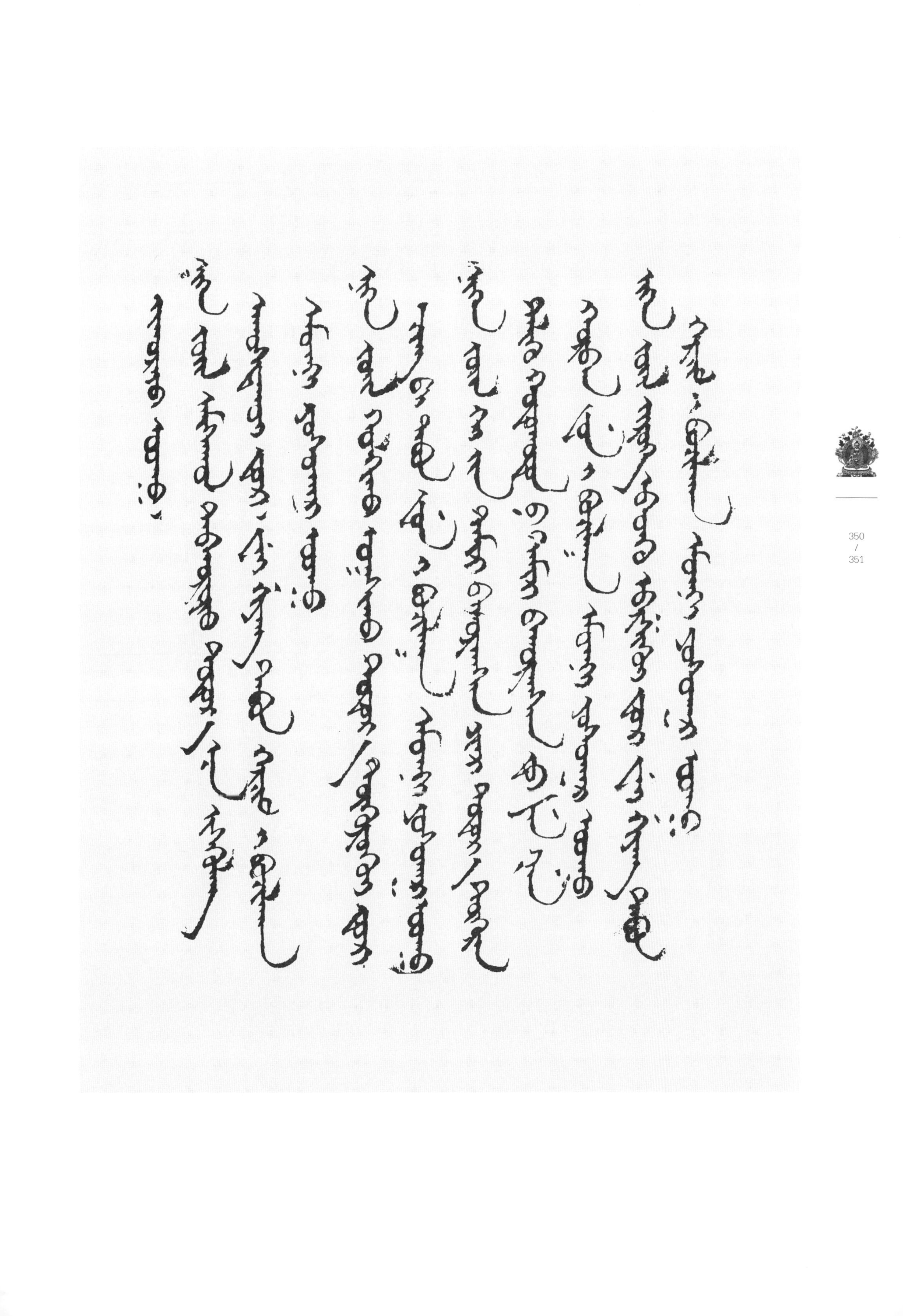

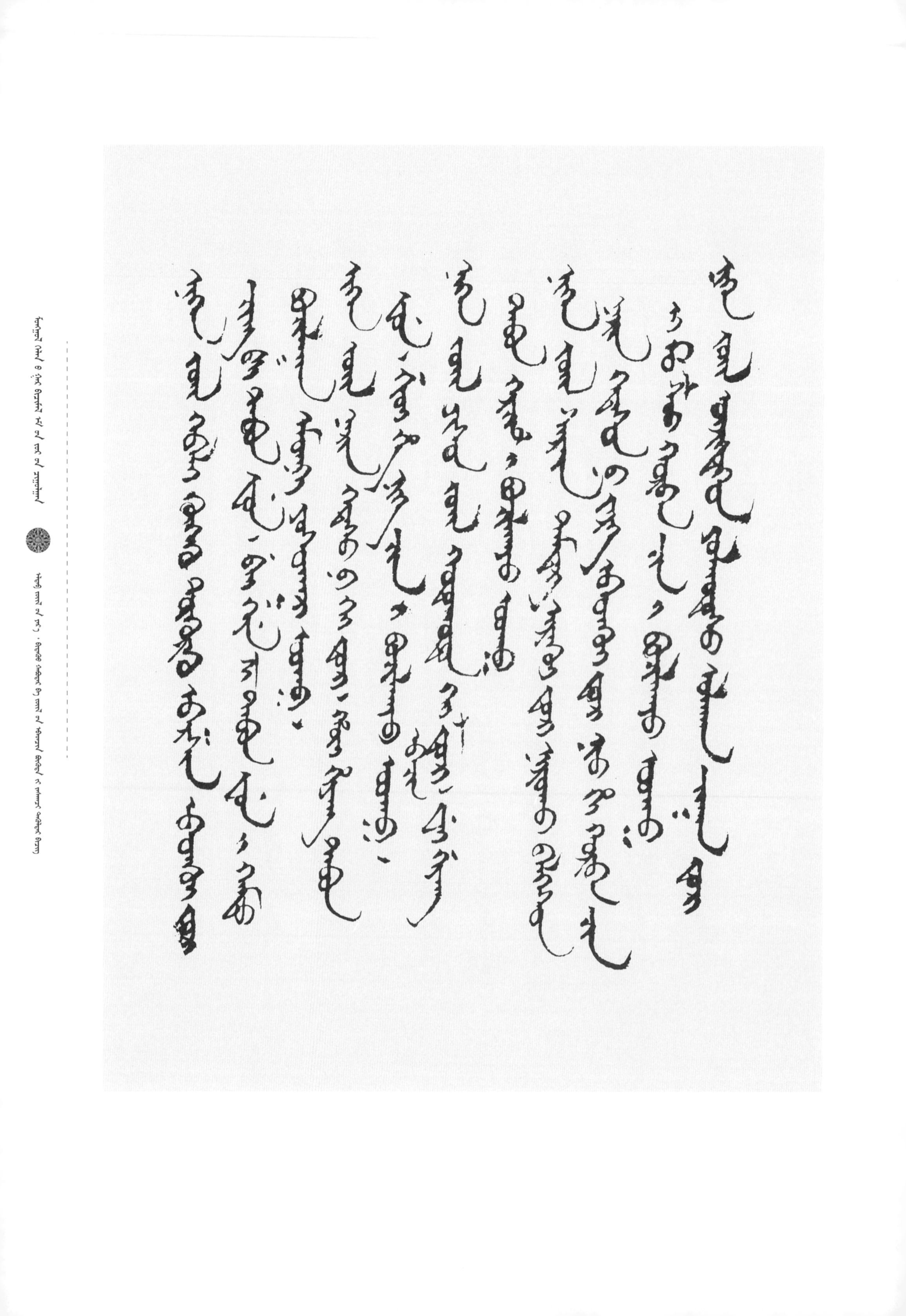

[illegible]

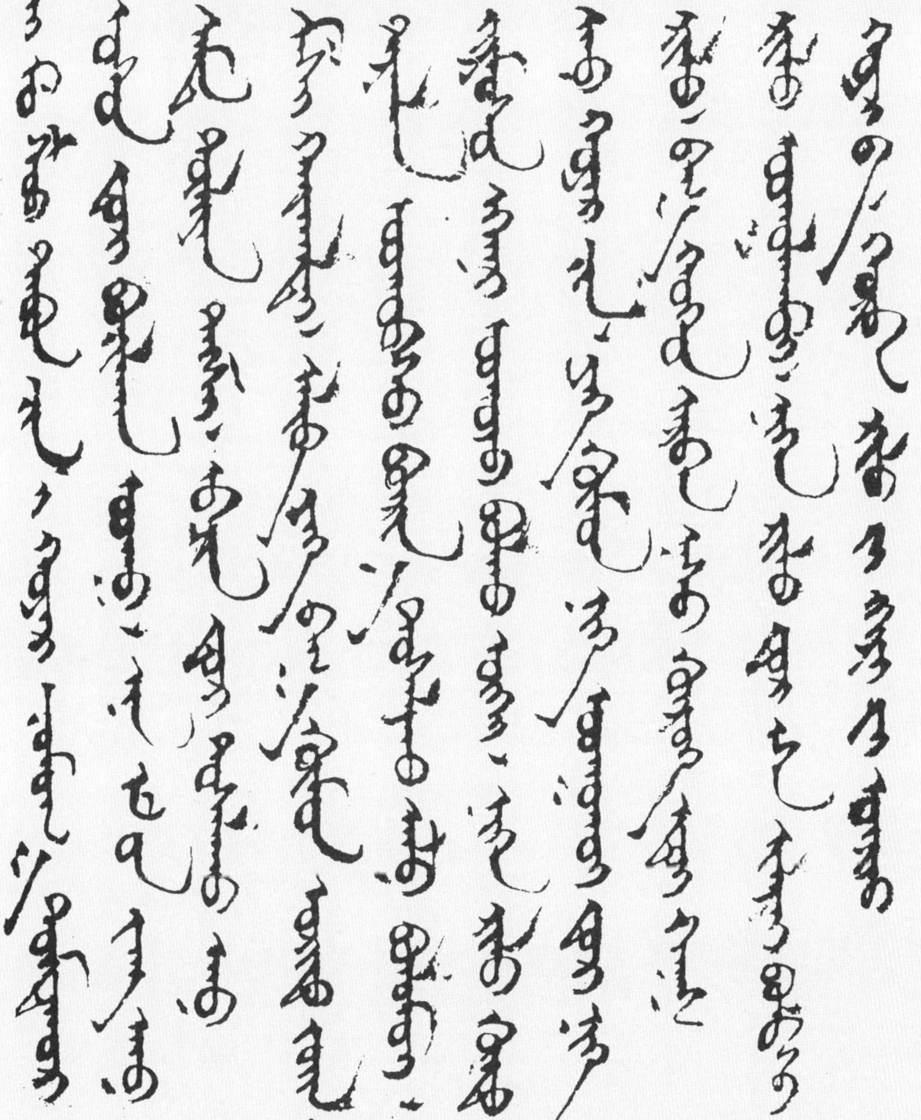

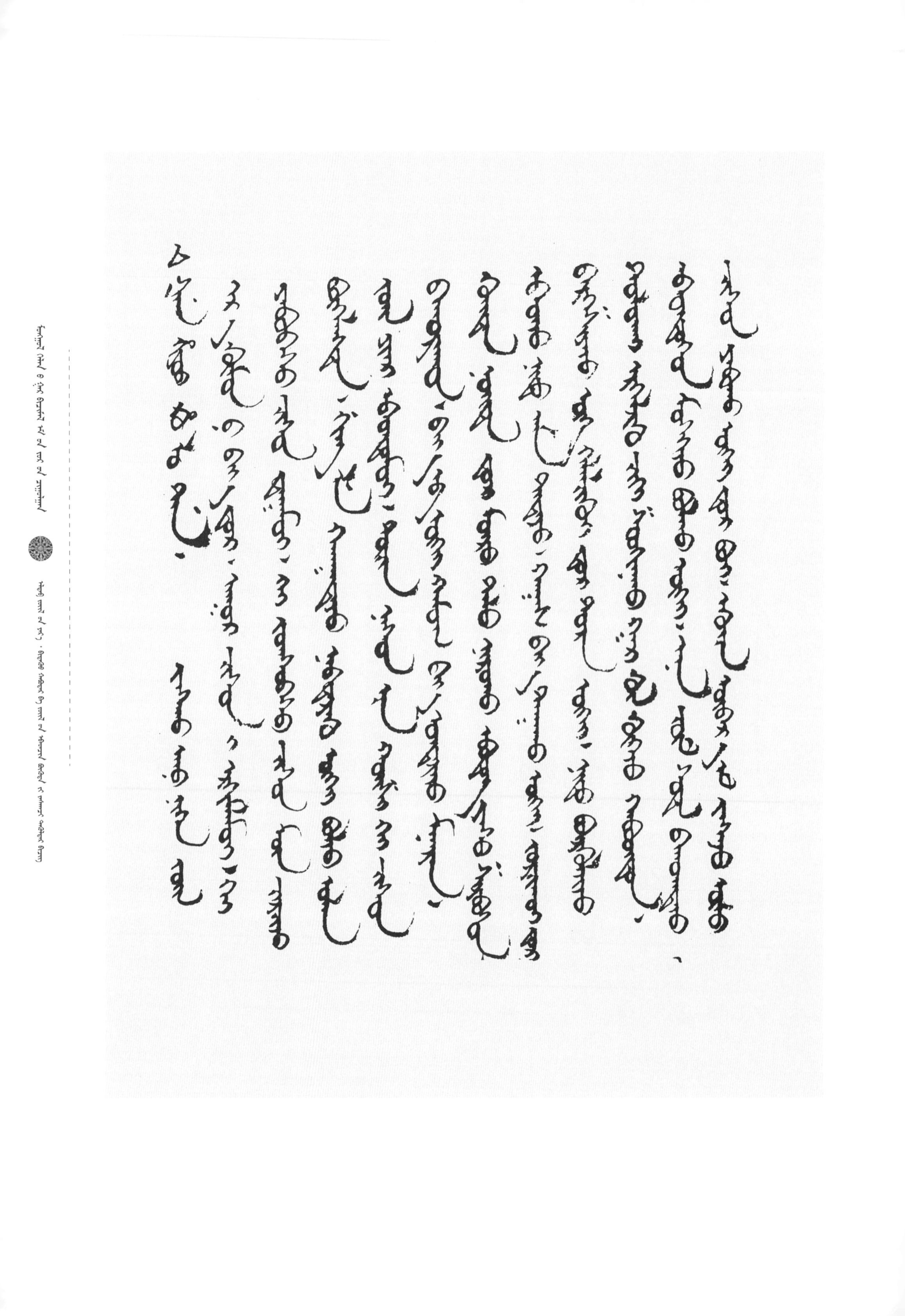

[illegible]

[illegible]

[illegible]

[illegible]

[illegible]

[illegible]

[illegible]

[illegible]

[illegible]

[illegible]

[illegible]

[illegible]

[illegible]

[illegible]

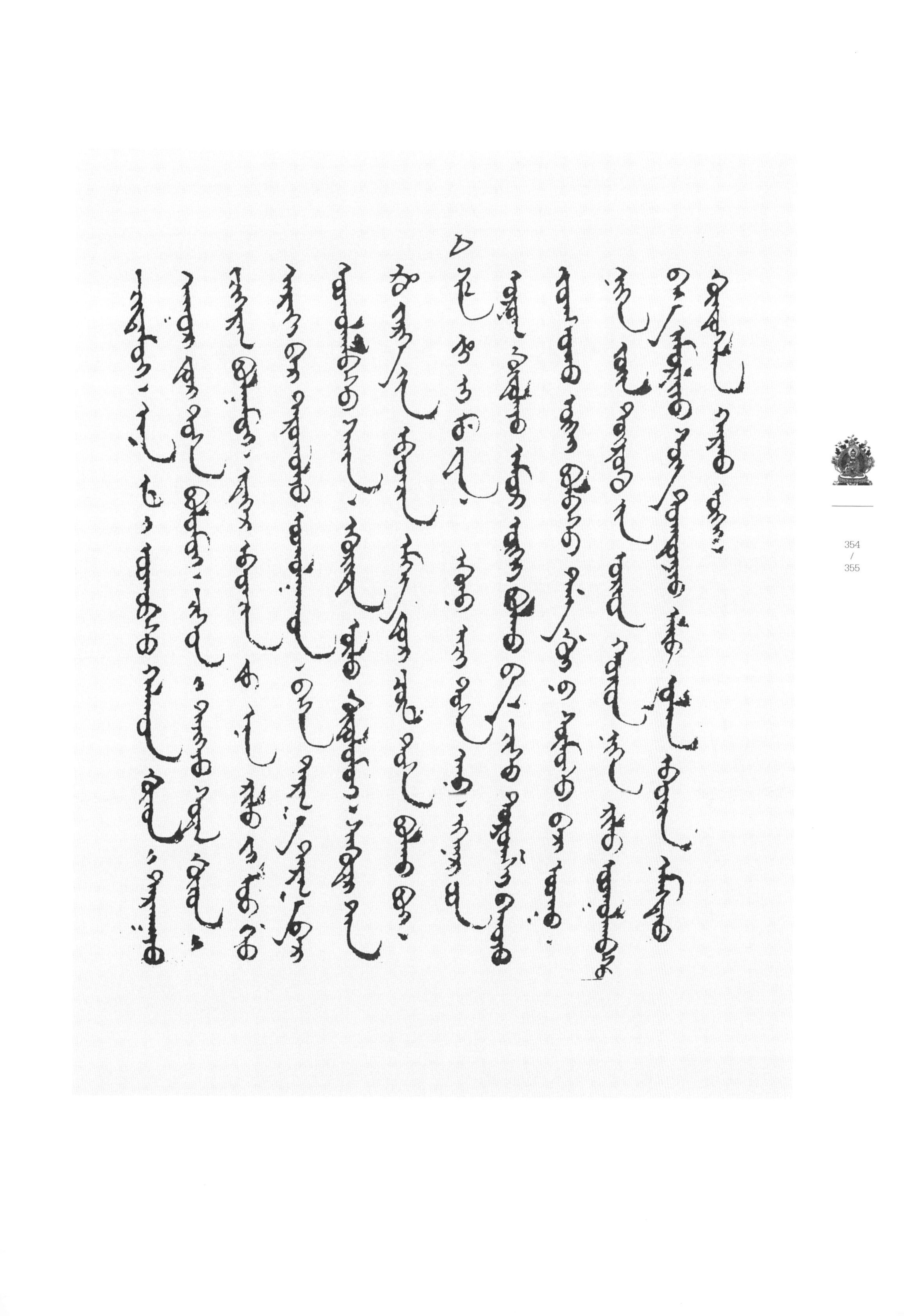

[illegible]

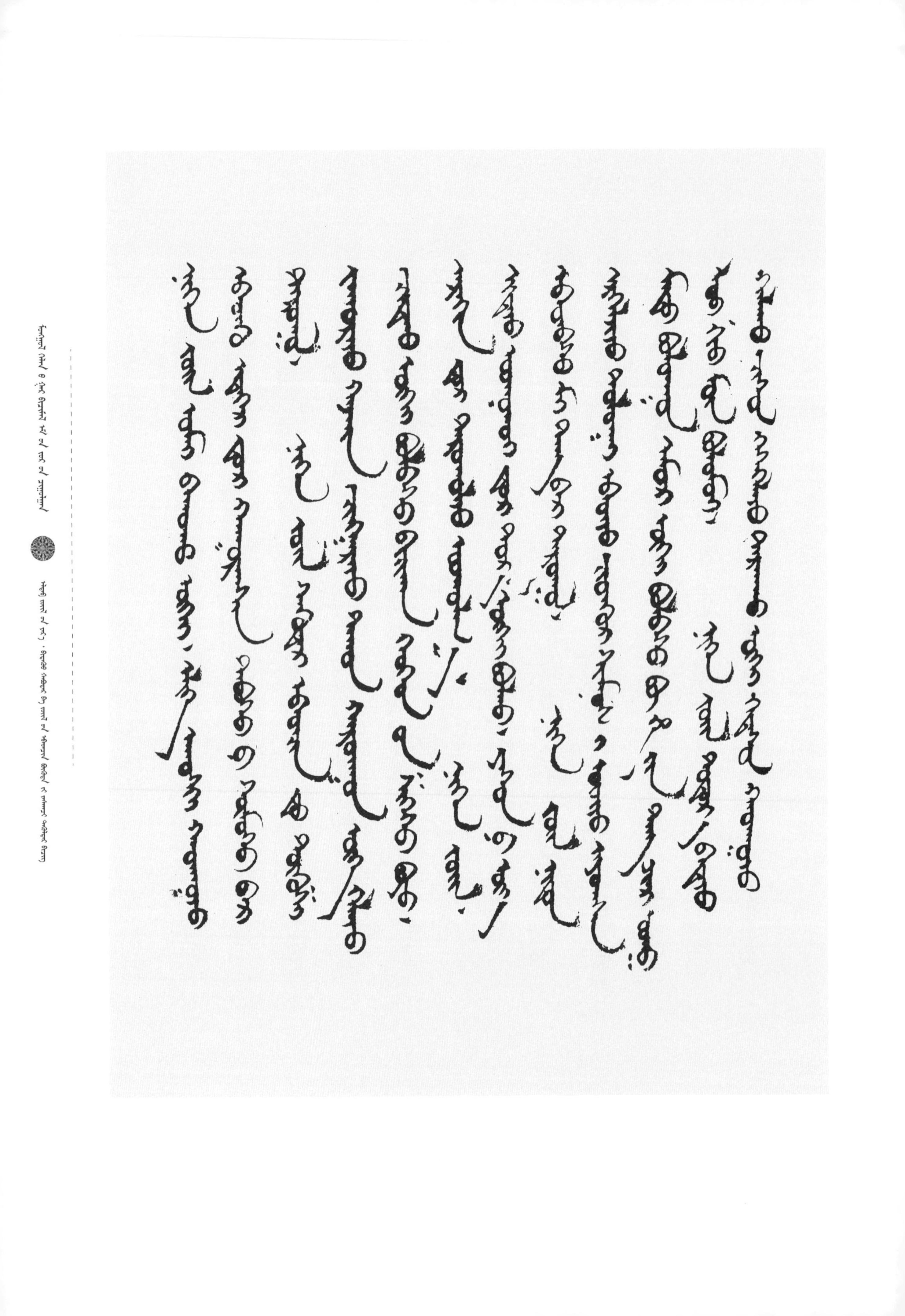

[illegible]

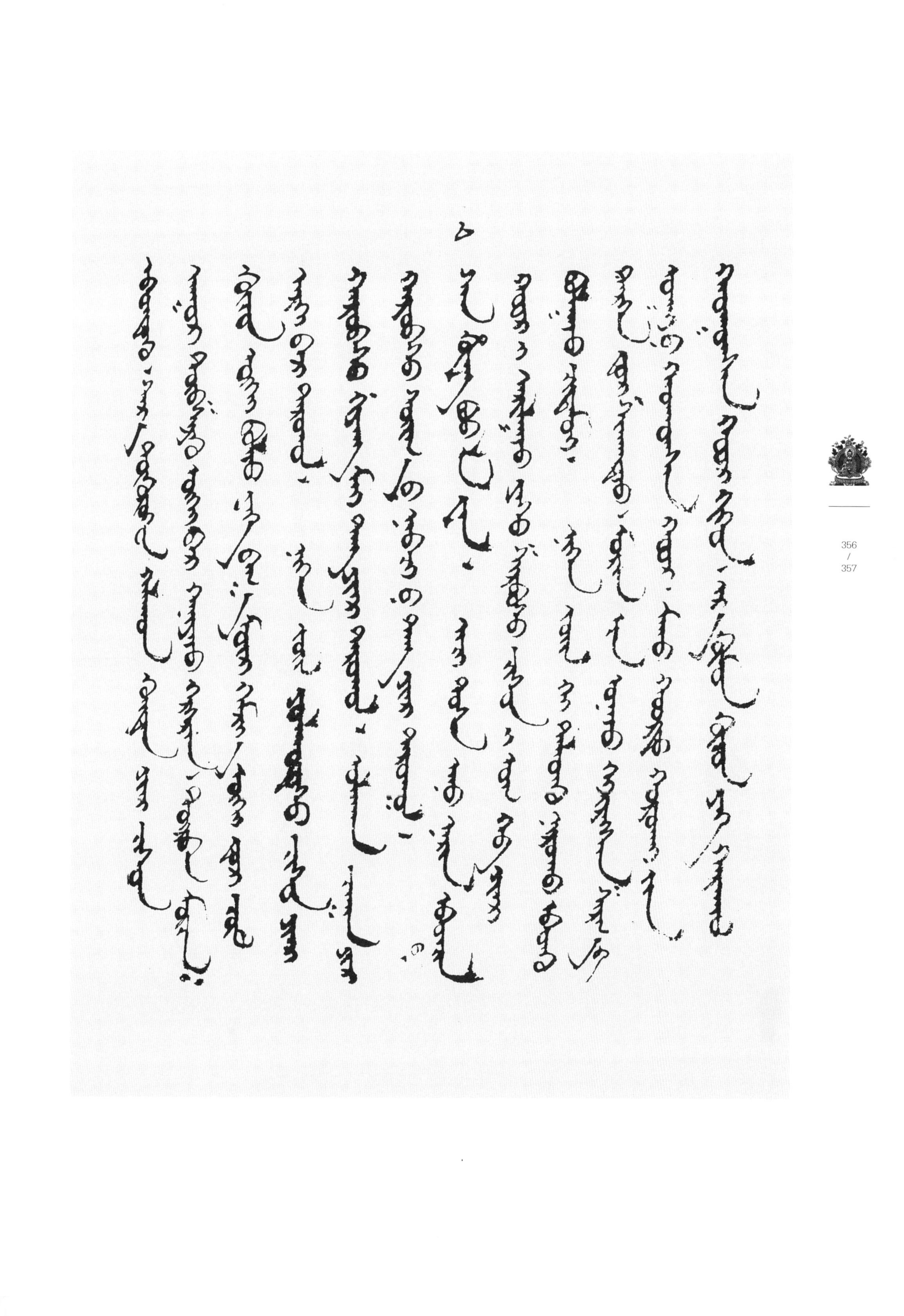

[illegible]

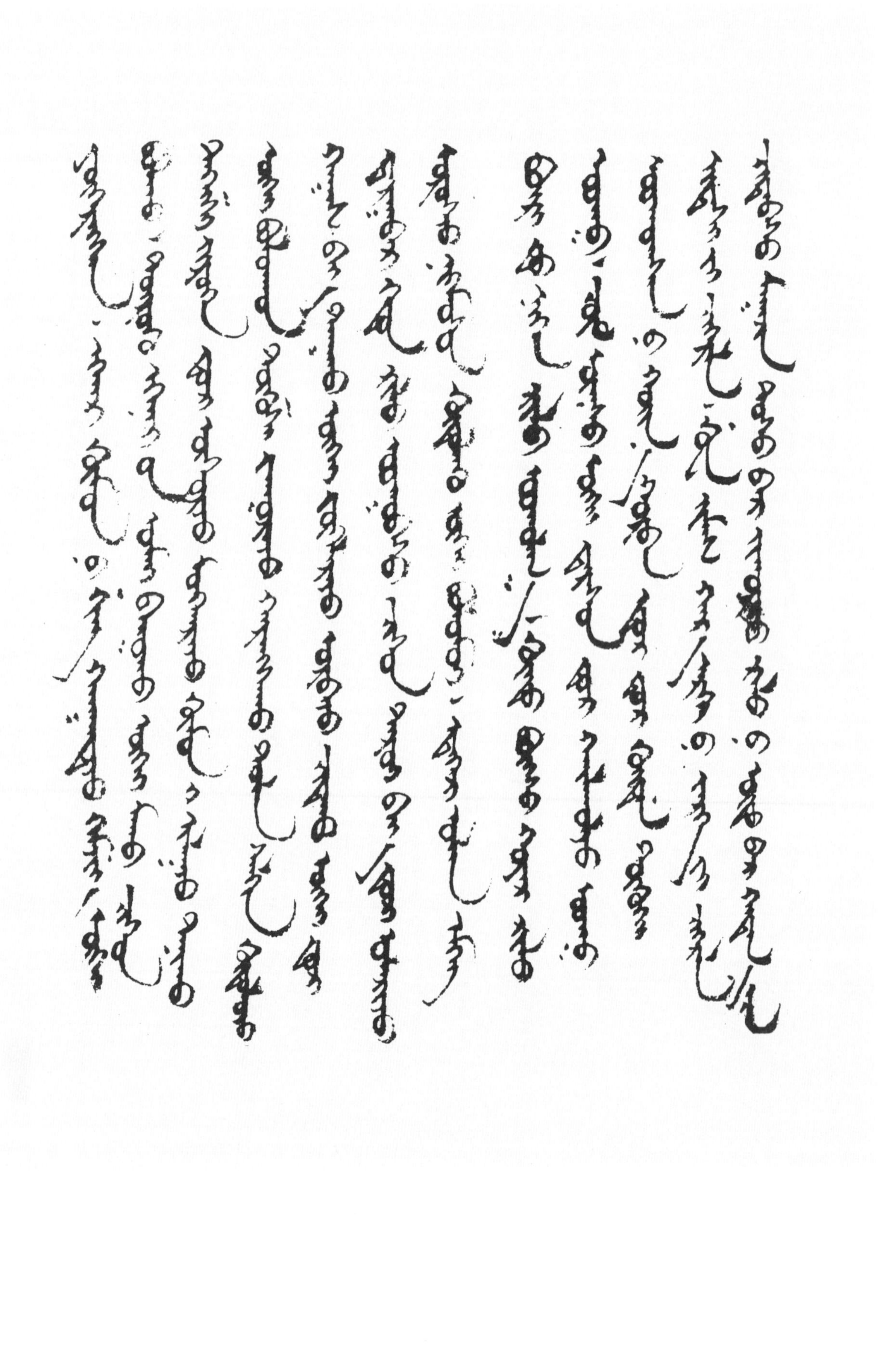

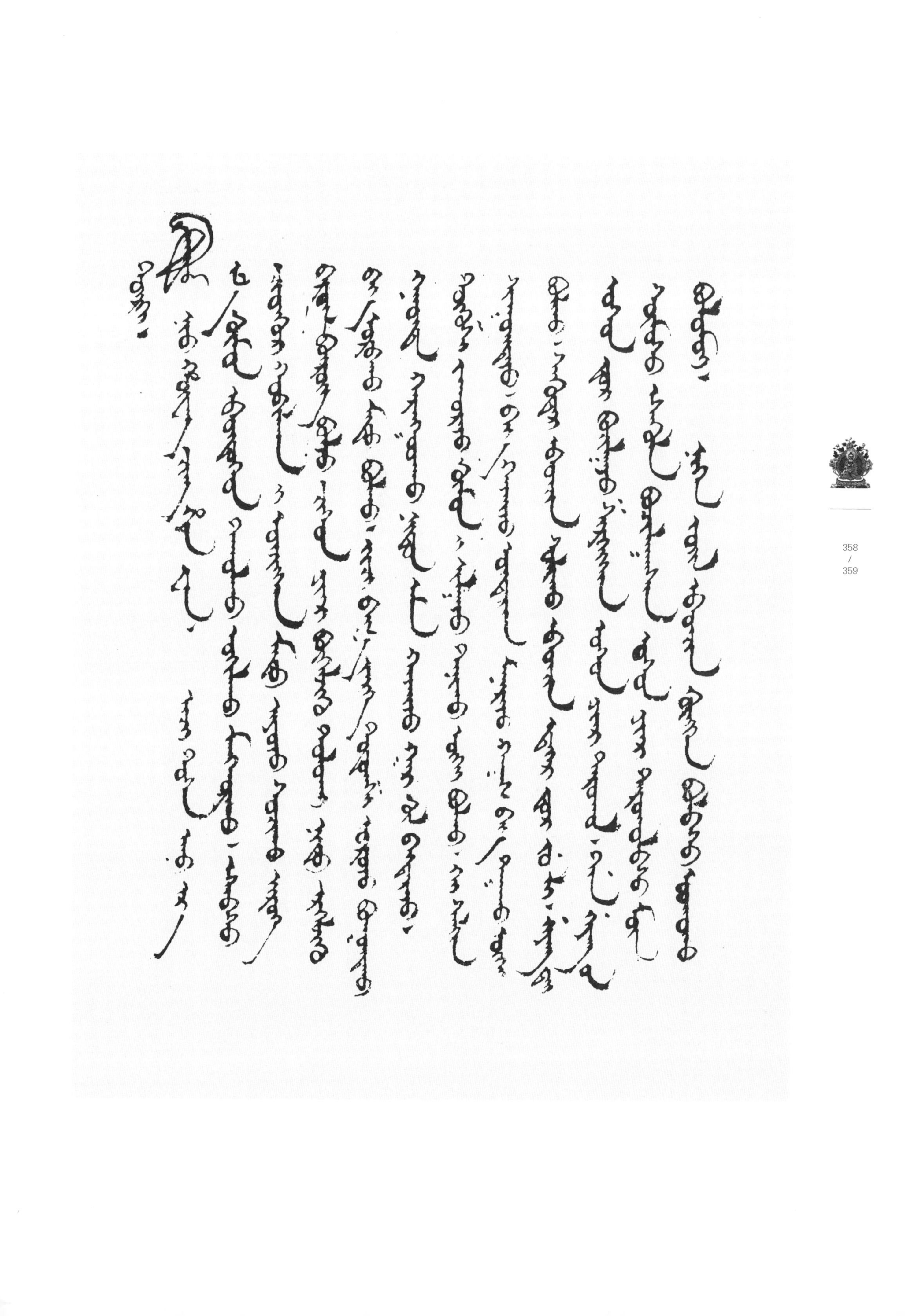

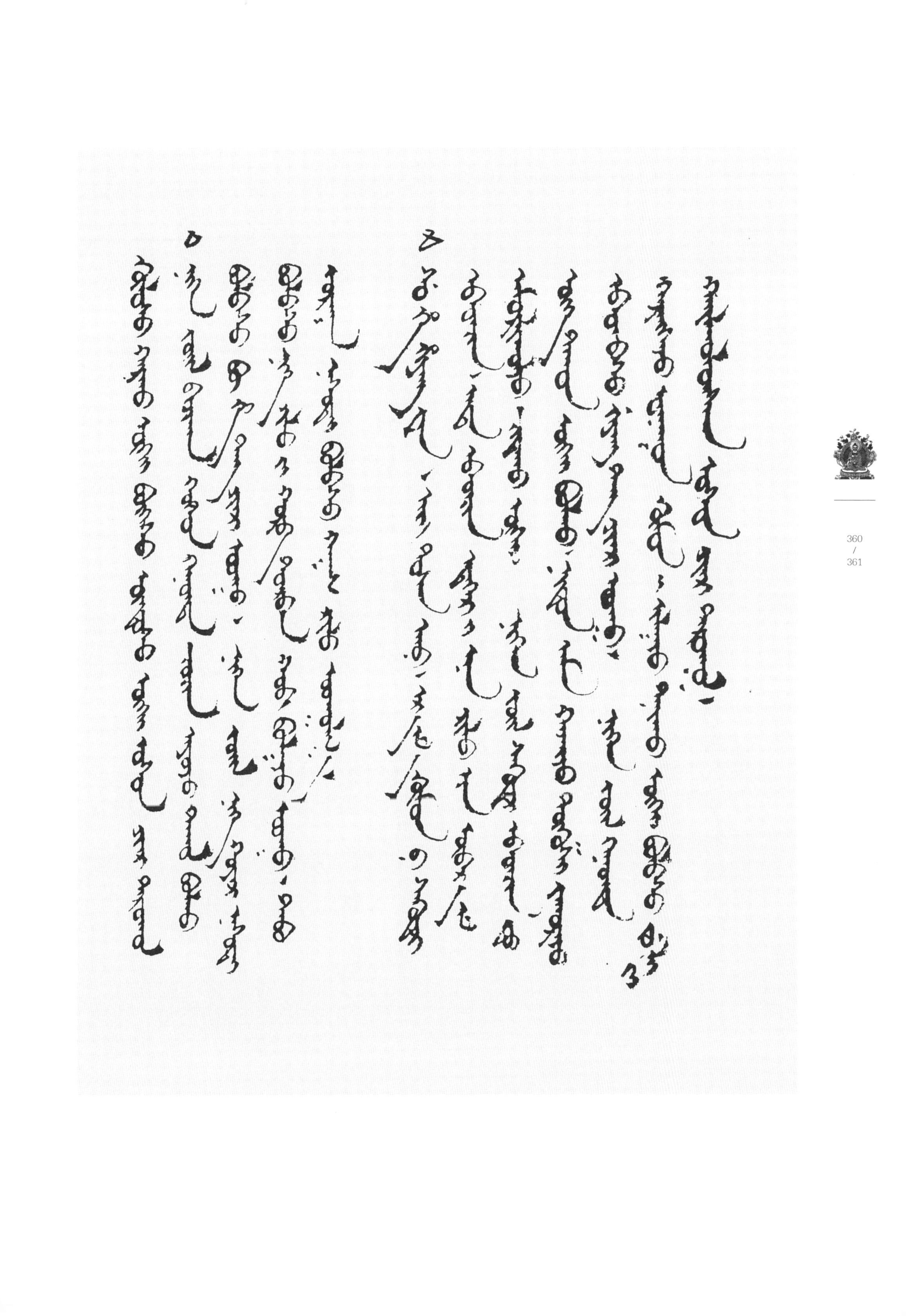

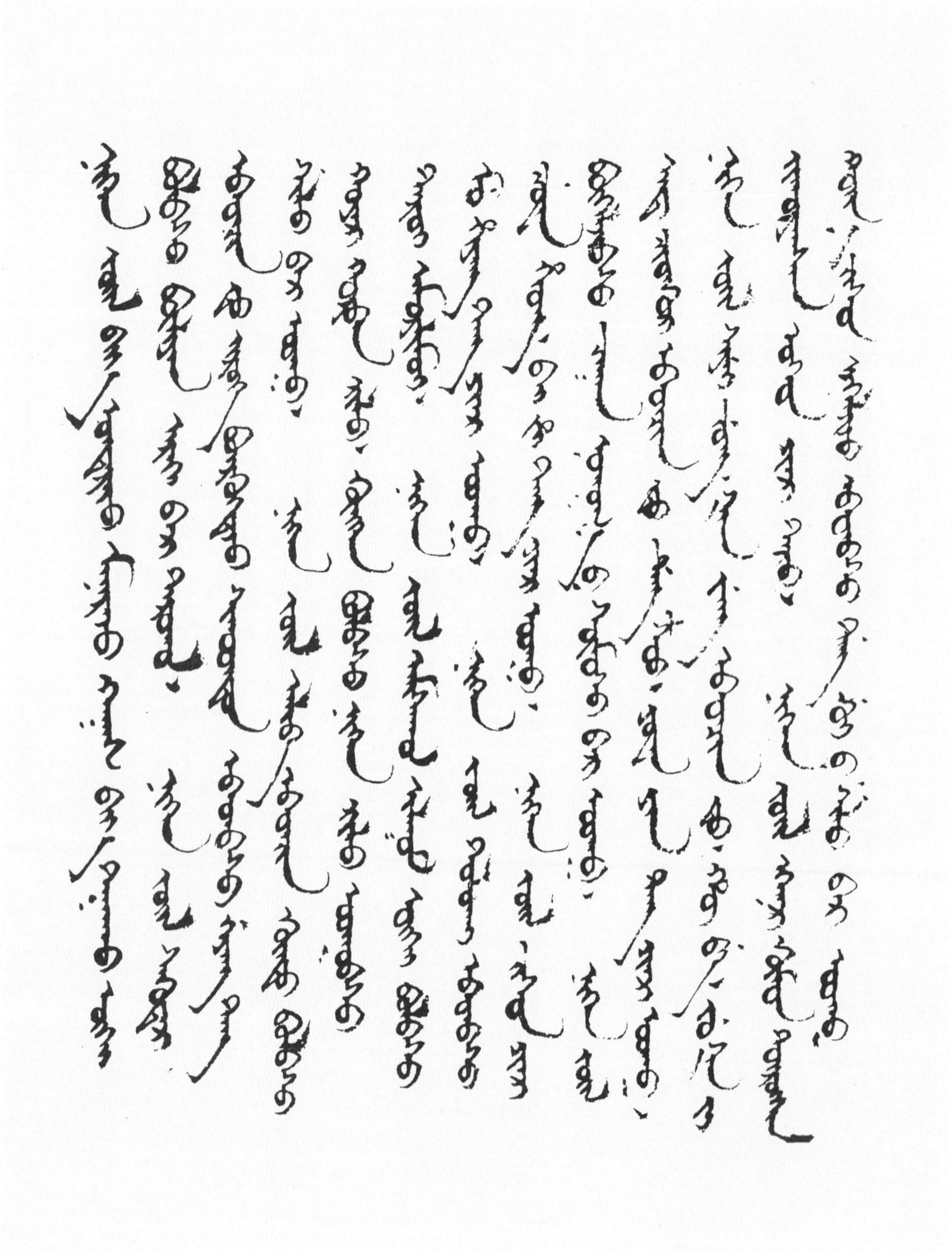

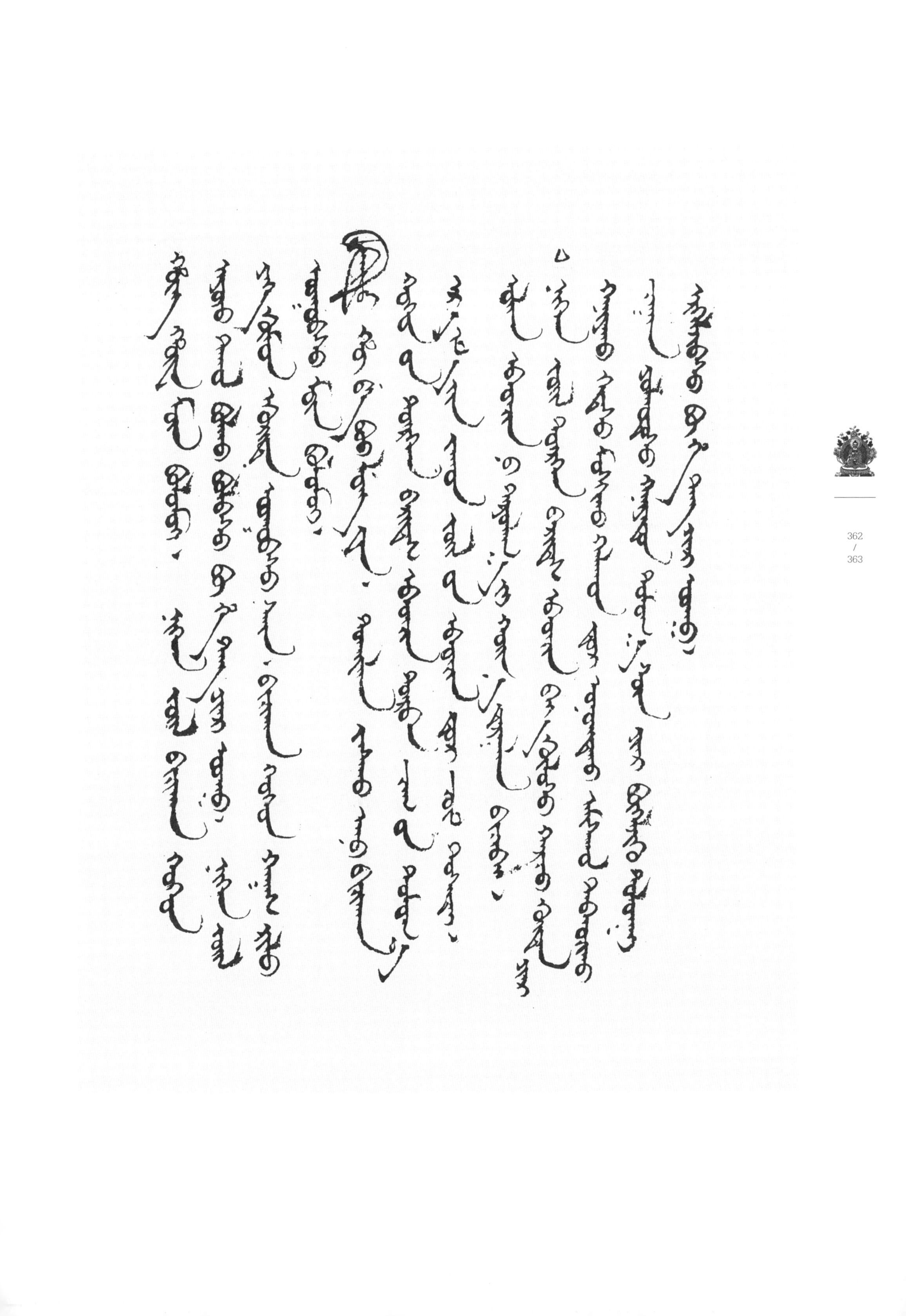

[illegible]

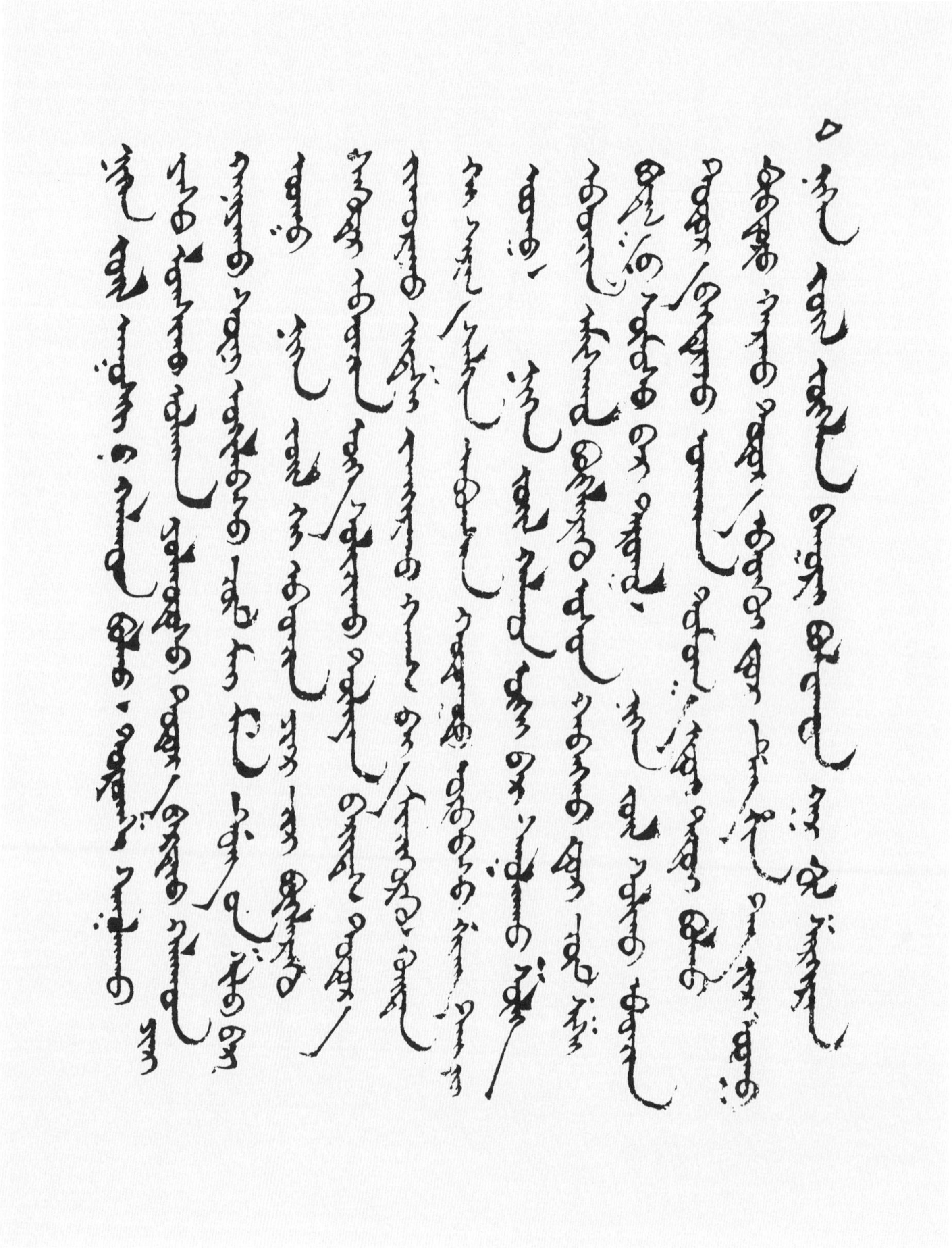

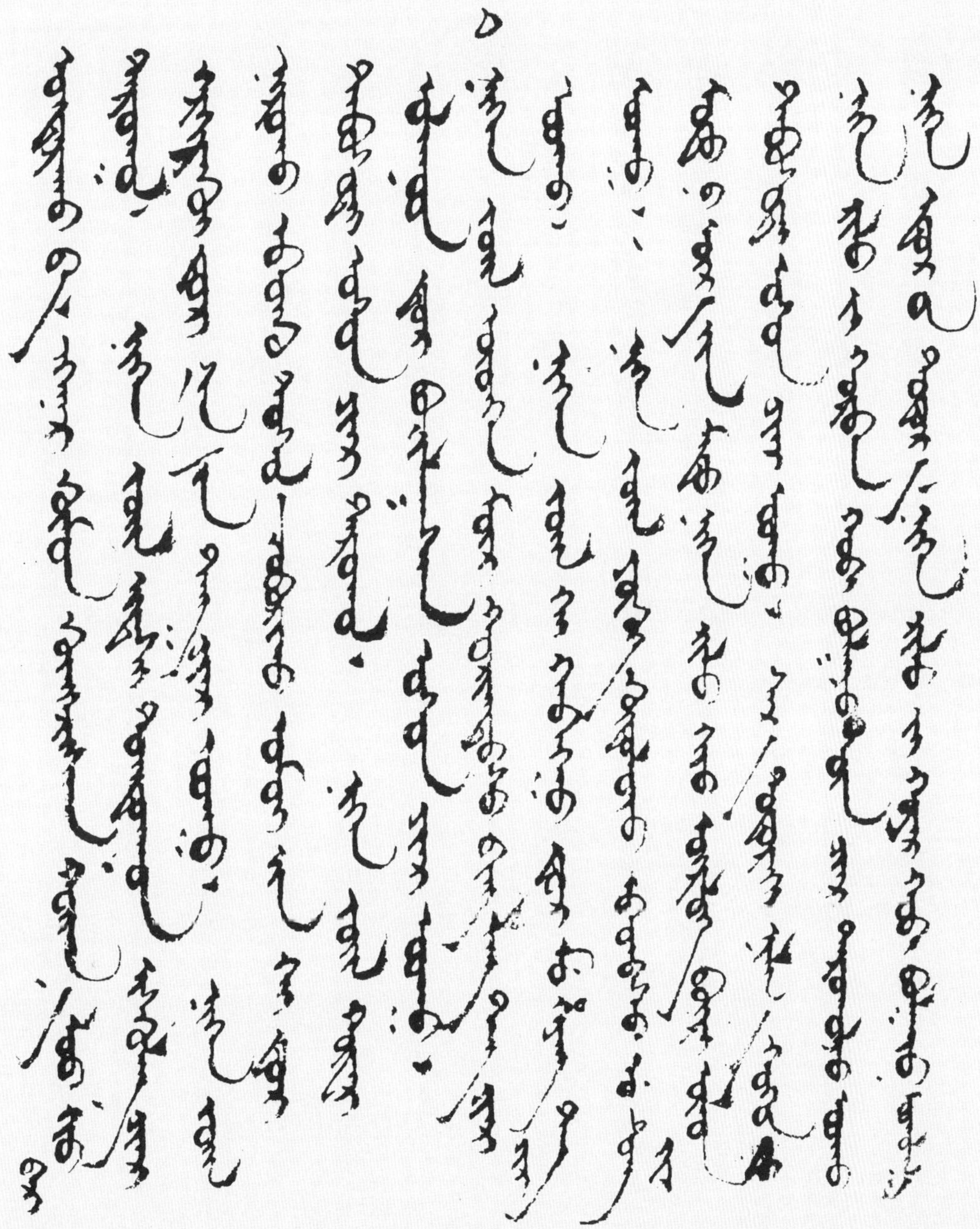

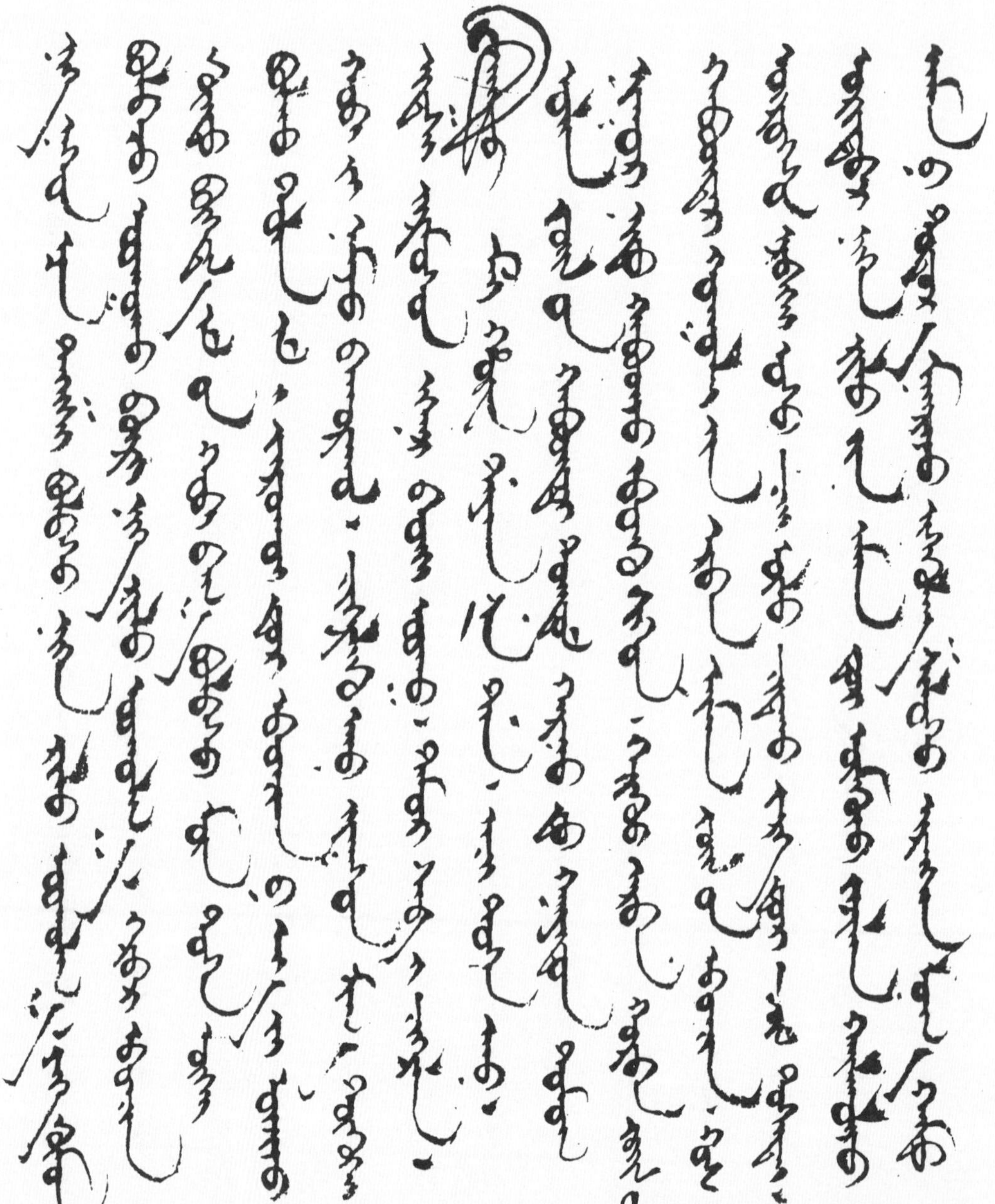

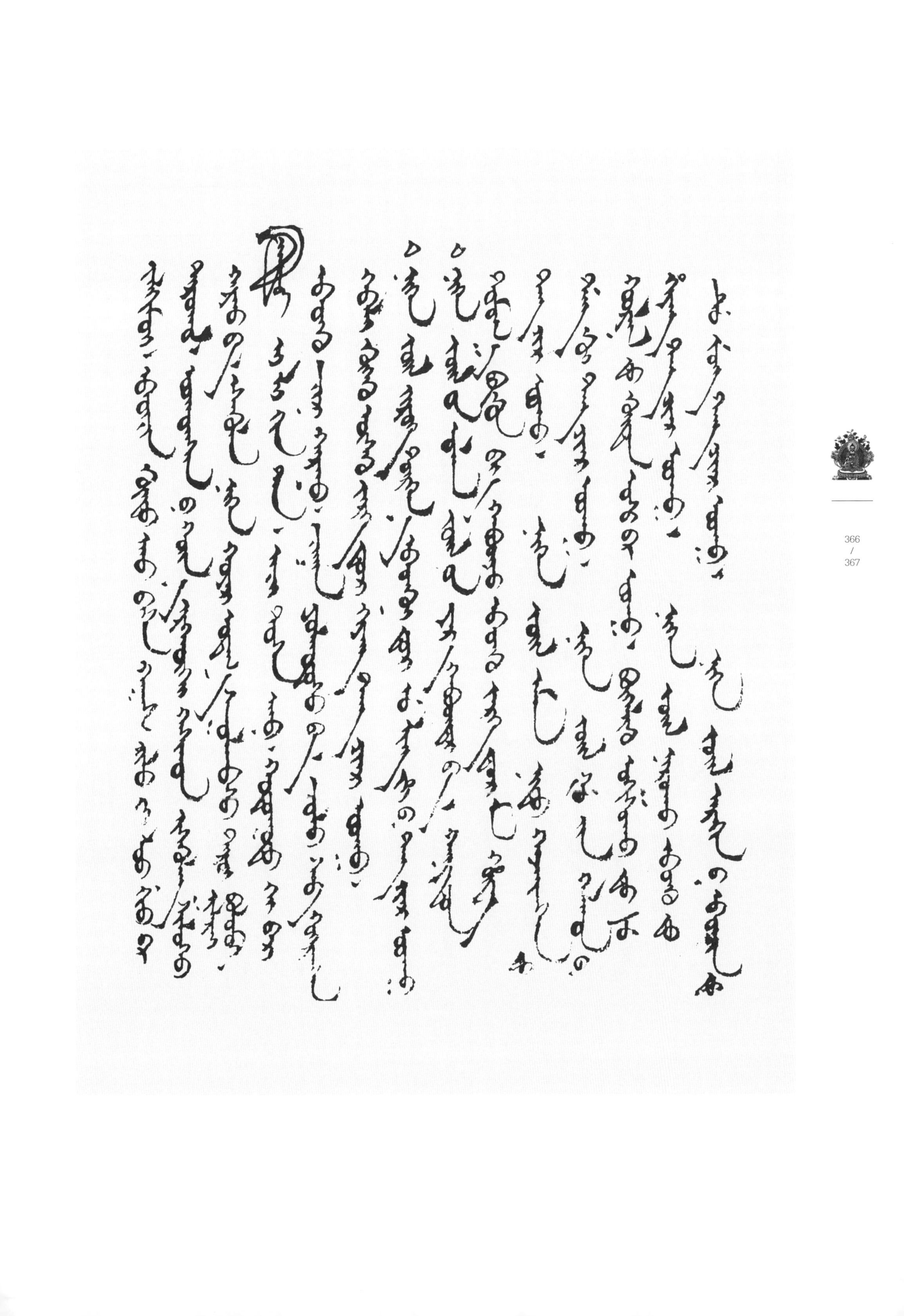

[illegible]

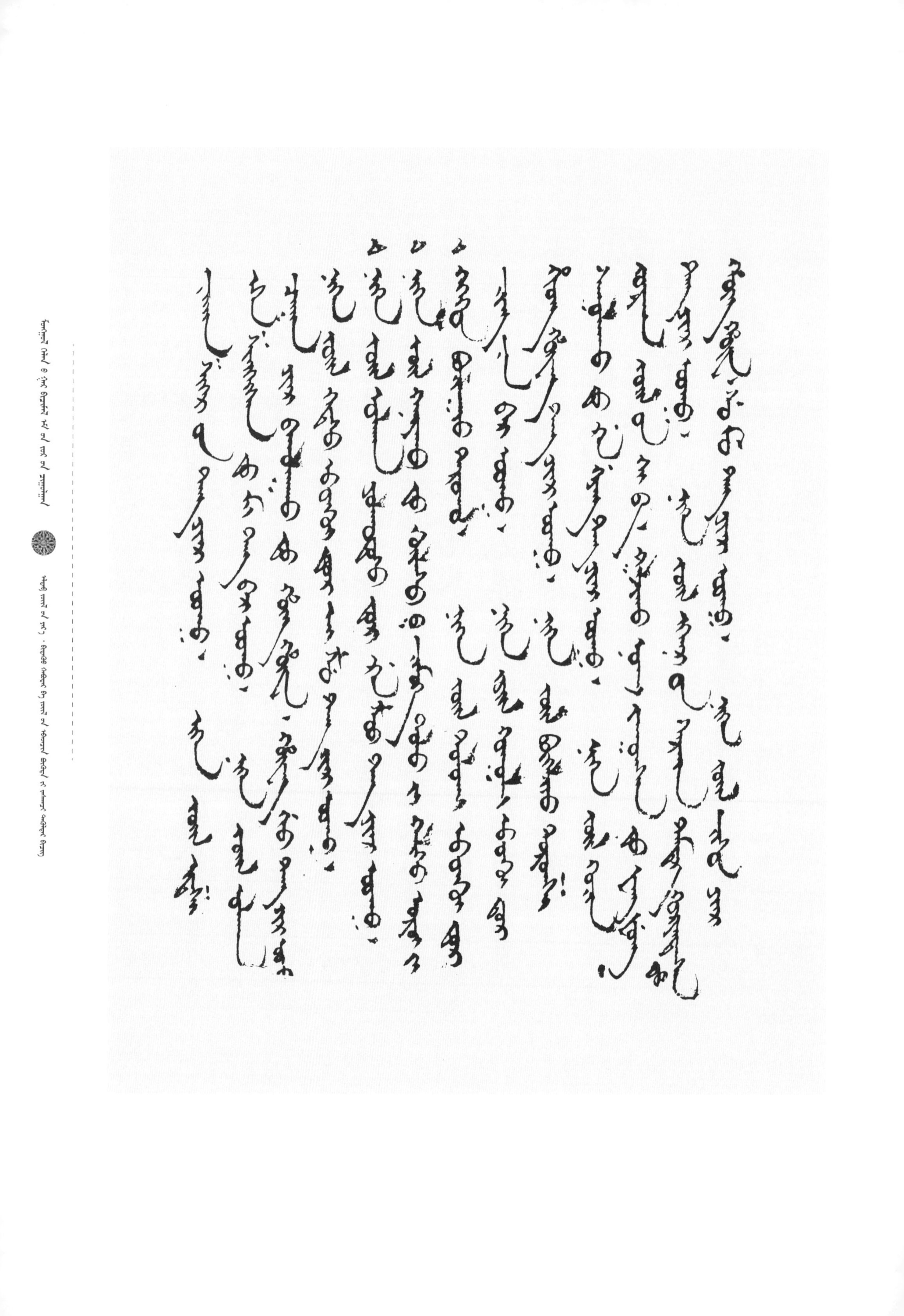

[illegible]

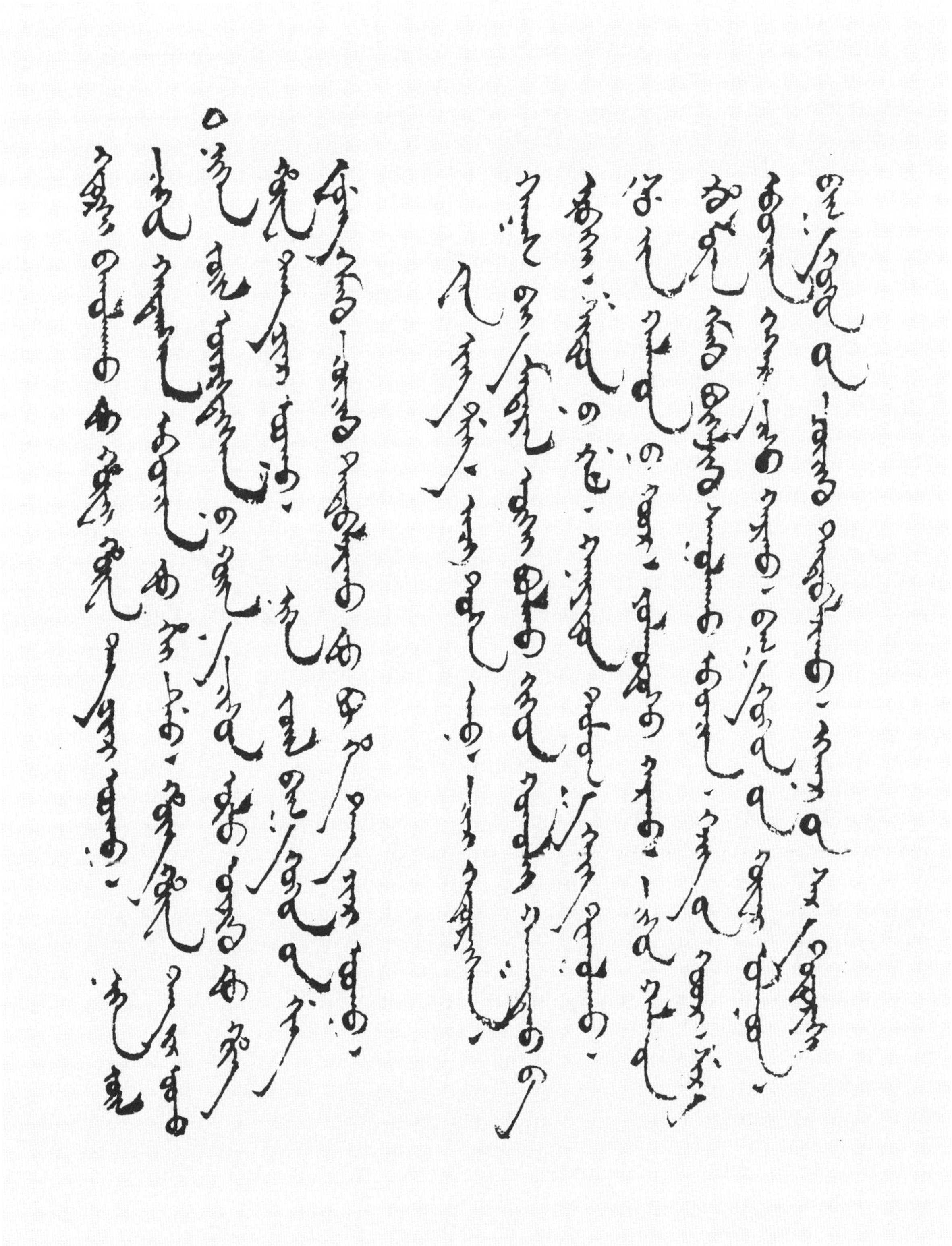

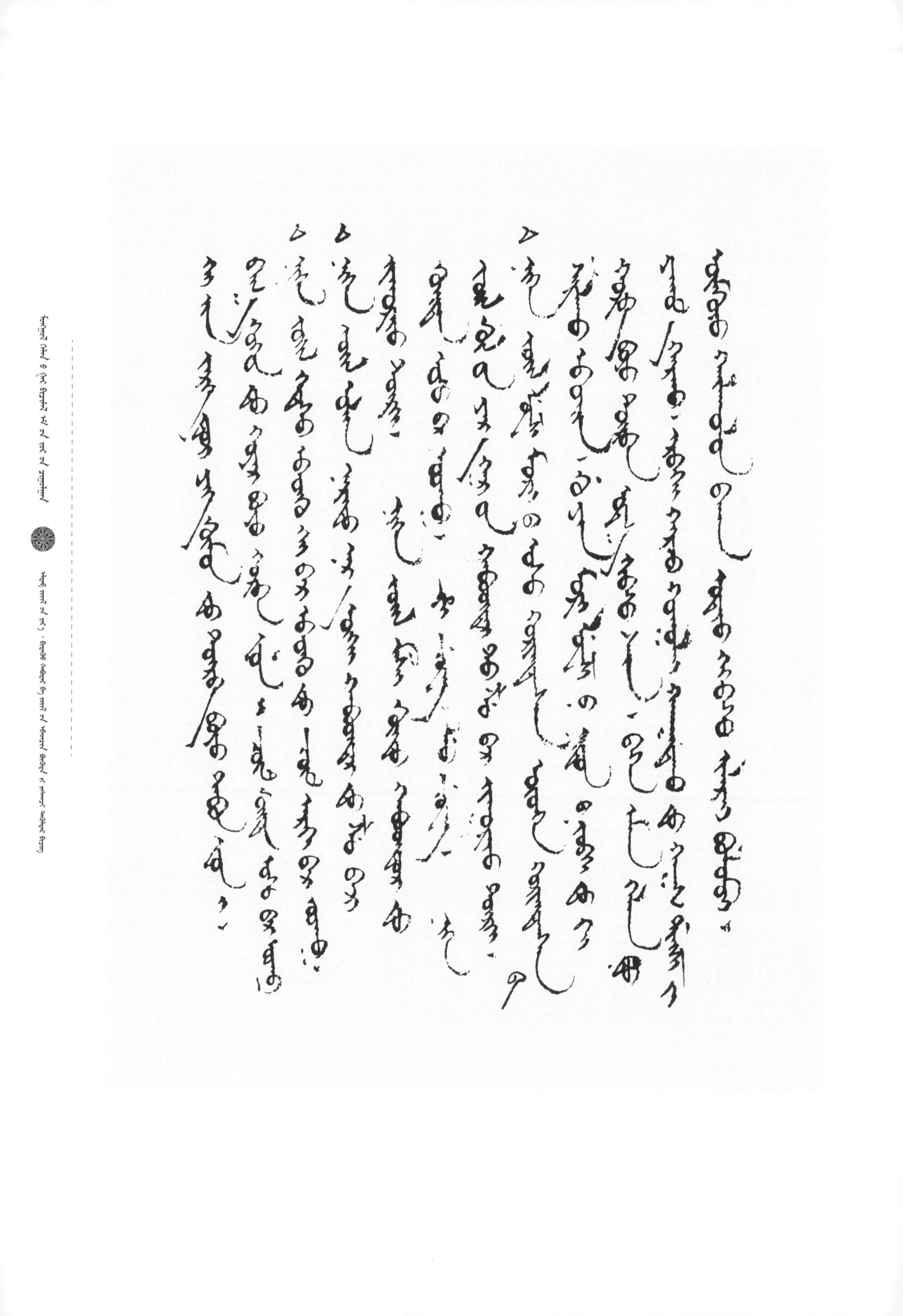

[illegible]

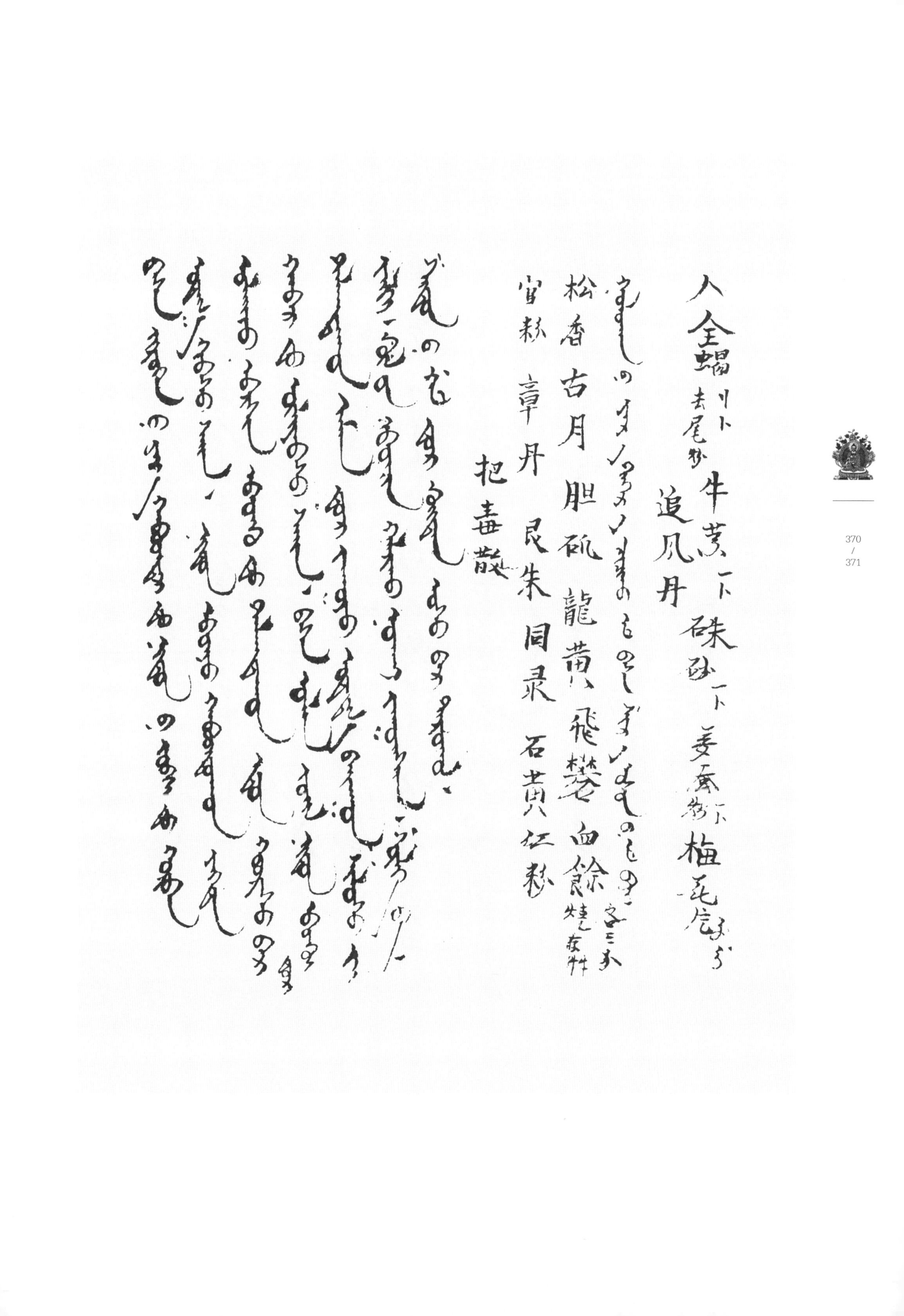

八全蝎リト去尾炒 牛黄一卜 硃砂一卜 姜蚕炒一卜 梅花片

追风丹

松香 古月 胆矾 龍黄 飛礬 血餘燒存性

官粉 章丹 艮朱 同录 石黄 紅粉

把毒散

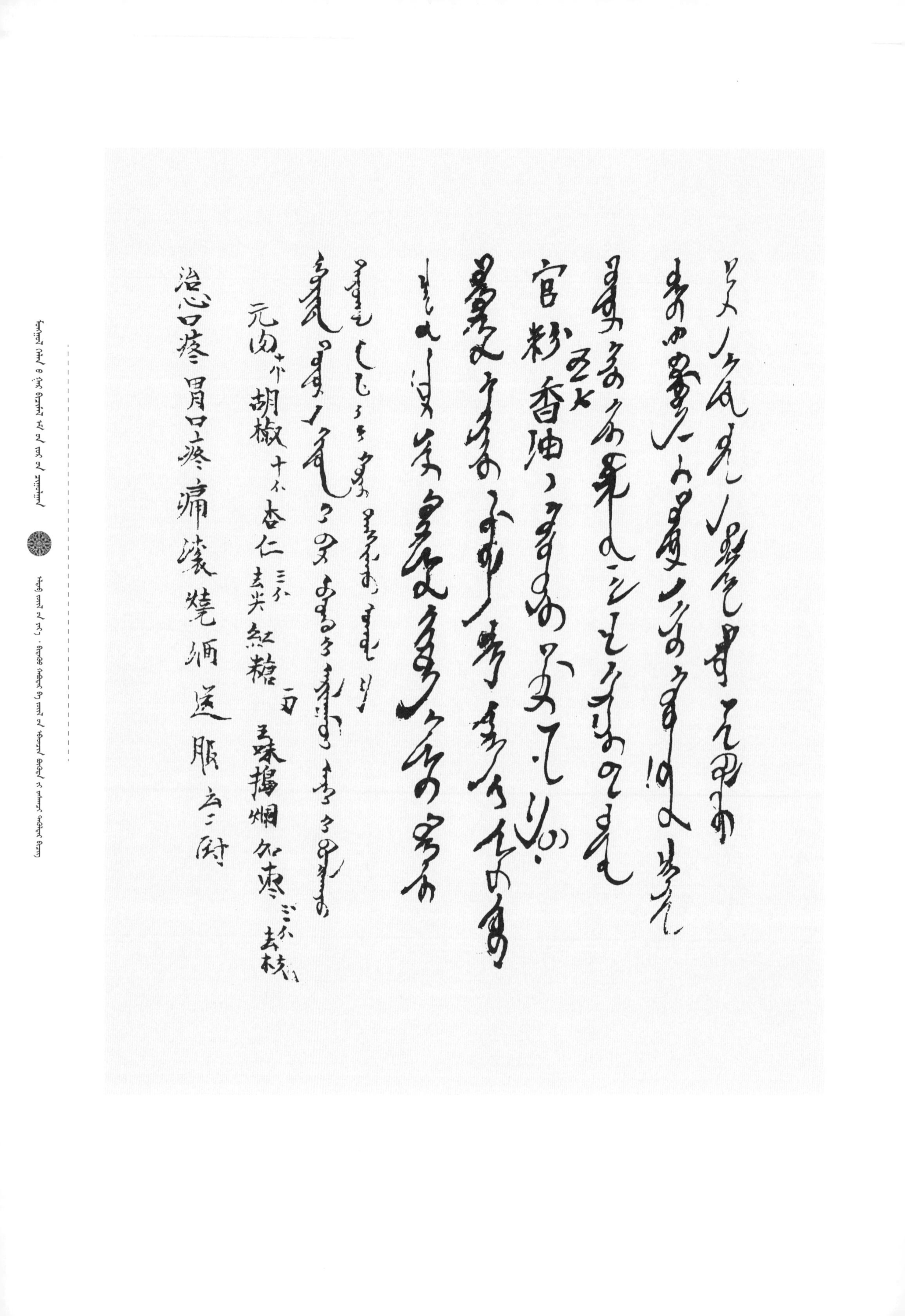

宫粉五钱 香油

元肉十个 胡椒十个 杏仁三个去尖 紅糖一两 三味搗爛 加枣三个去核

治心口疼 胃口上疼 痛壞 燒酒送服 五二付

治[illegible]

各色

元參桔梗双花共有[illegible]

[illegible]

[illegible]六分

水調開去查澄清共為細末

火燒七次入乳內沾其出研細井

[illegible]

爐甘石[illegible]乾梅花元之八熊膽之卜

[illegible]散

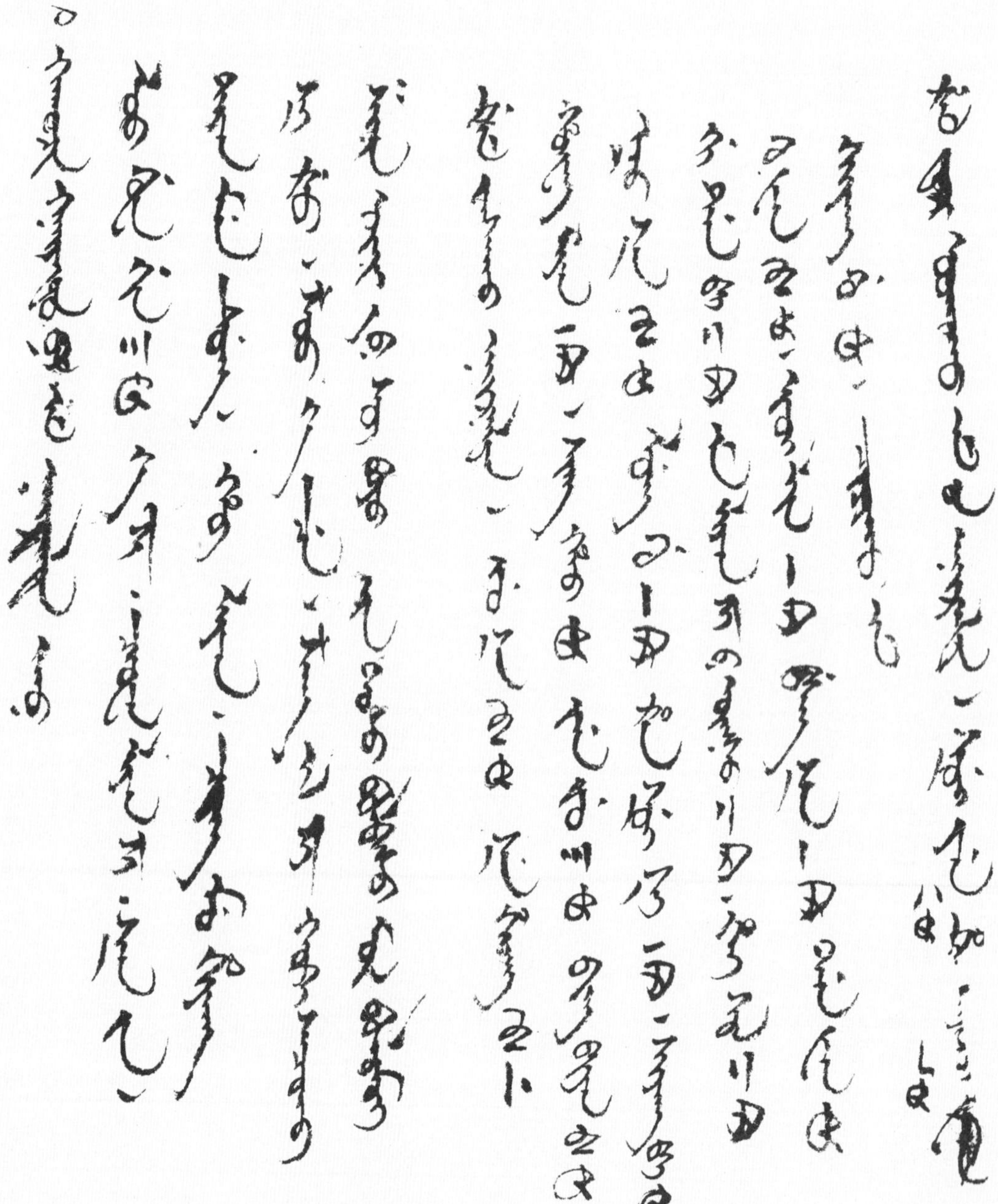

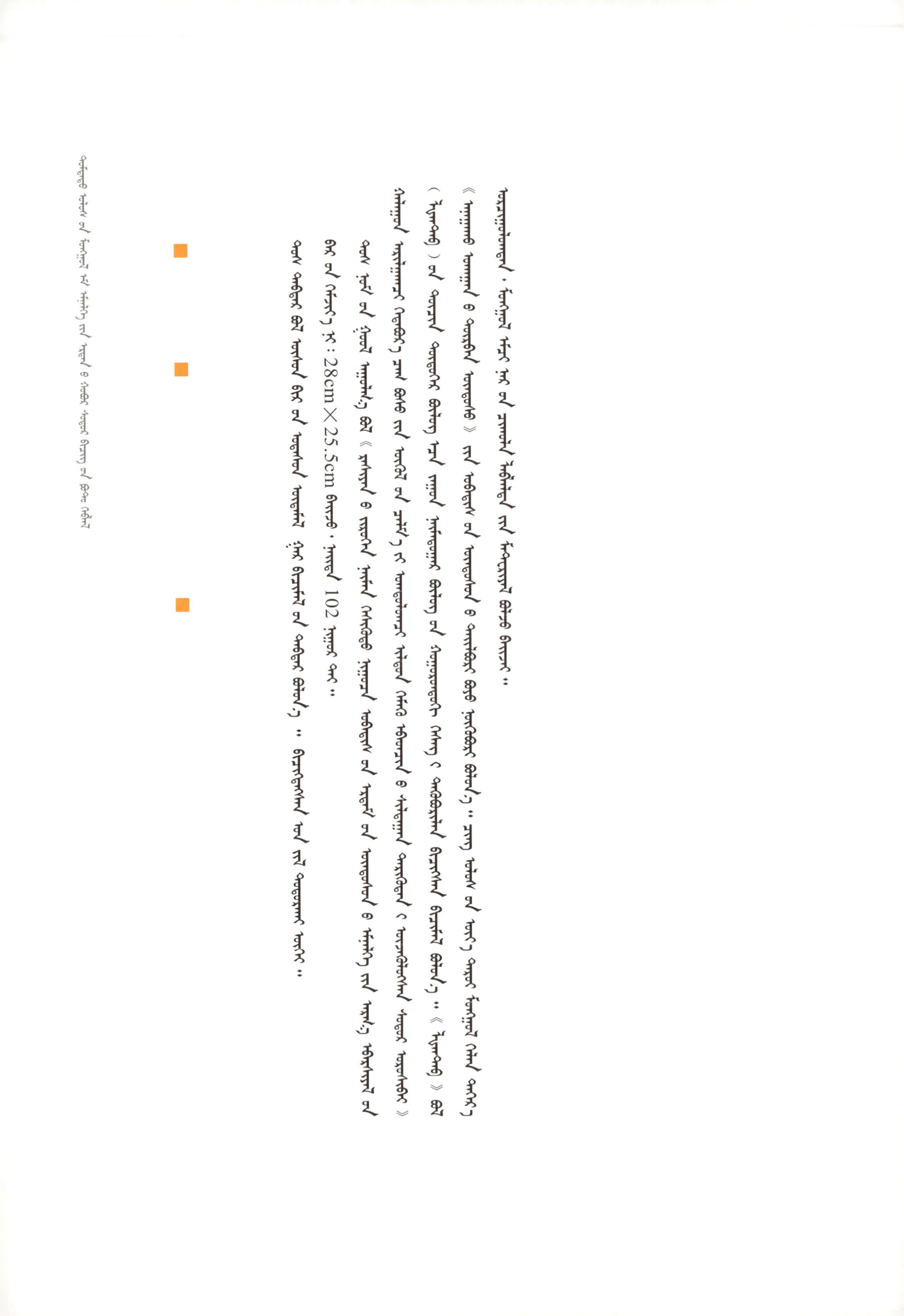

ᠪᠣᠳᠣ ᠶᠢᠨ ᠬᠡᠮᠵᠢᠶ᠎ᠡ : 28cm×25.5cm ᠪᠣᠯᠤᠨ᠎ᠠ · ᠨᠡᠢᠲᠡ 102 ᠨᠢᠭᠤᠷ ᠲᠠᠢ ::

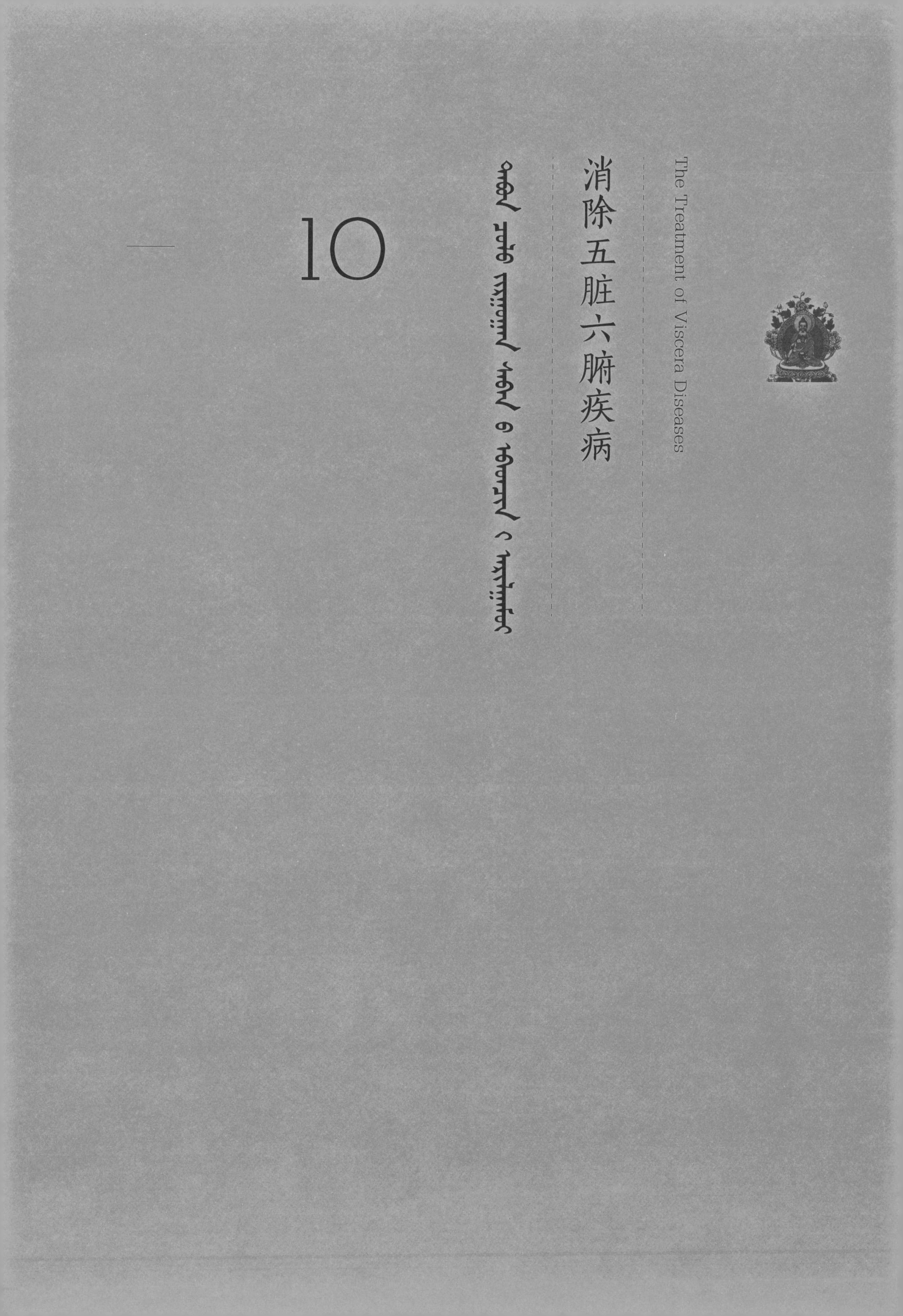

10

消除五脏六腑疾病

The Treatment of Viscera Diseases

[illegible]

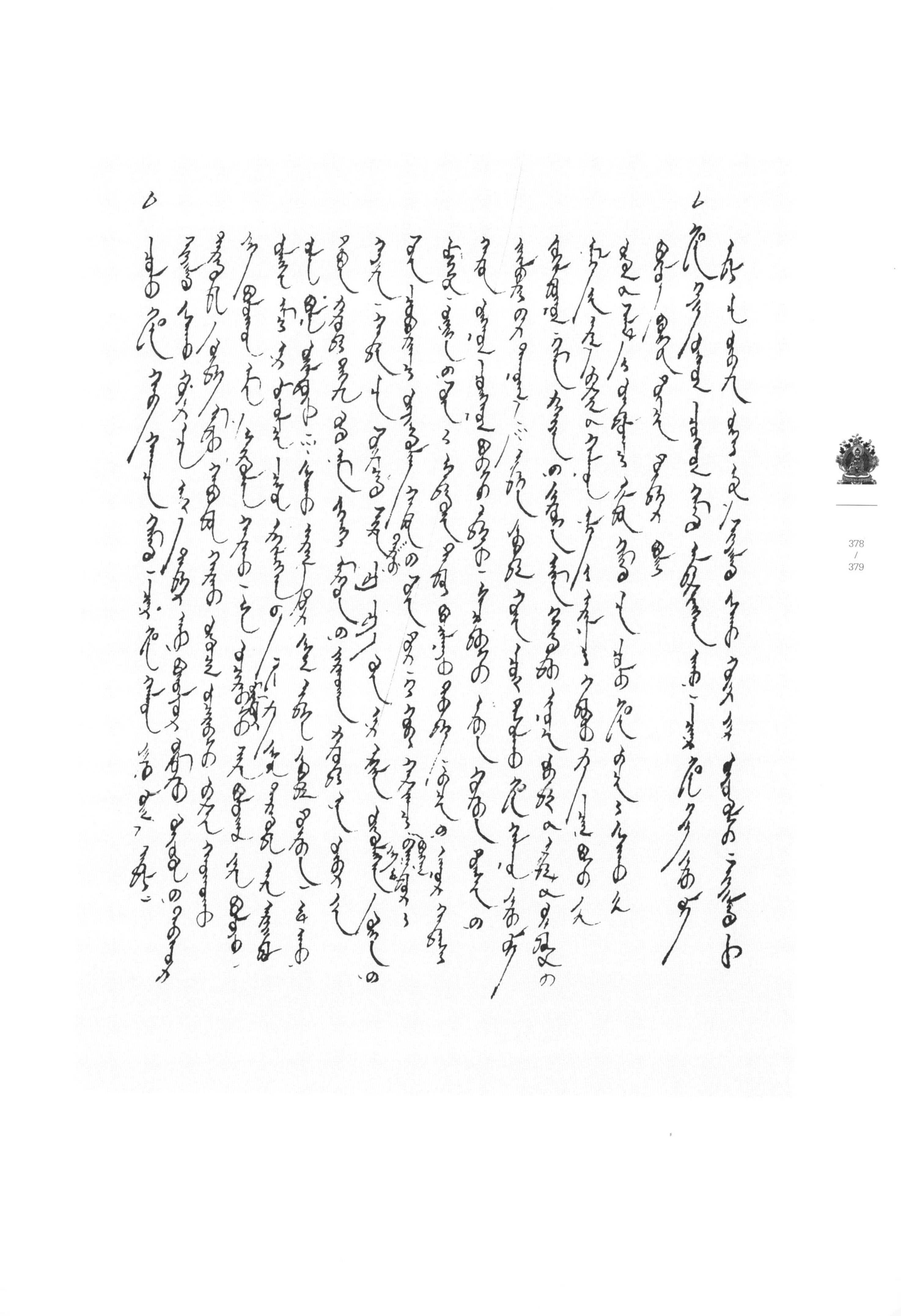

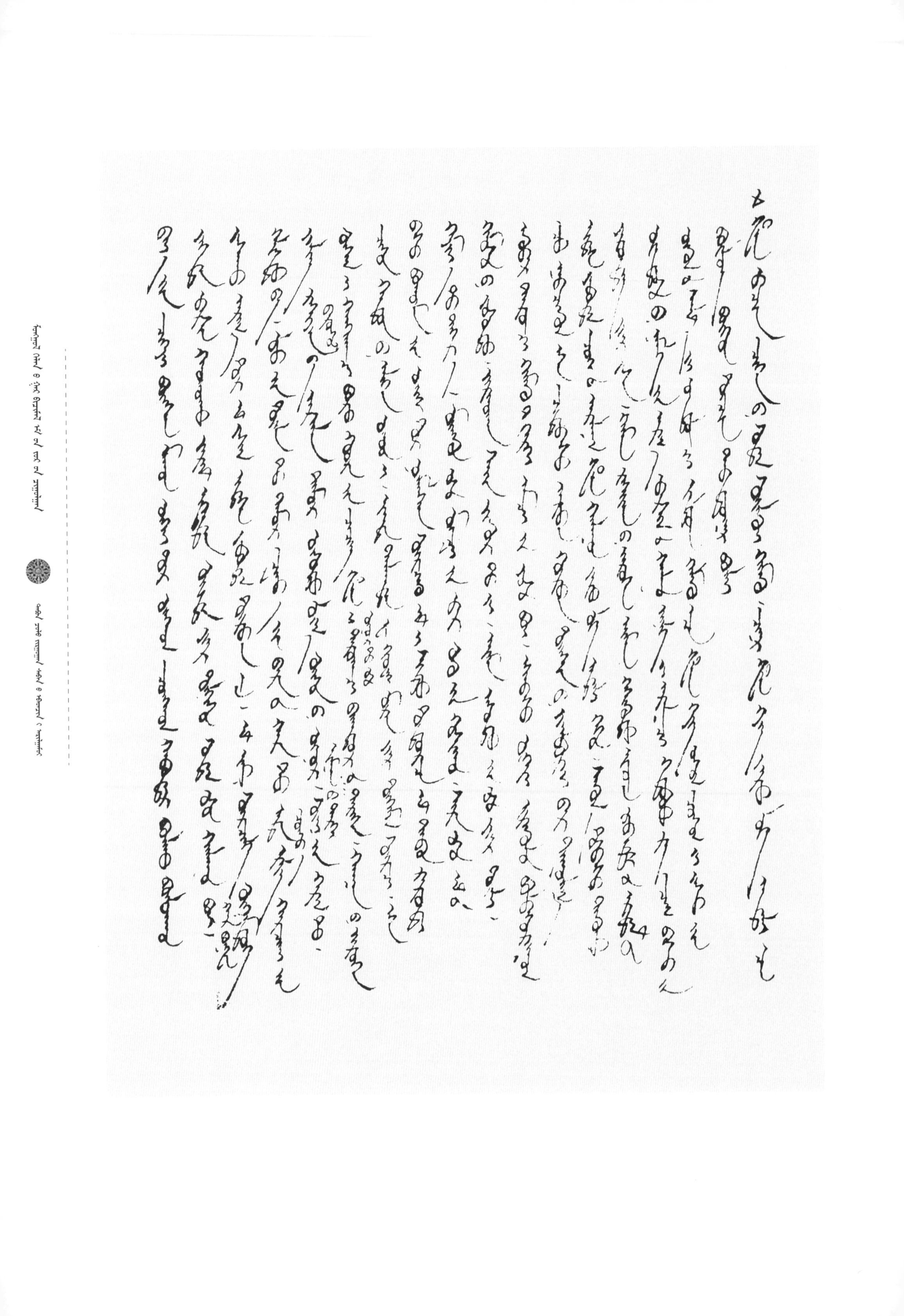

[illegible]

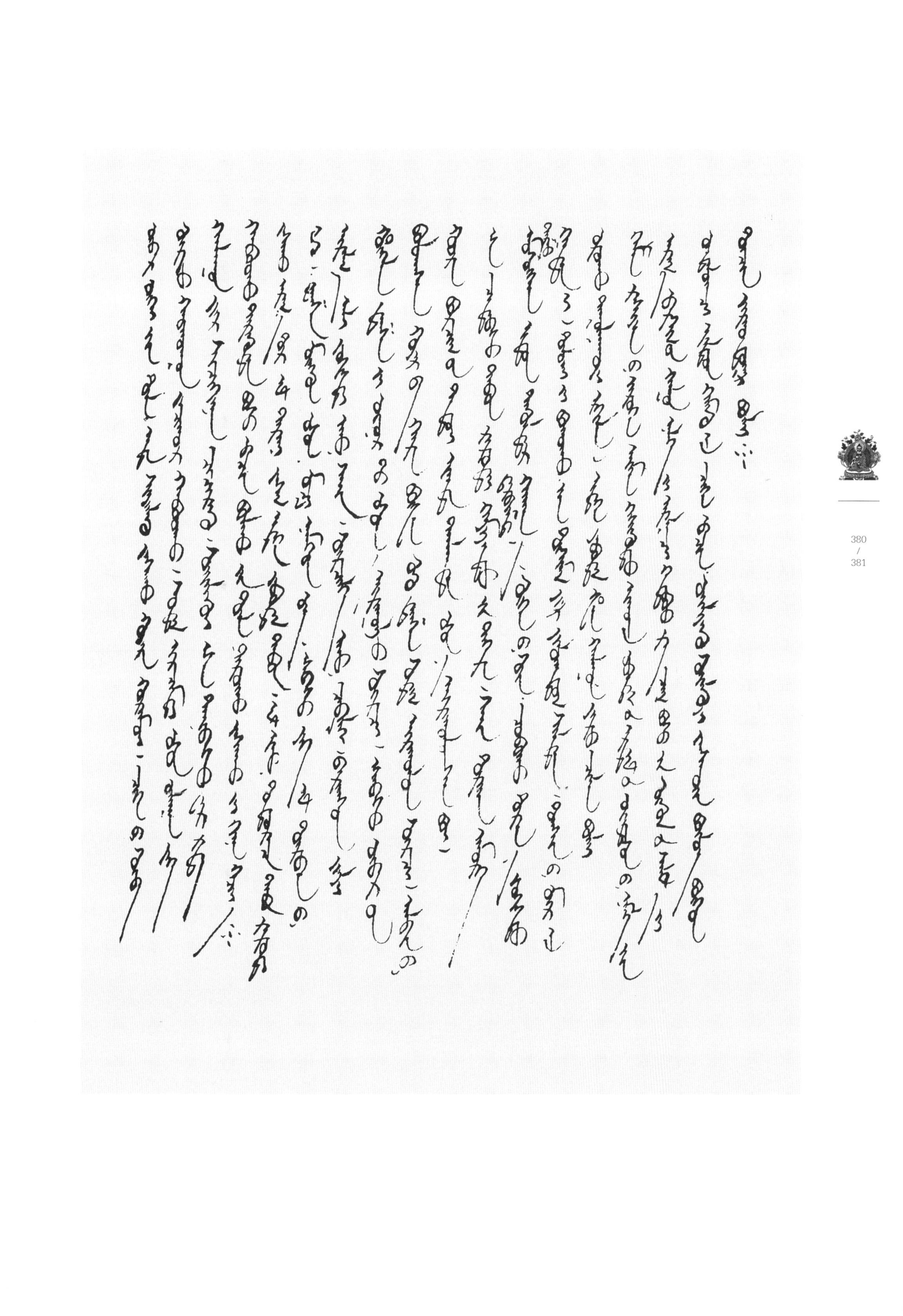

[illegible]

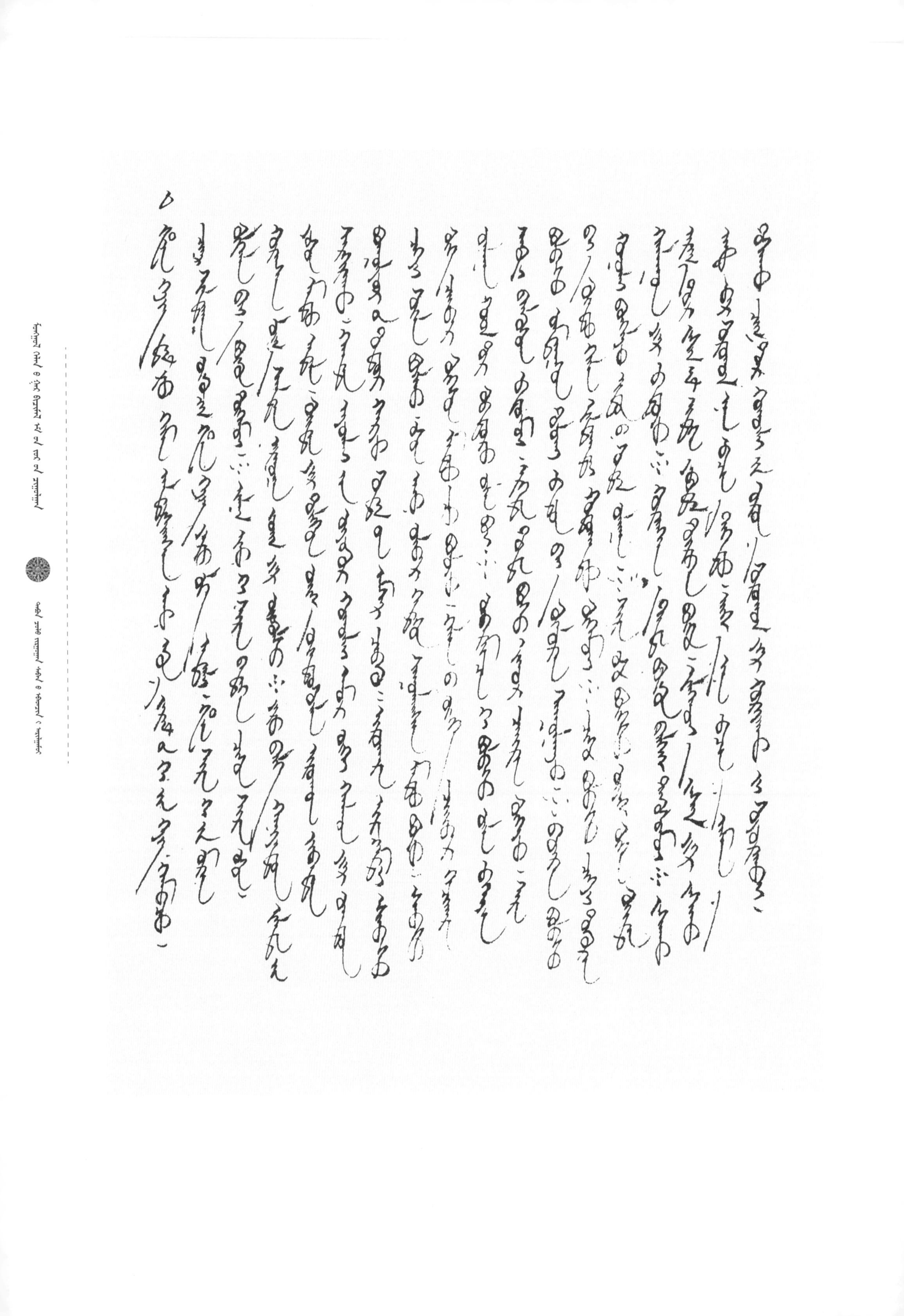

[illegible]

[illegible]

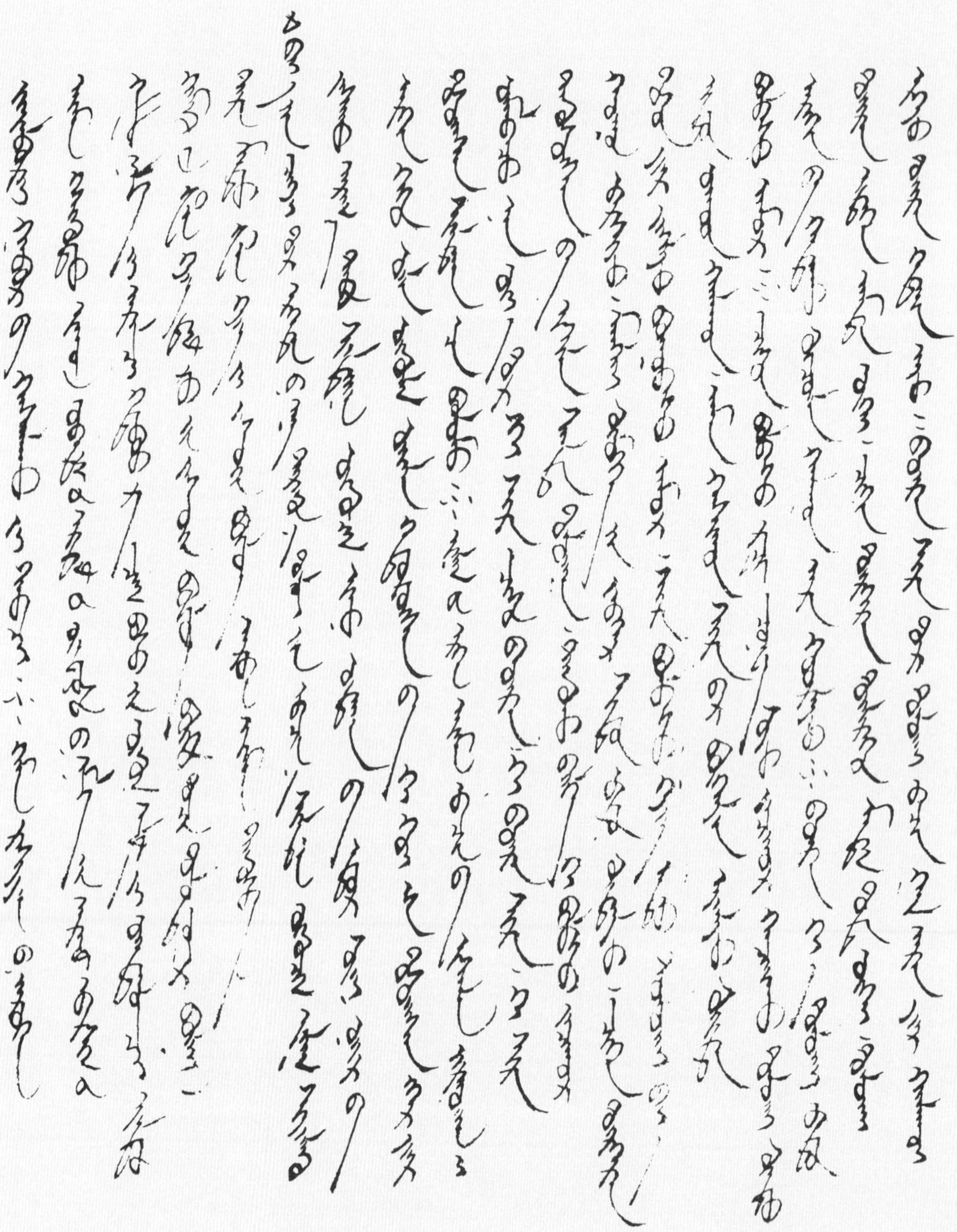

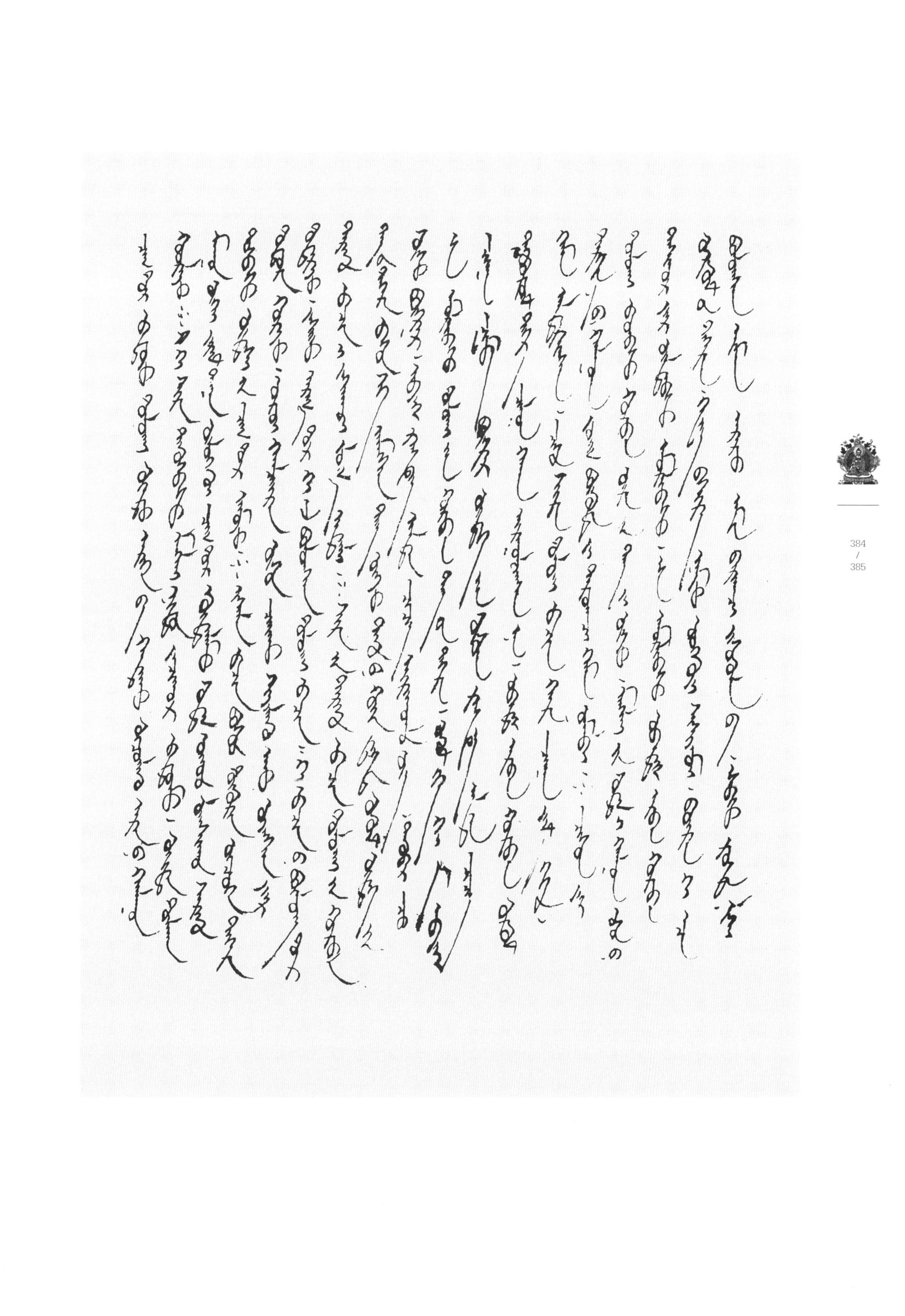

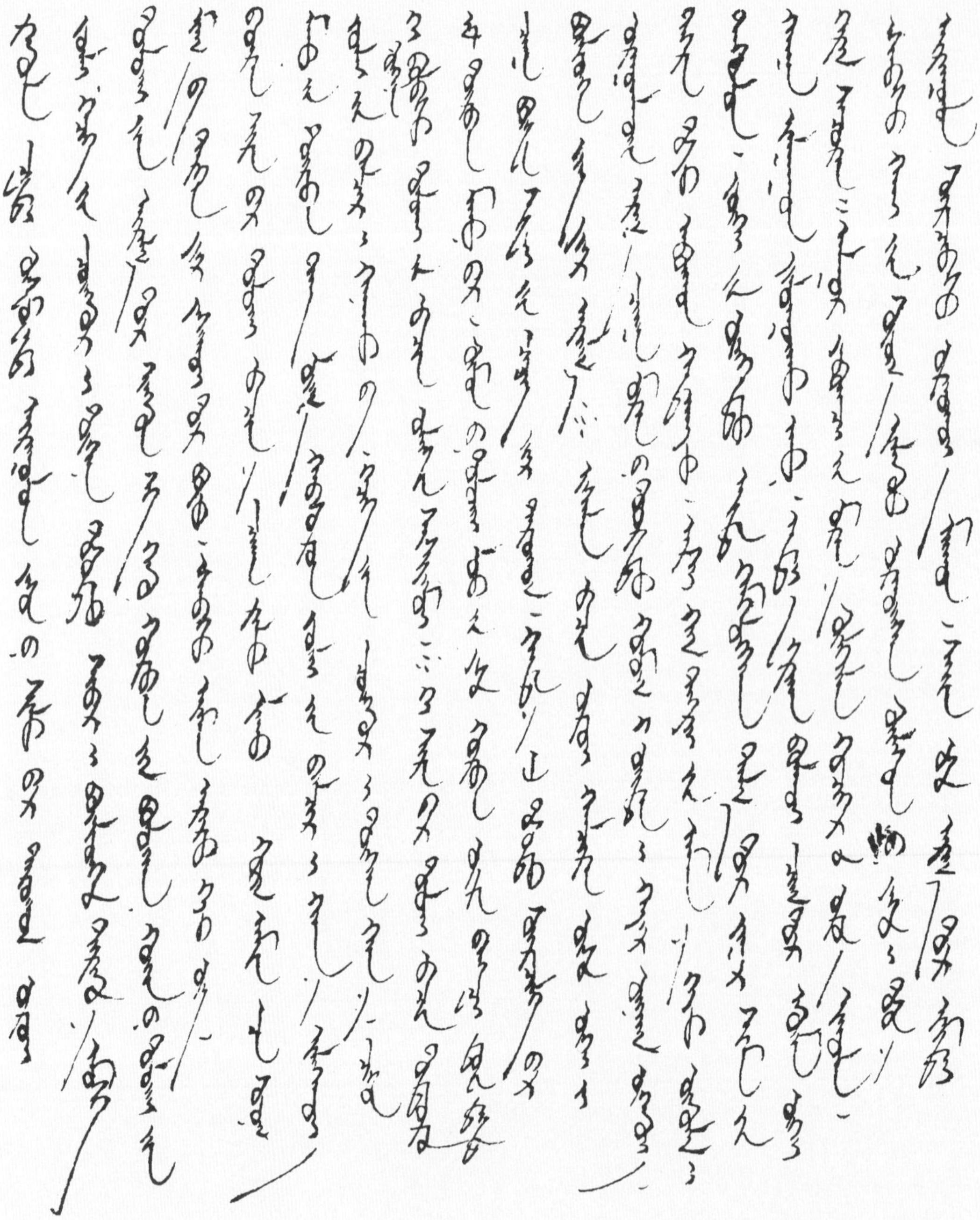

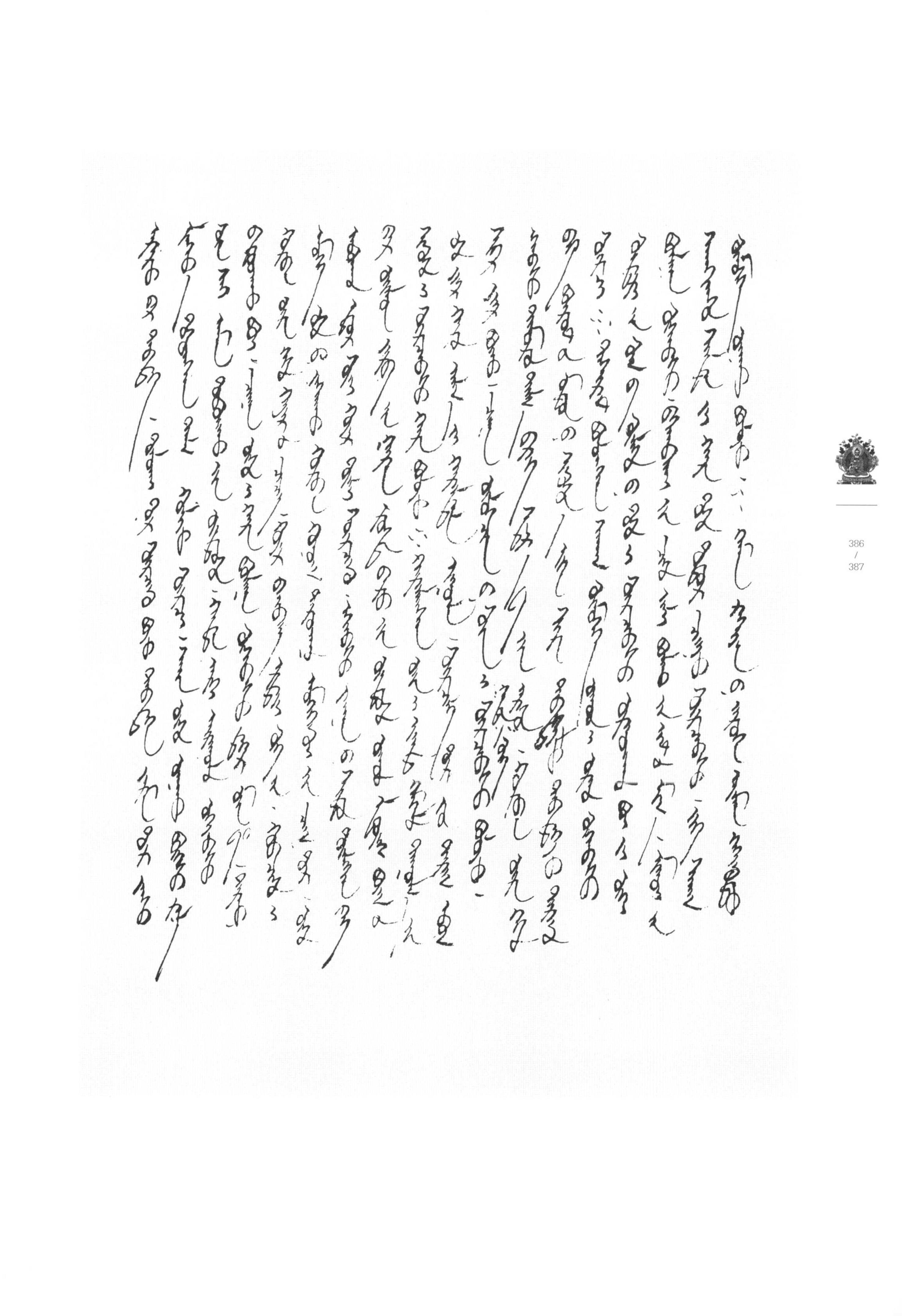

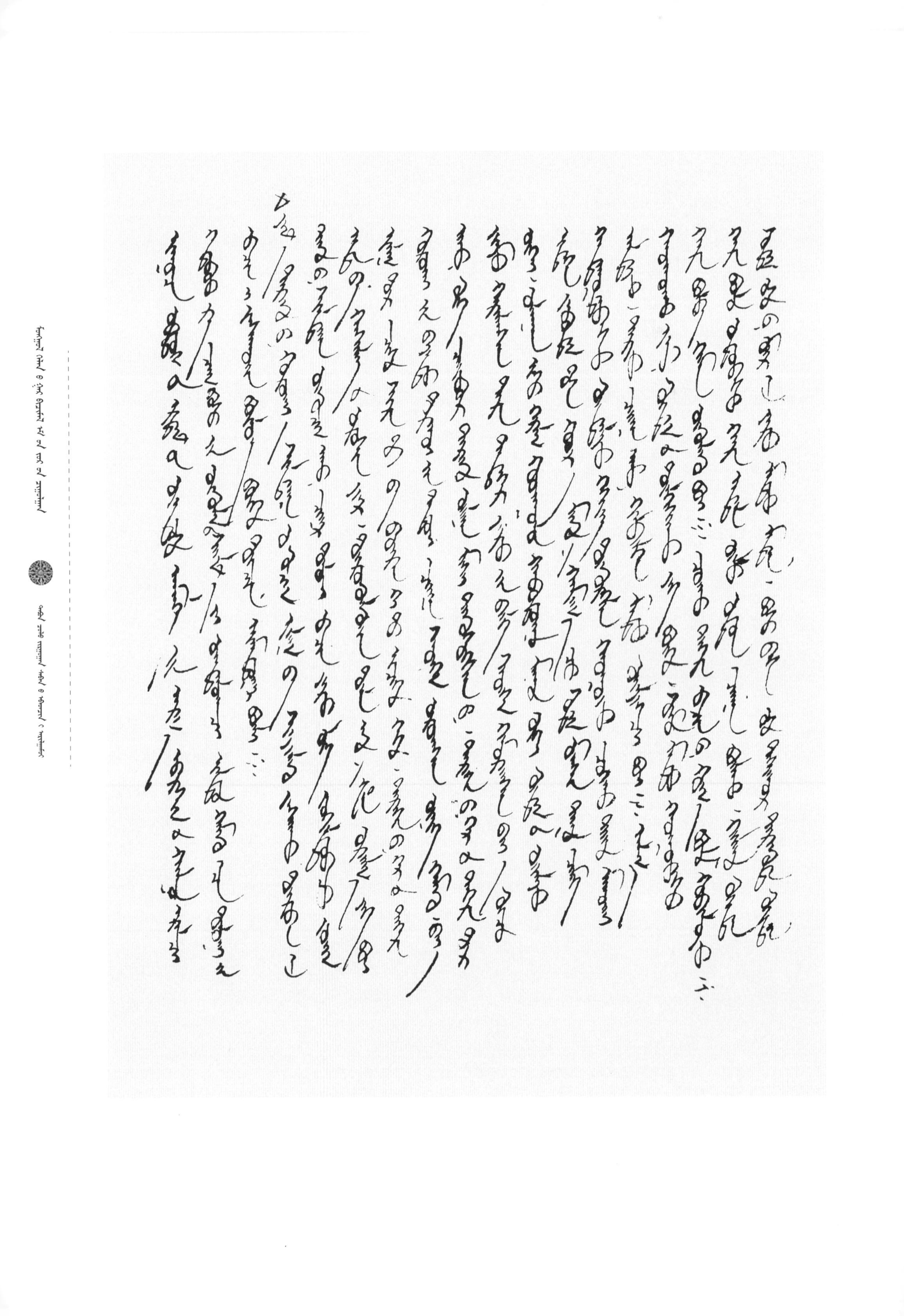

[illegible]

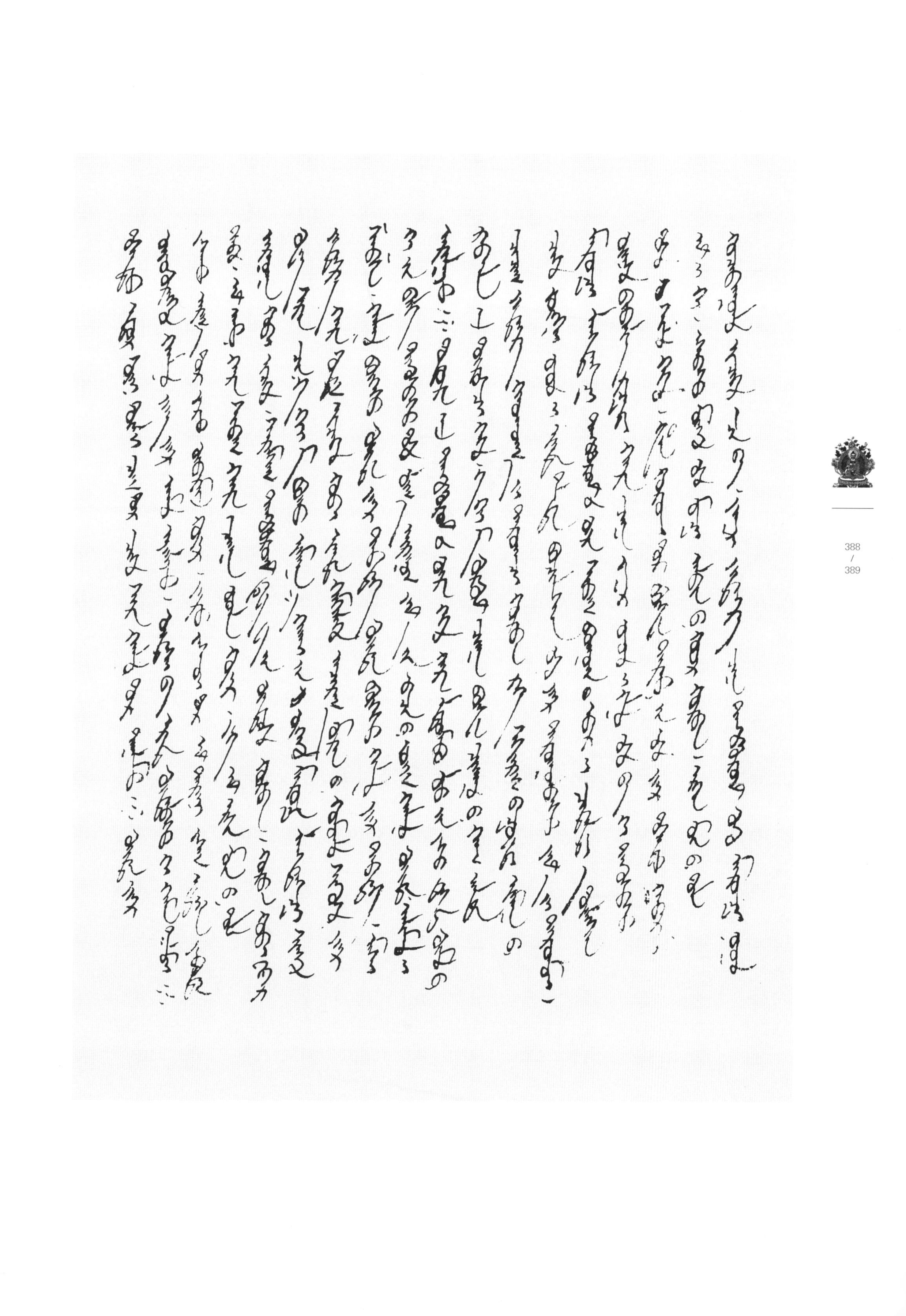

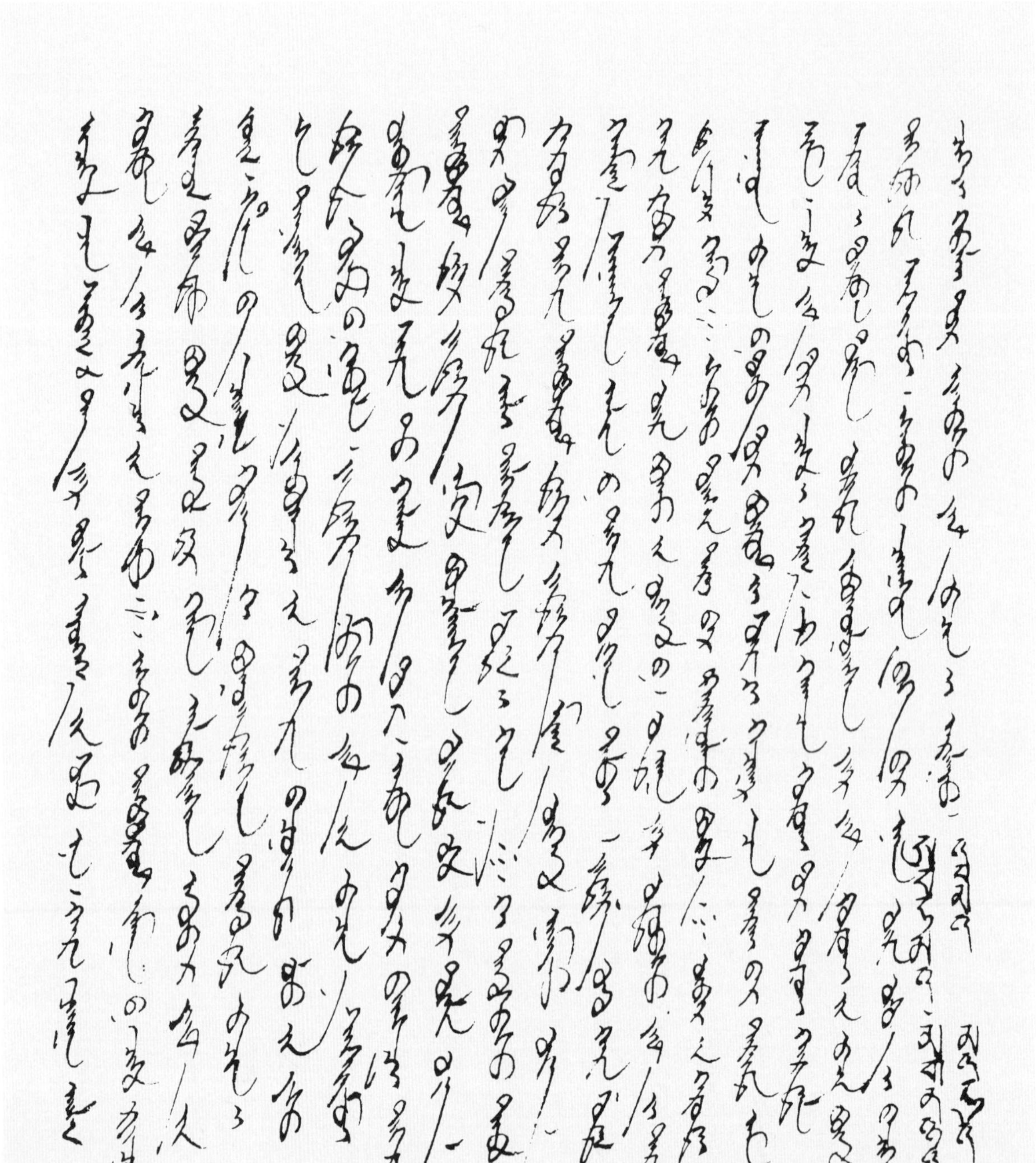

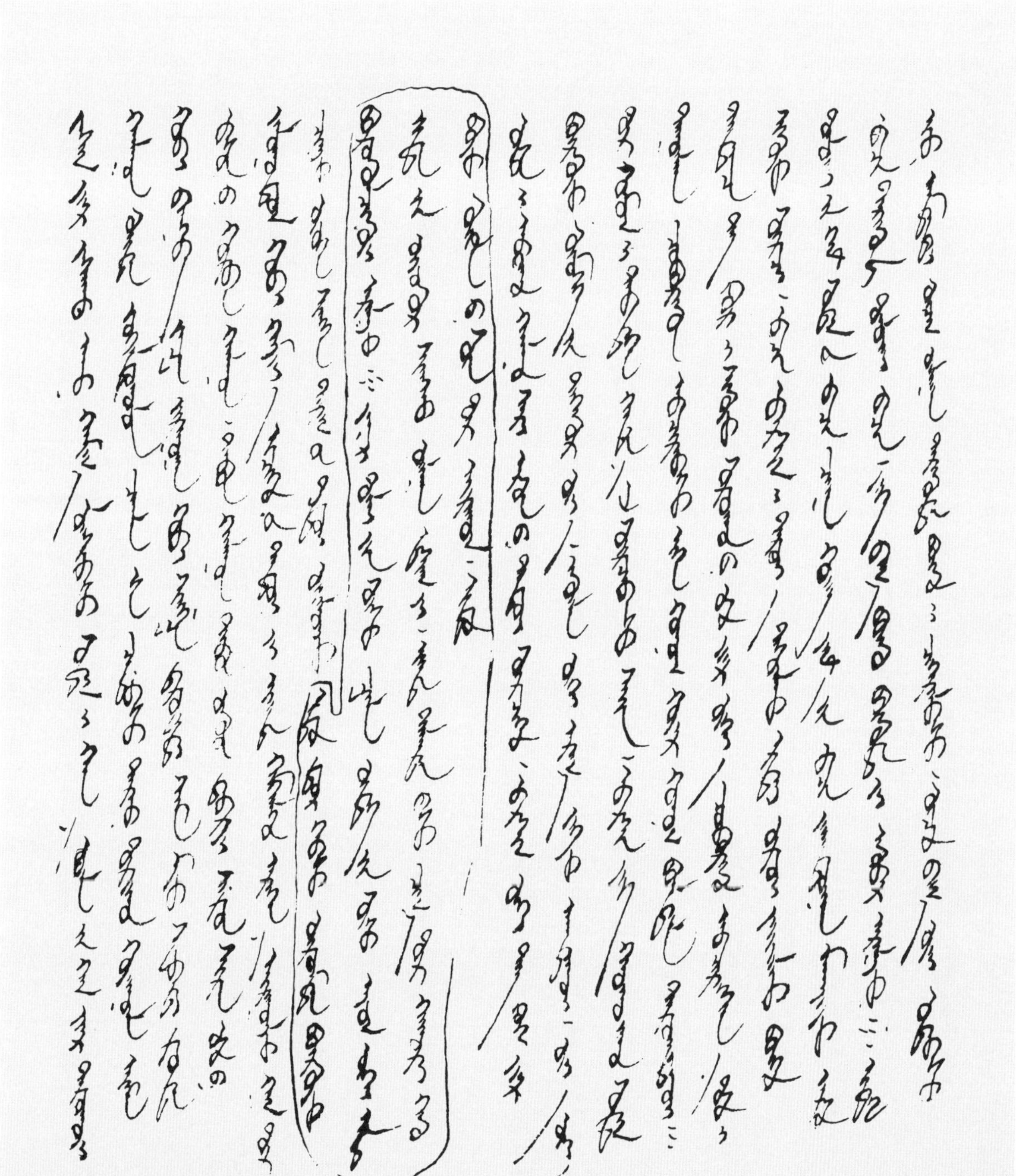

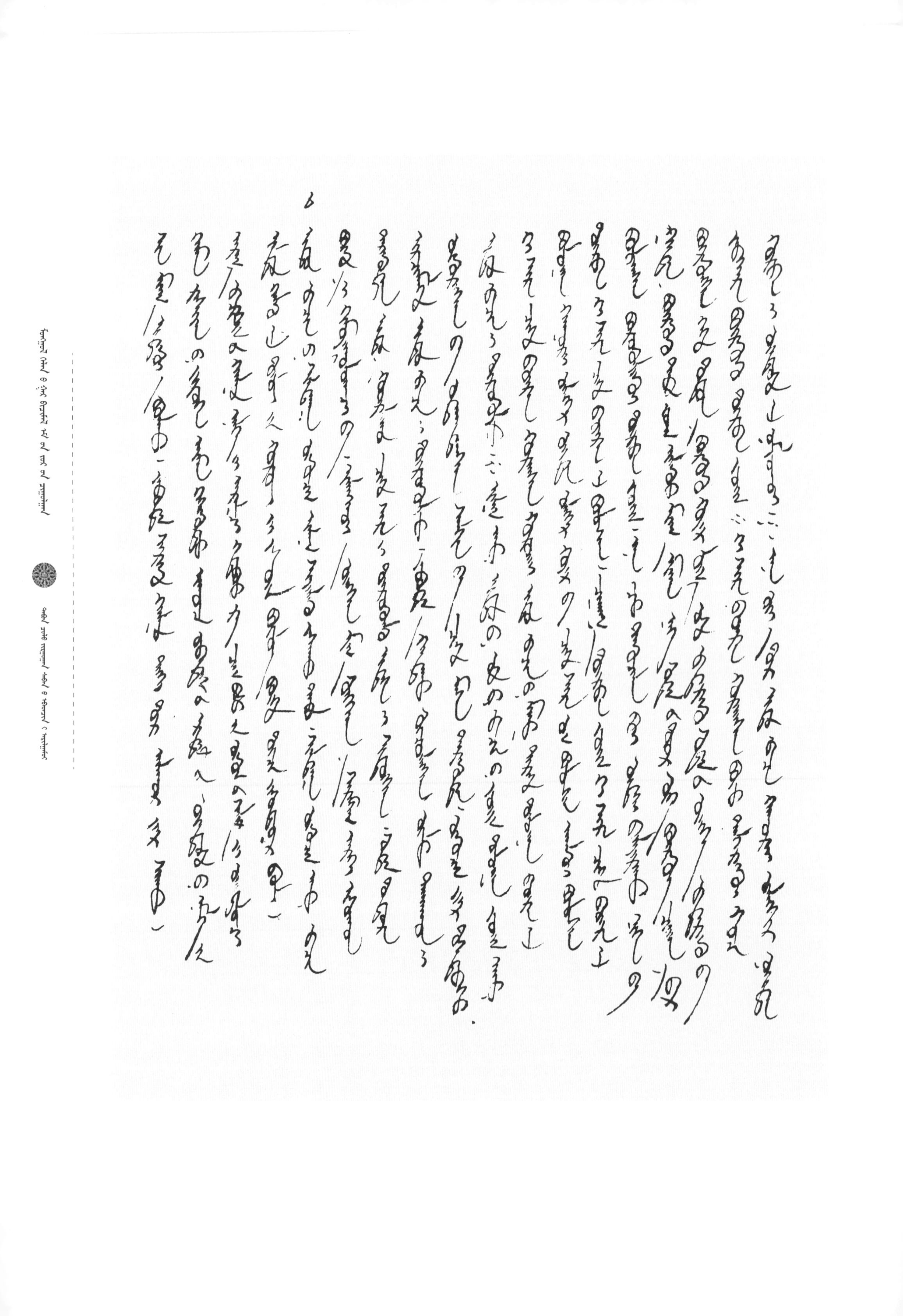

[illegible]

[illegible]

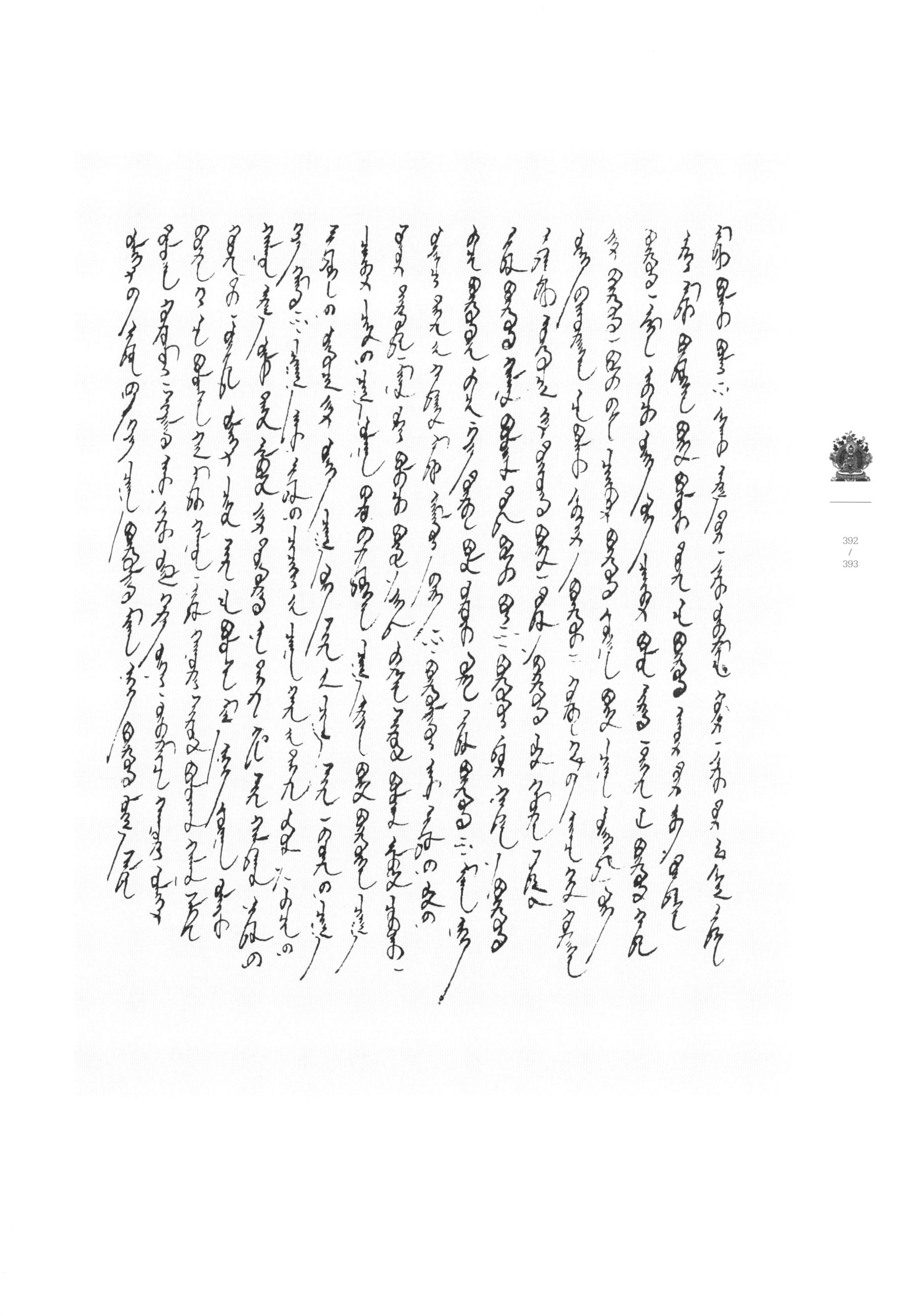

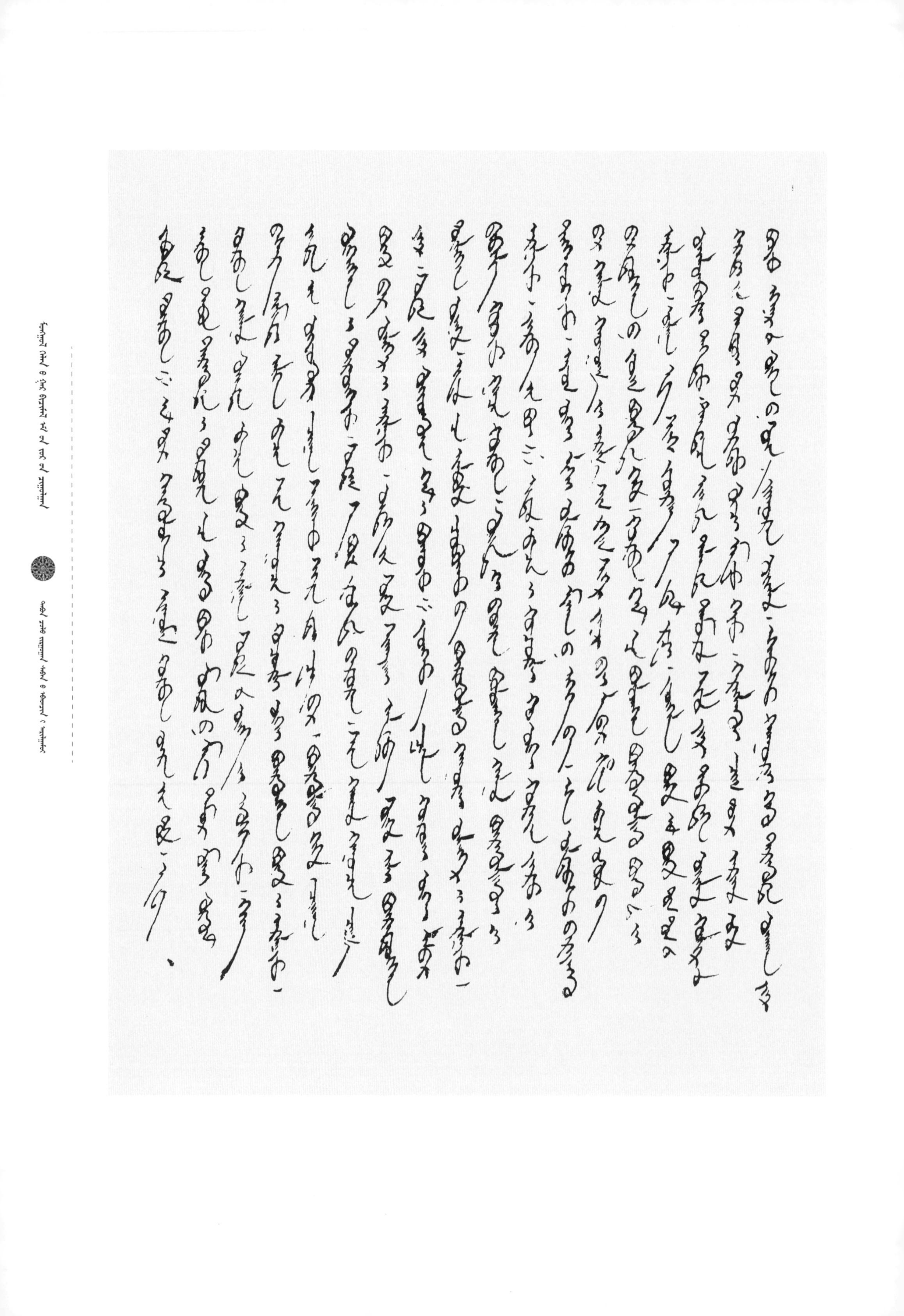

[illegible]

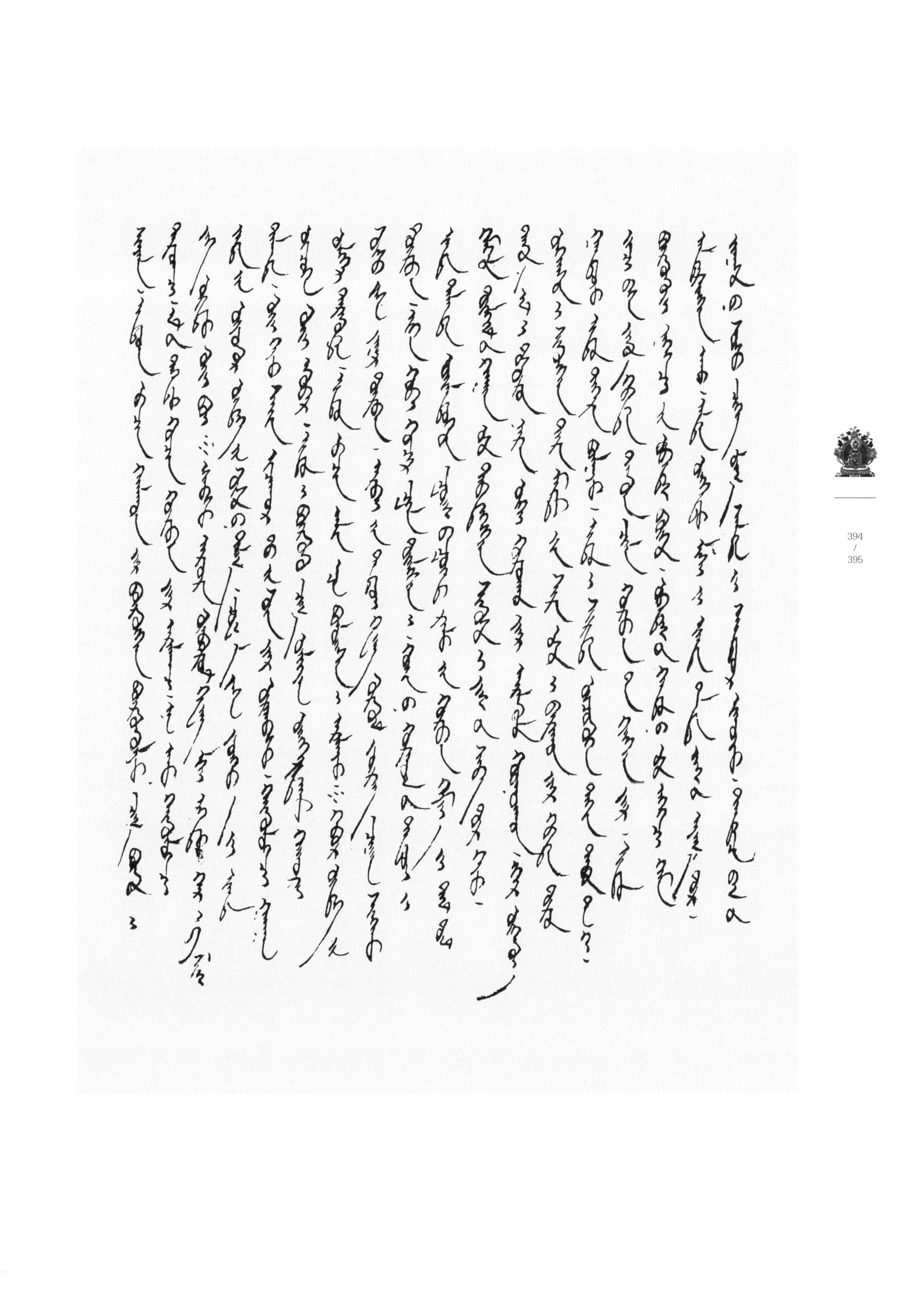

[illegible]

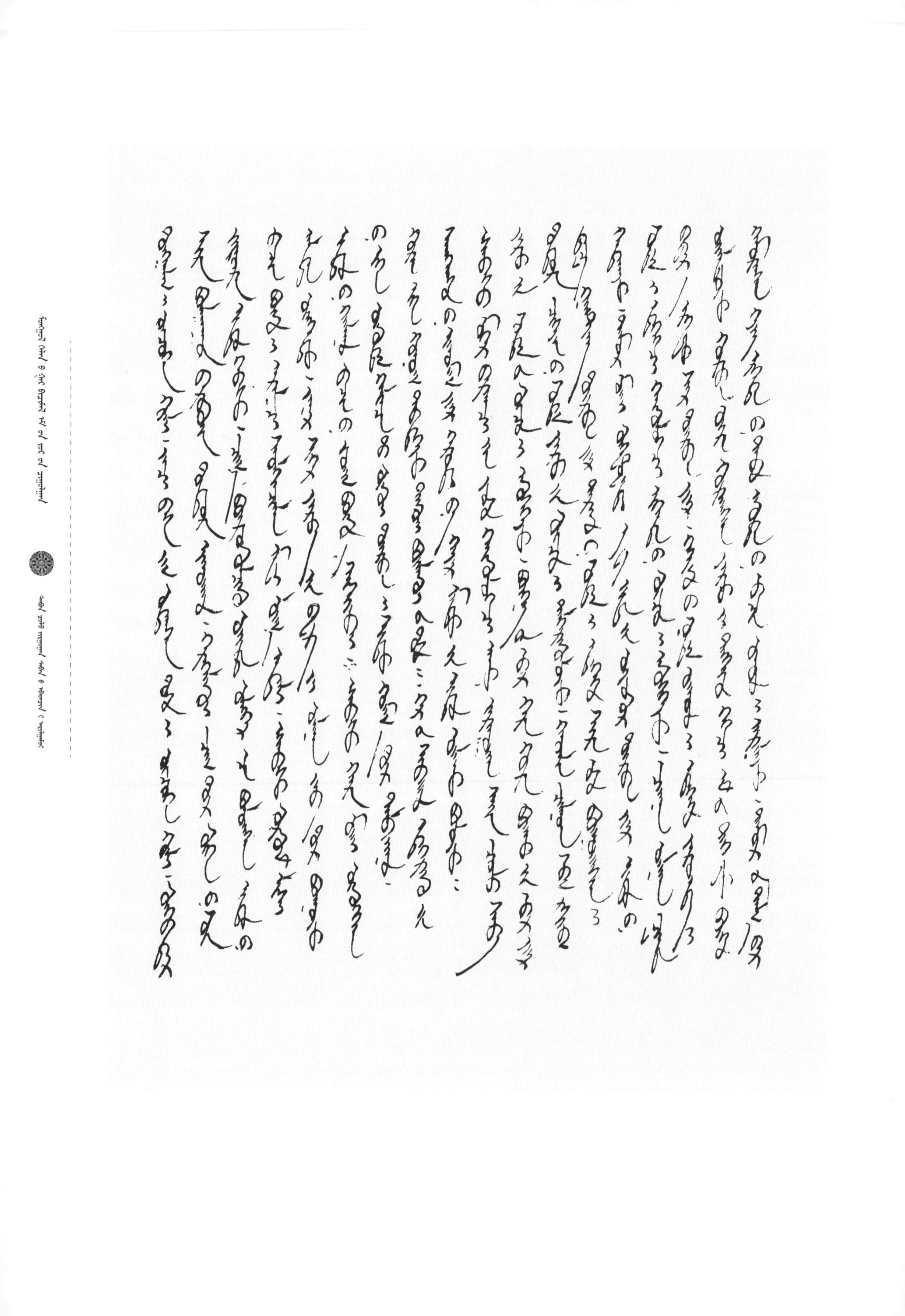

[illegible]

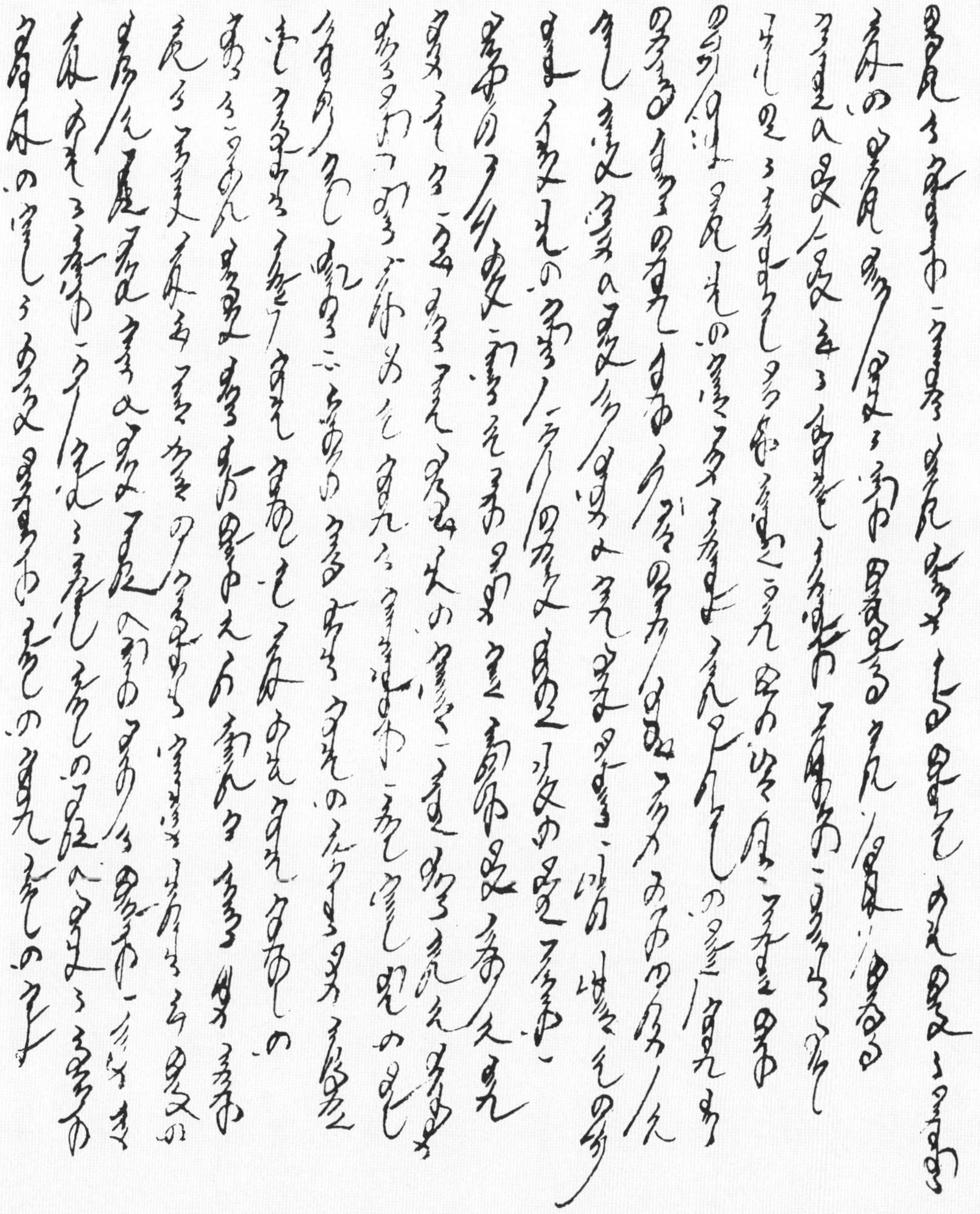

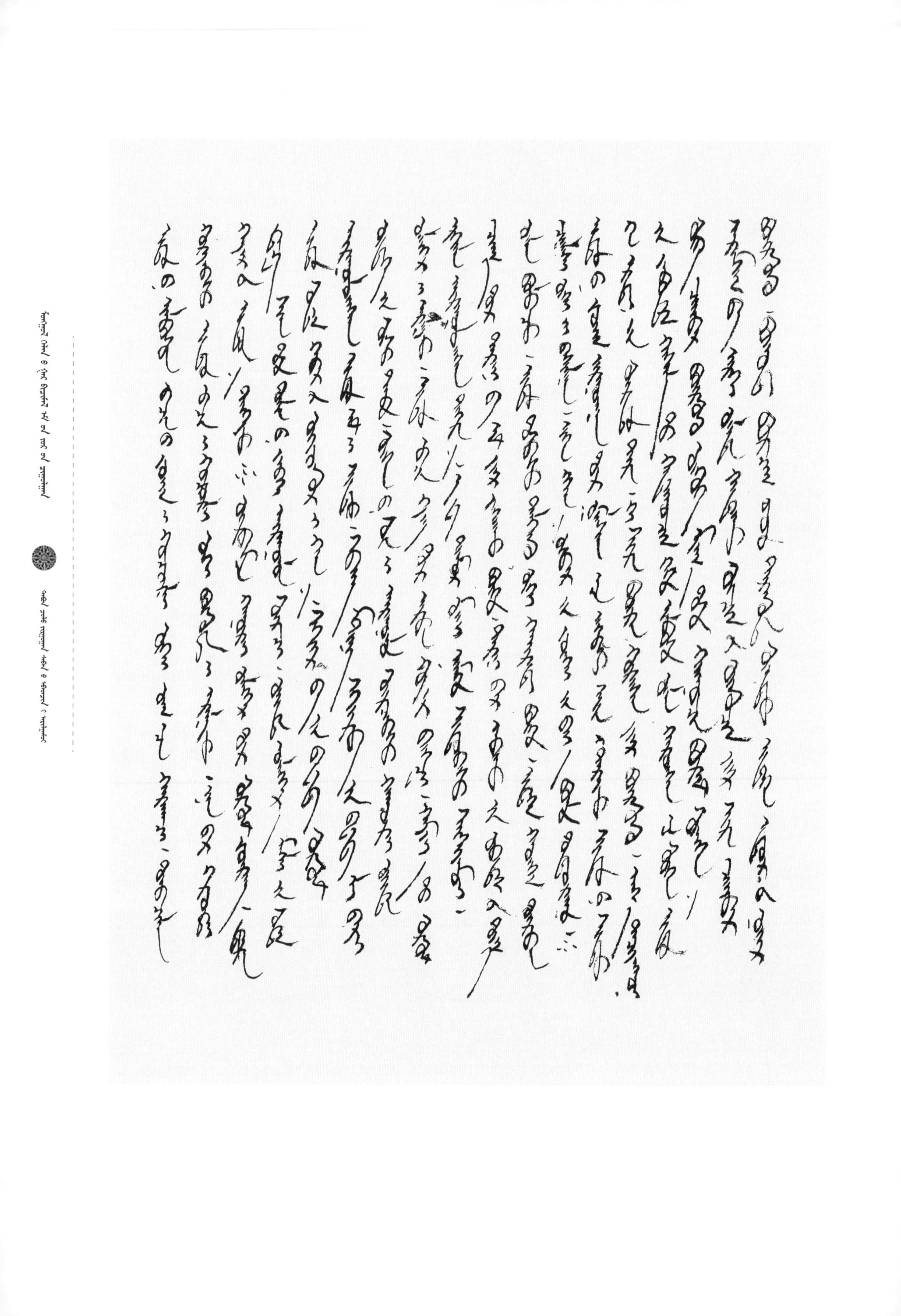

[illegible]
[illegible]
[illegible]
[illegible]
[illegible]
[illegible]
[illegible]
[illegible]
[illegible]
[illegible]
[illegible]
[illegible]
[illegible]
[illegible]
[illegible]

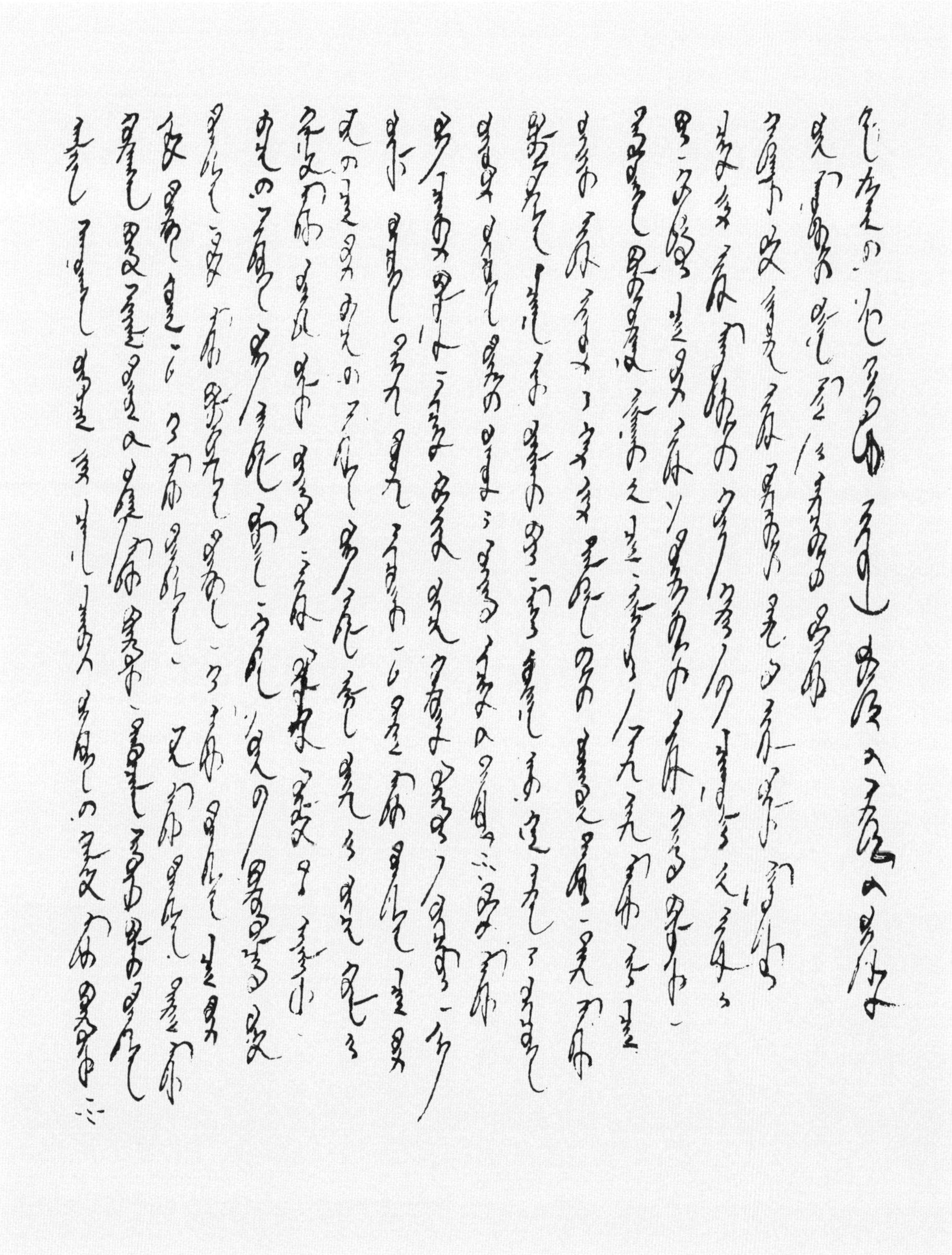

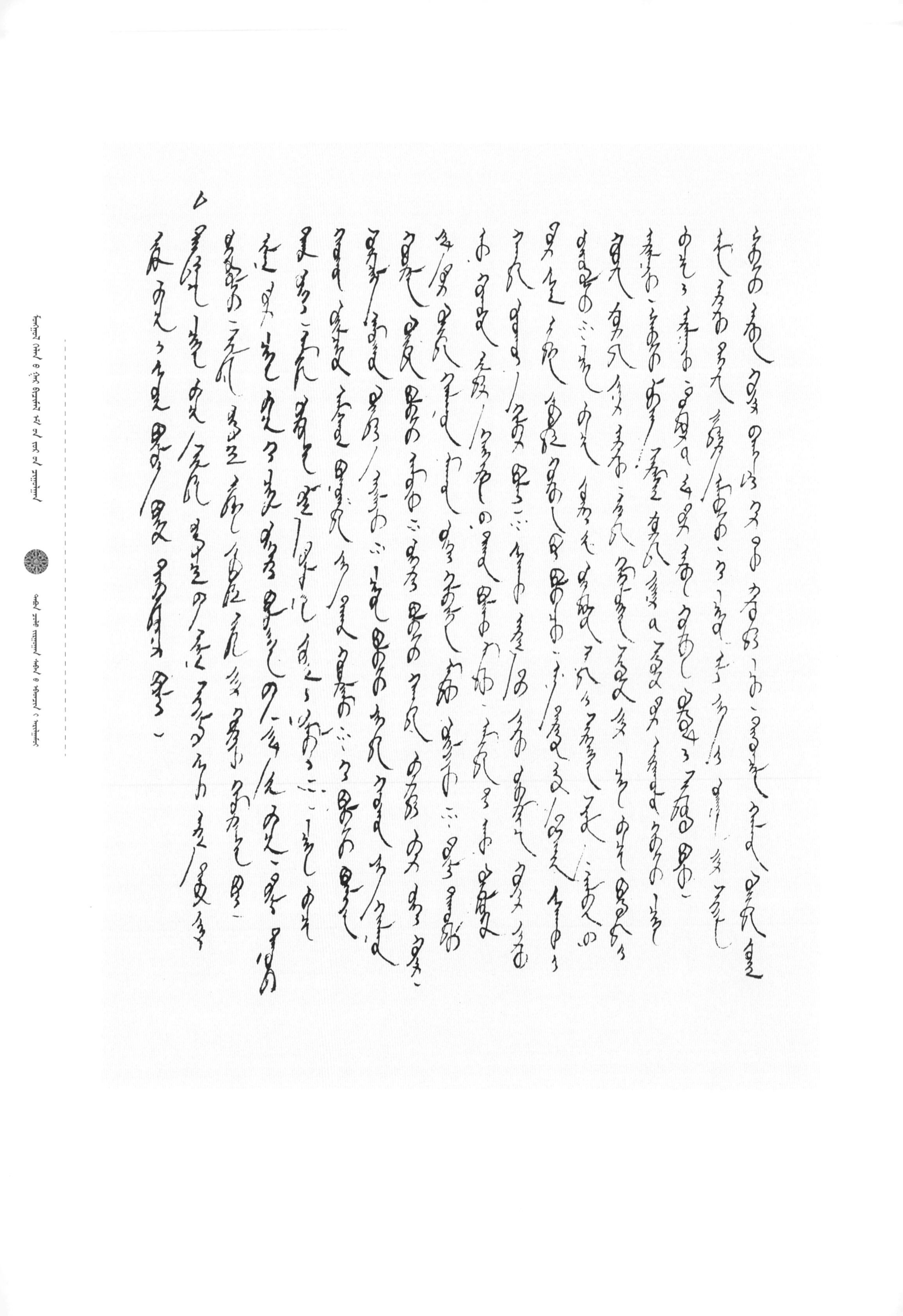

[illegible]

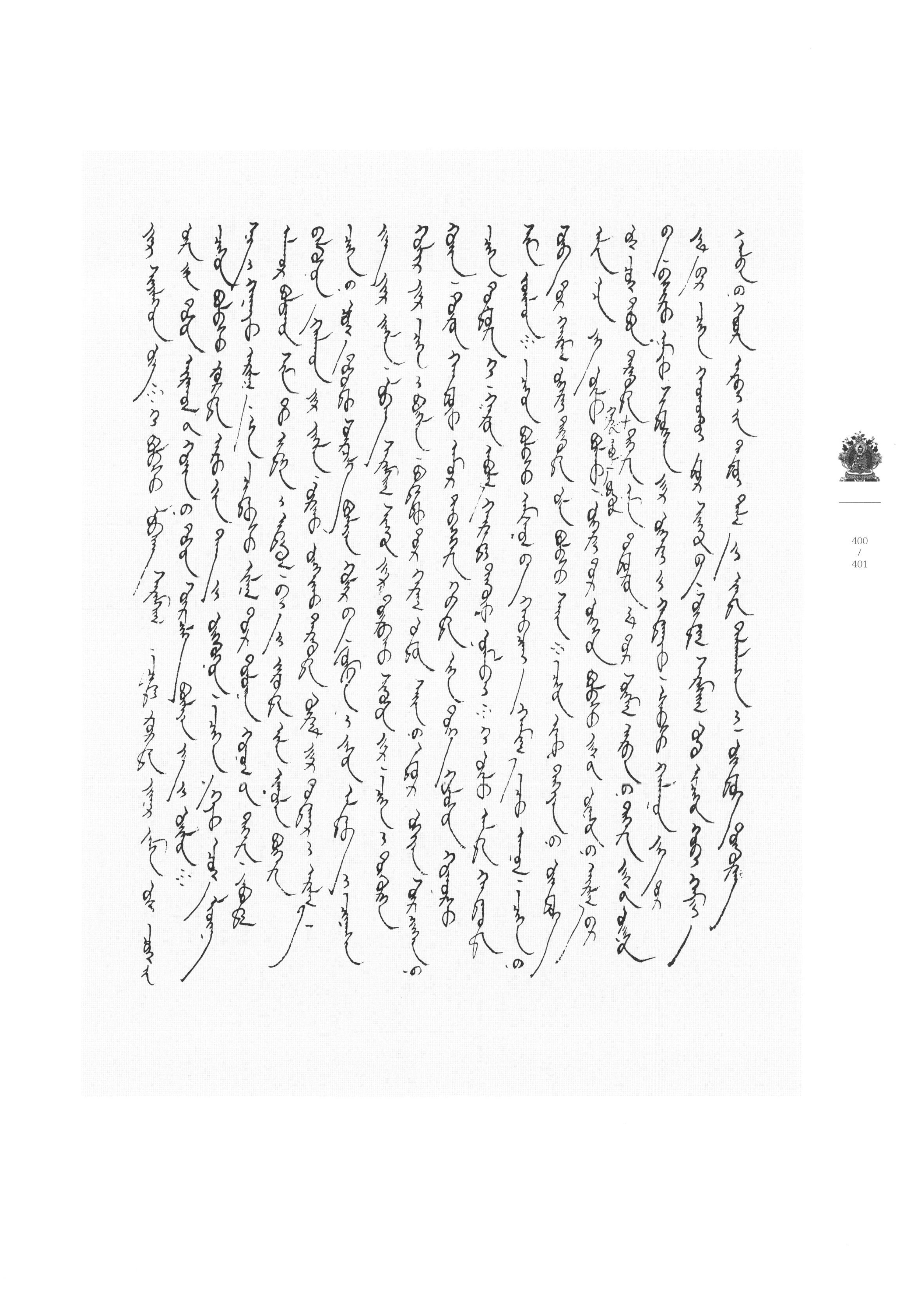

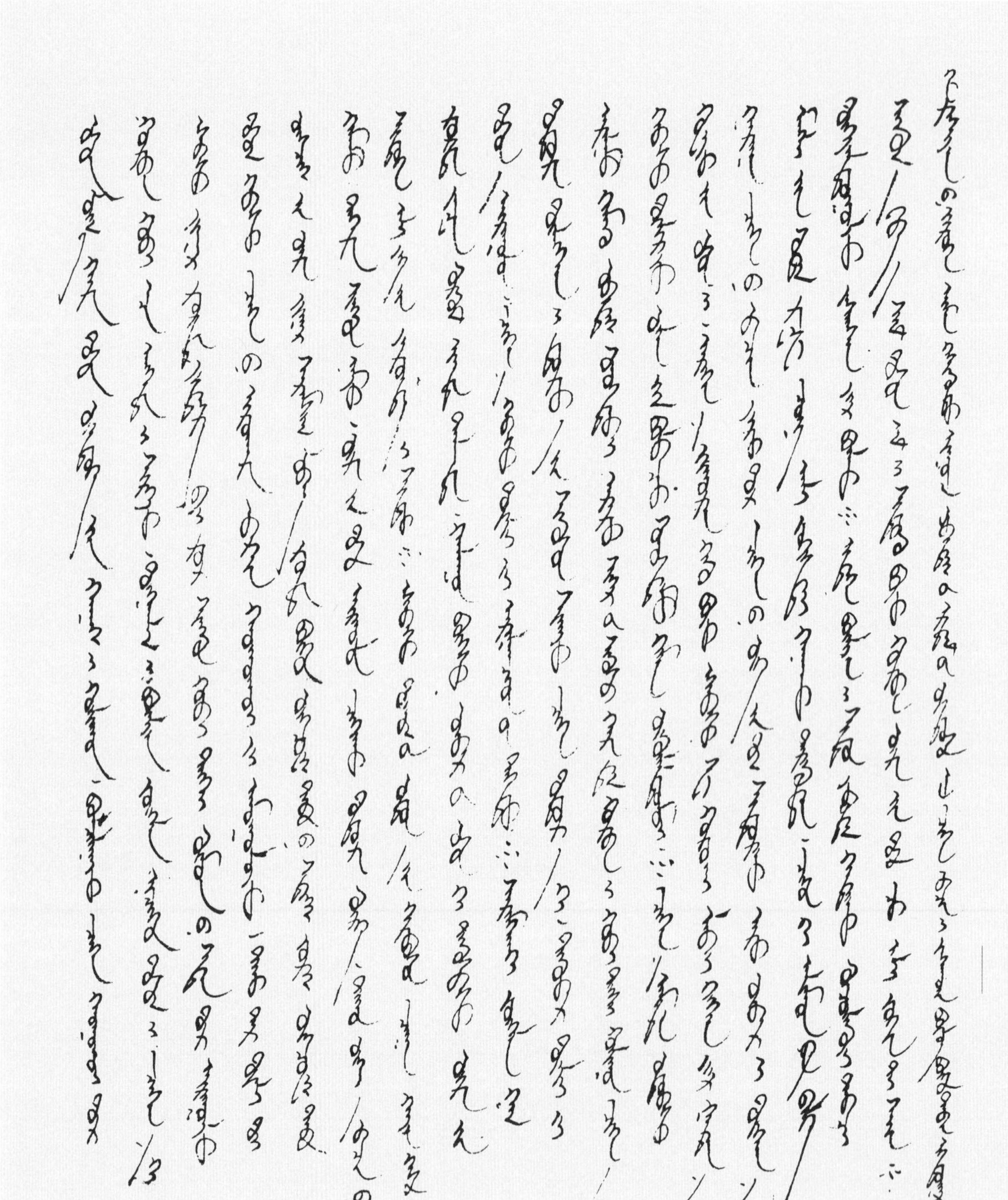

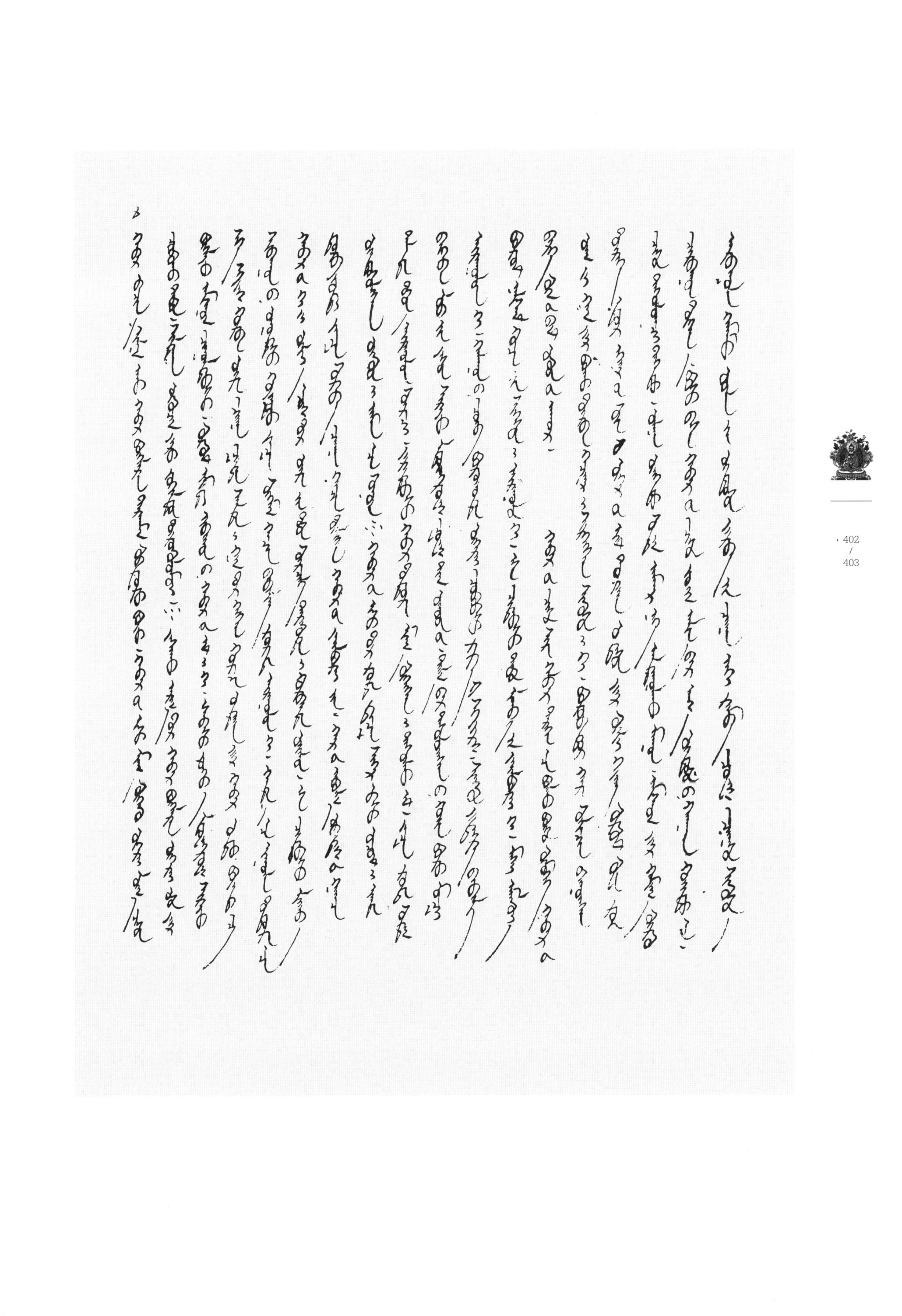

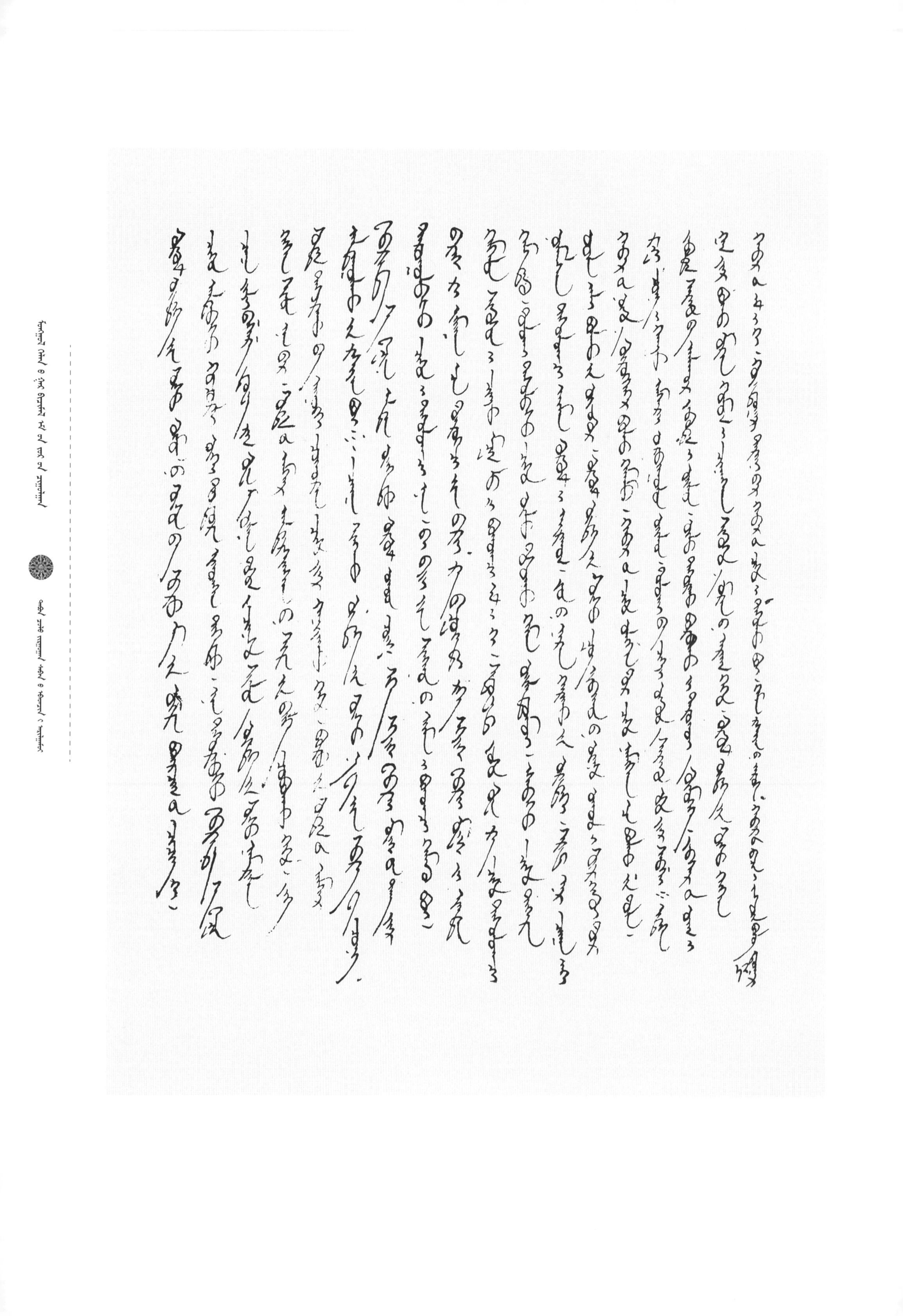

[illegible]
[illegible]
[illegible]
[illegible]
[illegible]
[illegible]
[illegible]
[illegible]
[illegible]
[illegible]
[illegible]
[illegible]
[illegible]
[illegible]
[illegible]
[illegible]

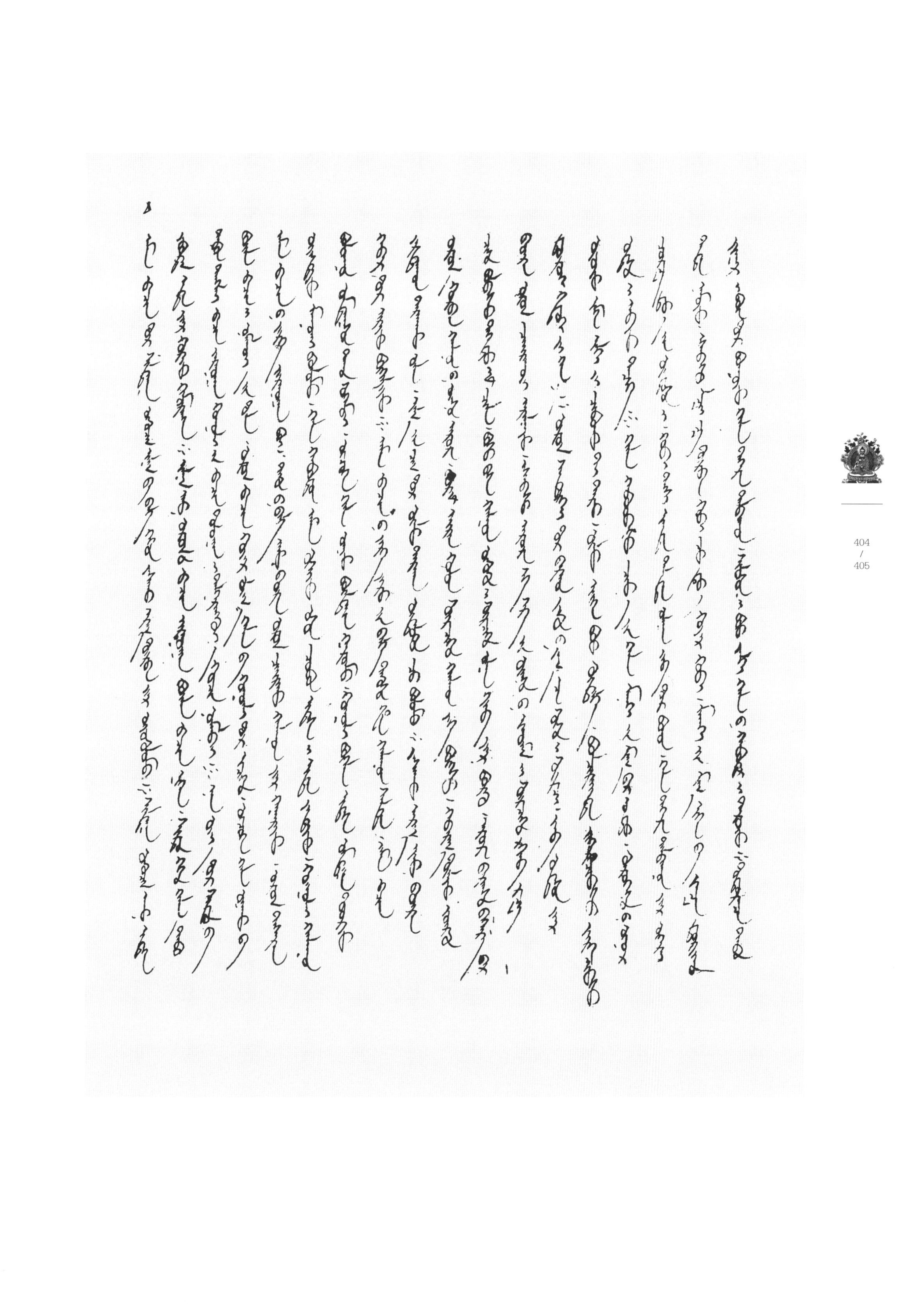

[illegible]

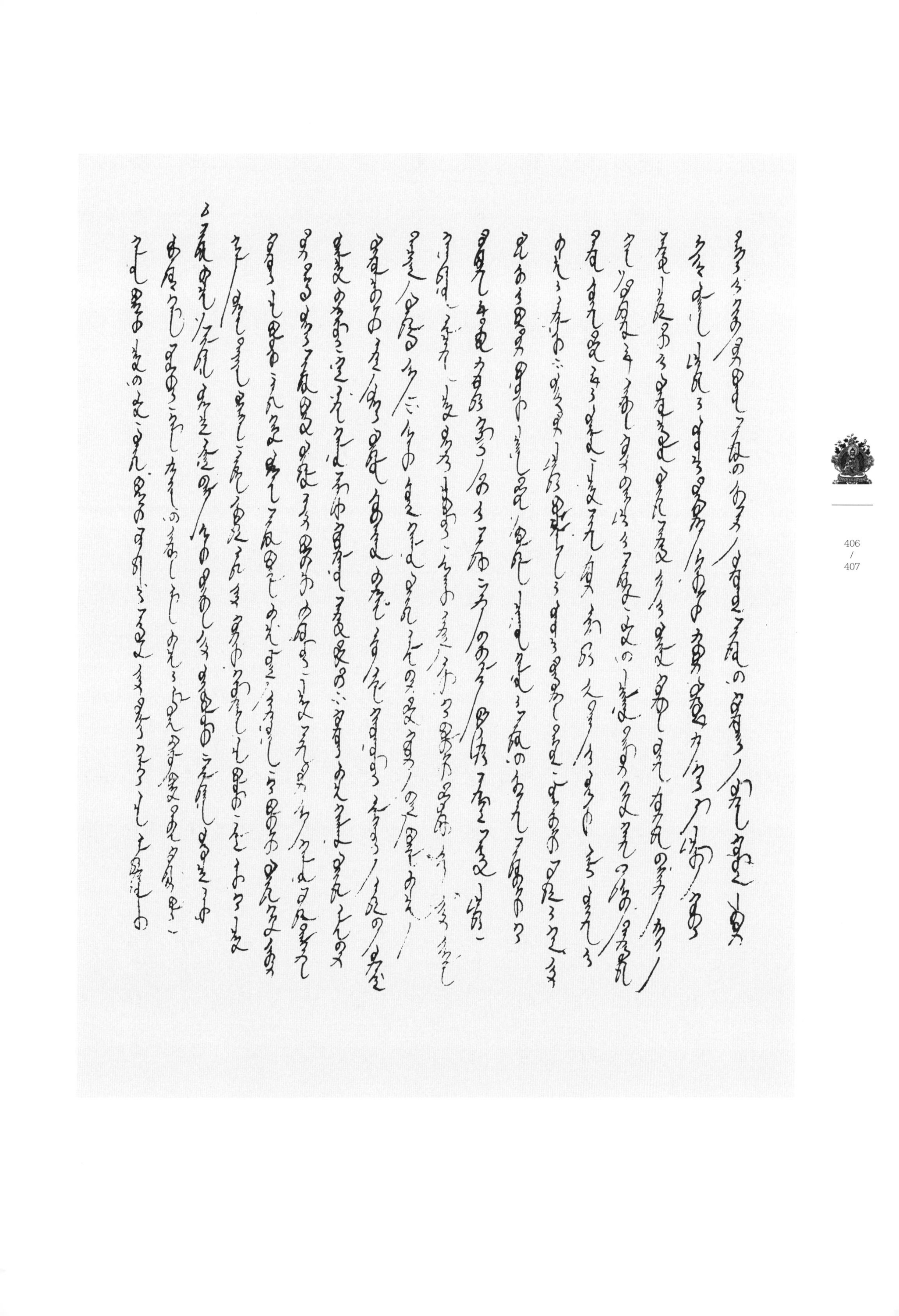

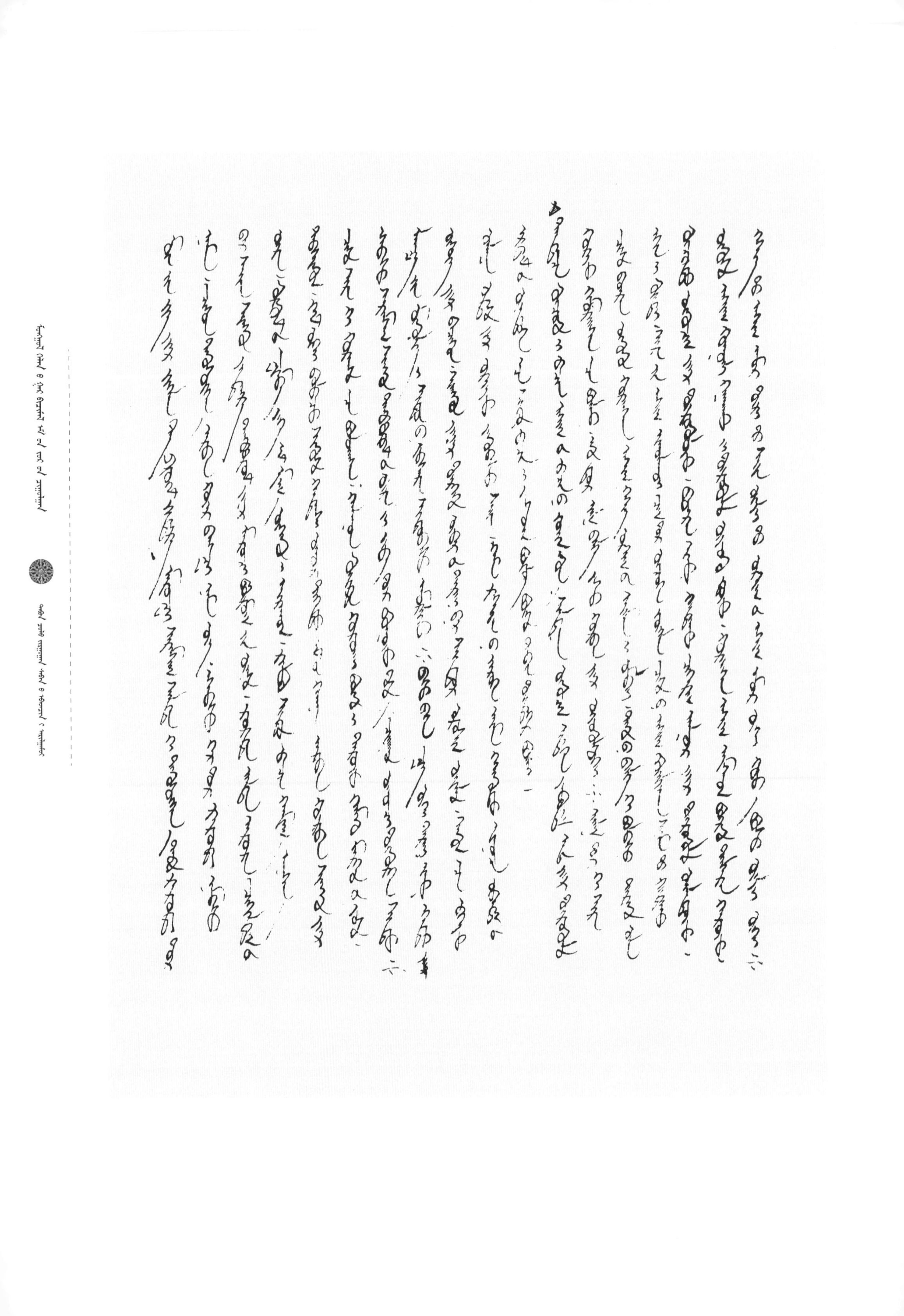

[illegible]

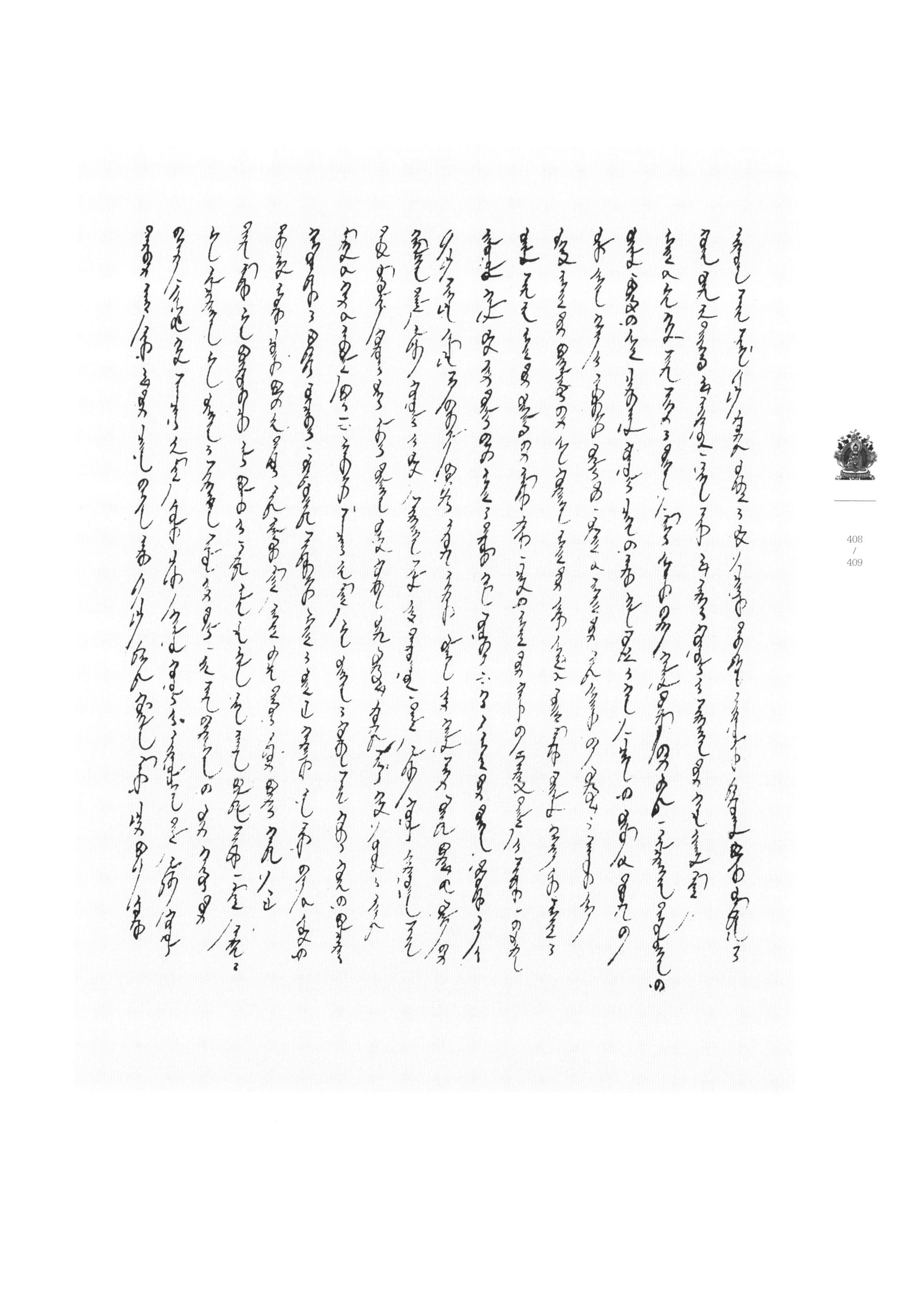

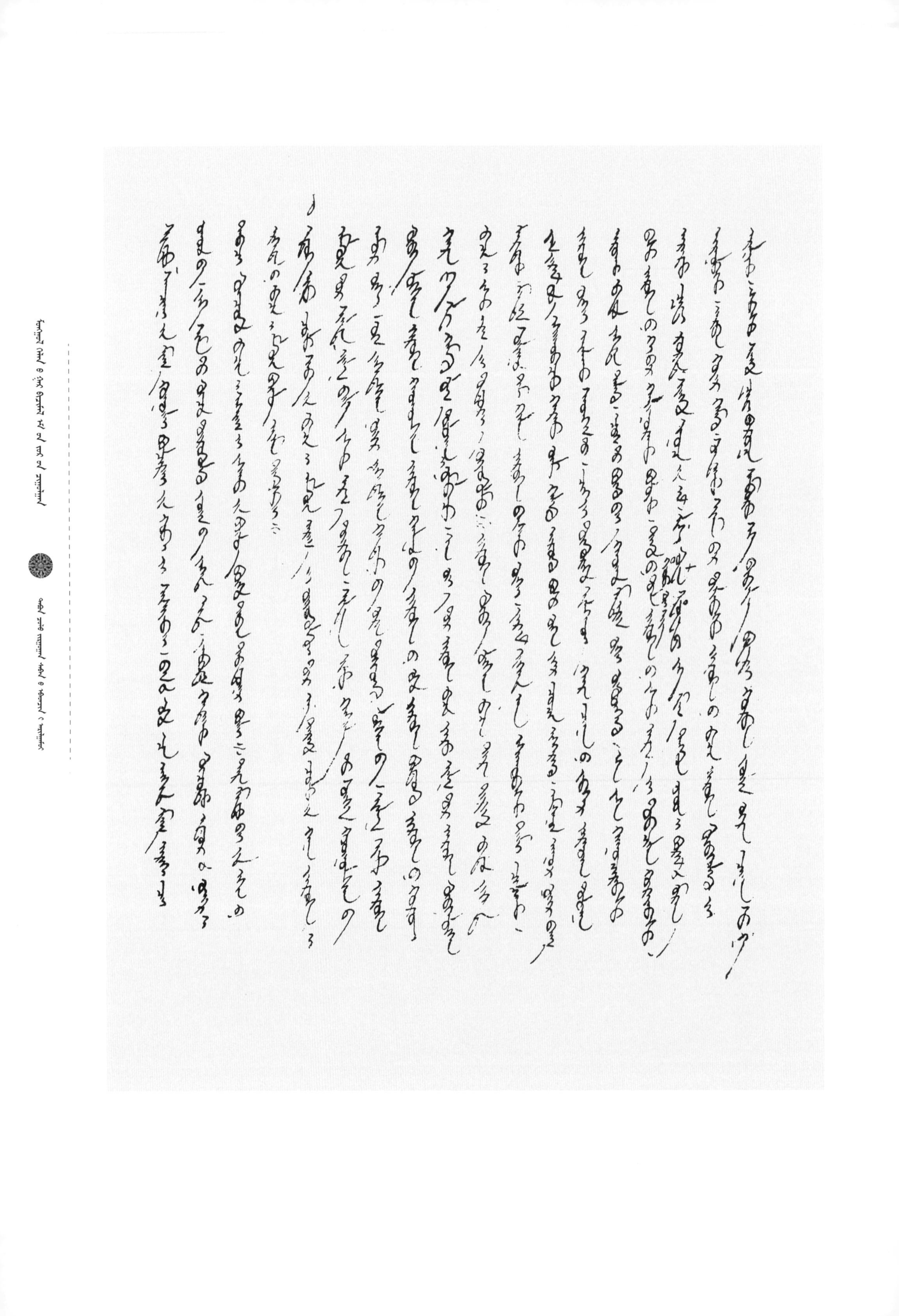

[illegible]

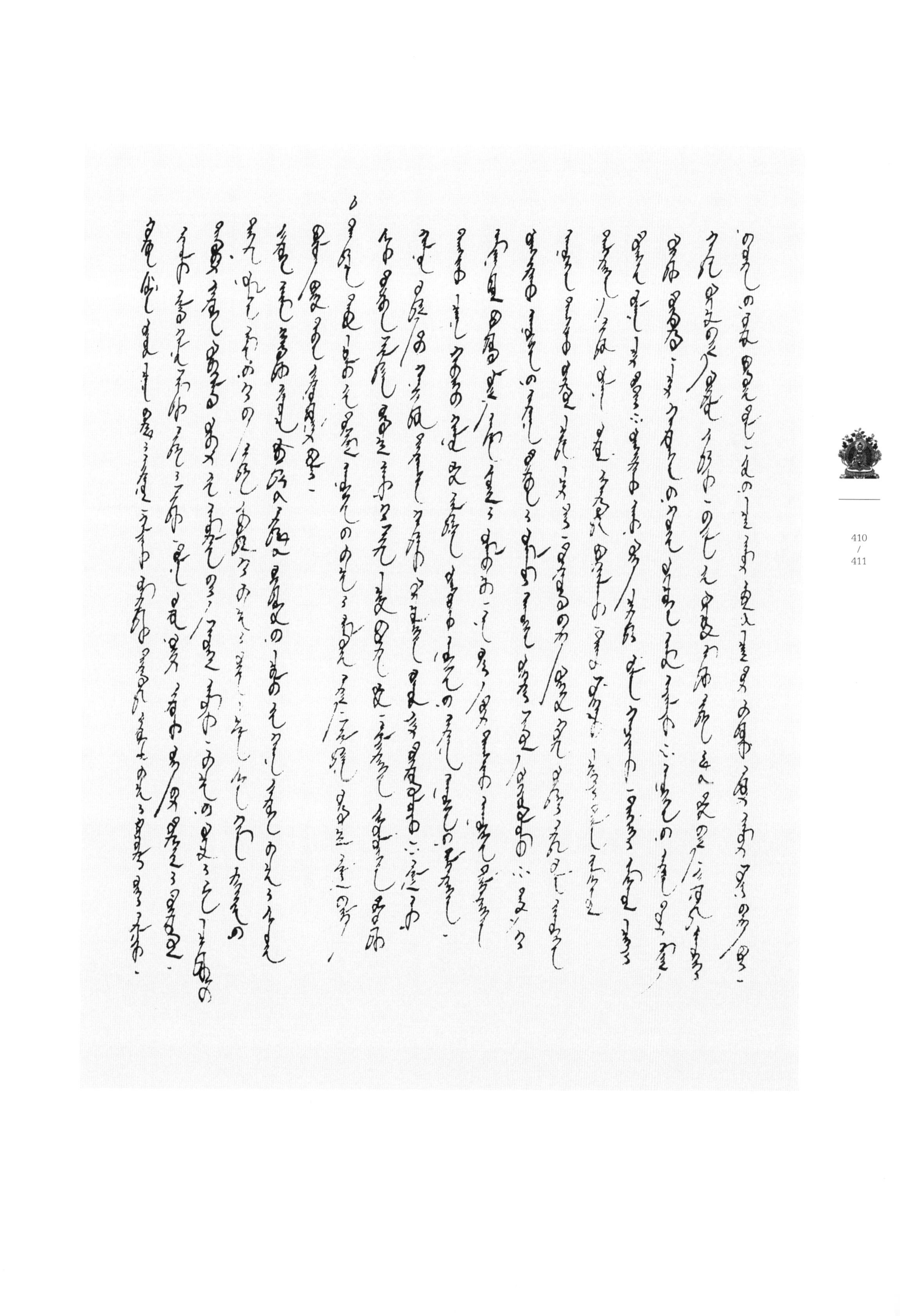

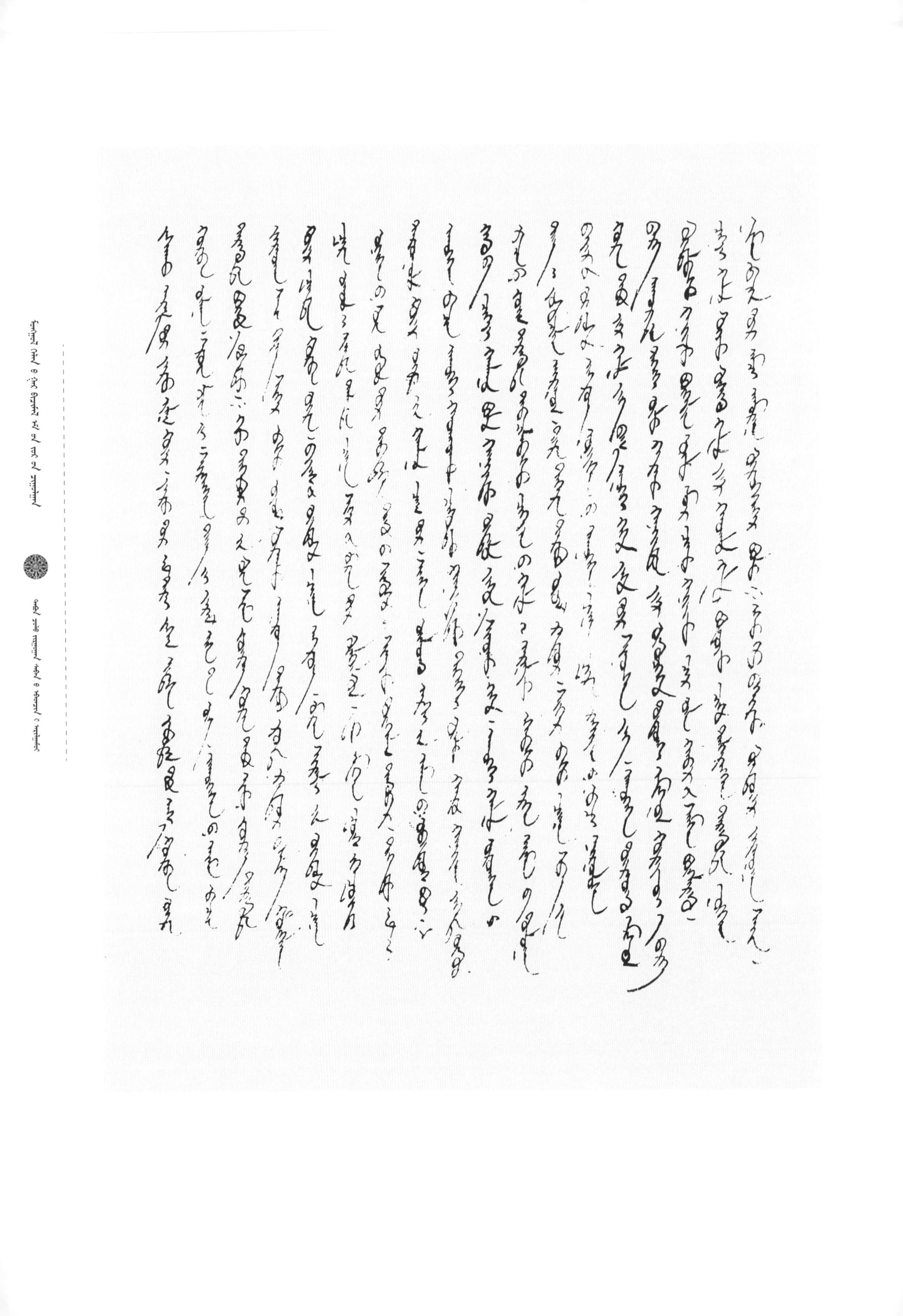

[illegible]

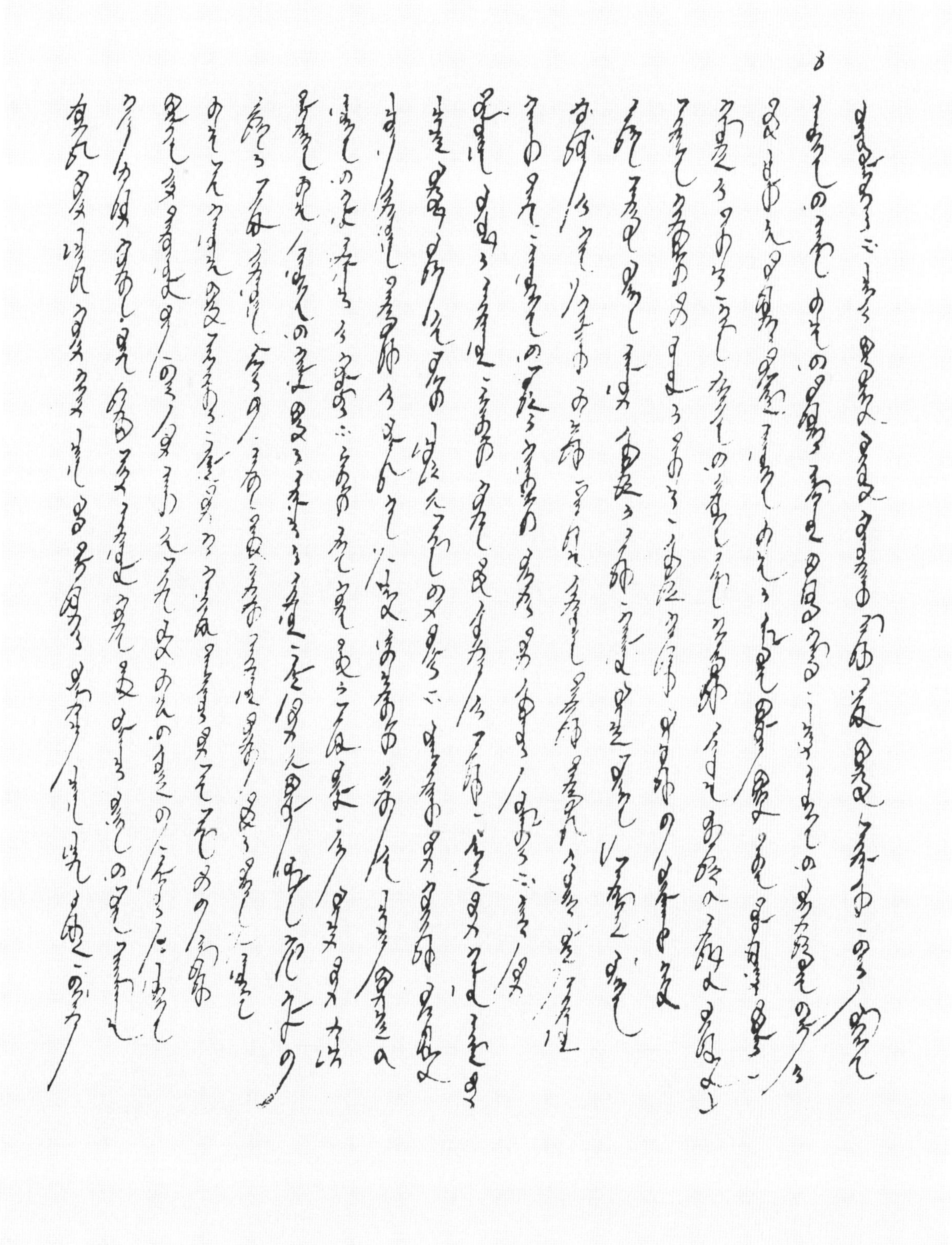

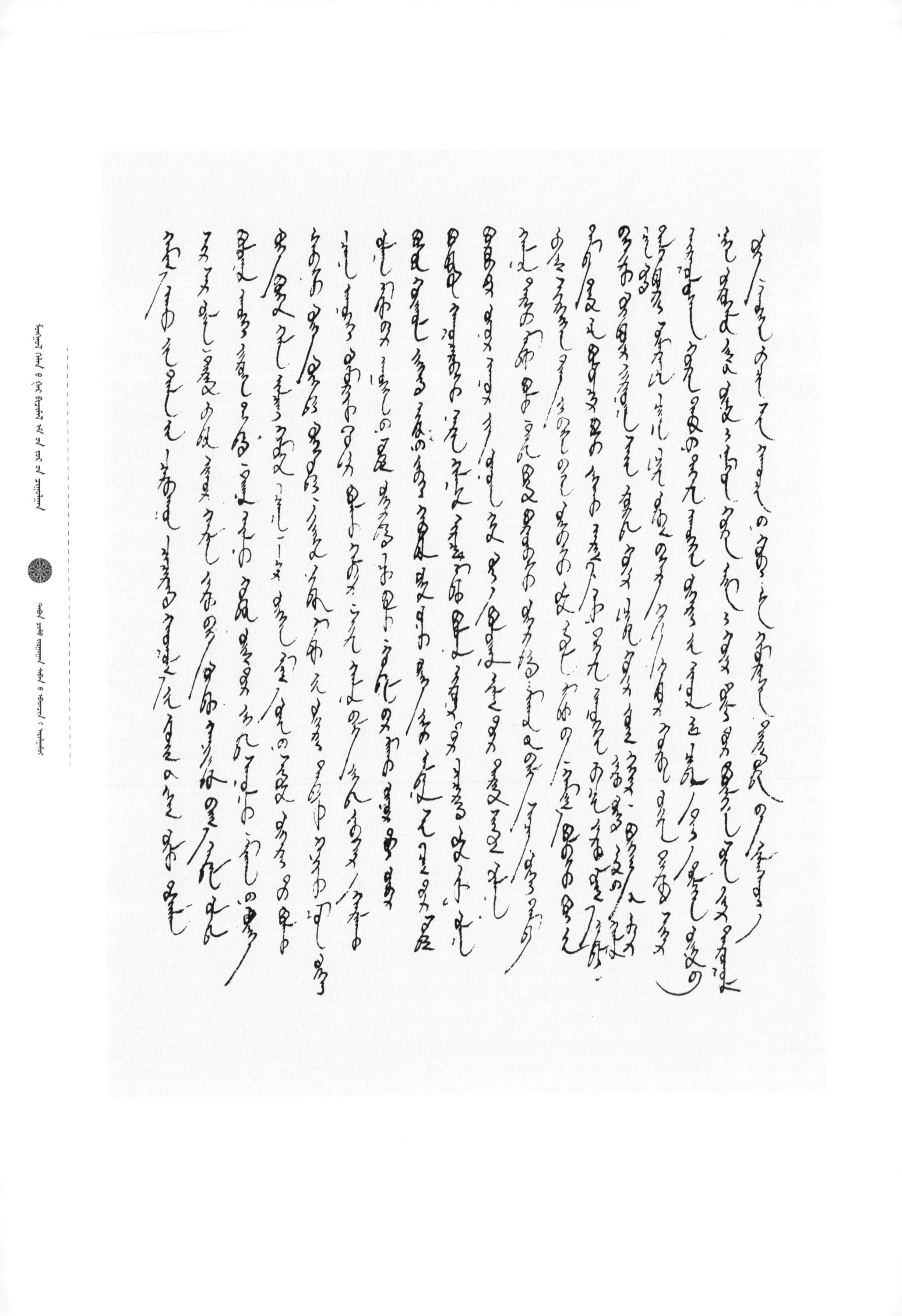

[illegible]

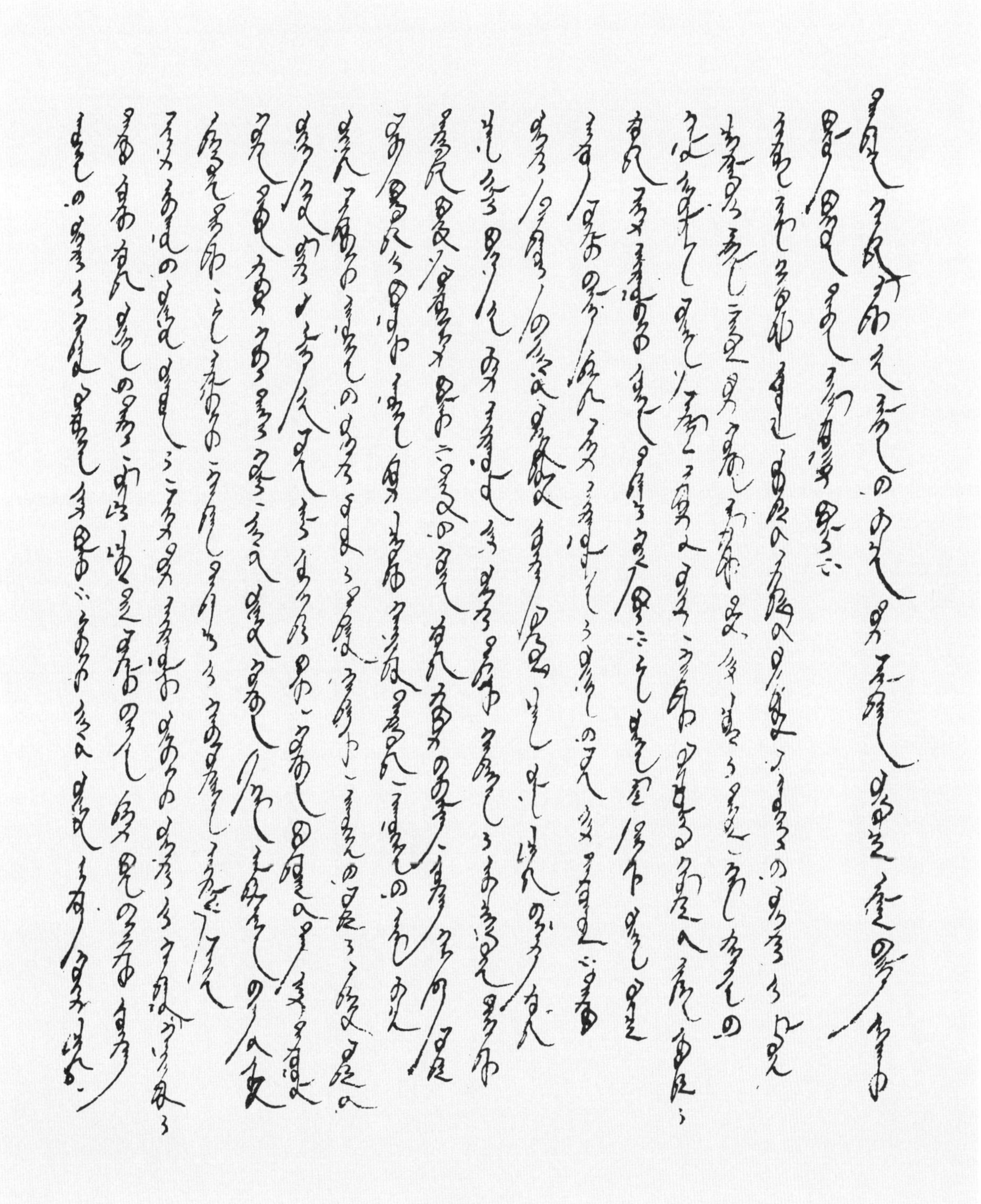

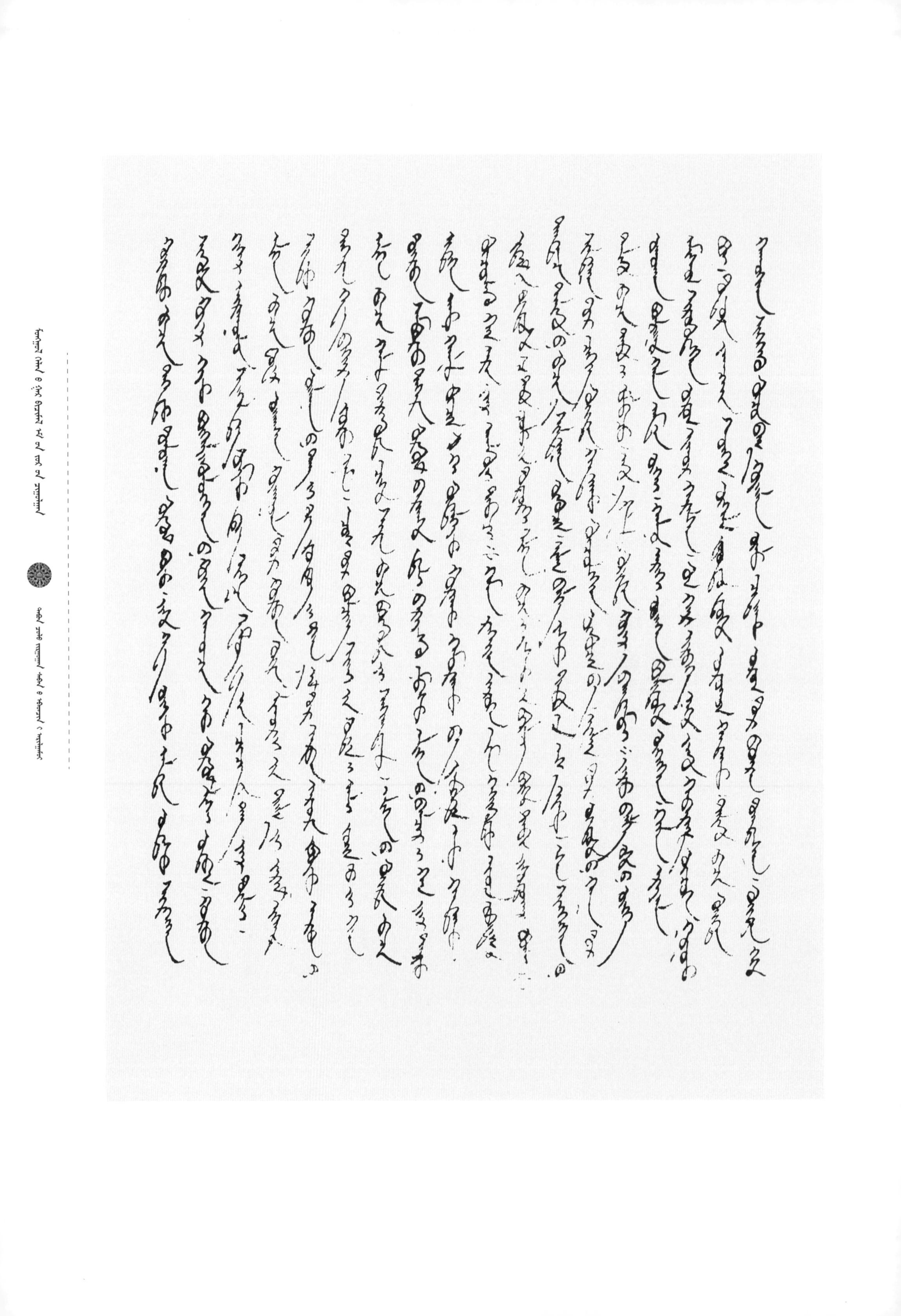

[illegible]

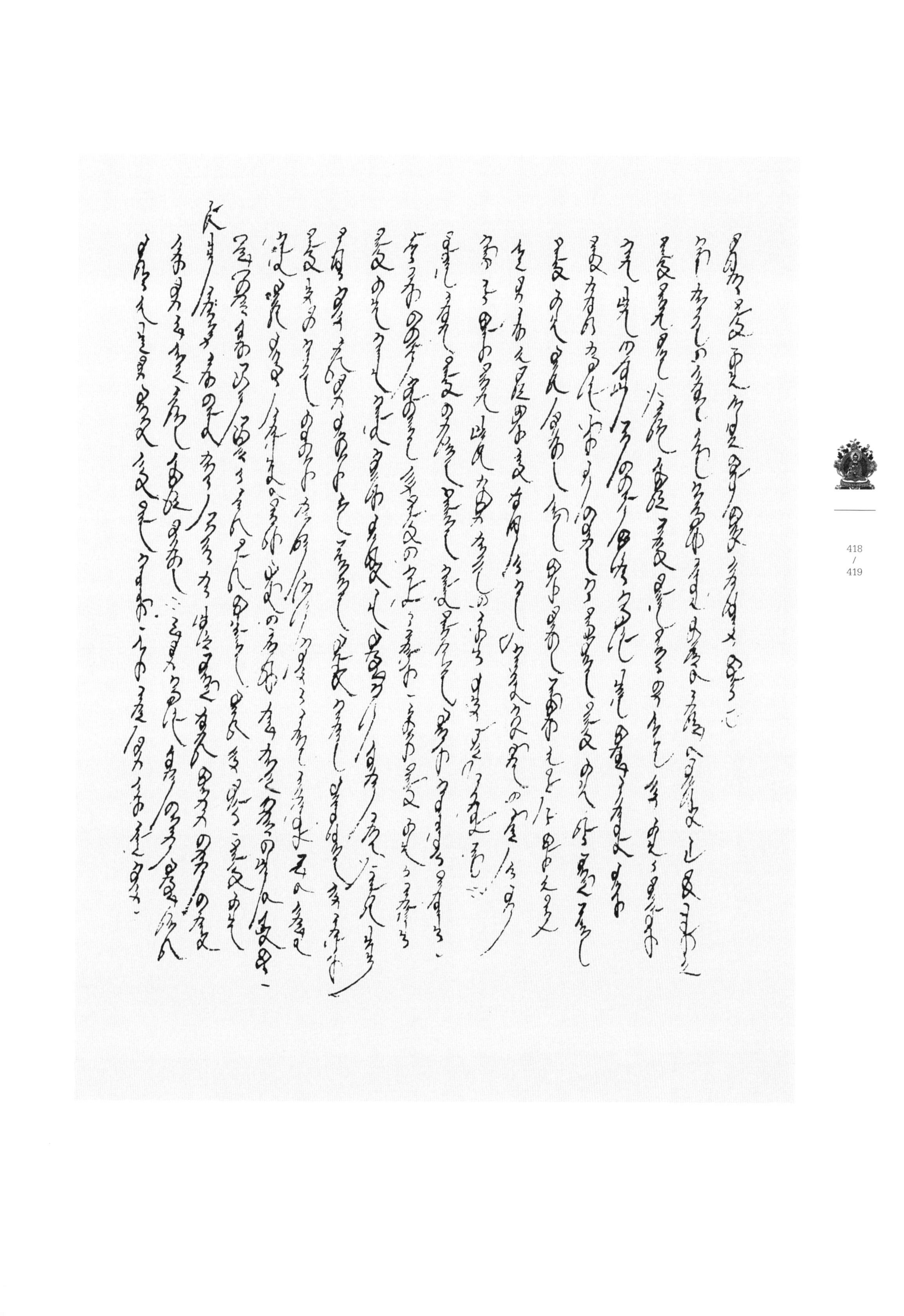

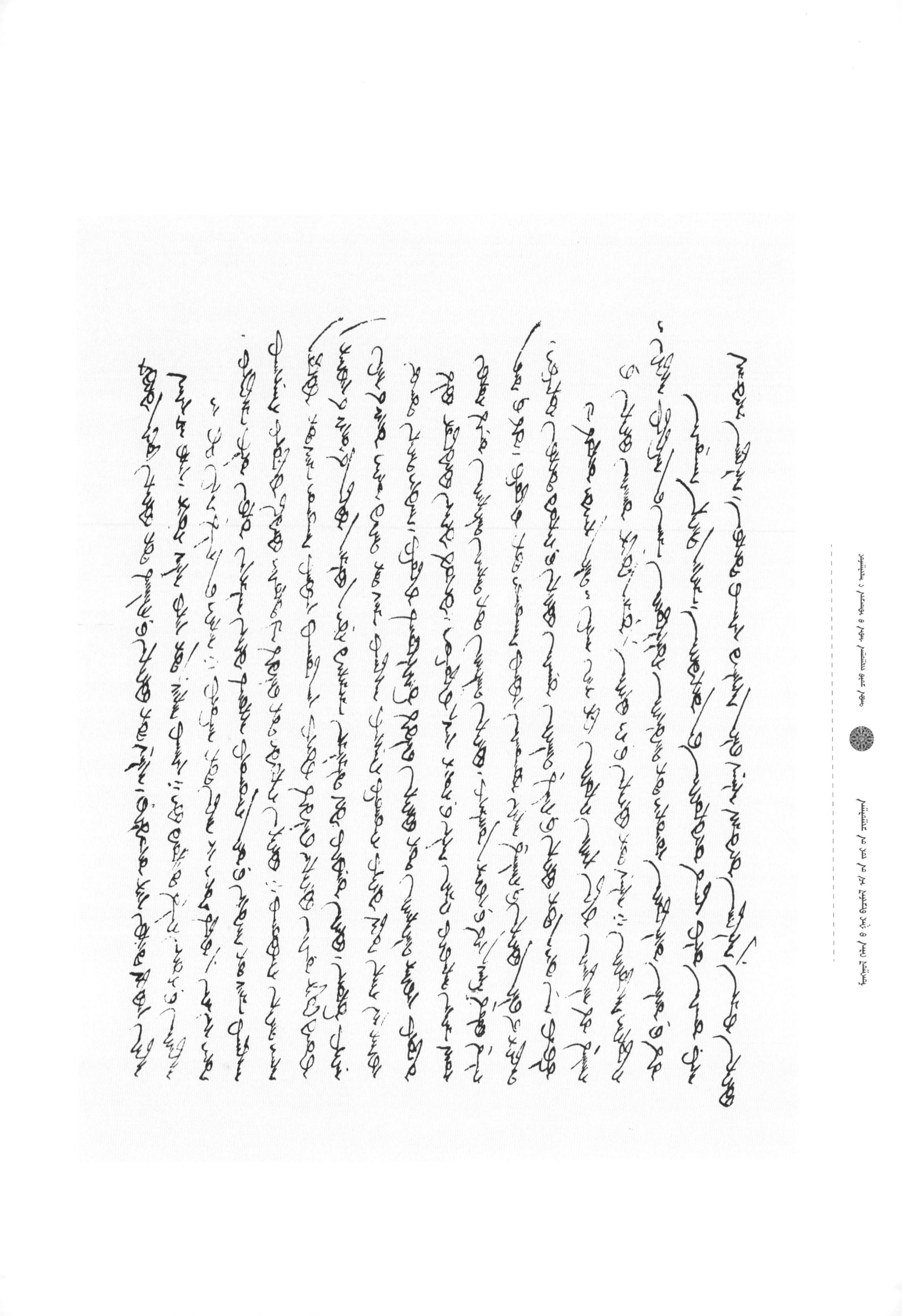

[illegible]
[illegible]
[illegible]
[illegible]
[illegible]
[illegible]
[illegible]
[illegible]
[illegible]
[illegible]
[illegible]
[illegible]
[illegible]
[illegible]
[illegible]
[illegible]
[illegible]
[illegible]

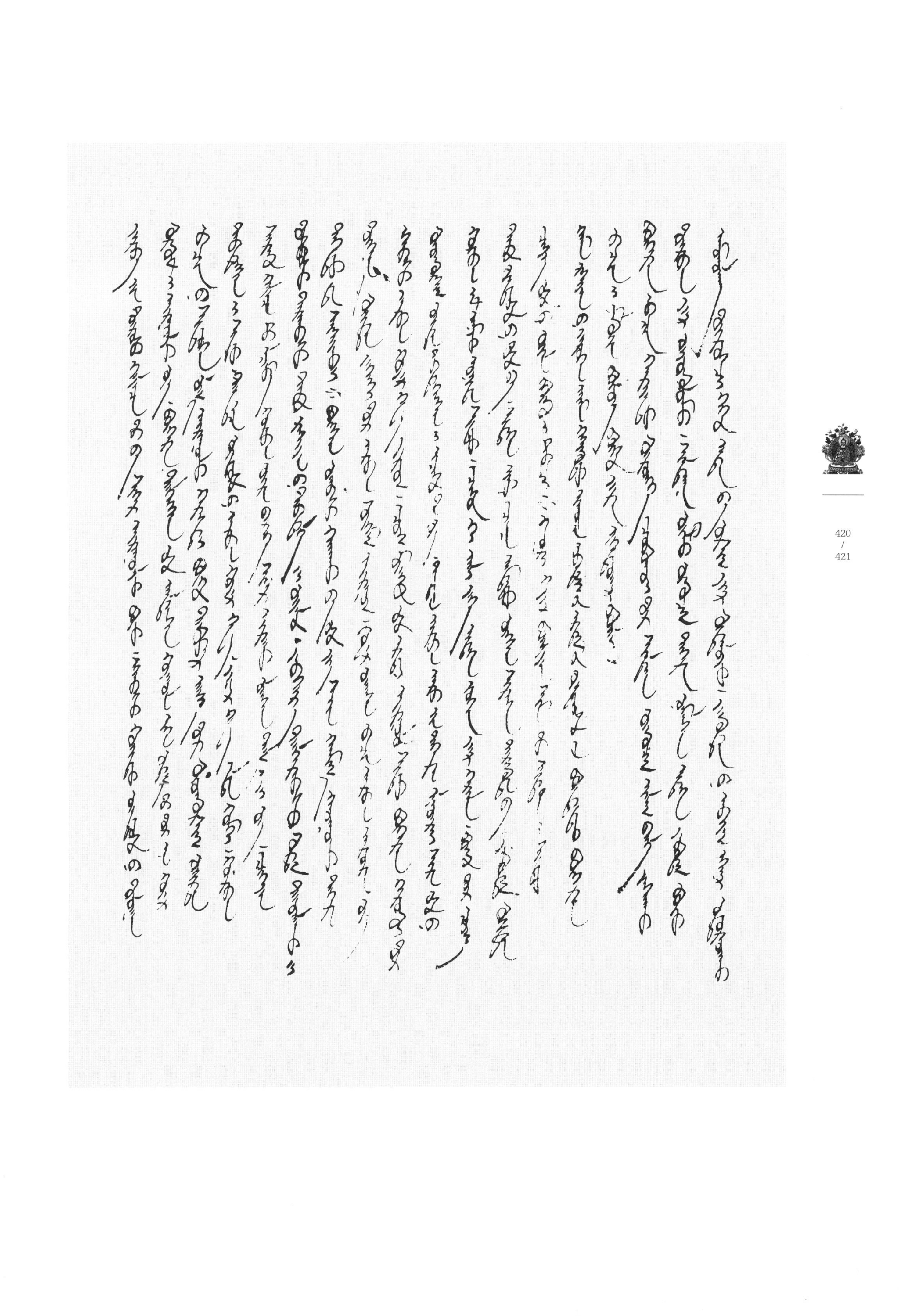

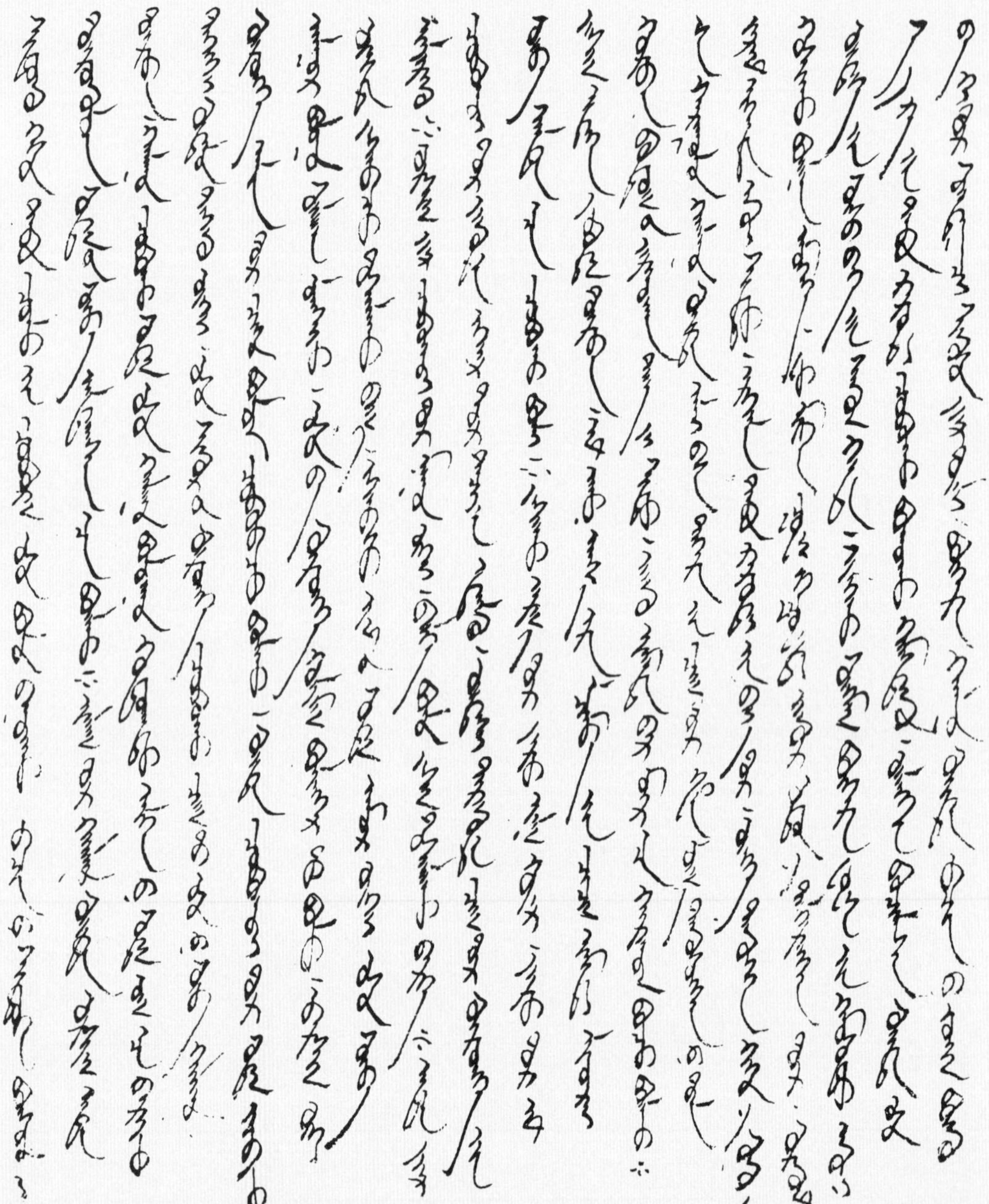

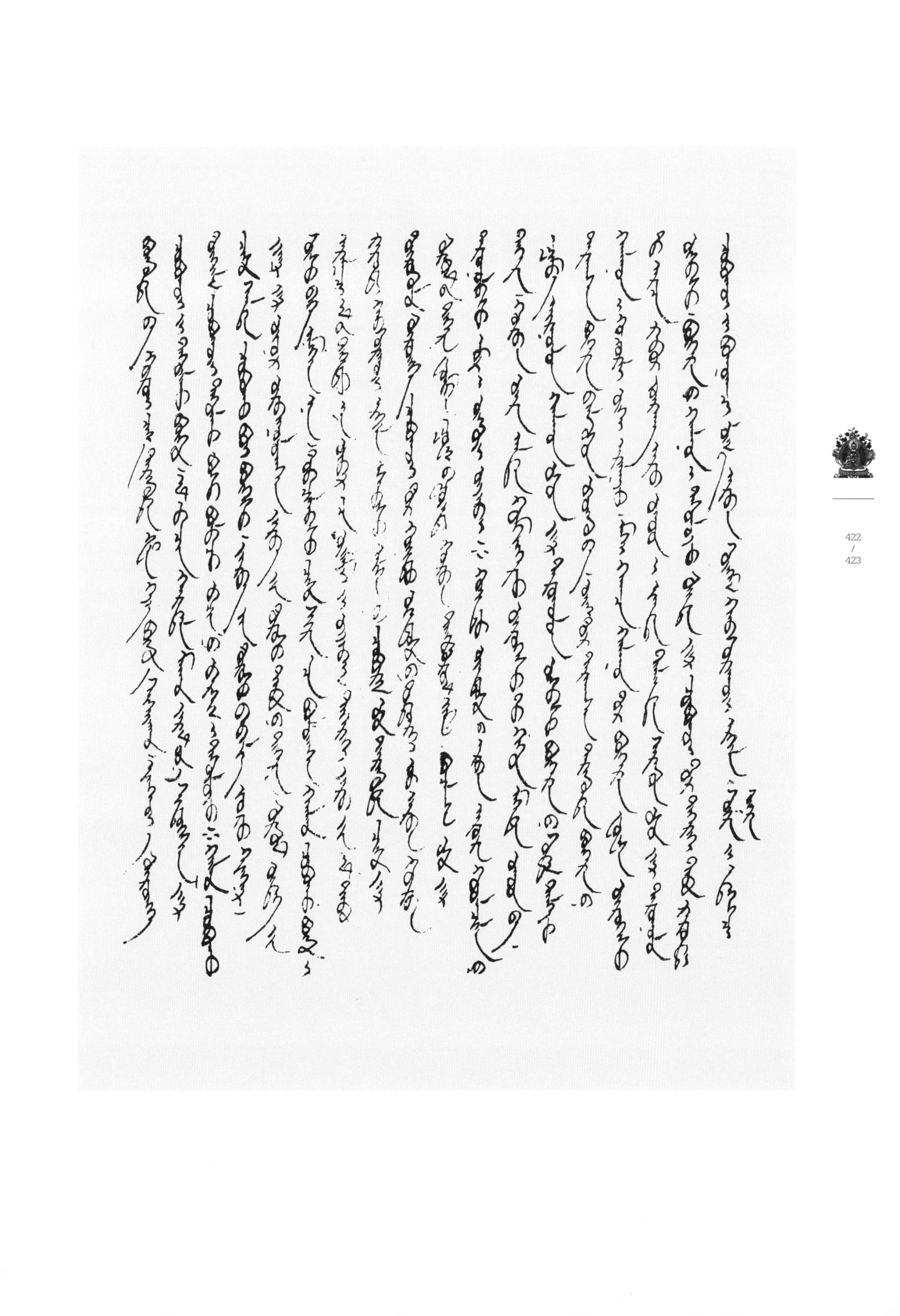

[illegible]

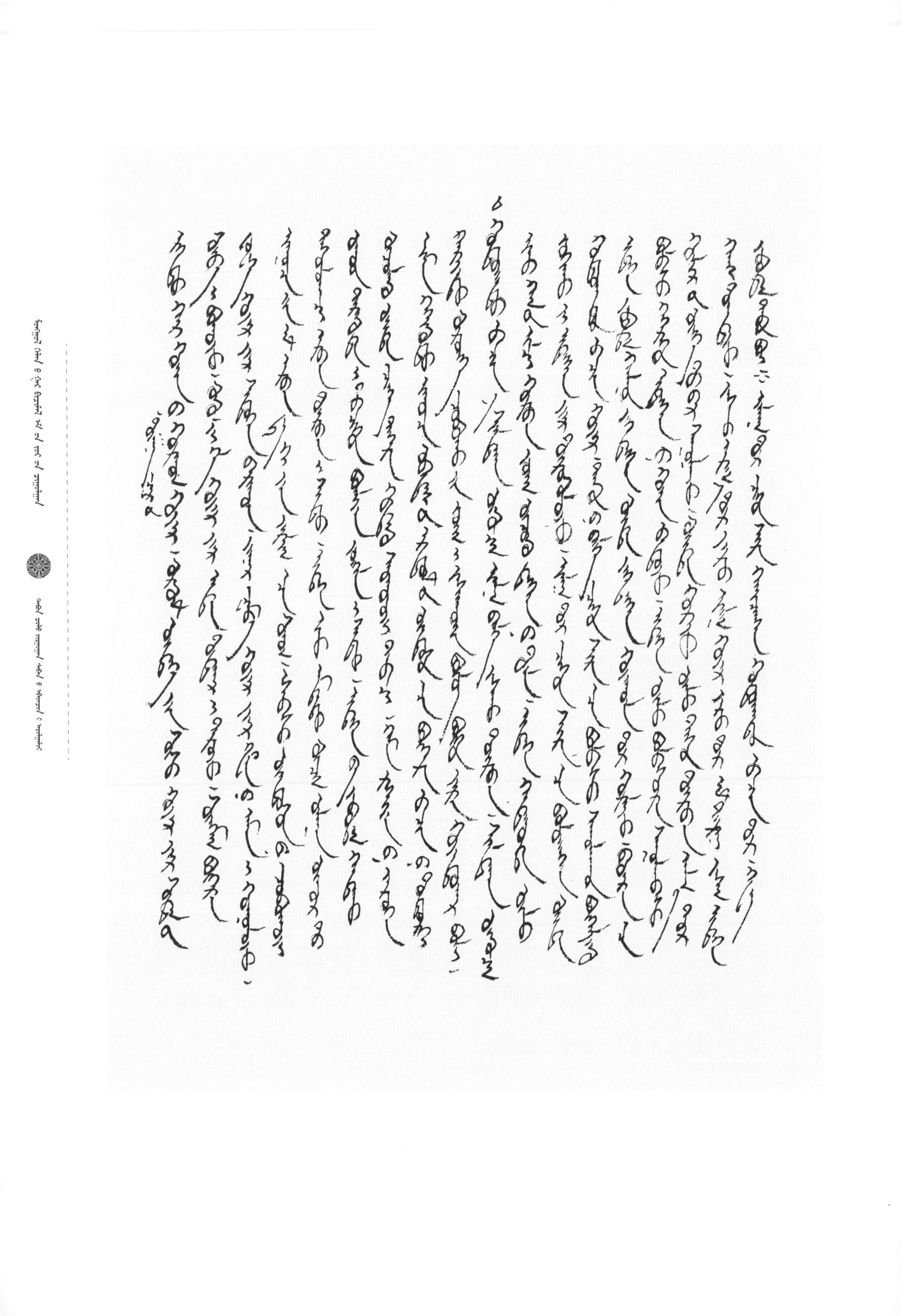

[illegible]

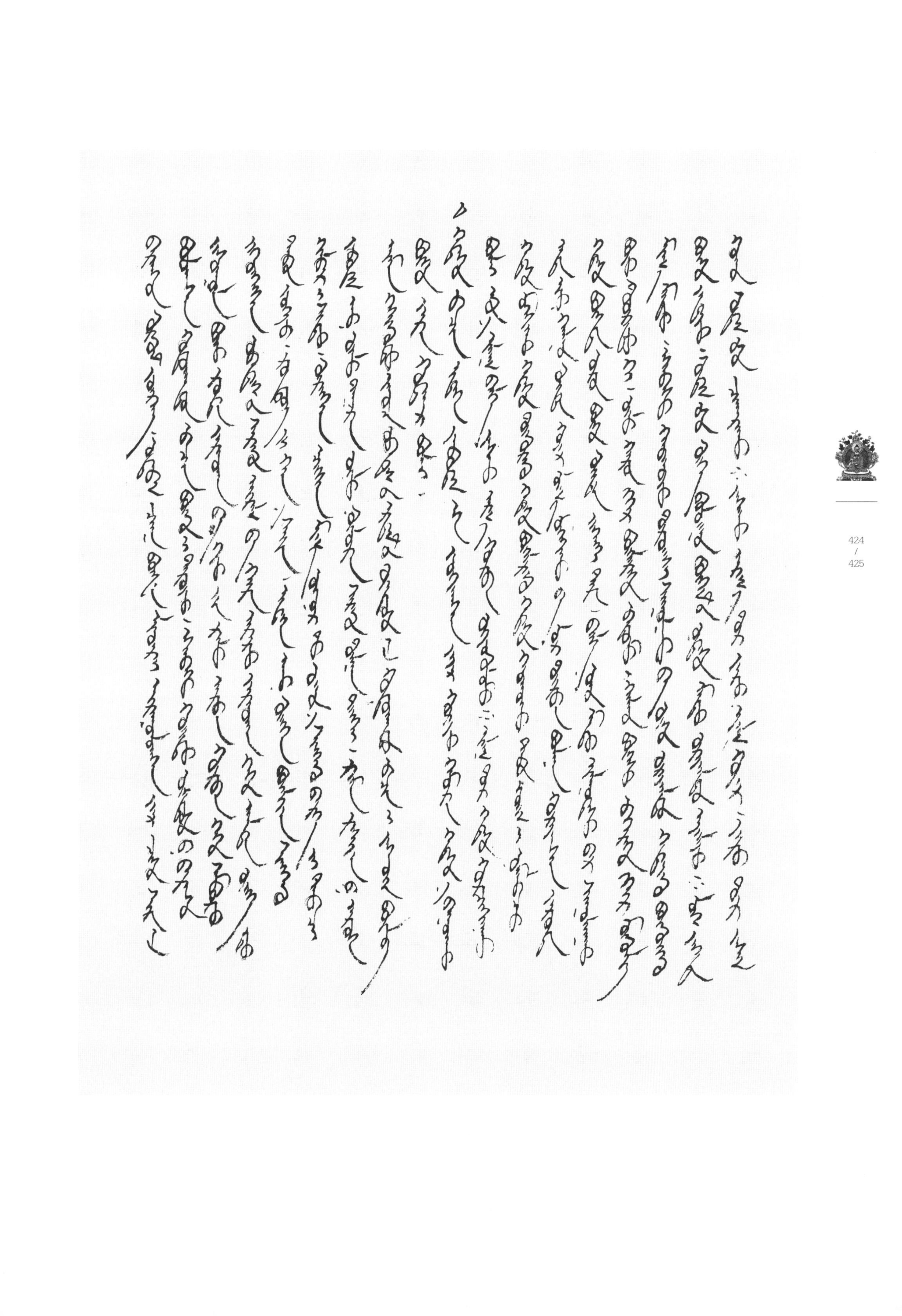

[illegible]

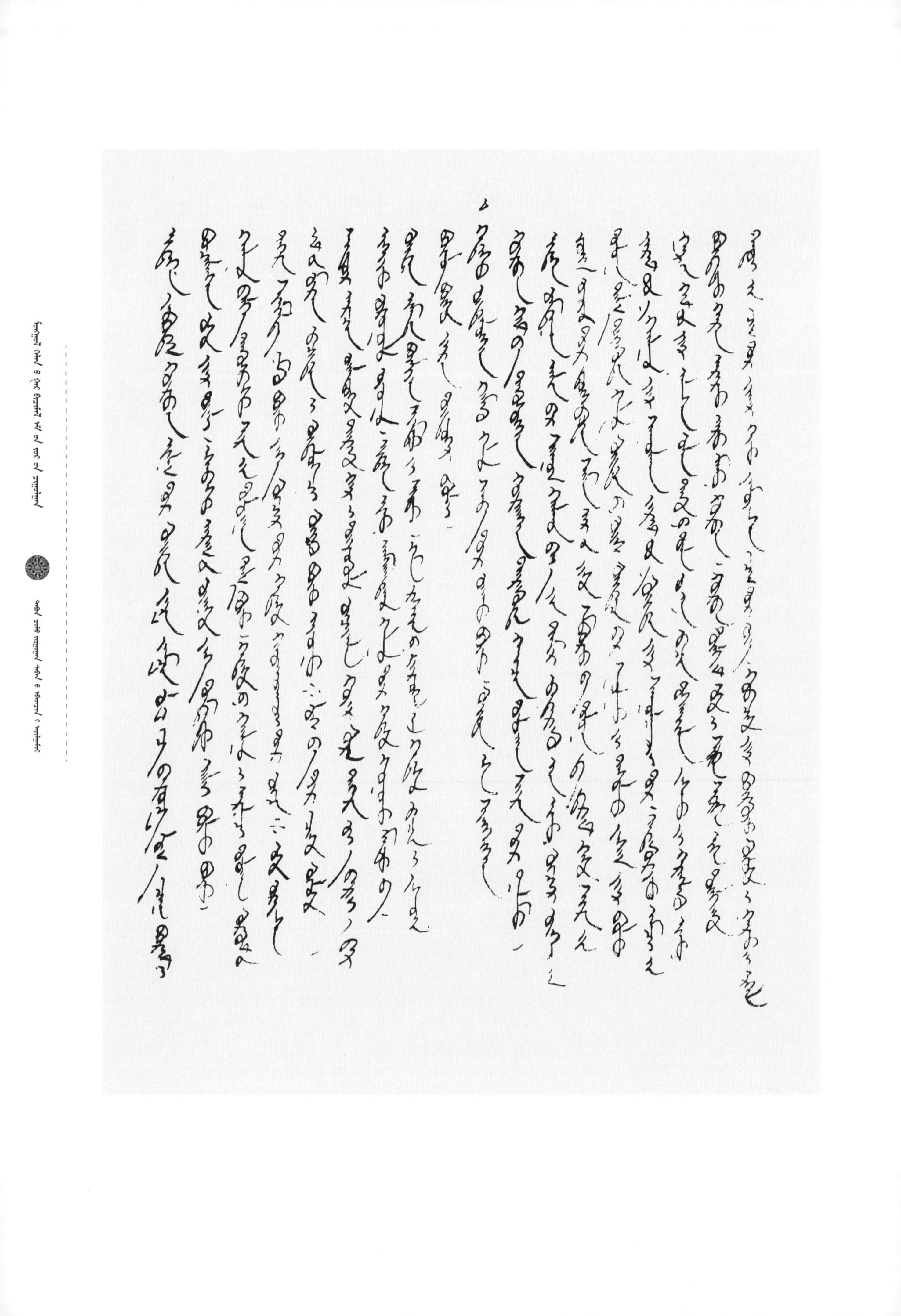

[illegible]

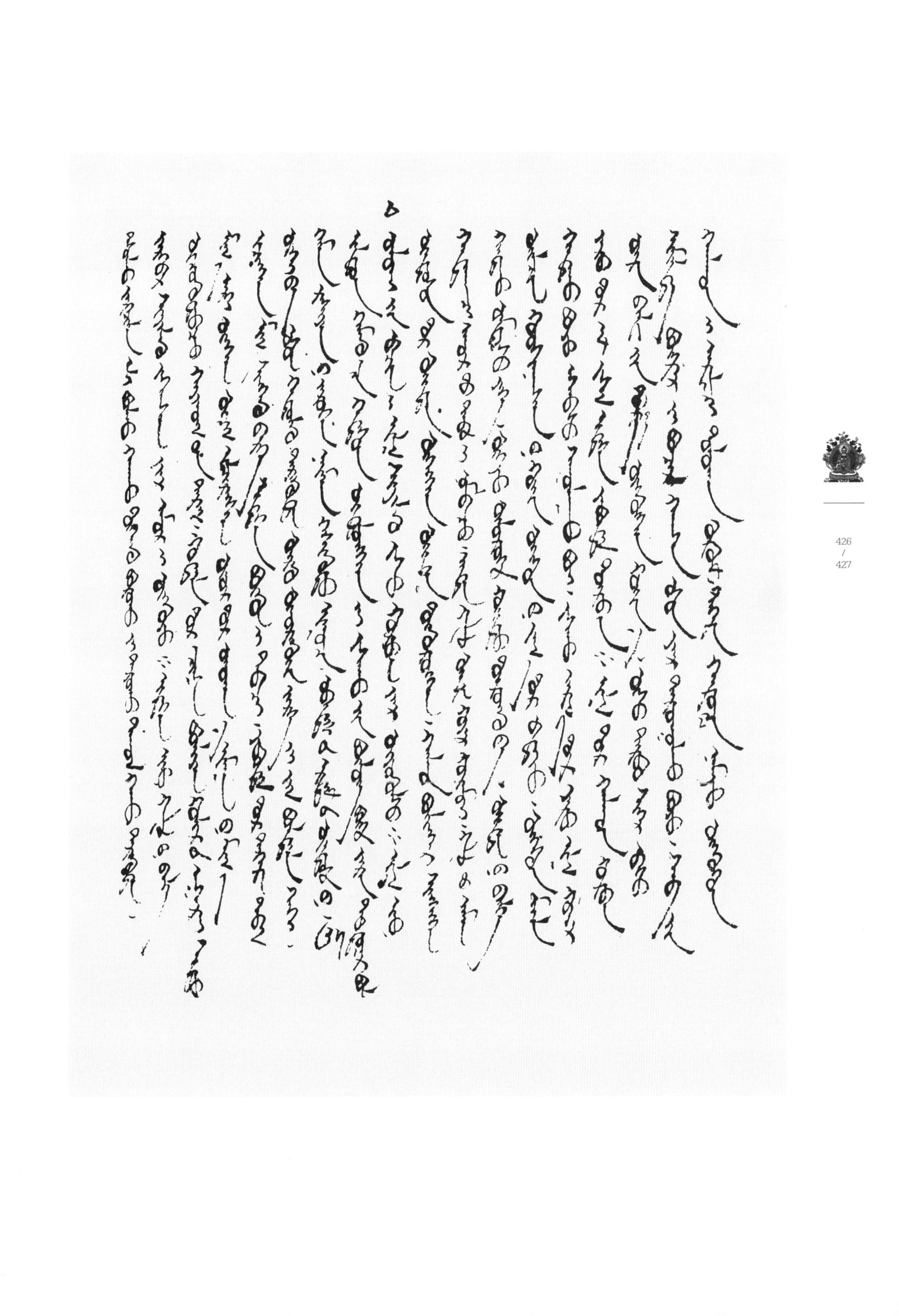

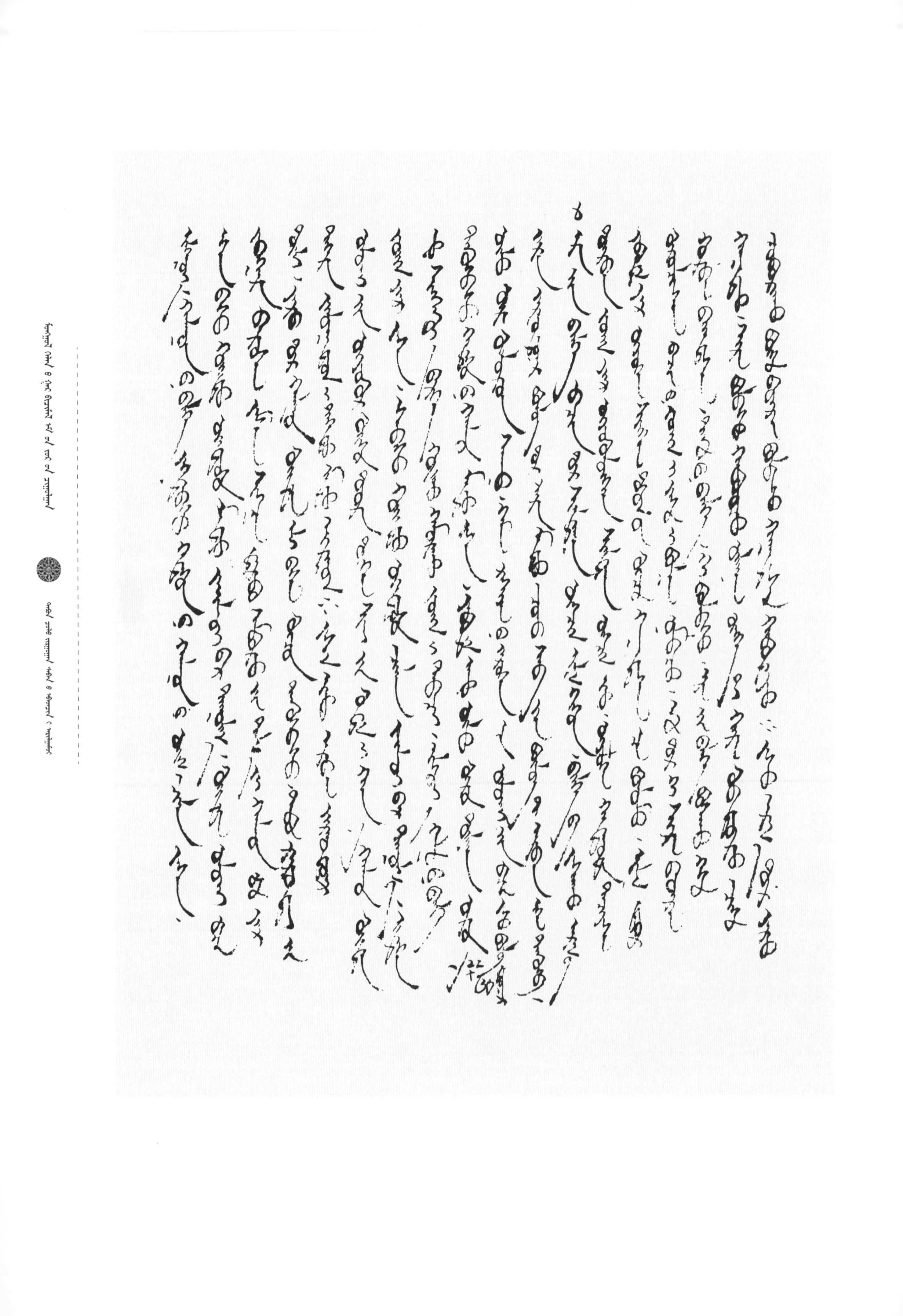

[illegible]
[illegible]
[illegible]
[illegible]
[illegible]
[illegible]
[illegible]
[illegible]
[illegible]
[illegible]
[illegible]
[illegible]
[illegible]
[illegible]
[illegible]
[illegible]
[illegible]
[illegible]
[illegible]

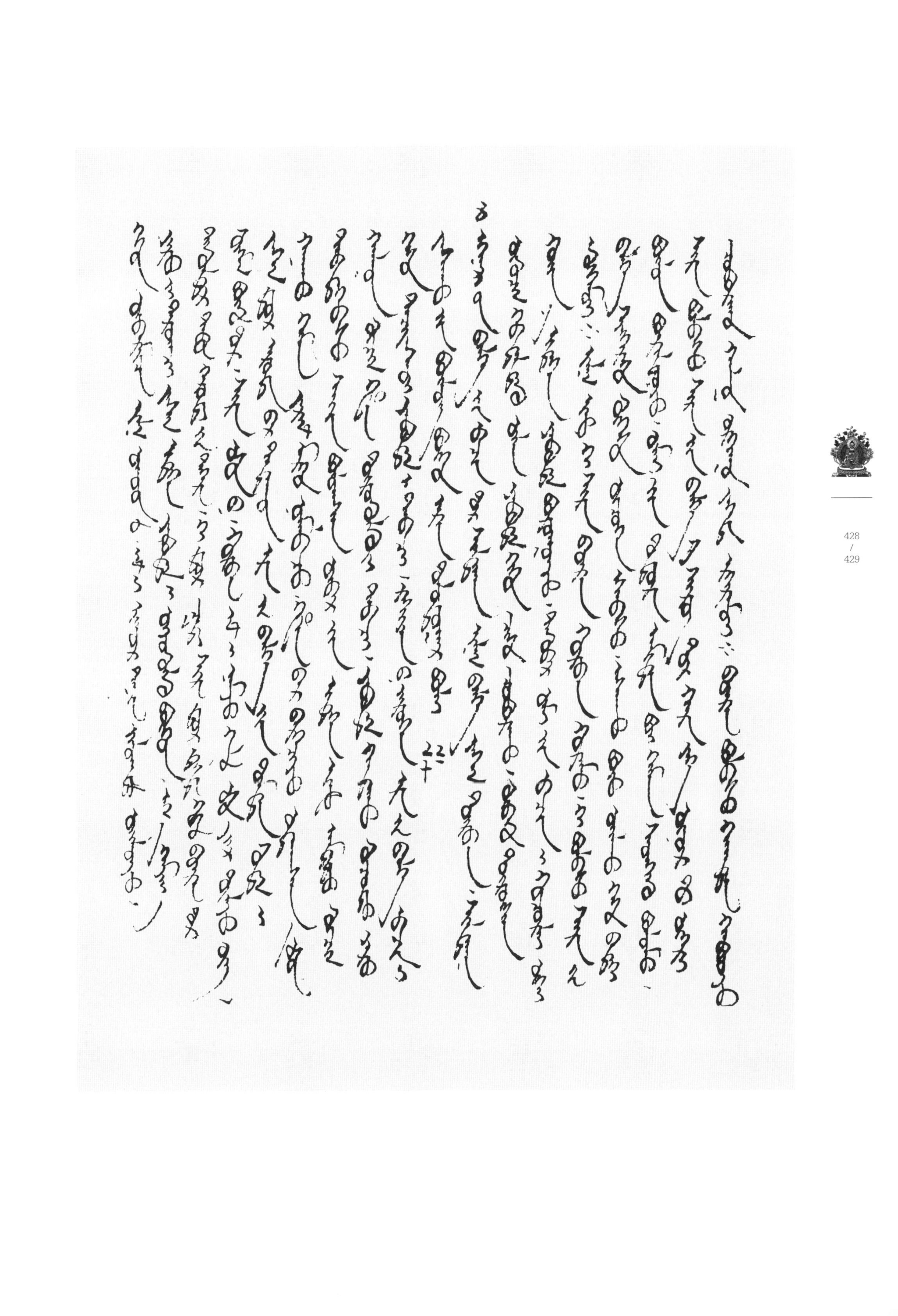

[illegible]

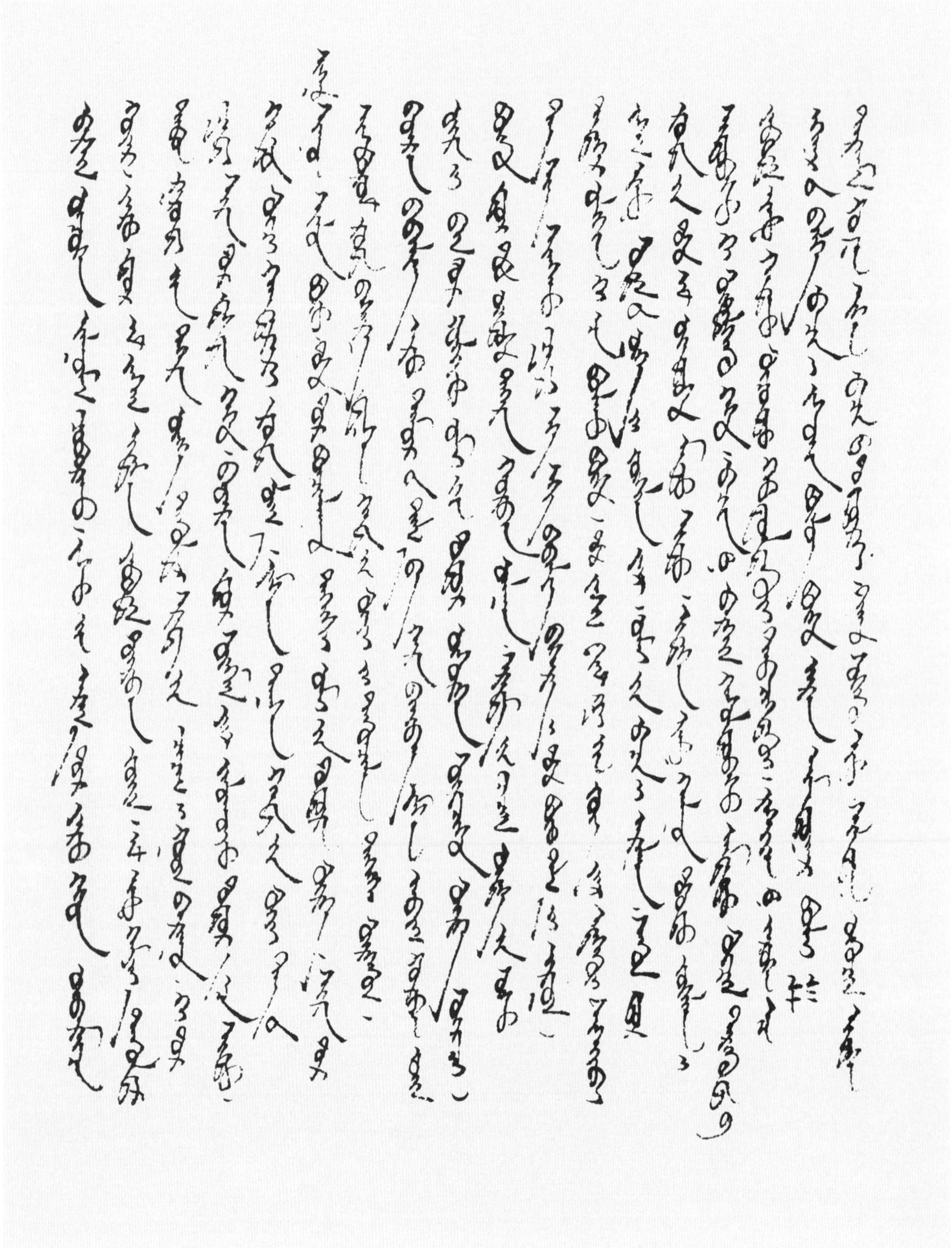

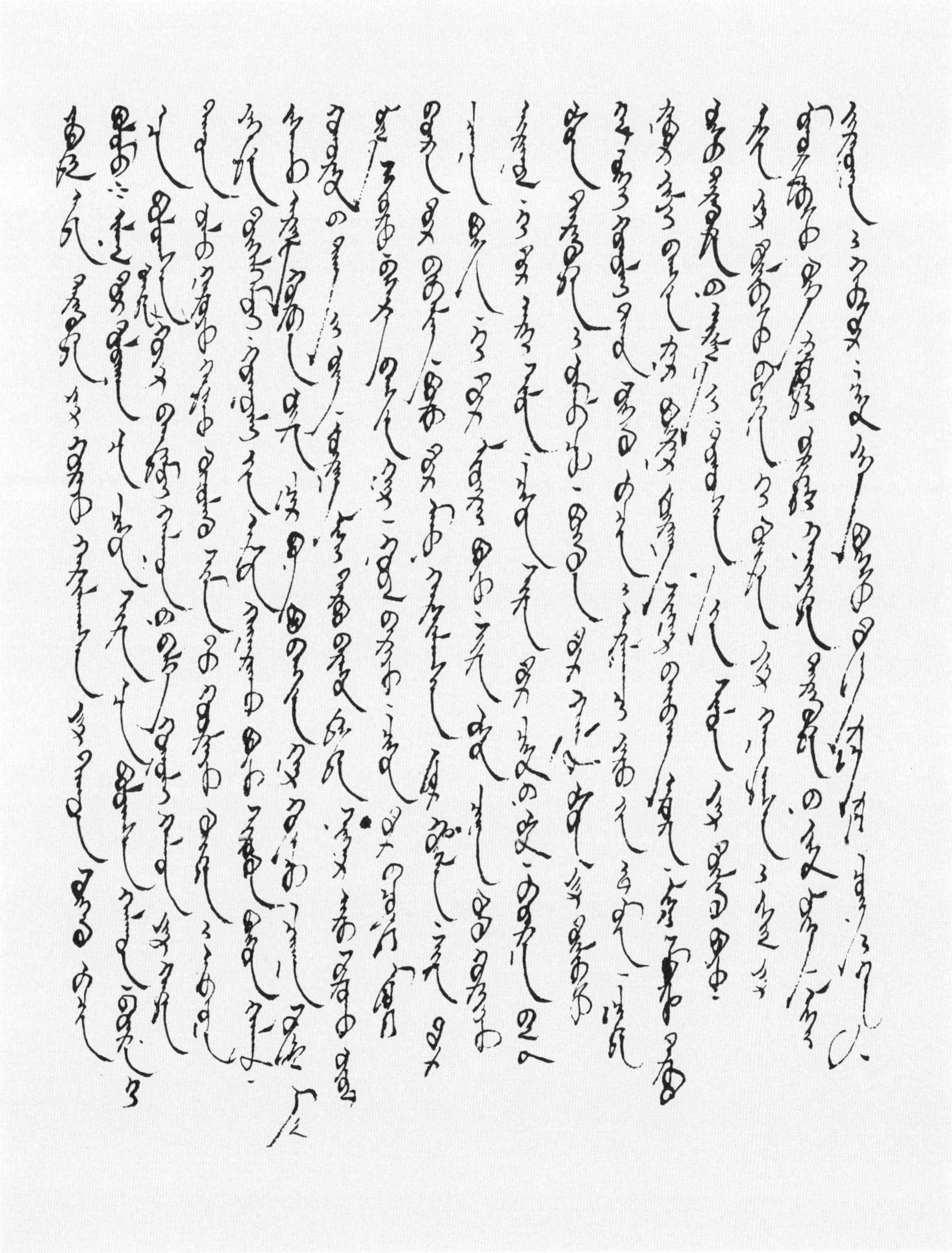

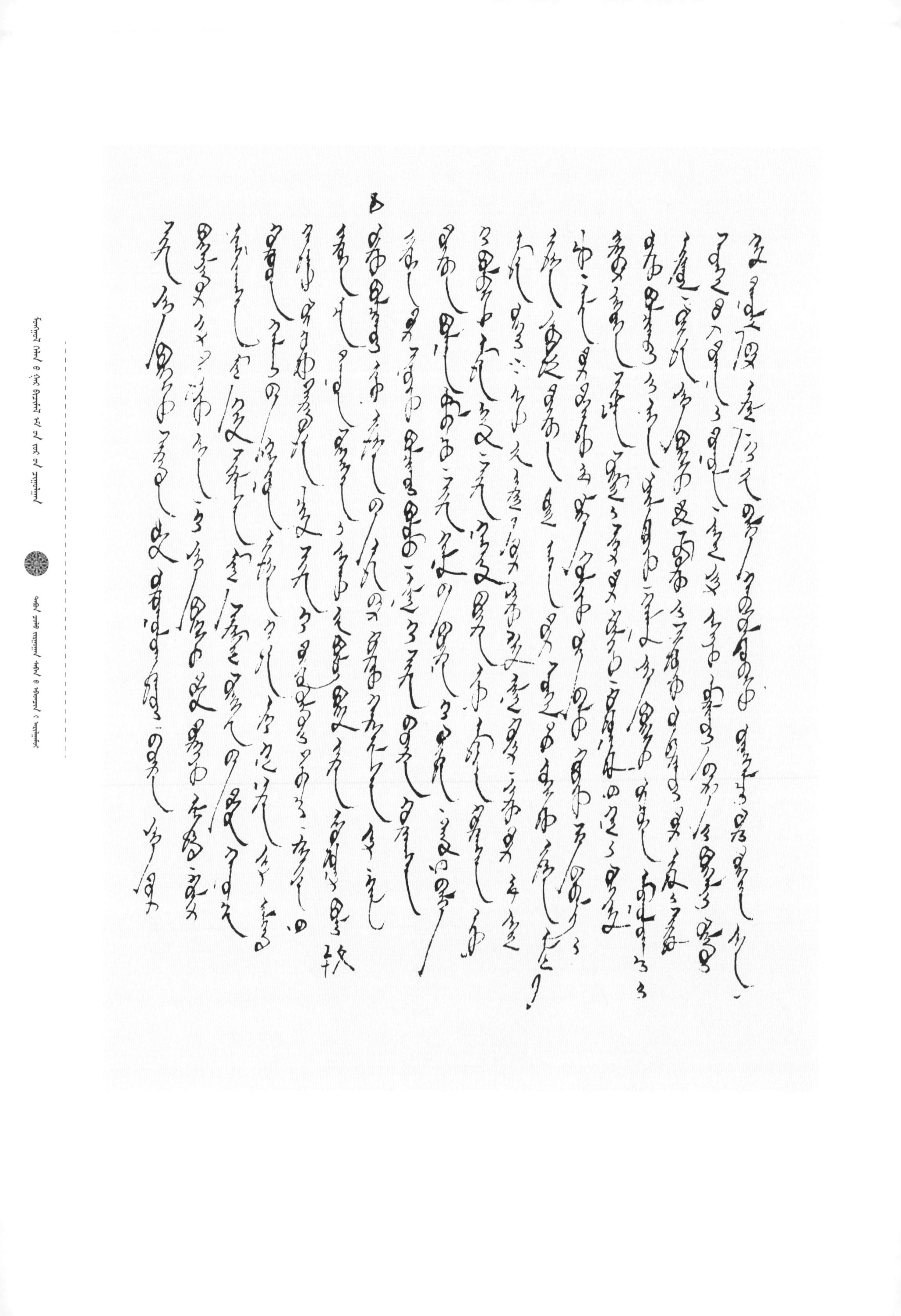

[illegible]

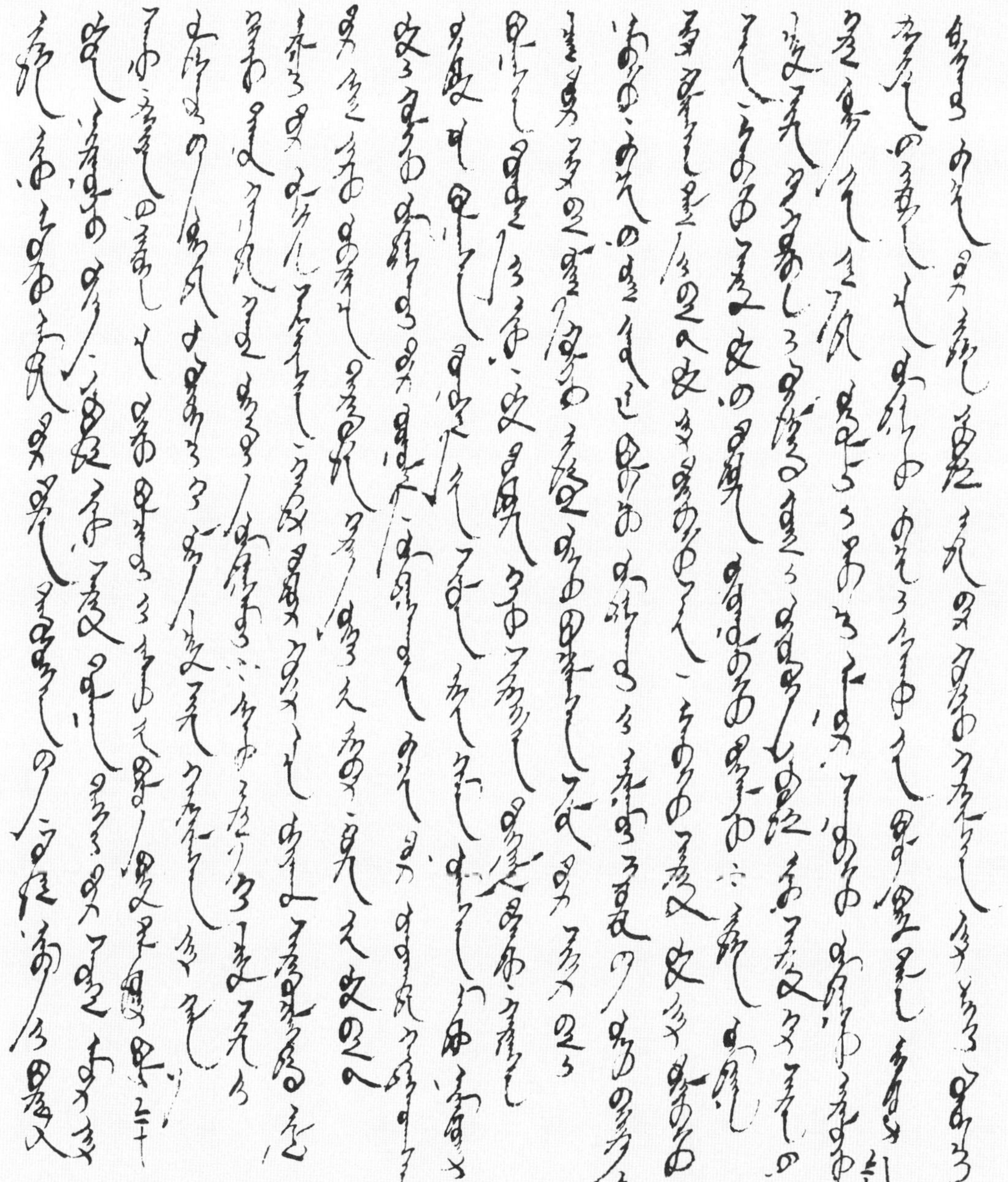

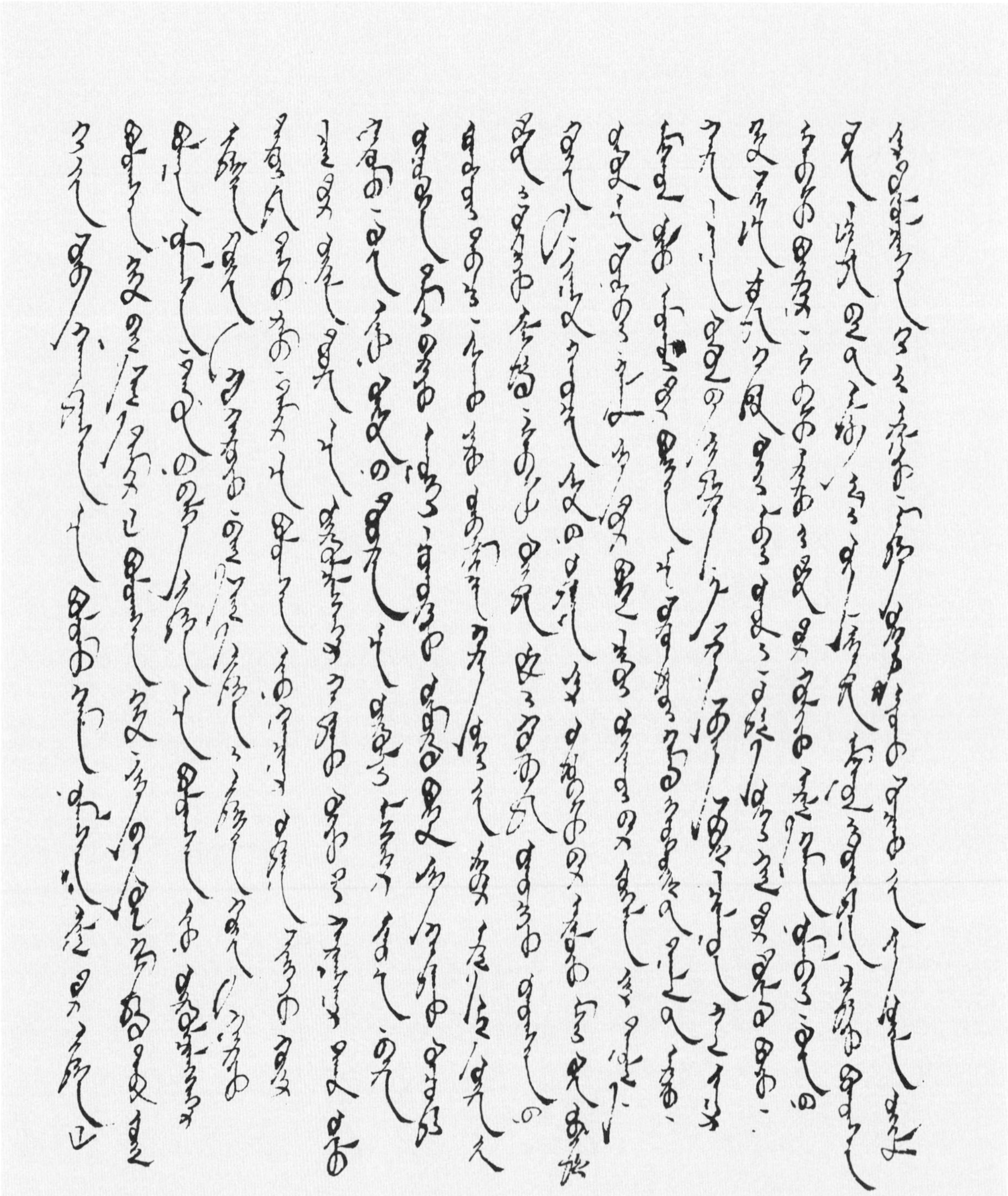

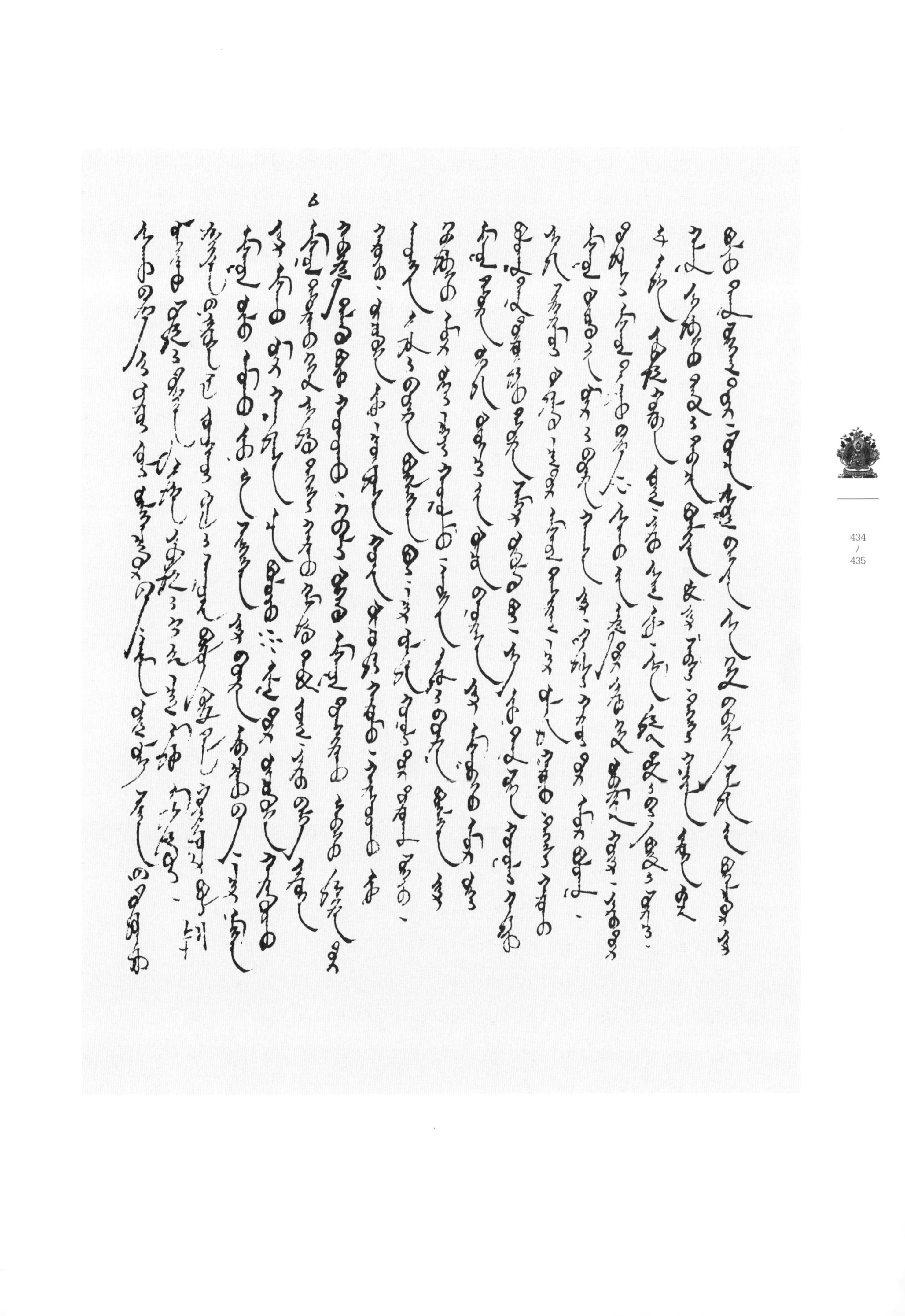

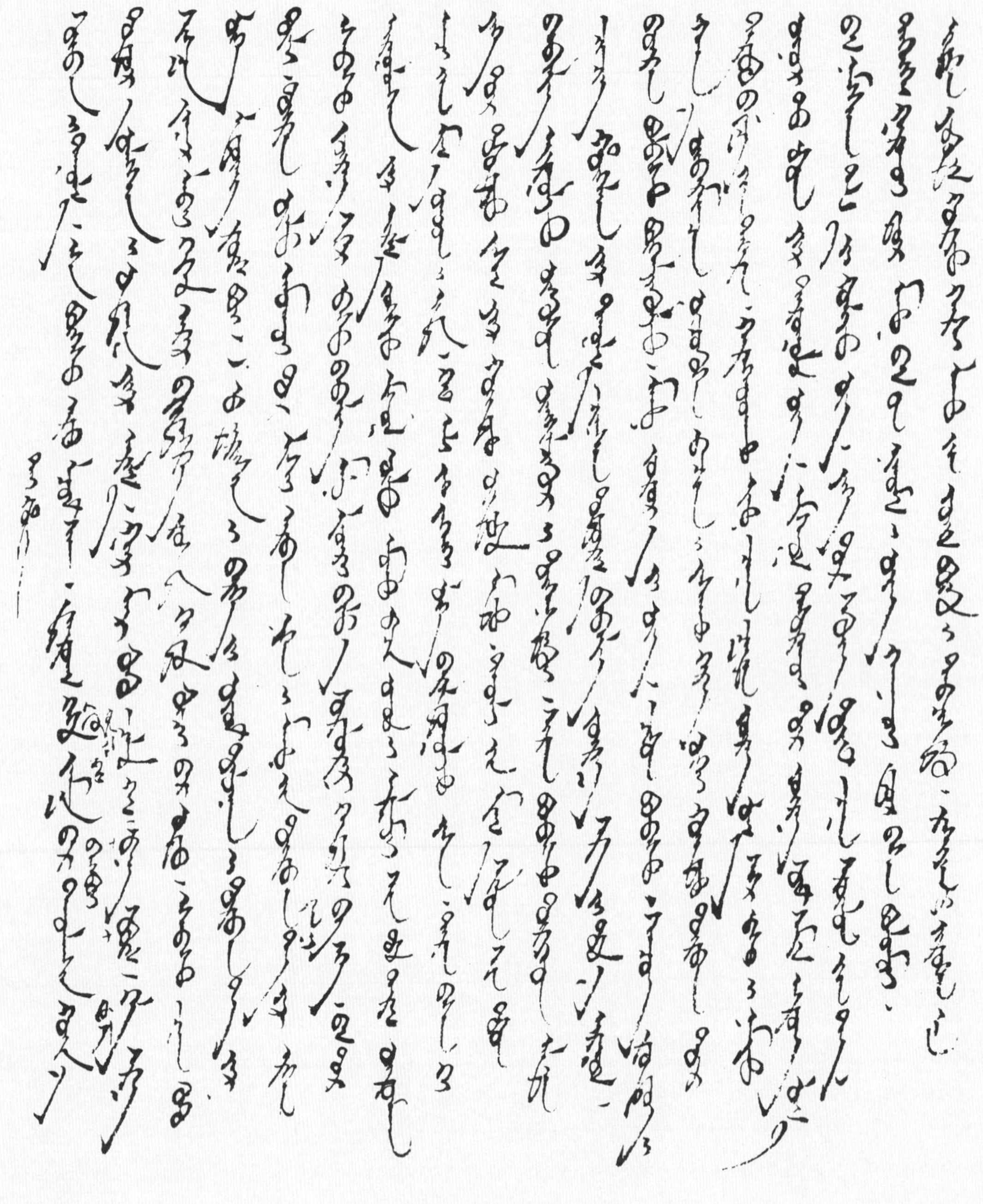

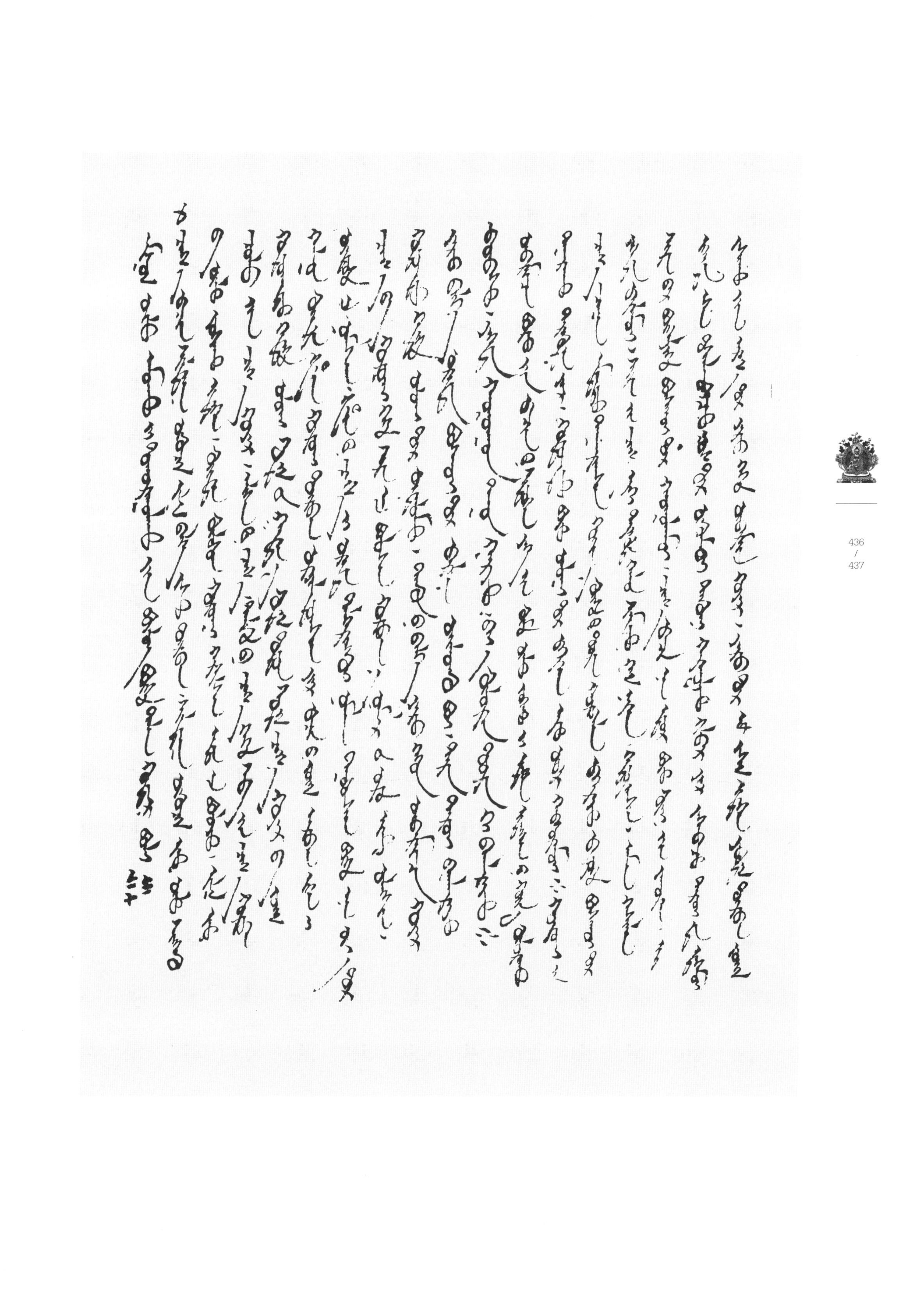

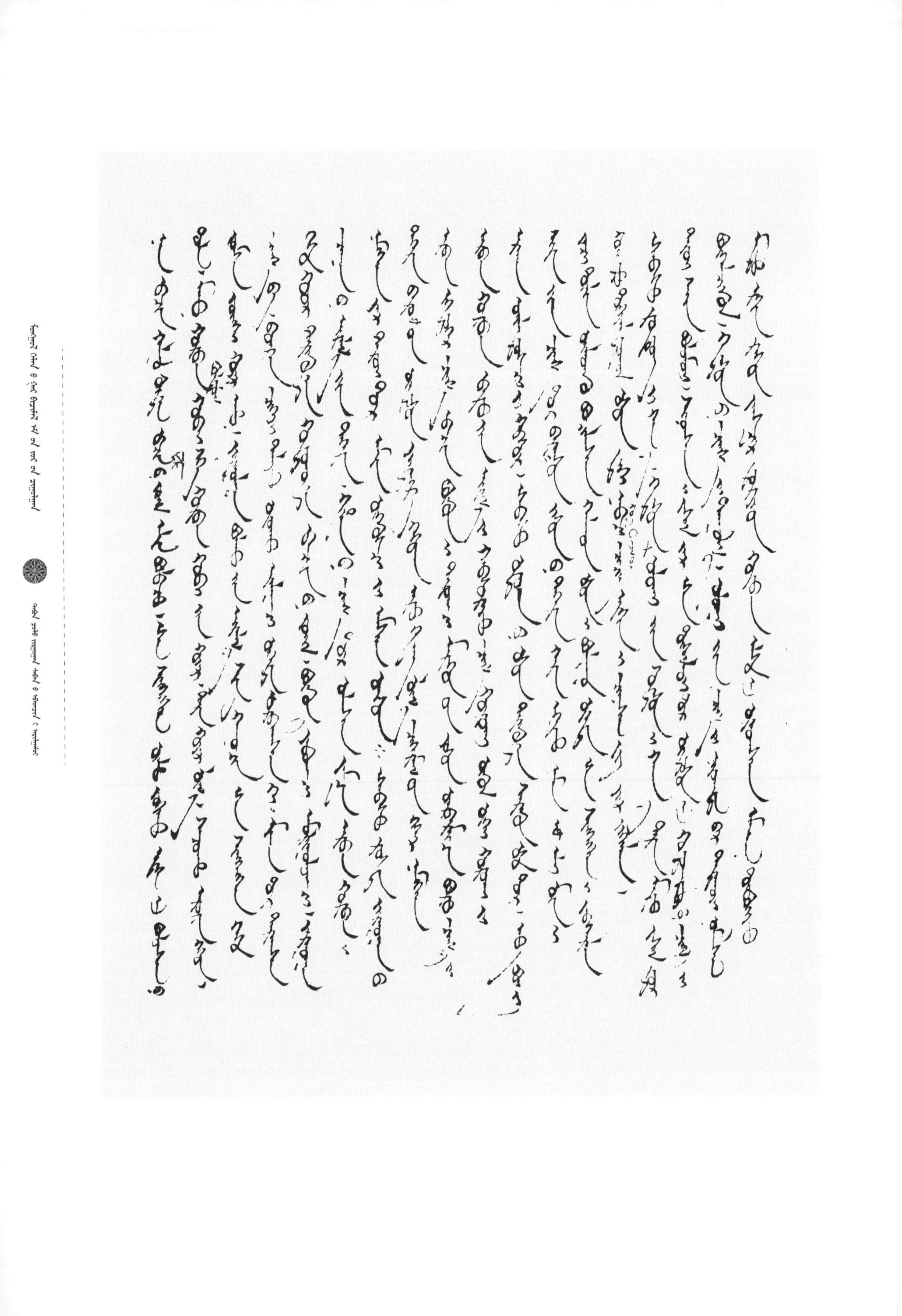

[illegible]

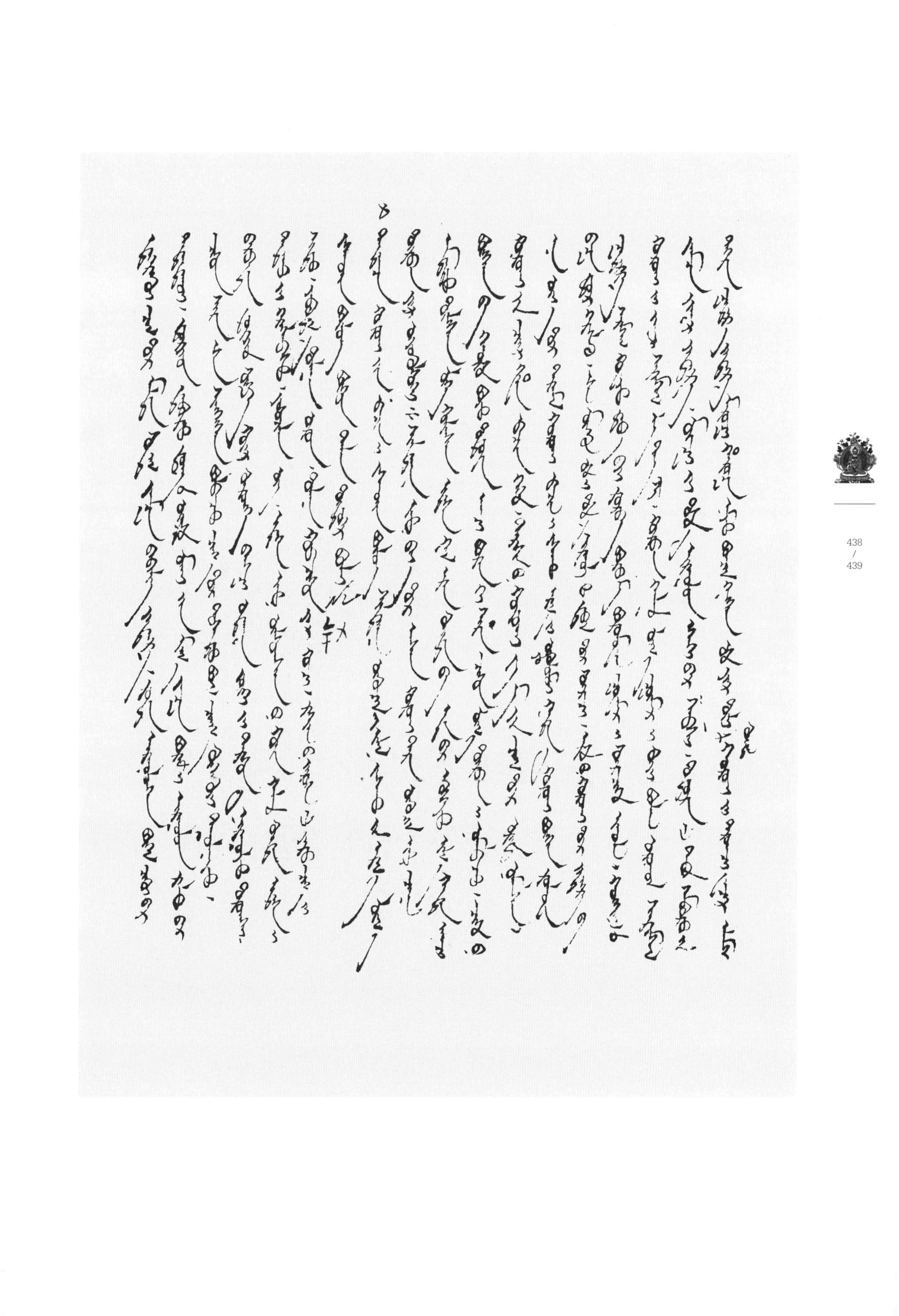

[illegible]

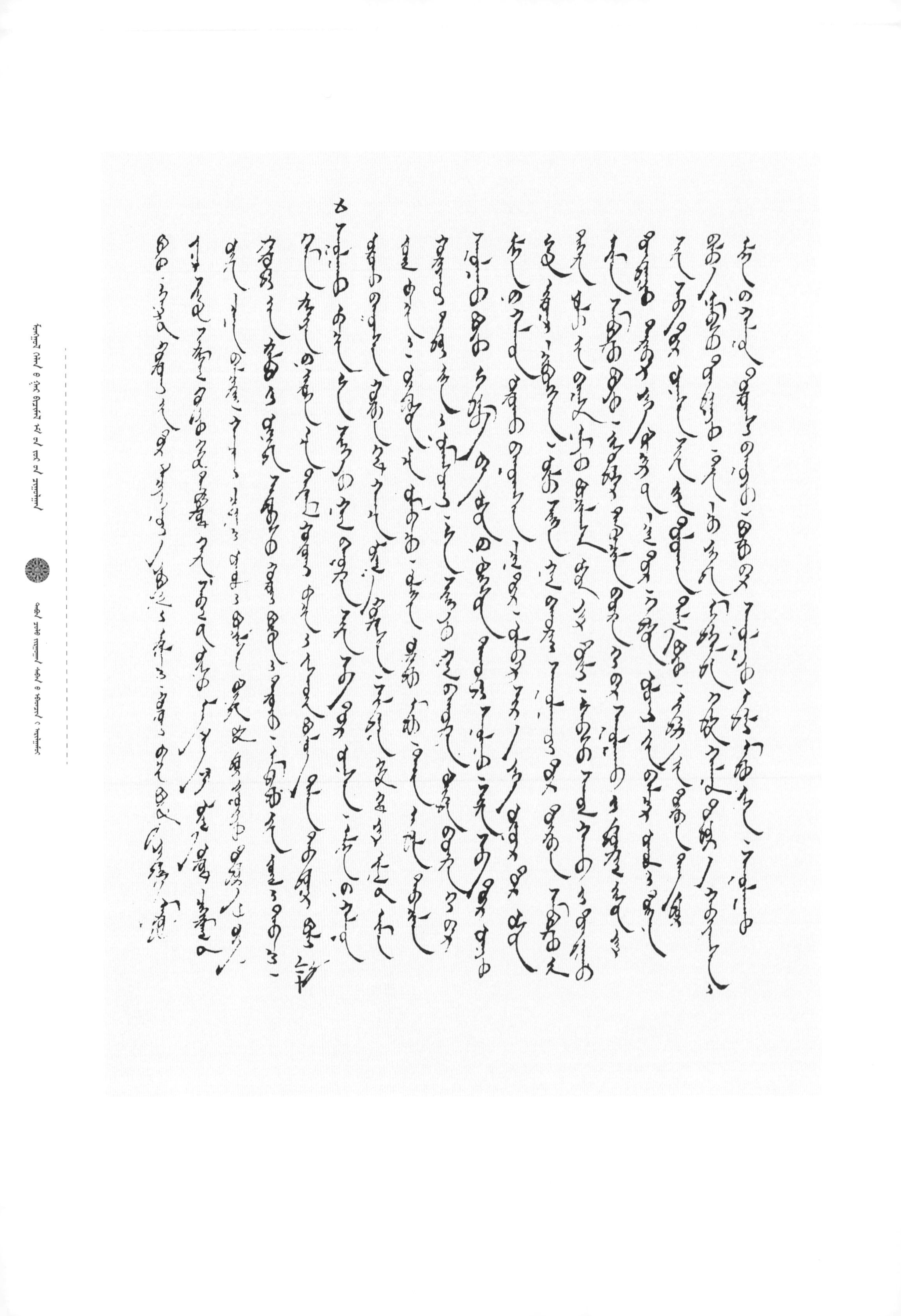

[illegible]

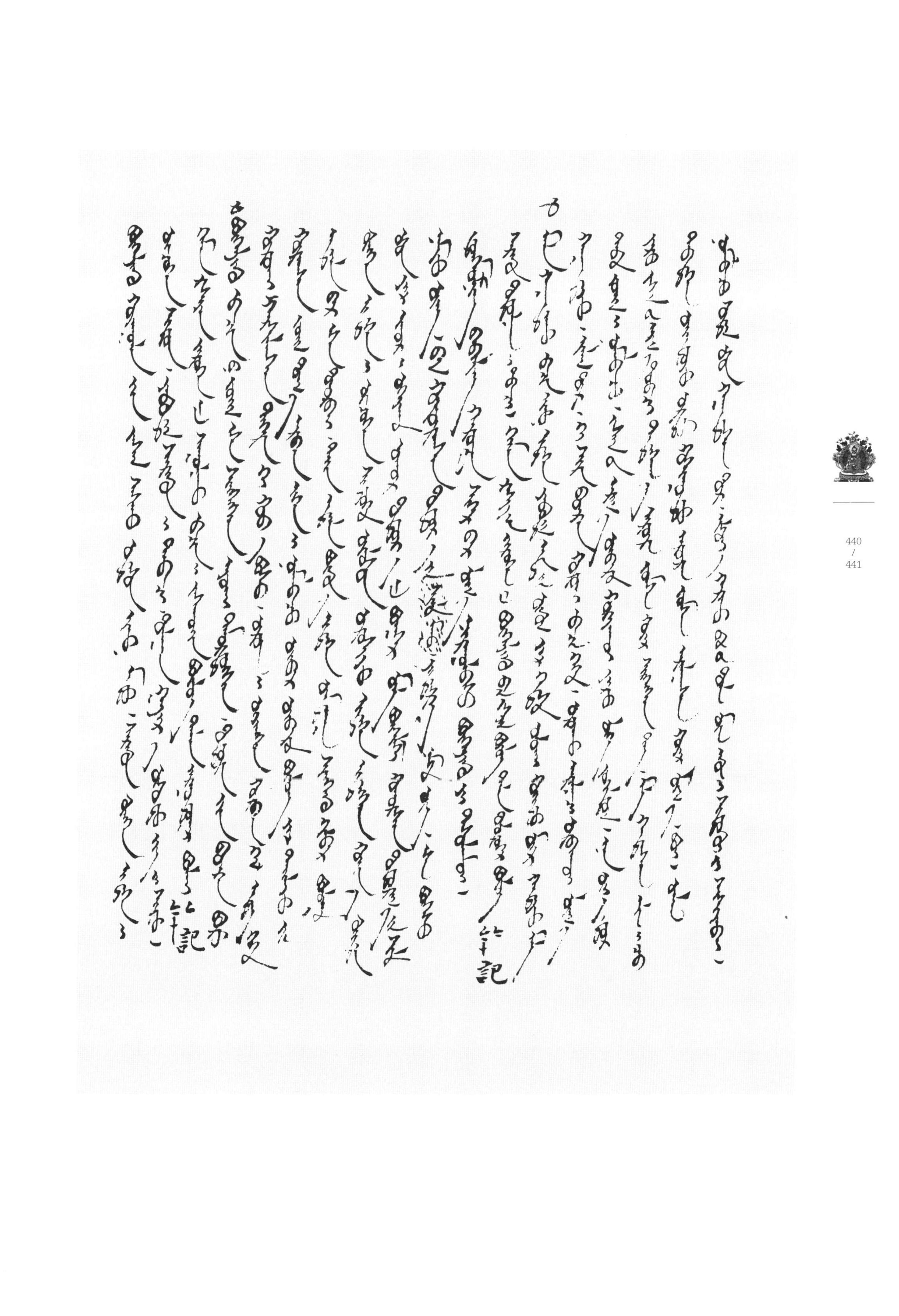

[illegible]

朱記

[illegible]

朱記

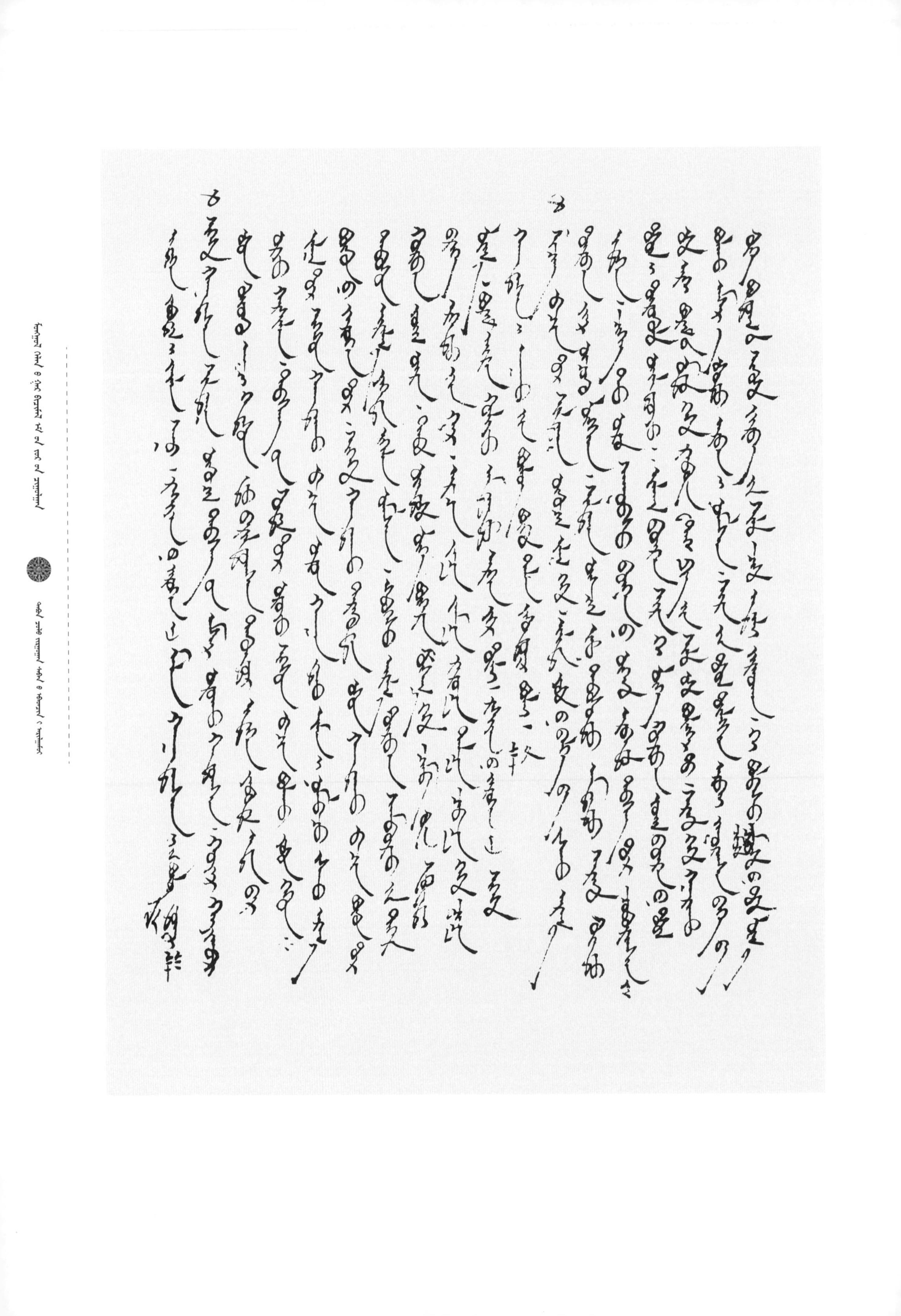

[illegible]

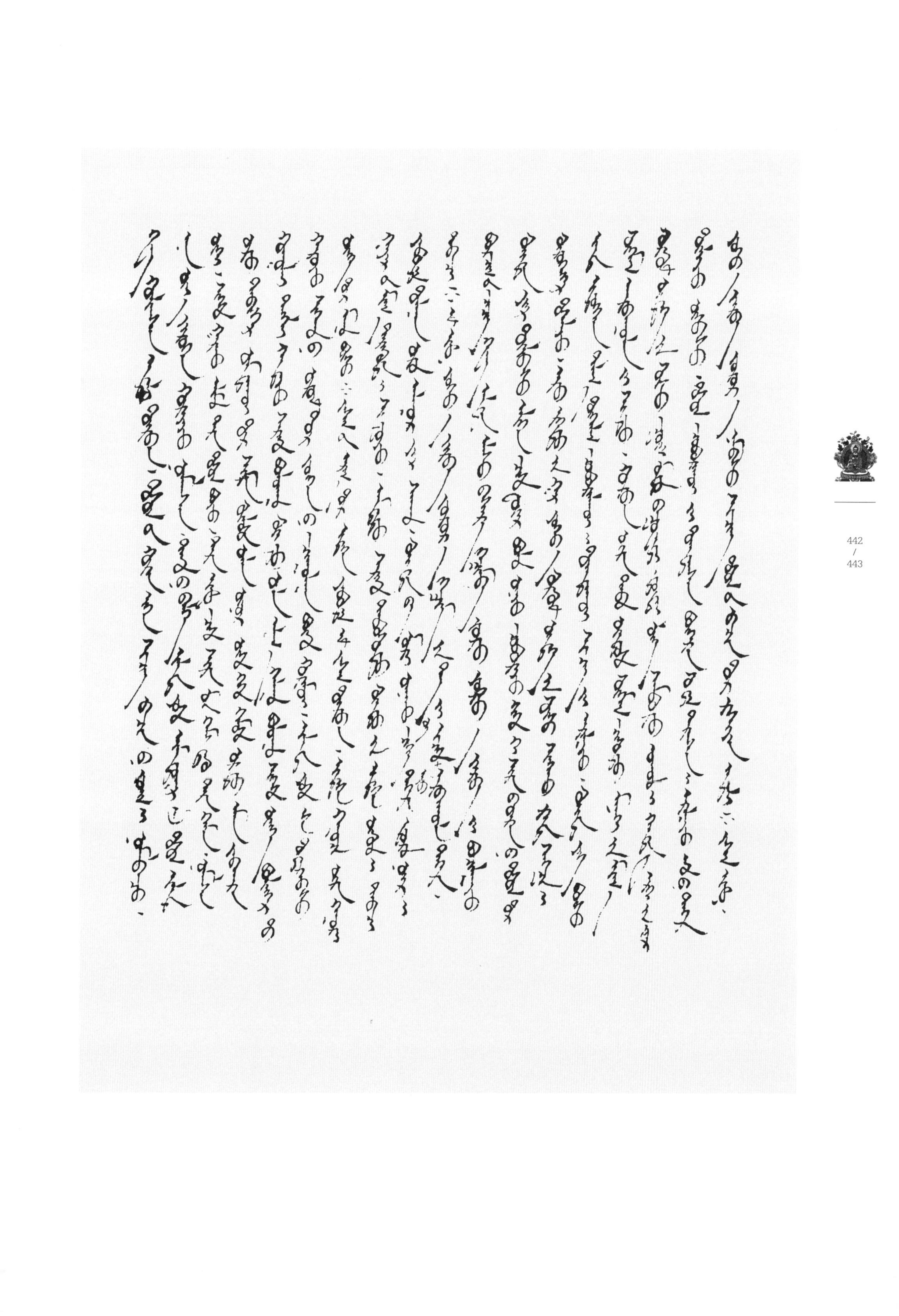

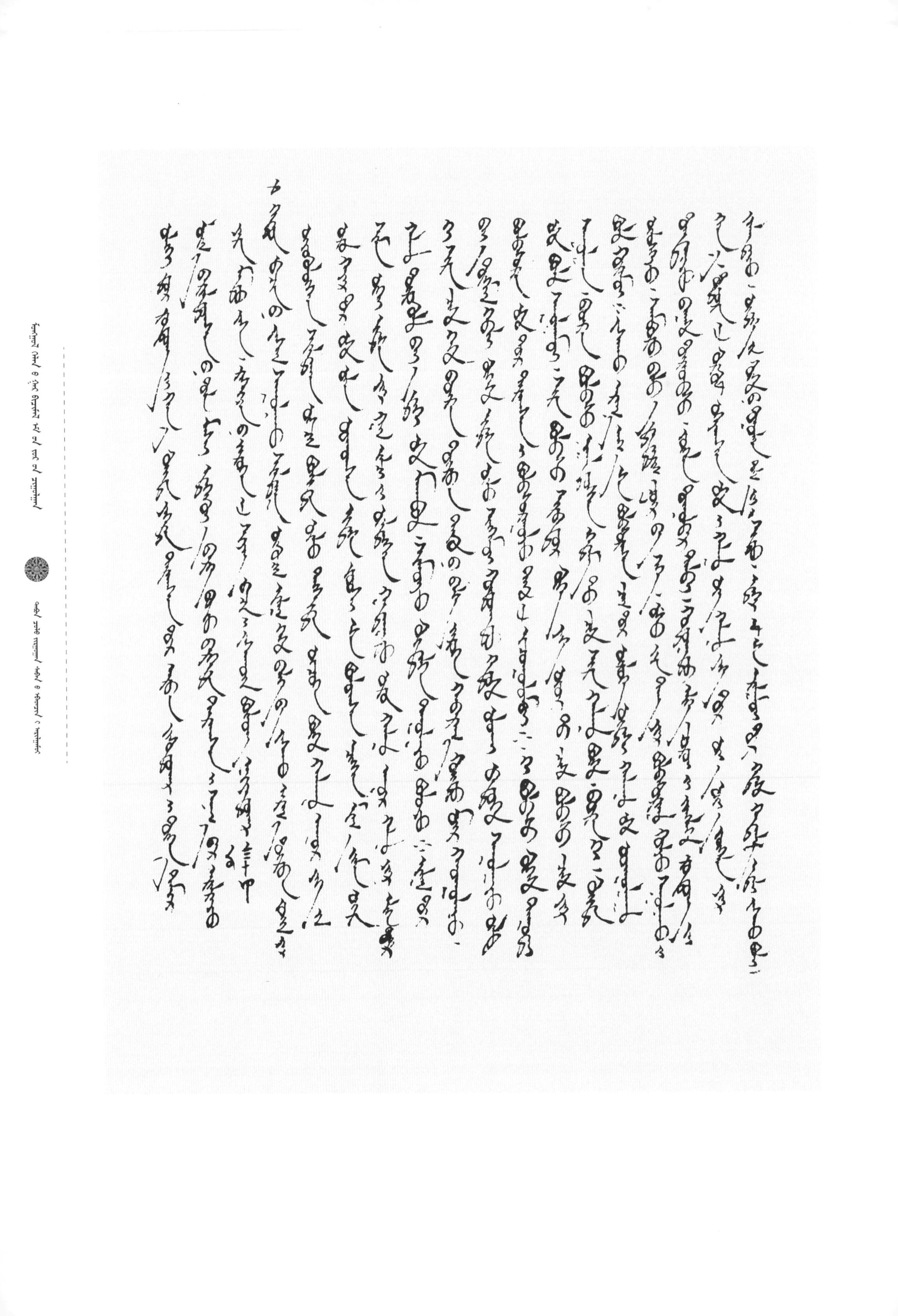

[illegible]
[illegible]
[illegible]
[illegible]
[illegible]
[illegible]
[illegible]
[illegible]
[illegible]
[illegible]
[illegible]
[illegible]
[illegible]
[illegible]
[illegible]
[illegible]
[illegible]
[illegible]
[illegible]

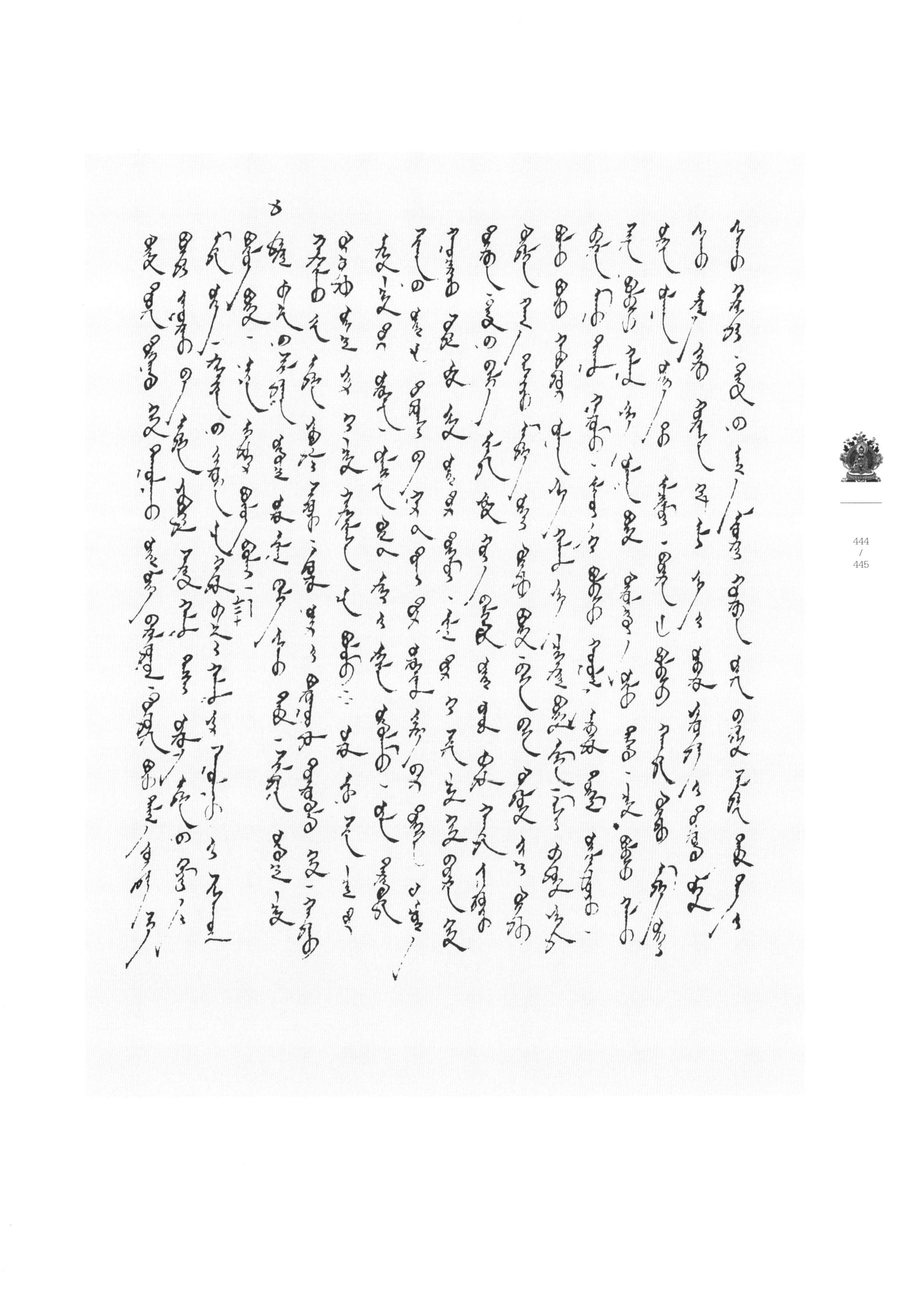

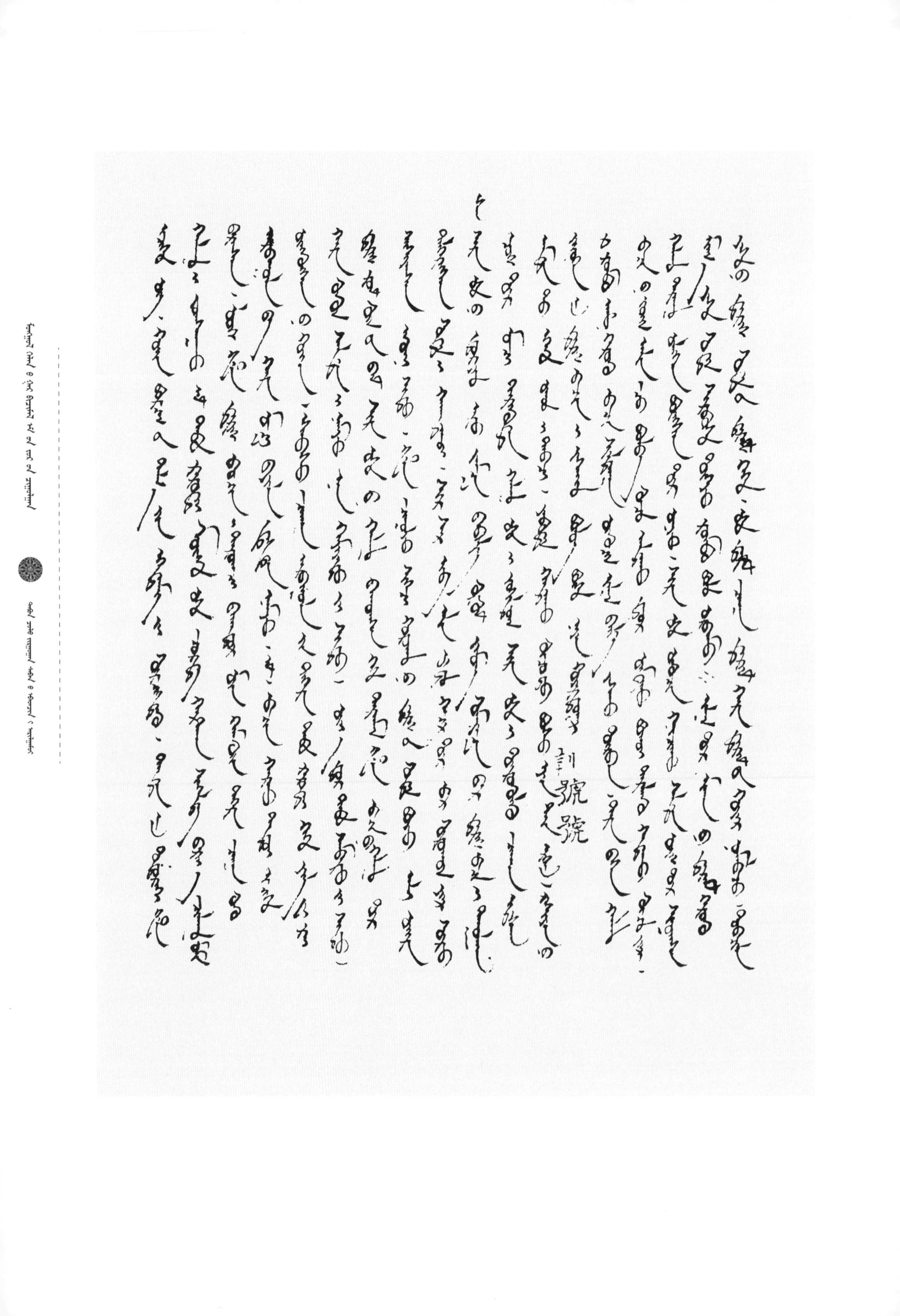

訓號
號

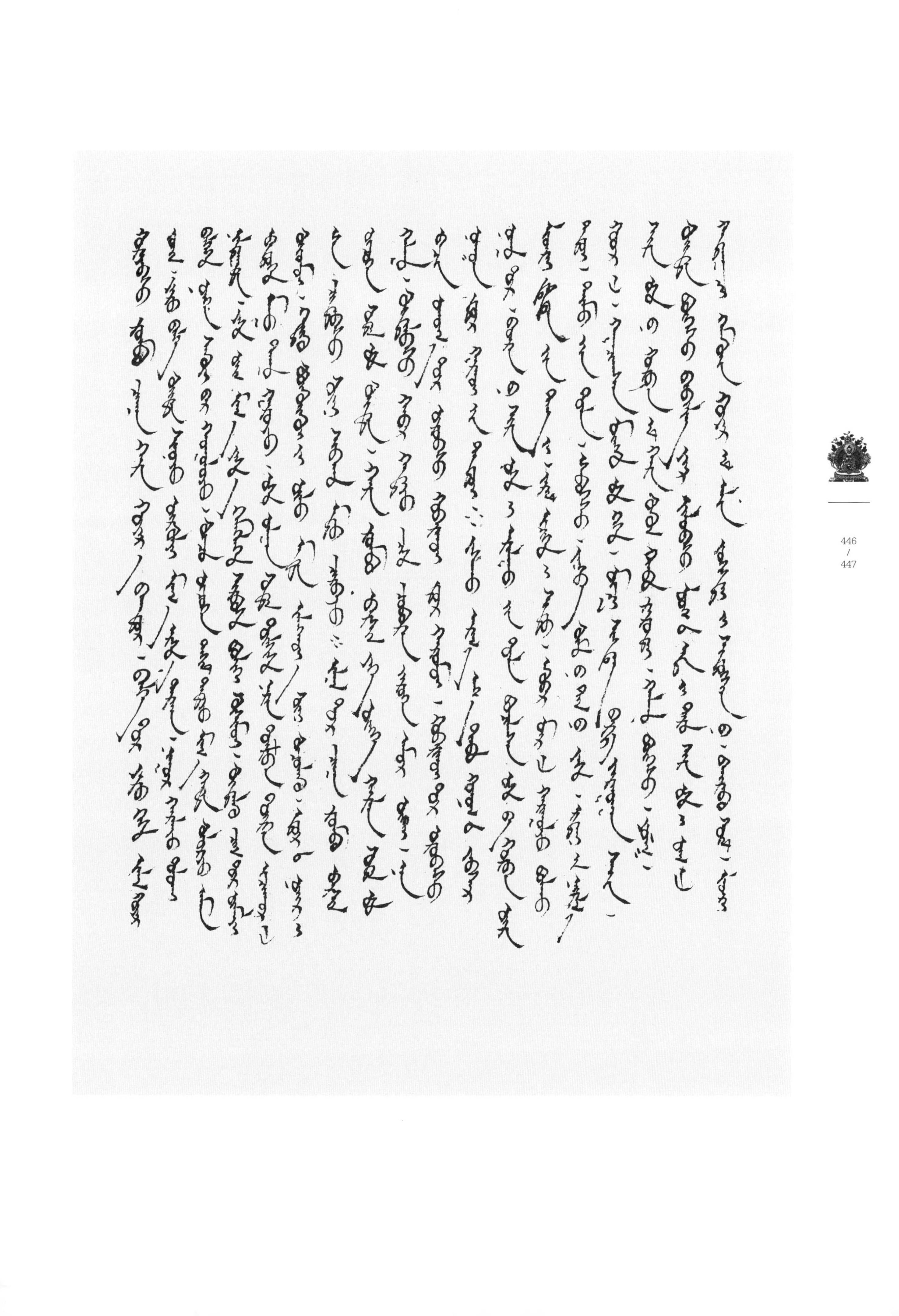

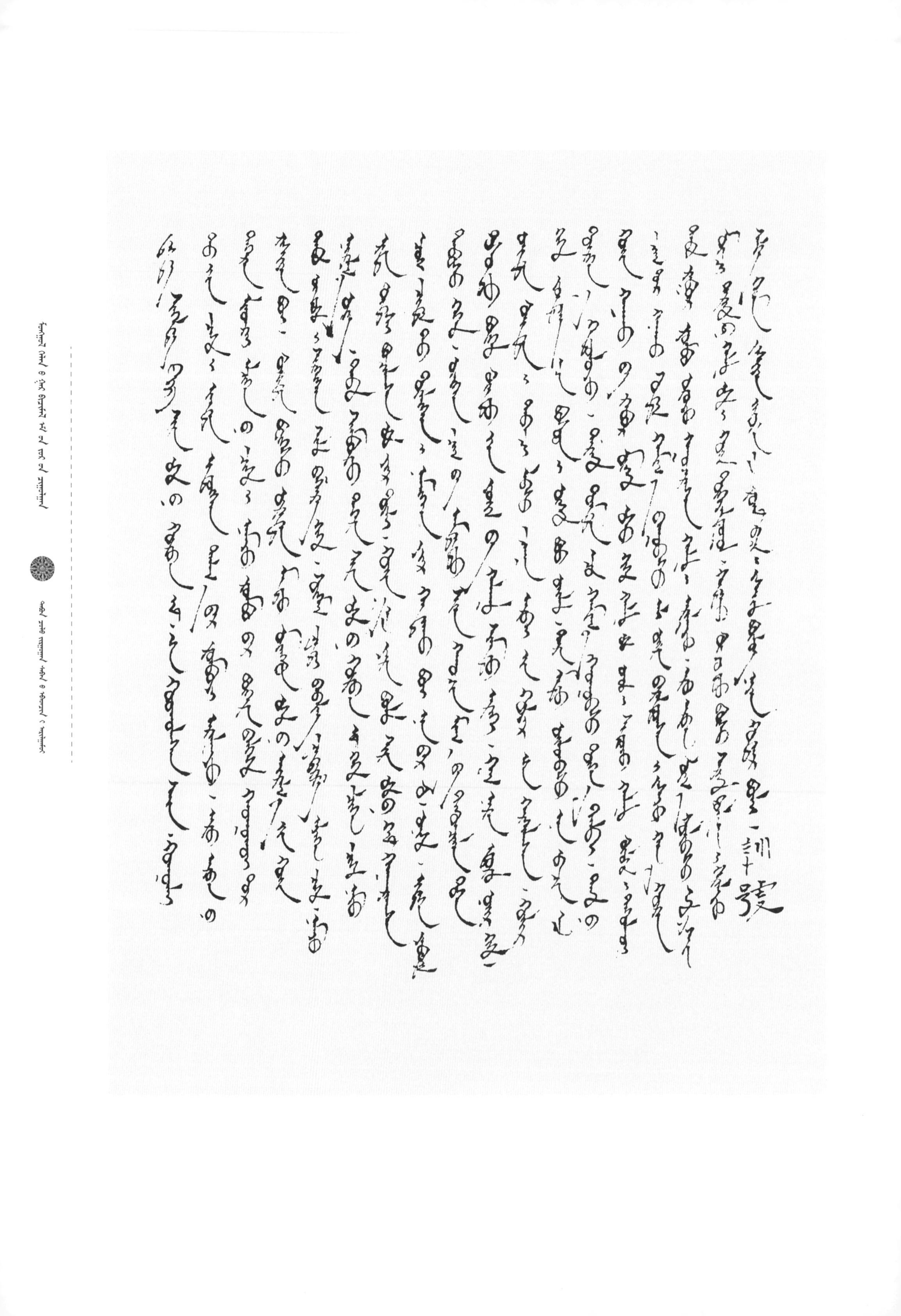

訓十號

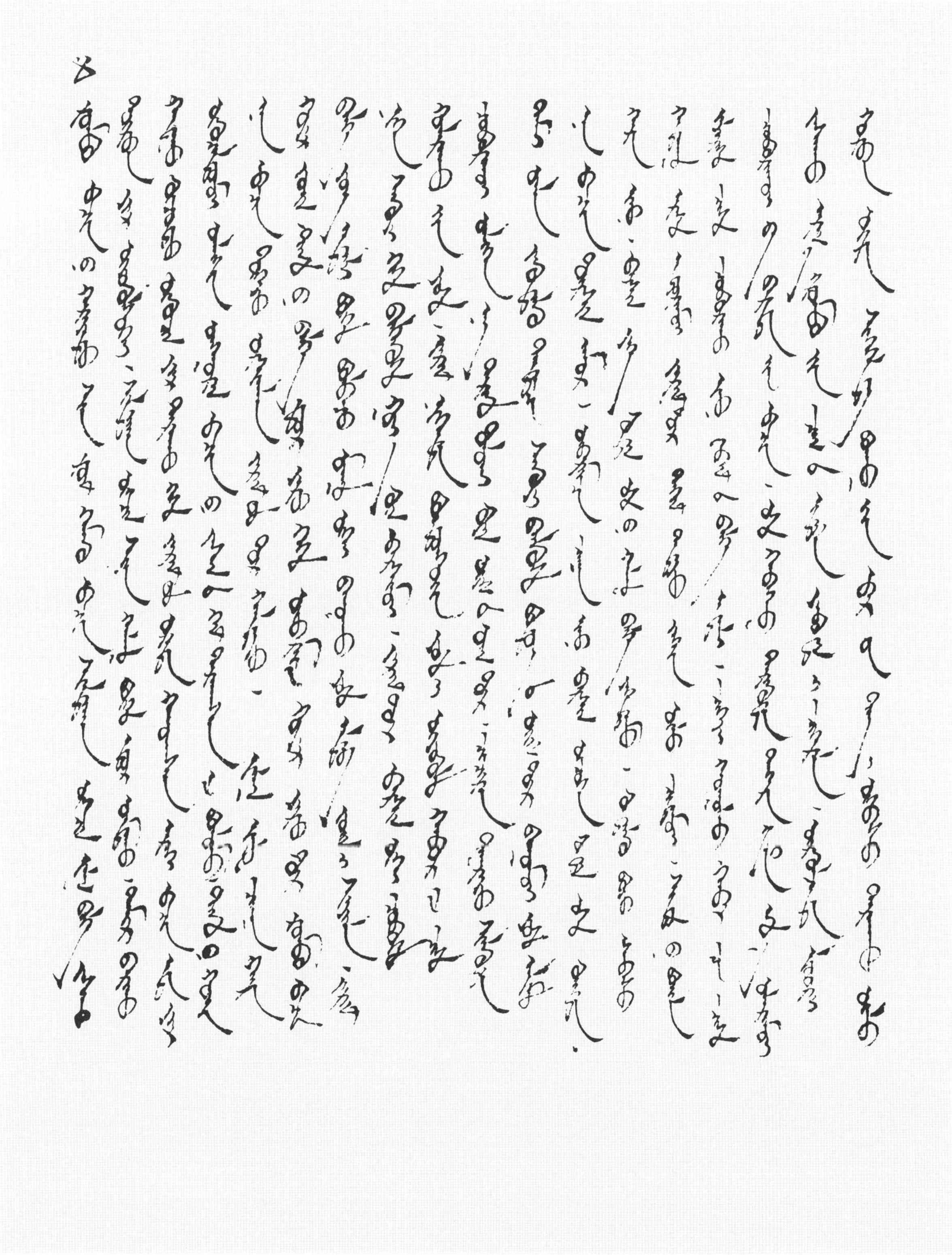

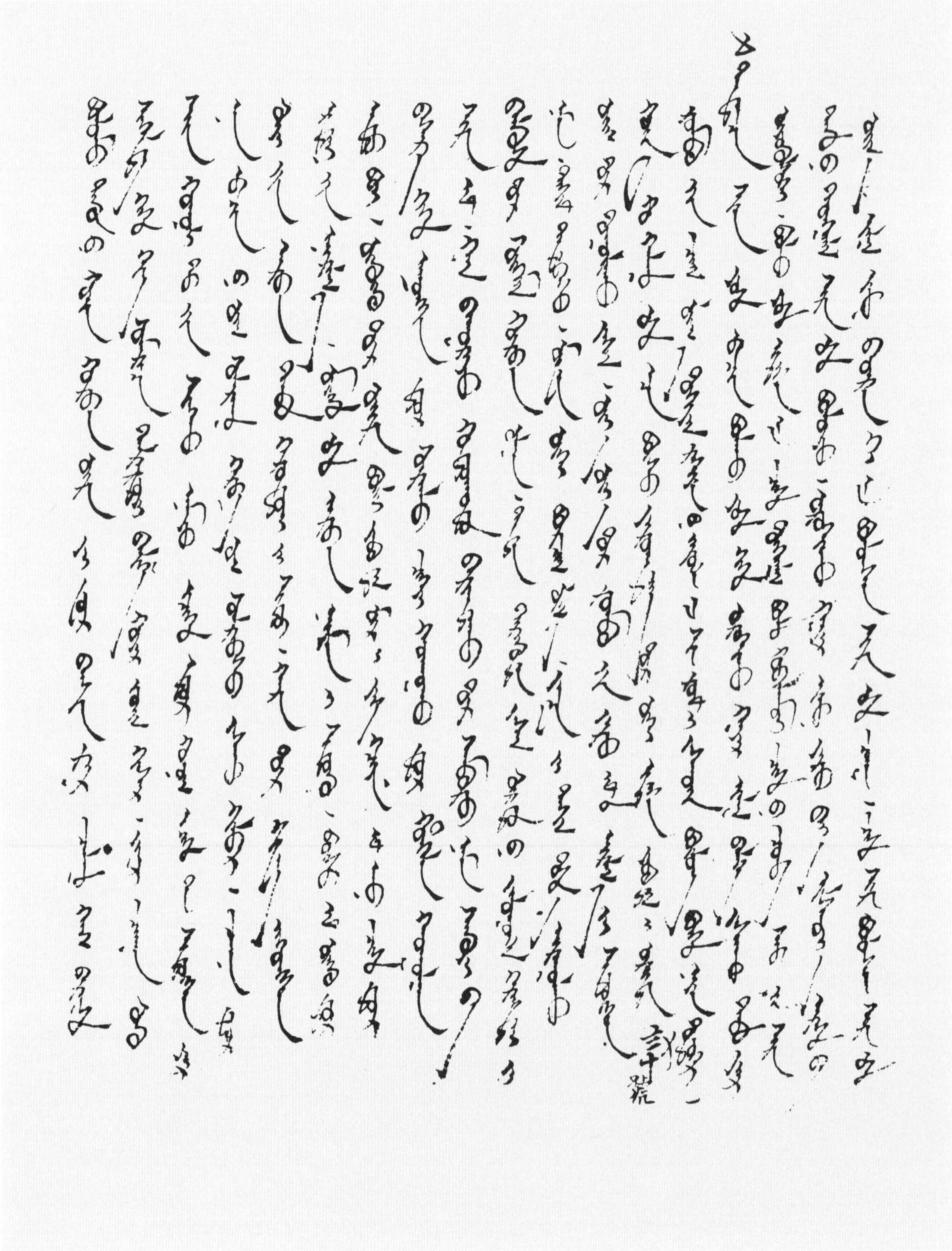

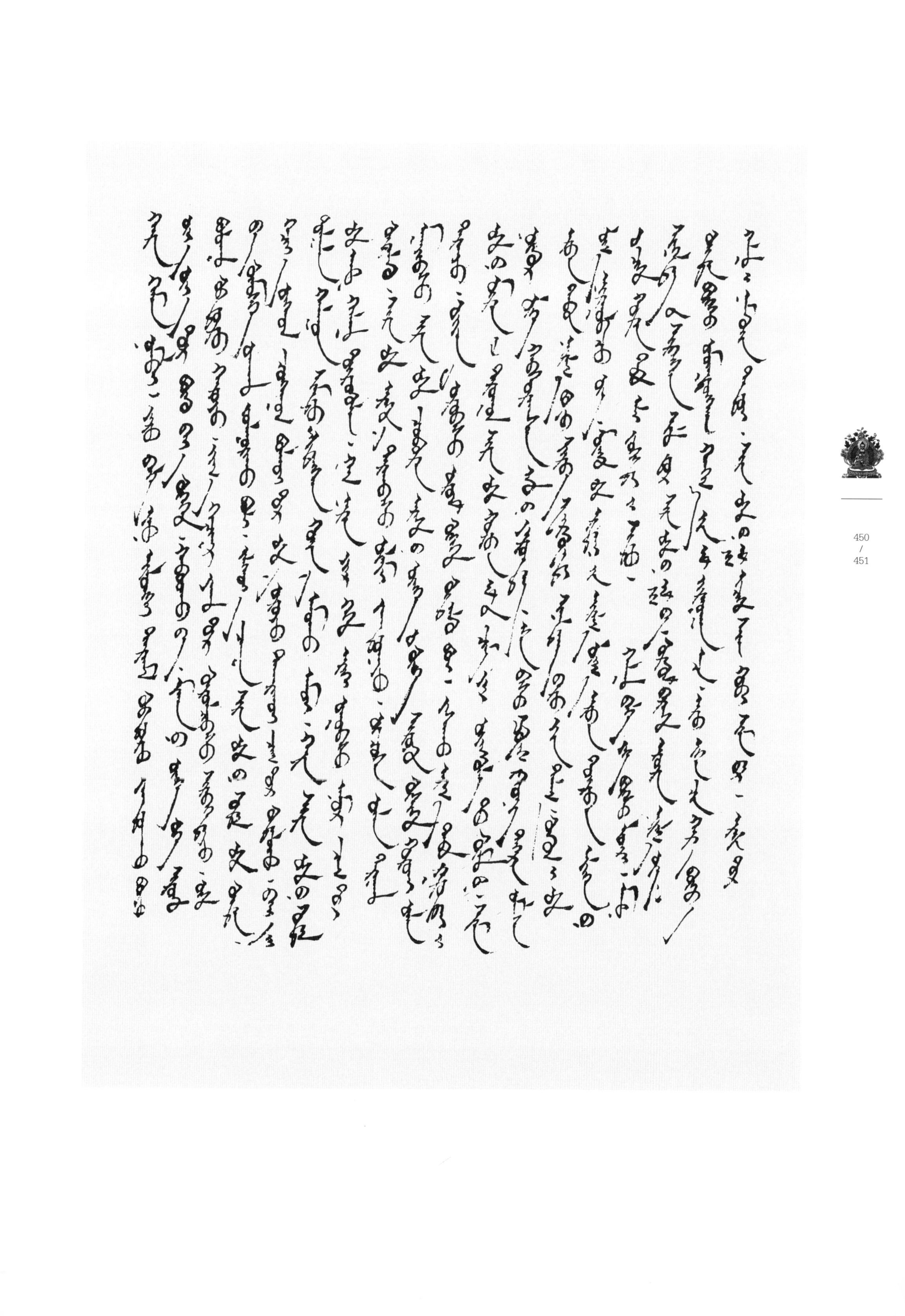

[illegible]

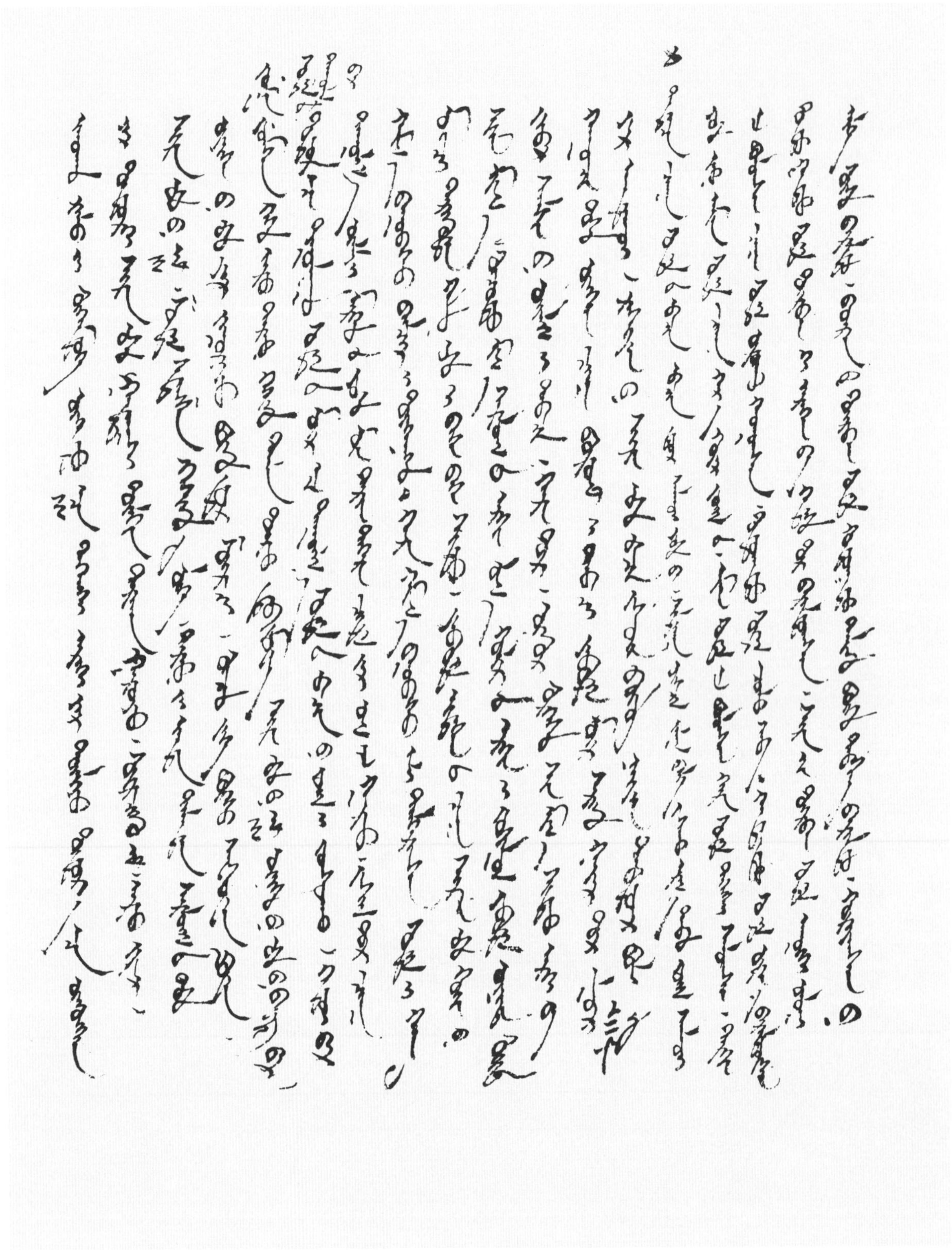
[illegible]

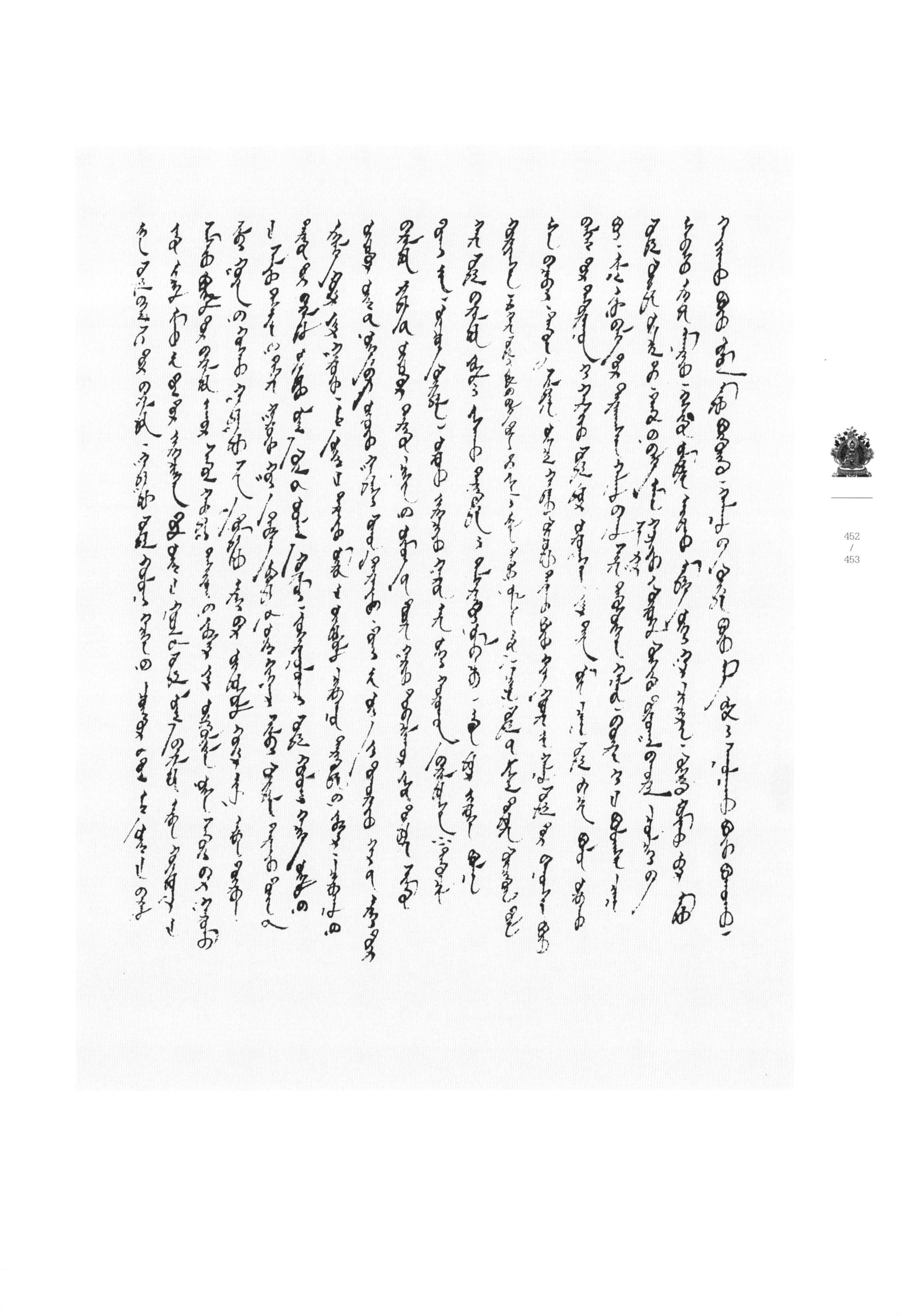

[illegible]

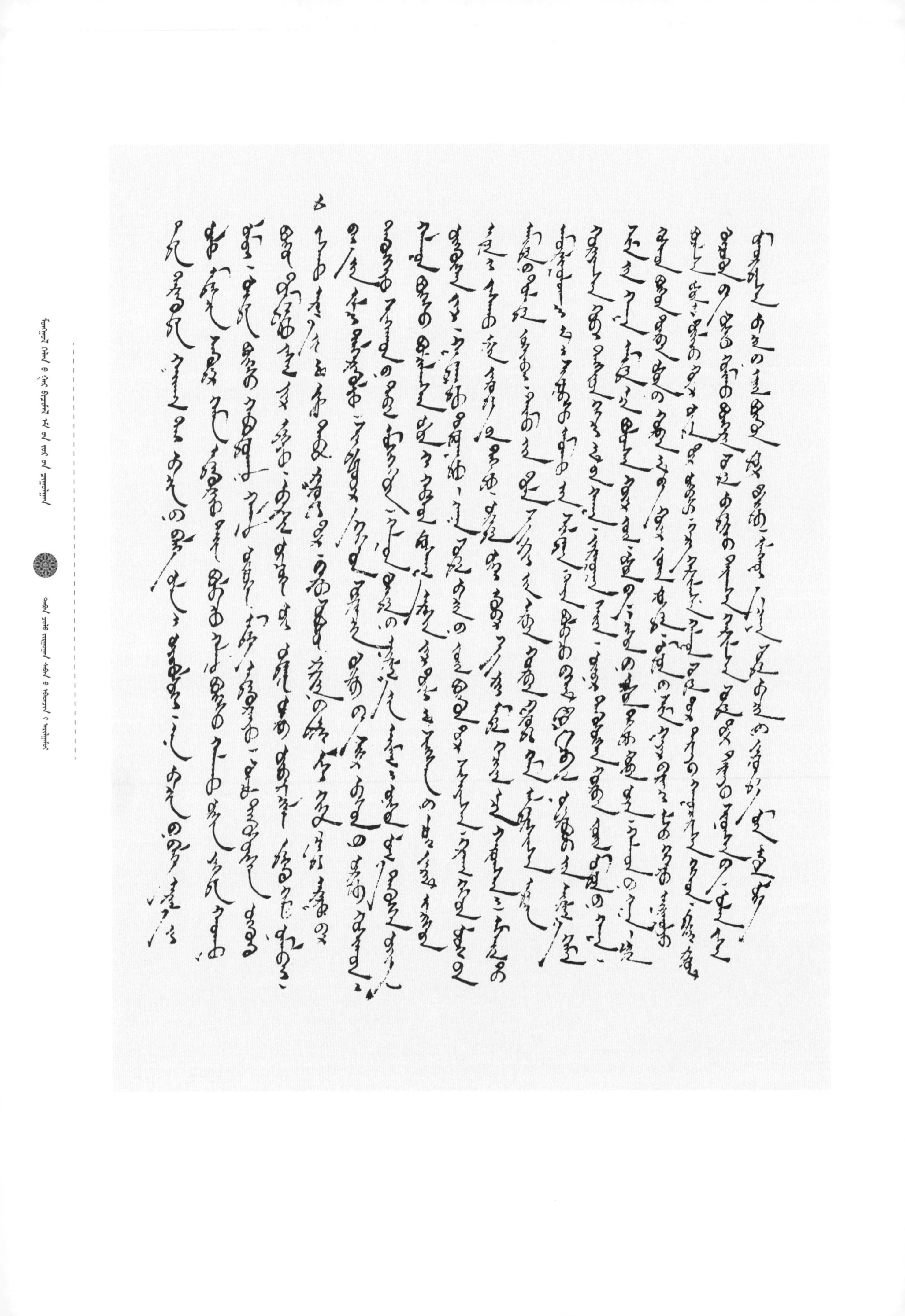

[illegible]

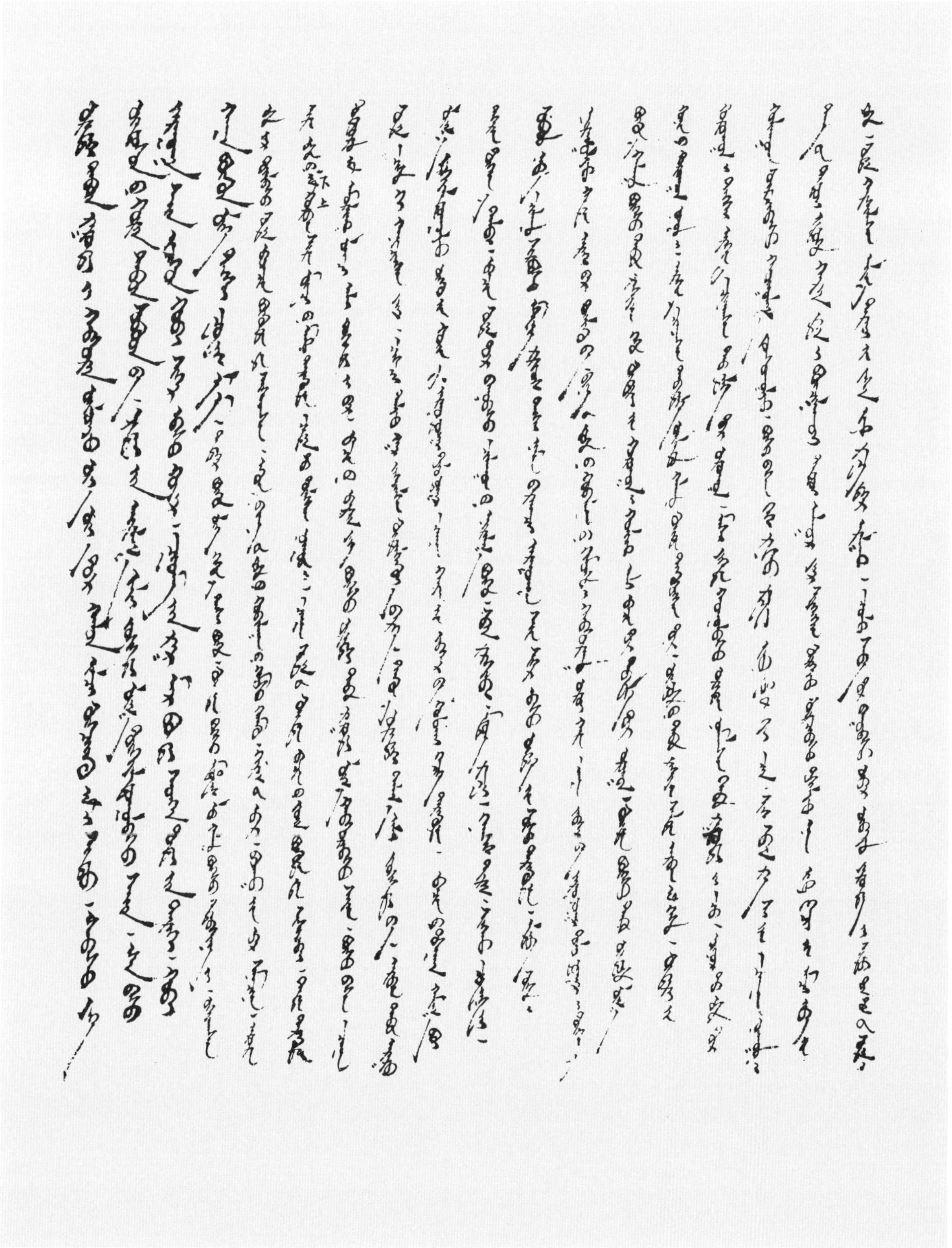

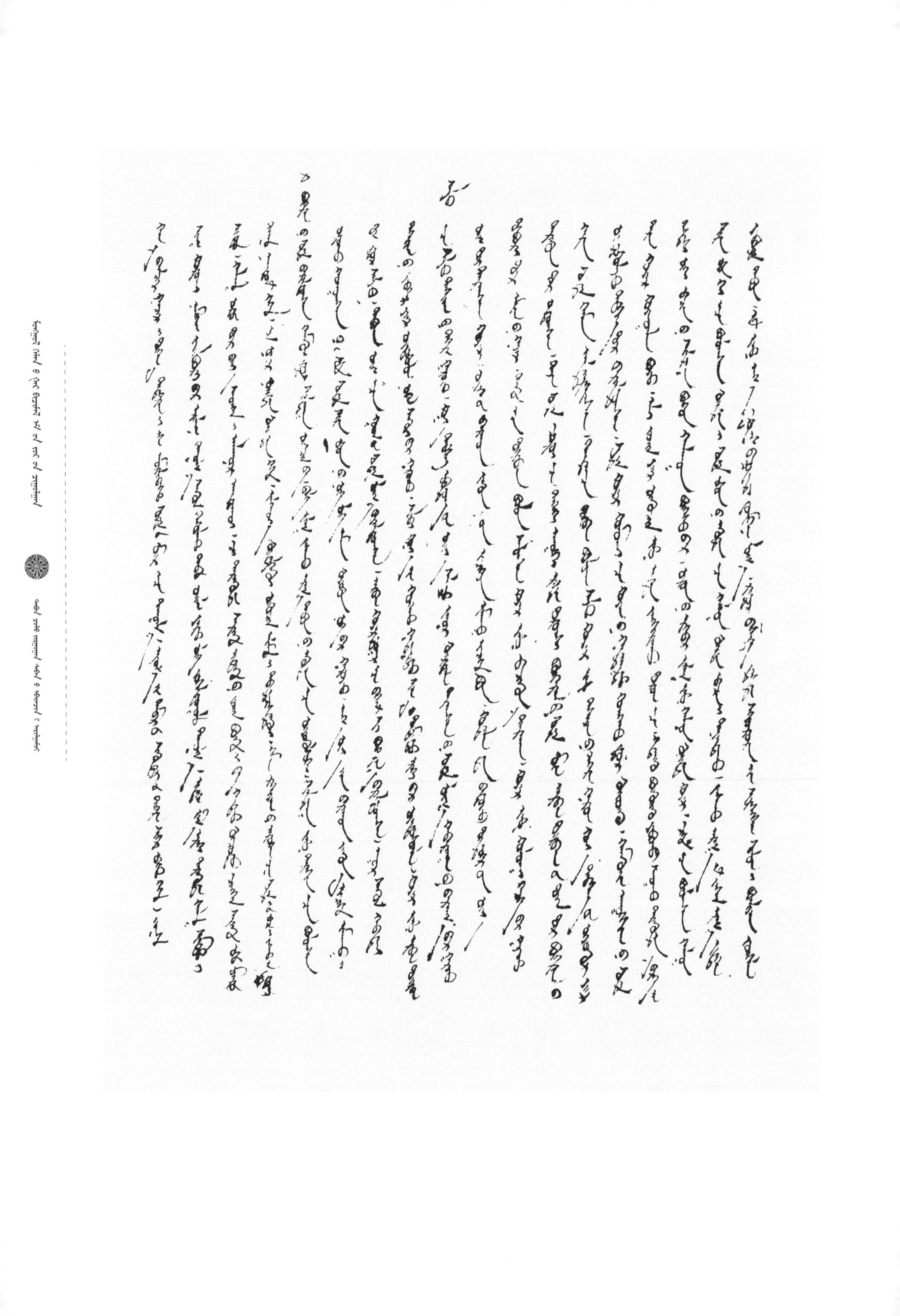

[illegible]

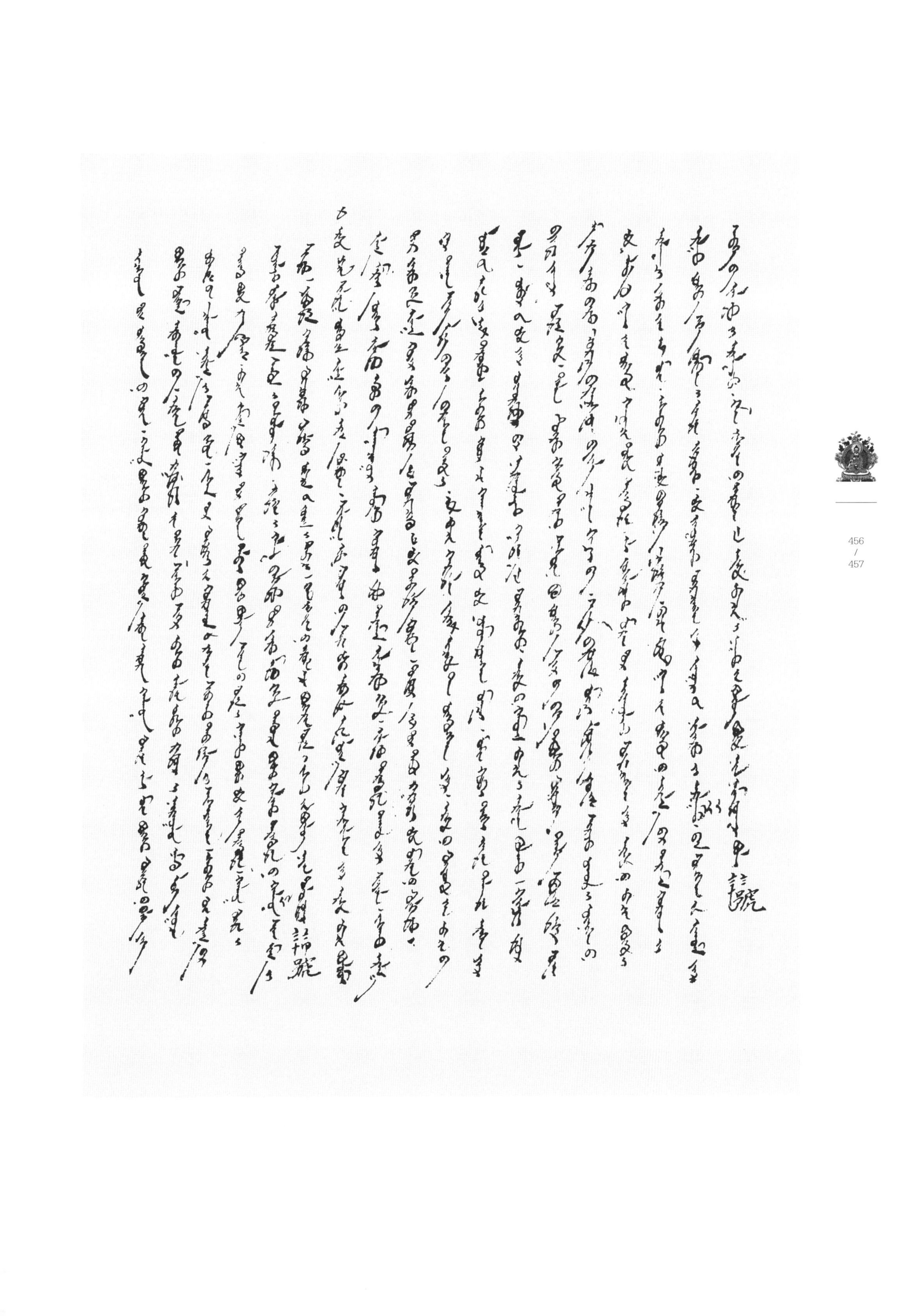

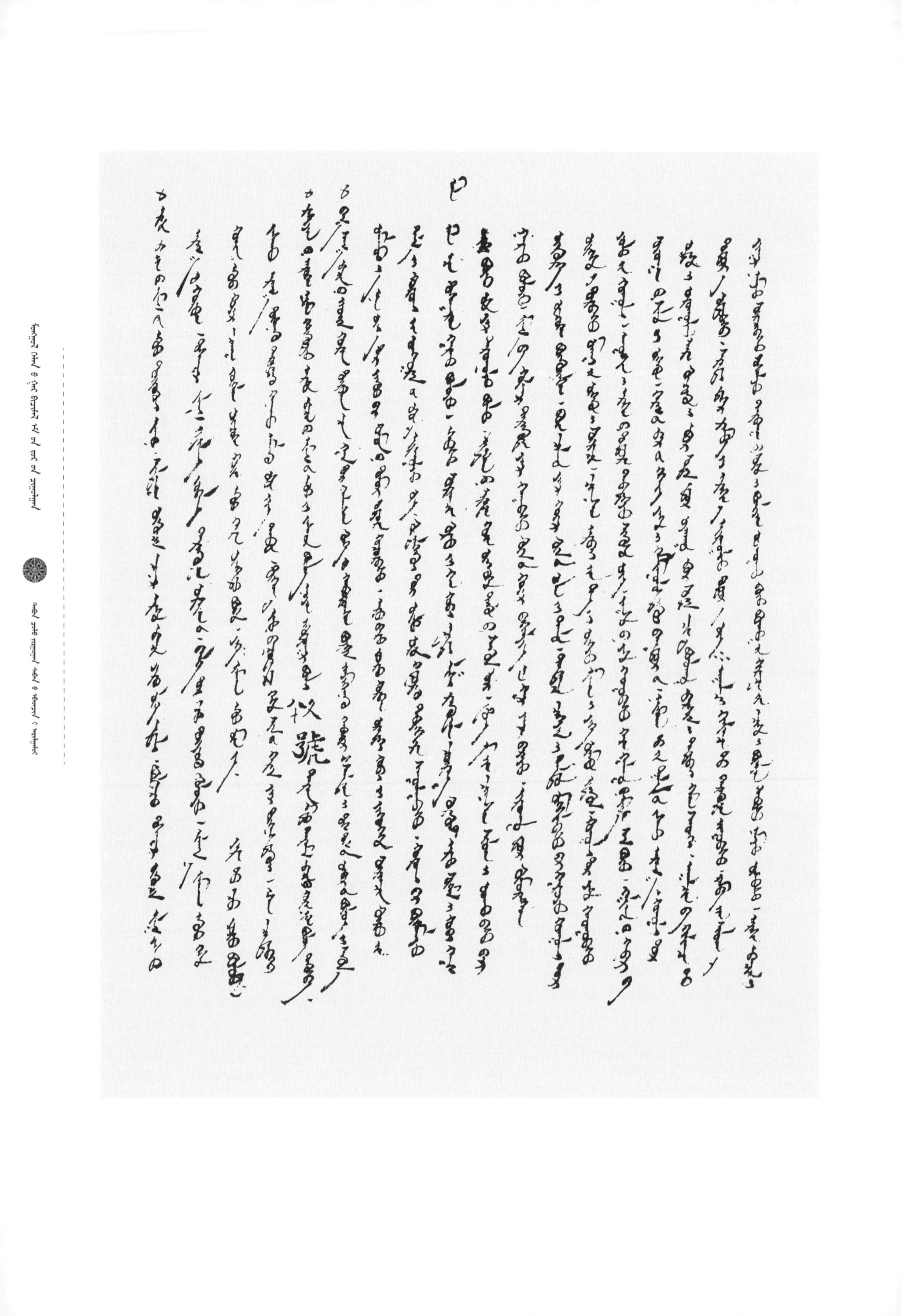

收號

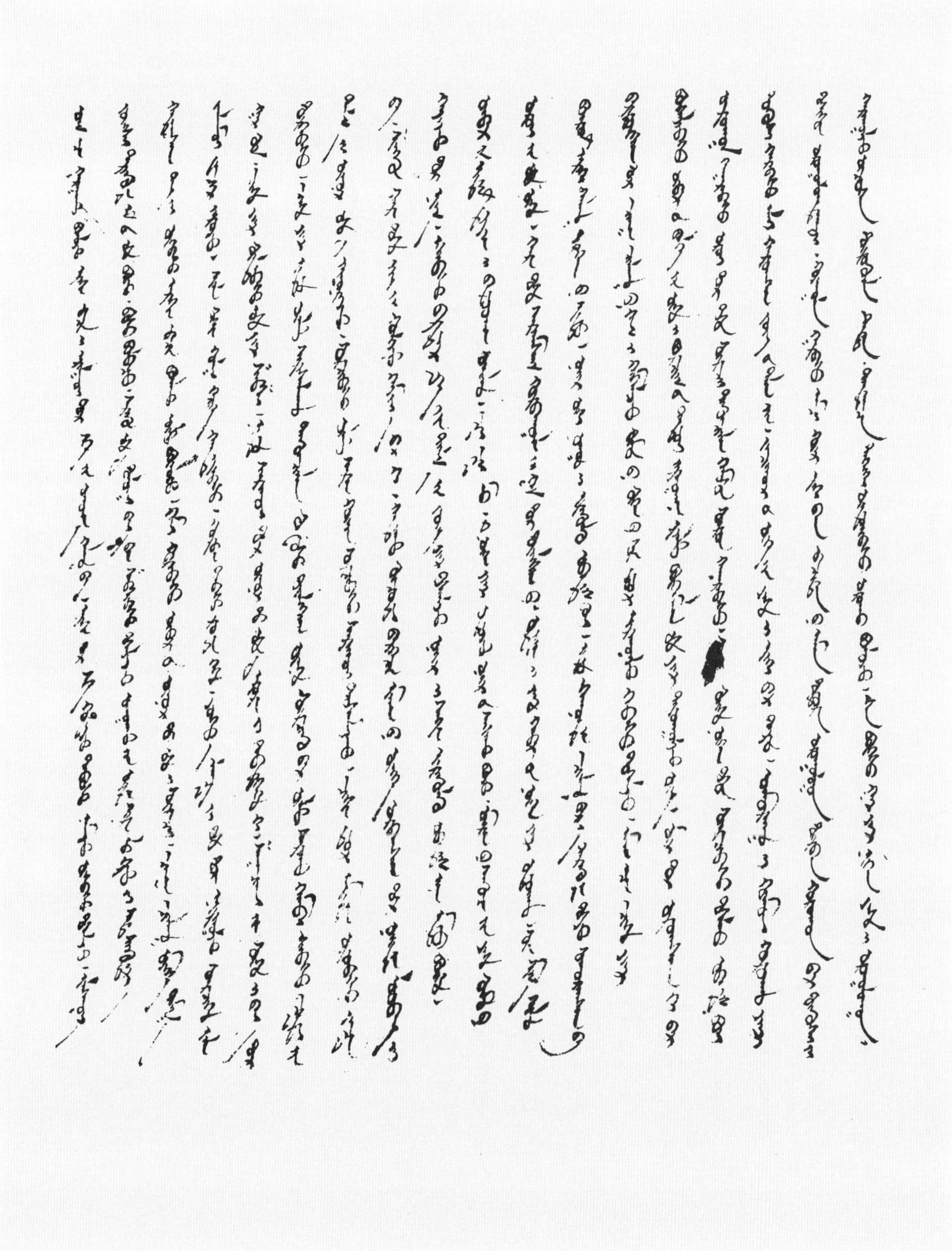

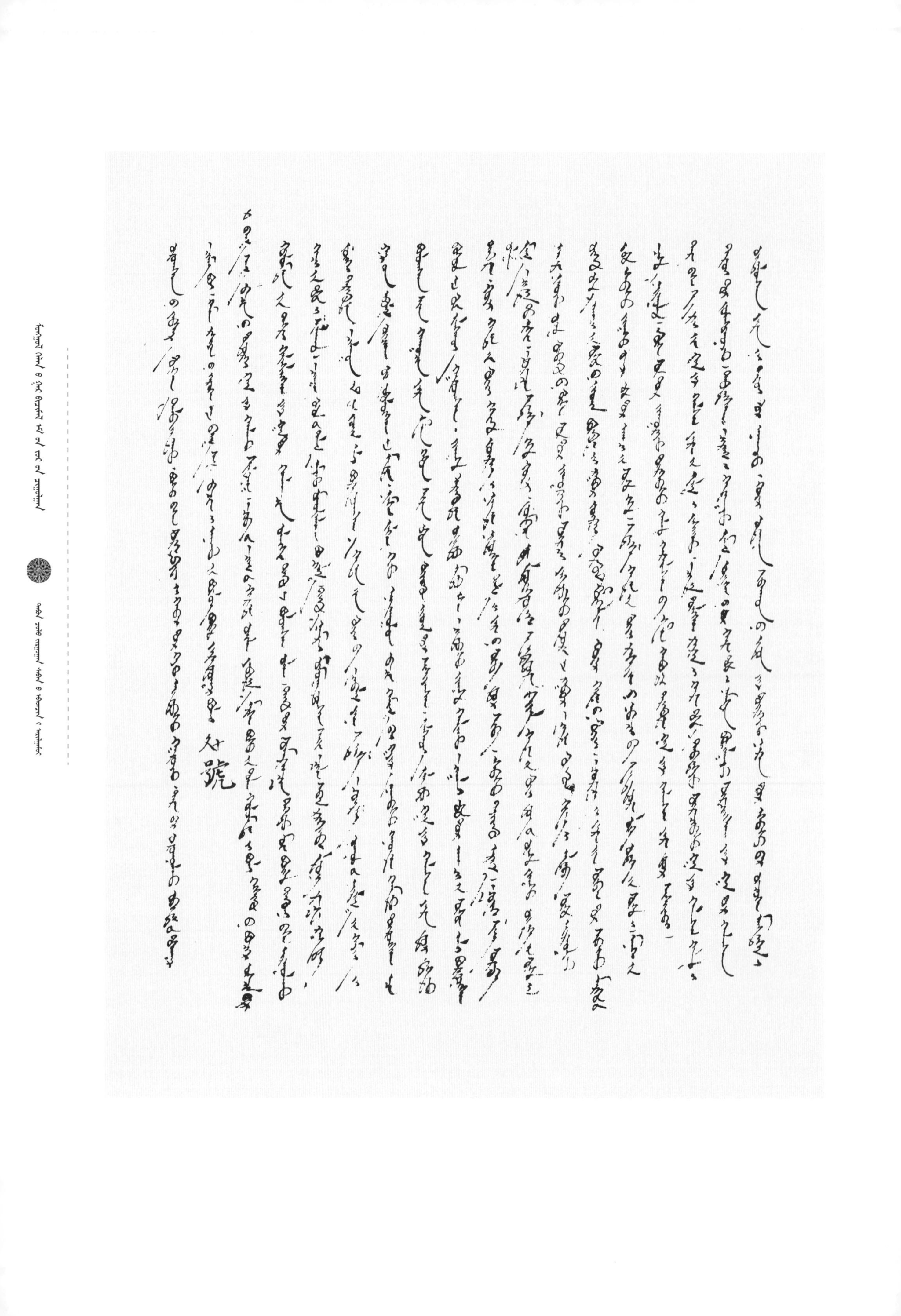

號

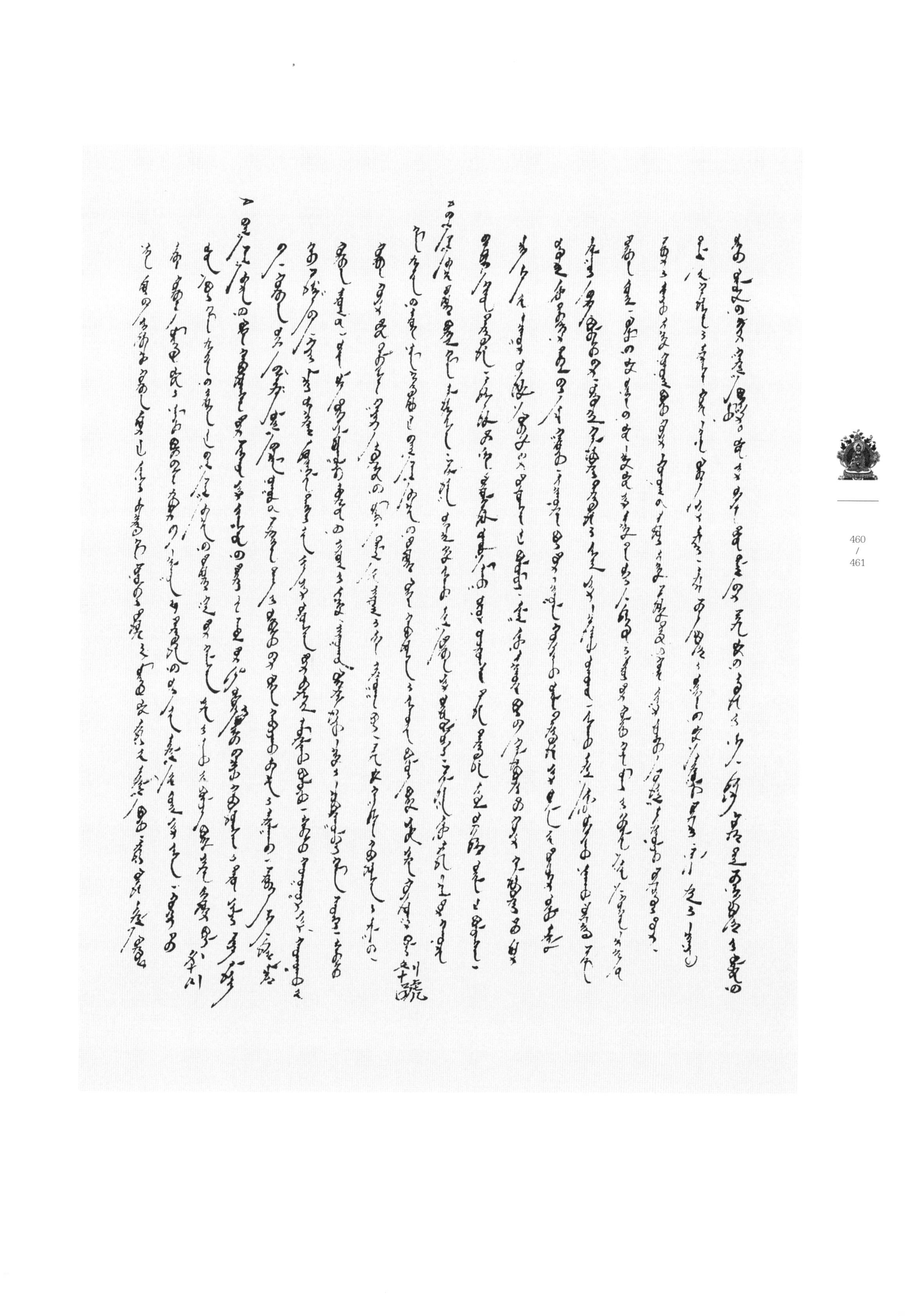

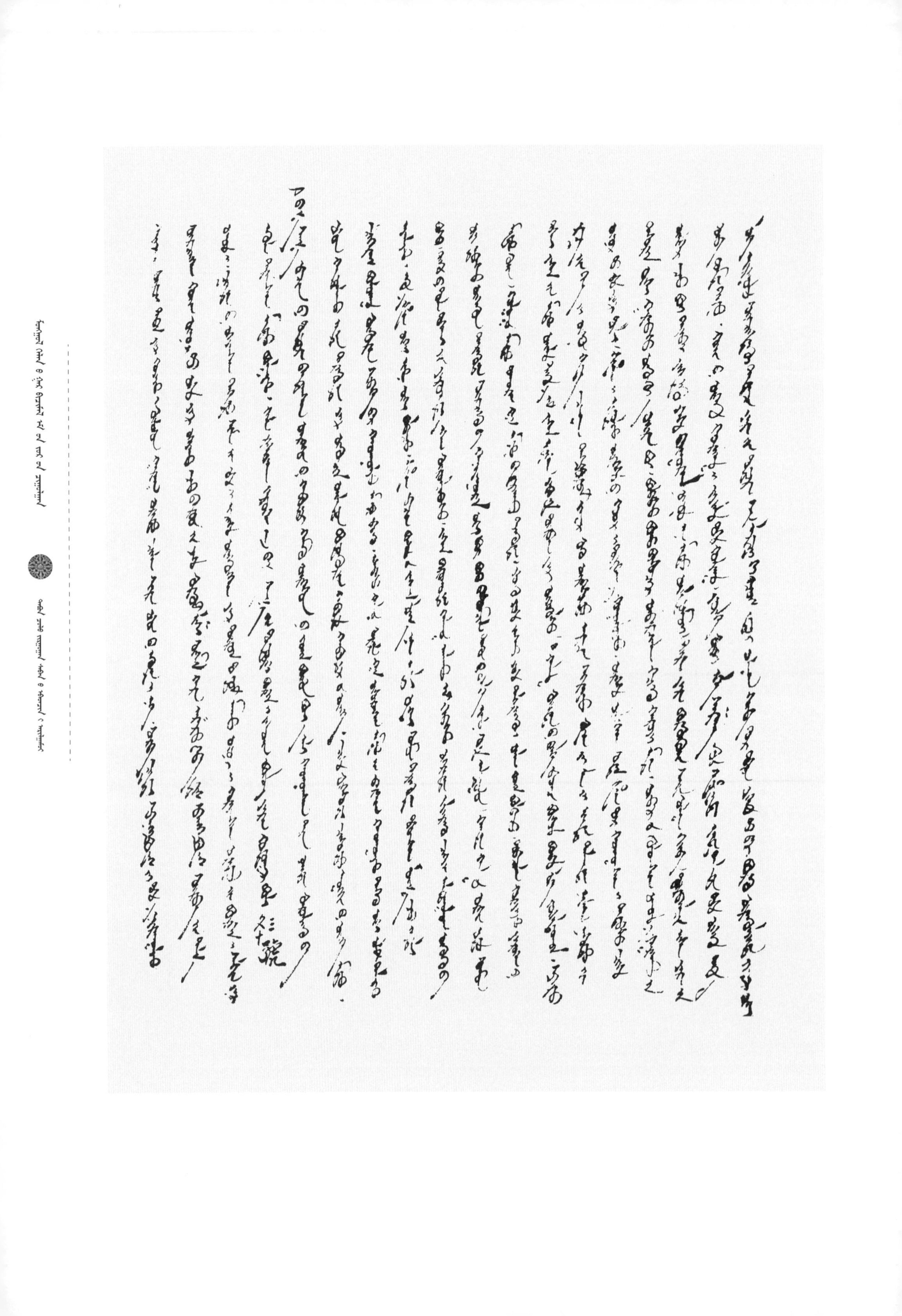

[illegible]

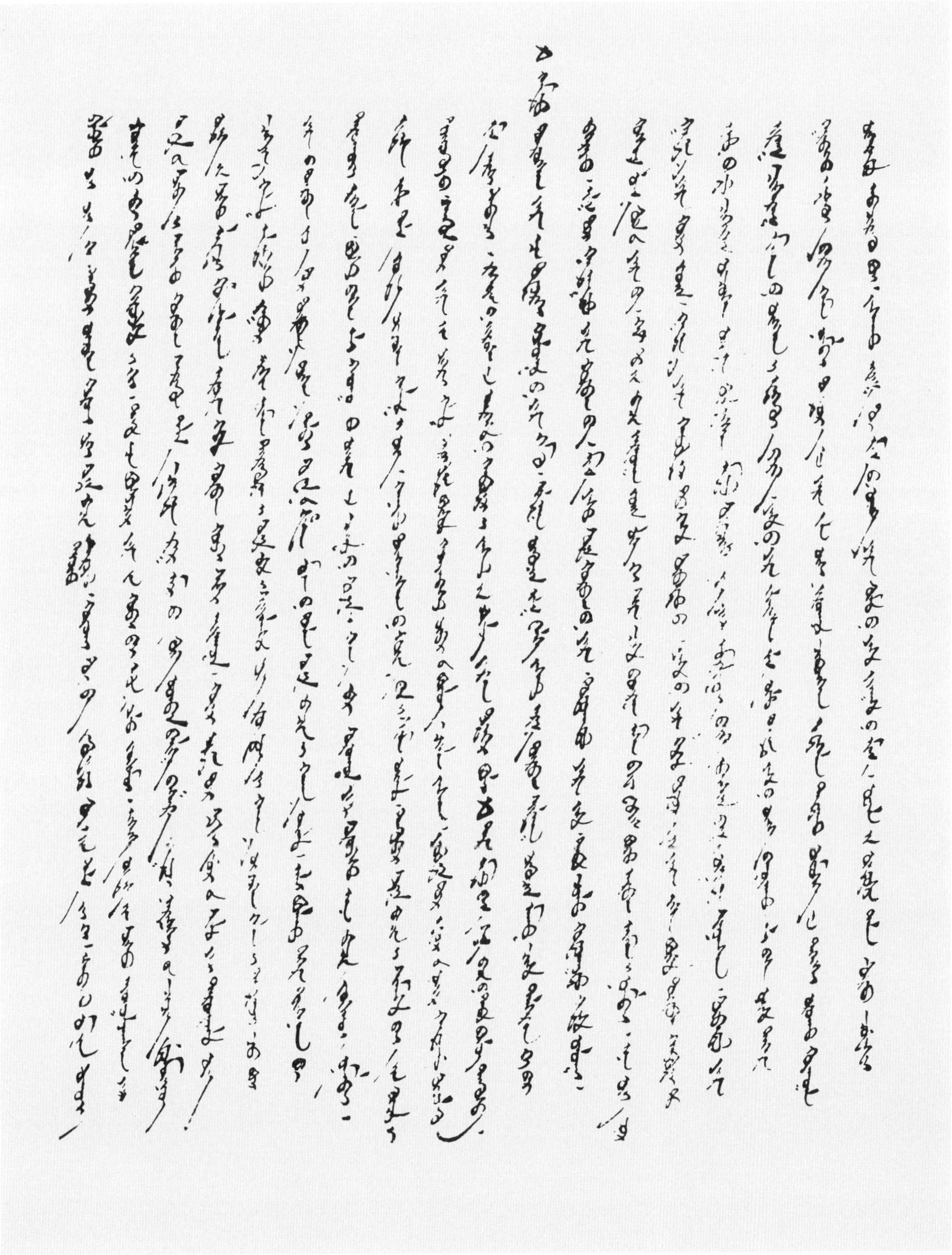

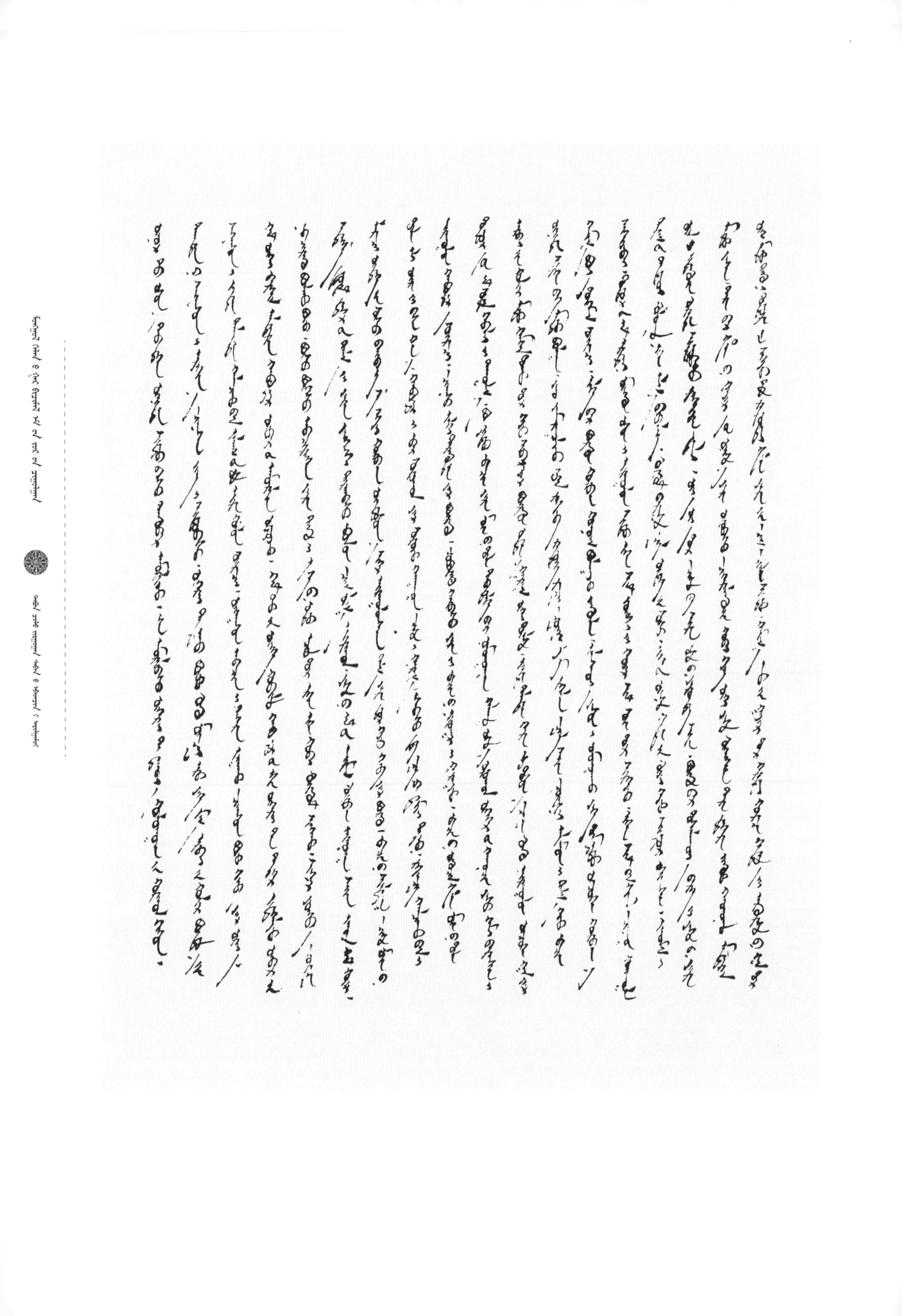

[illegible]

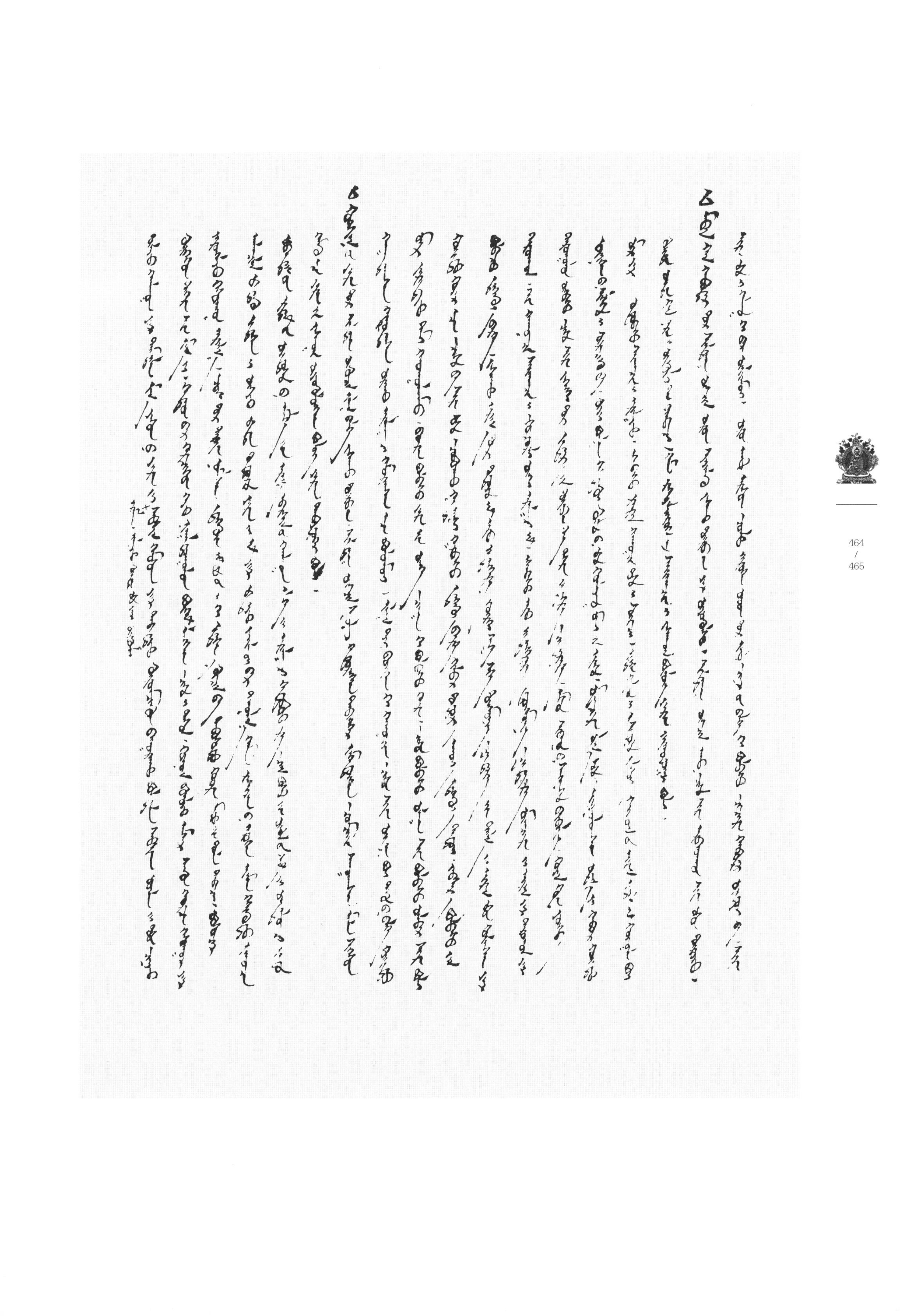

[illegible]

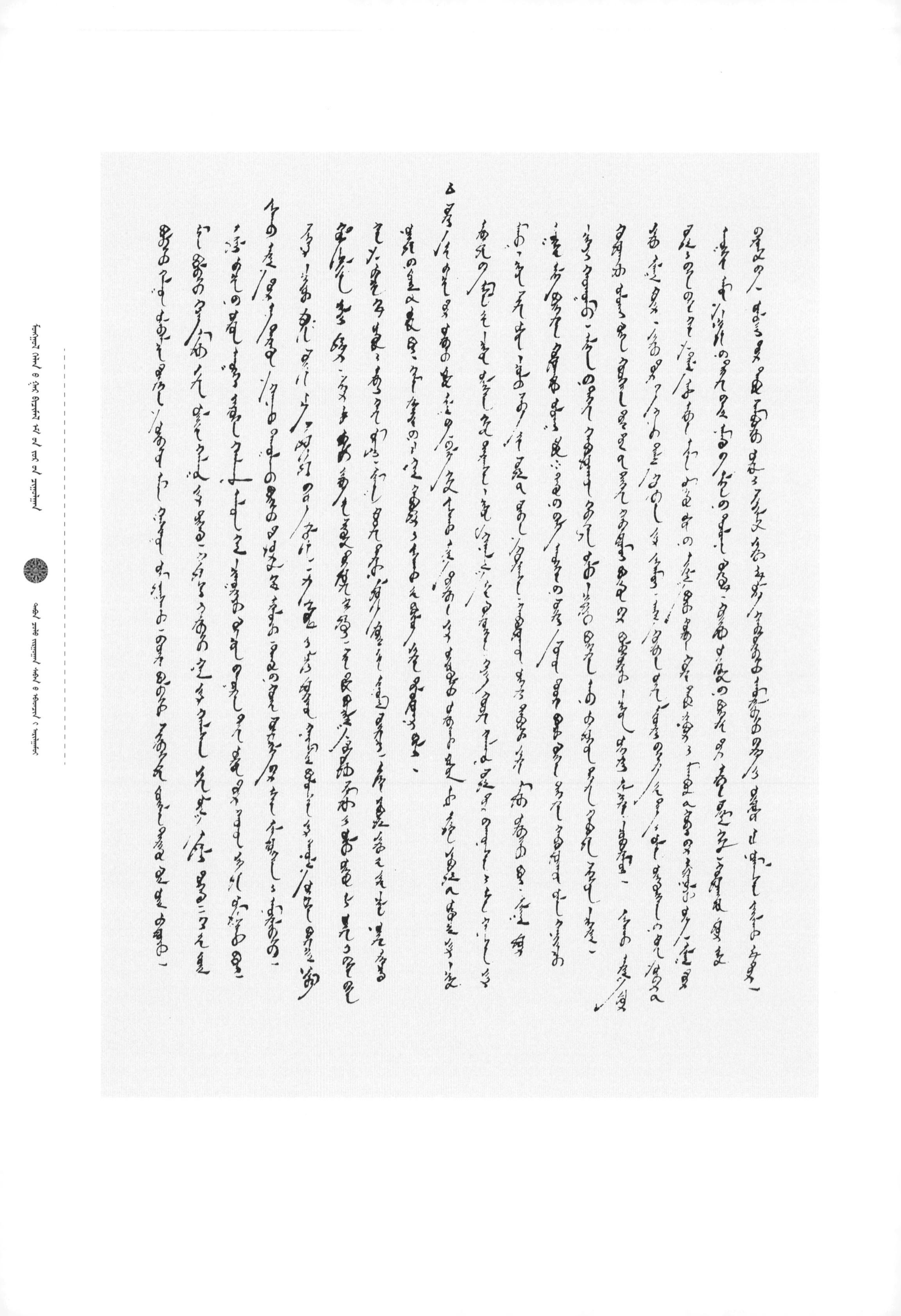

[illegible]

[illegible]

[illegible]

[illegible]

[illegible]

[illegible]

[illegible]

[illegible]

[illegible]

[illegible]

[illegible]

[illegible]

[illegible]

[illegible]

[illegible]

[illegible]

[illegible]

[illegible]

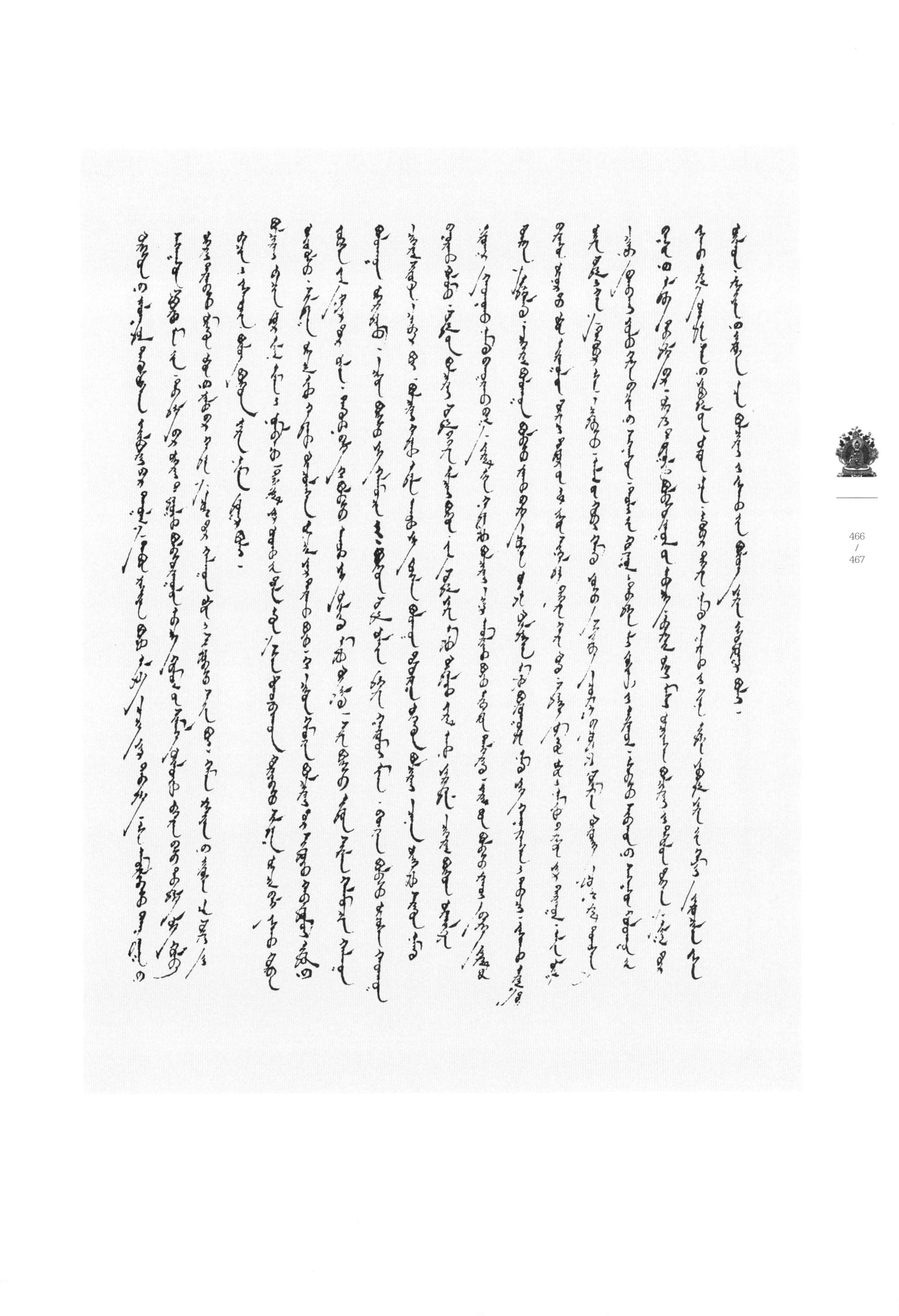

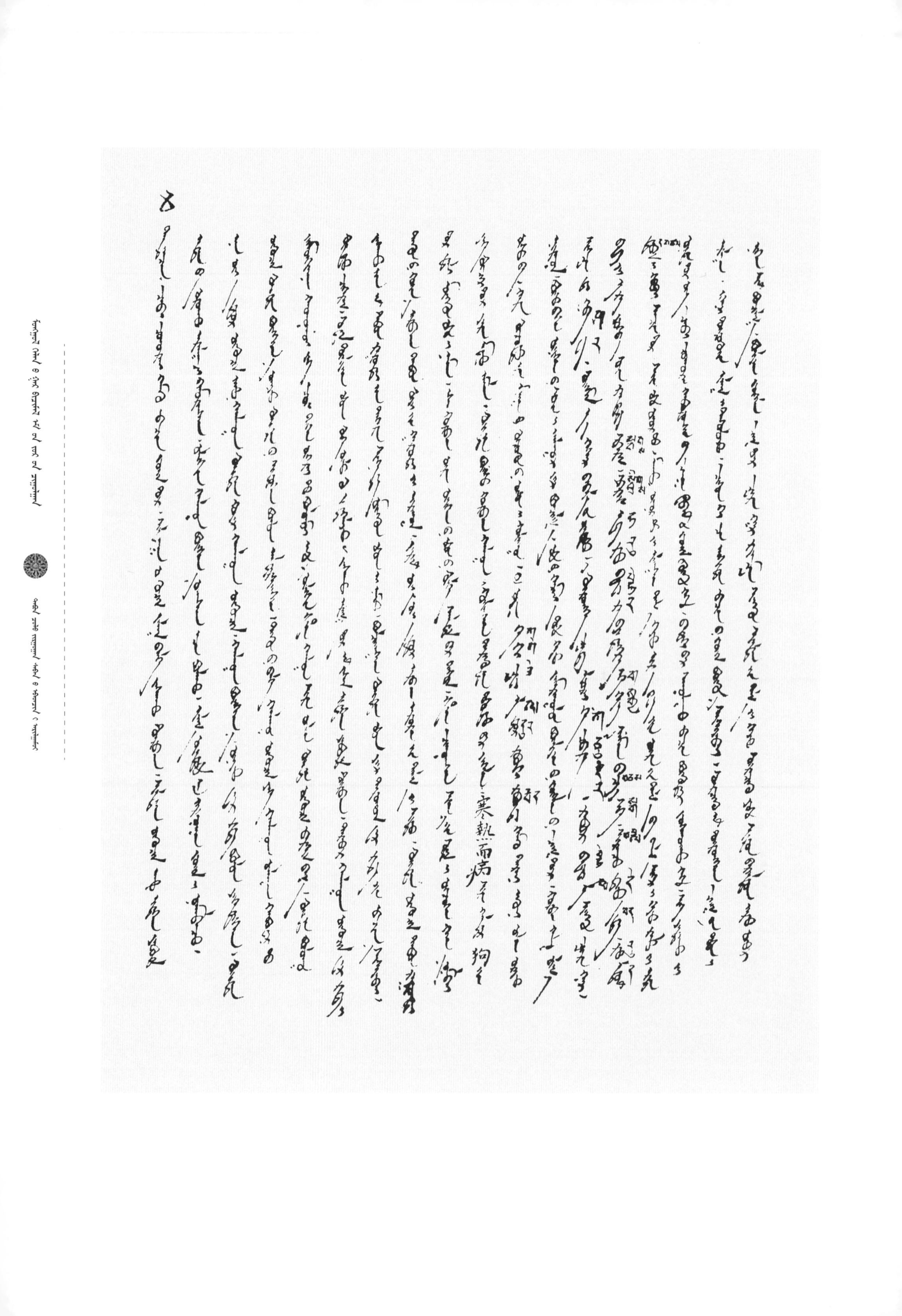

[illegible]

[illegible] 寒熱而病 [illegible] 狗 [illegible]

[illegible]

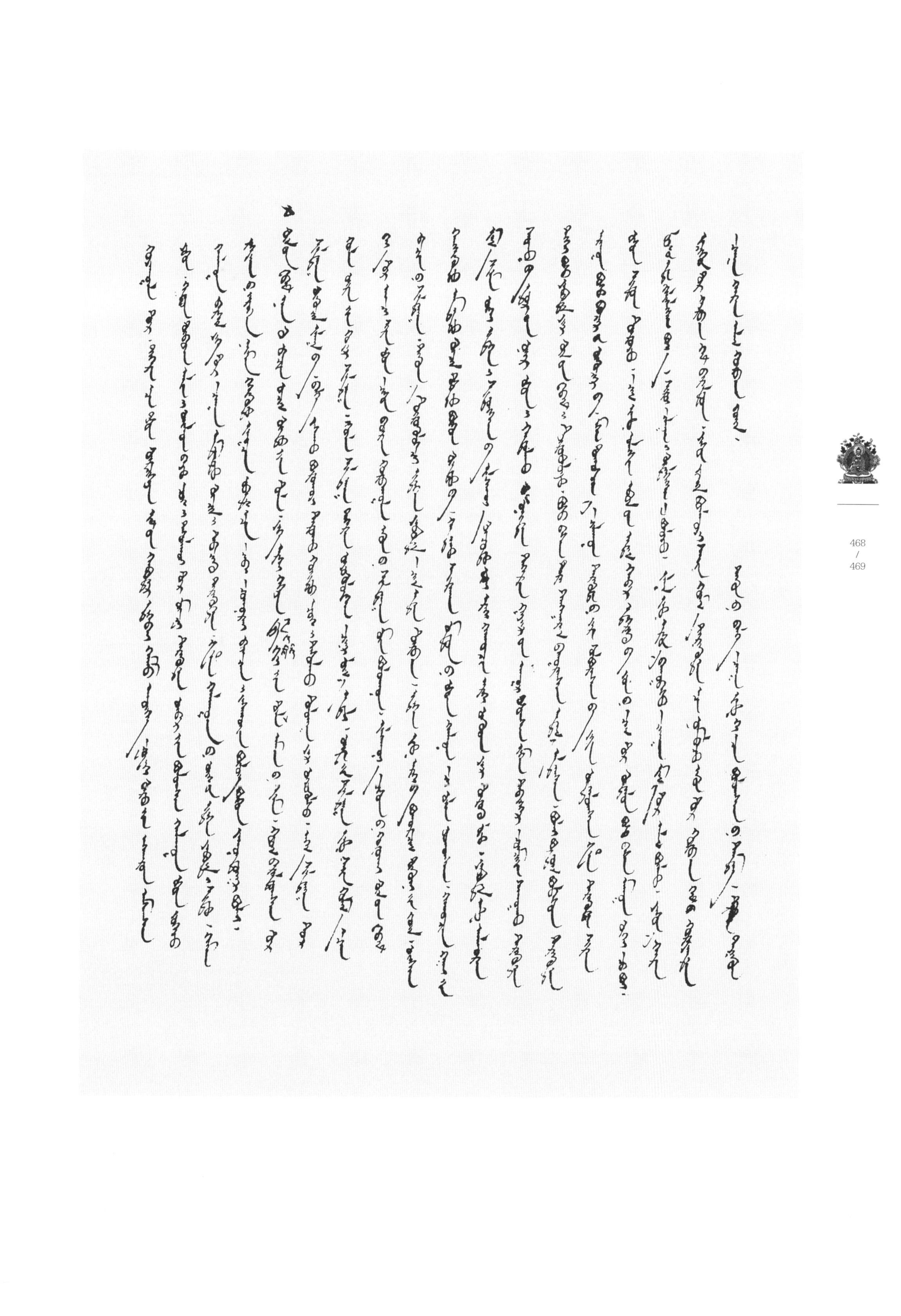

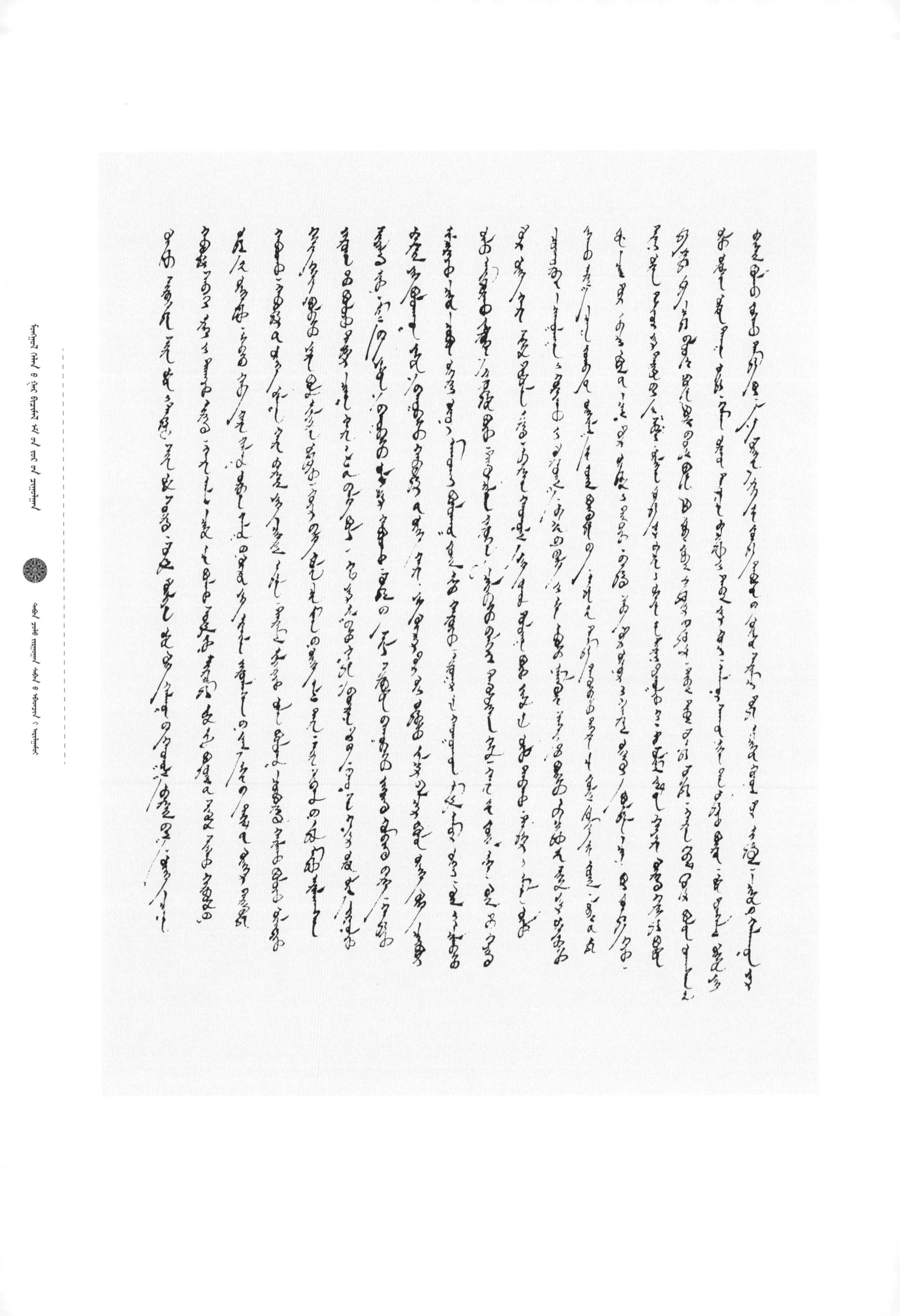

[illegible]

[illegible]
[illegible]
[illegible]
[illegible]
[illegible]
[illegible]
[illegible]
[illegible]
[illegible]
[illegible]
[illegible]
[illegible]
[illegible]
[illegible]
[illegible]
[illegible]
[illegible]
[illegible]

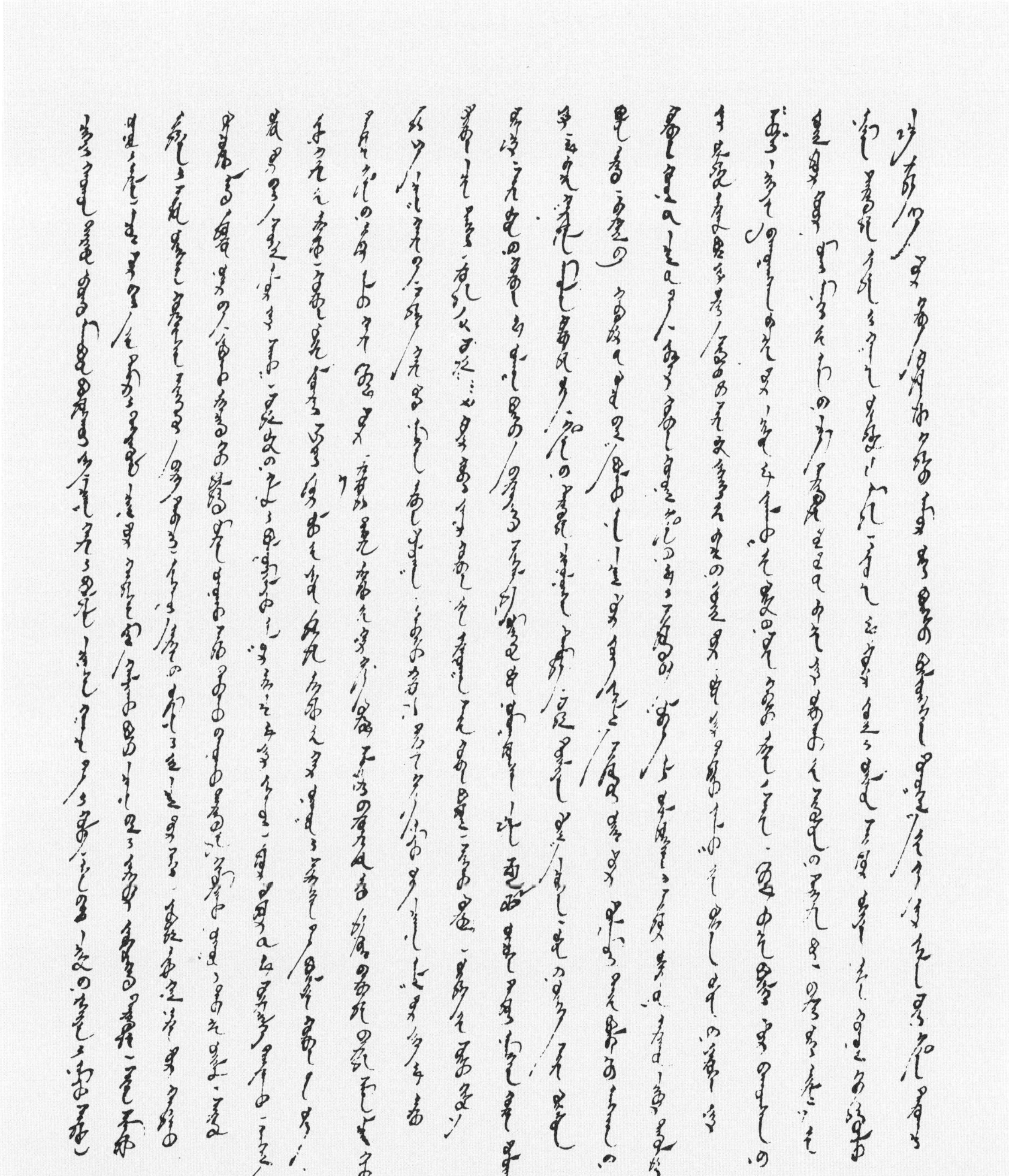

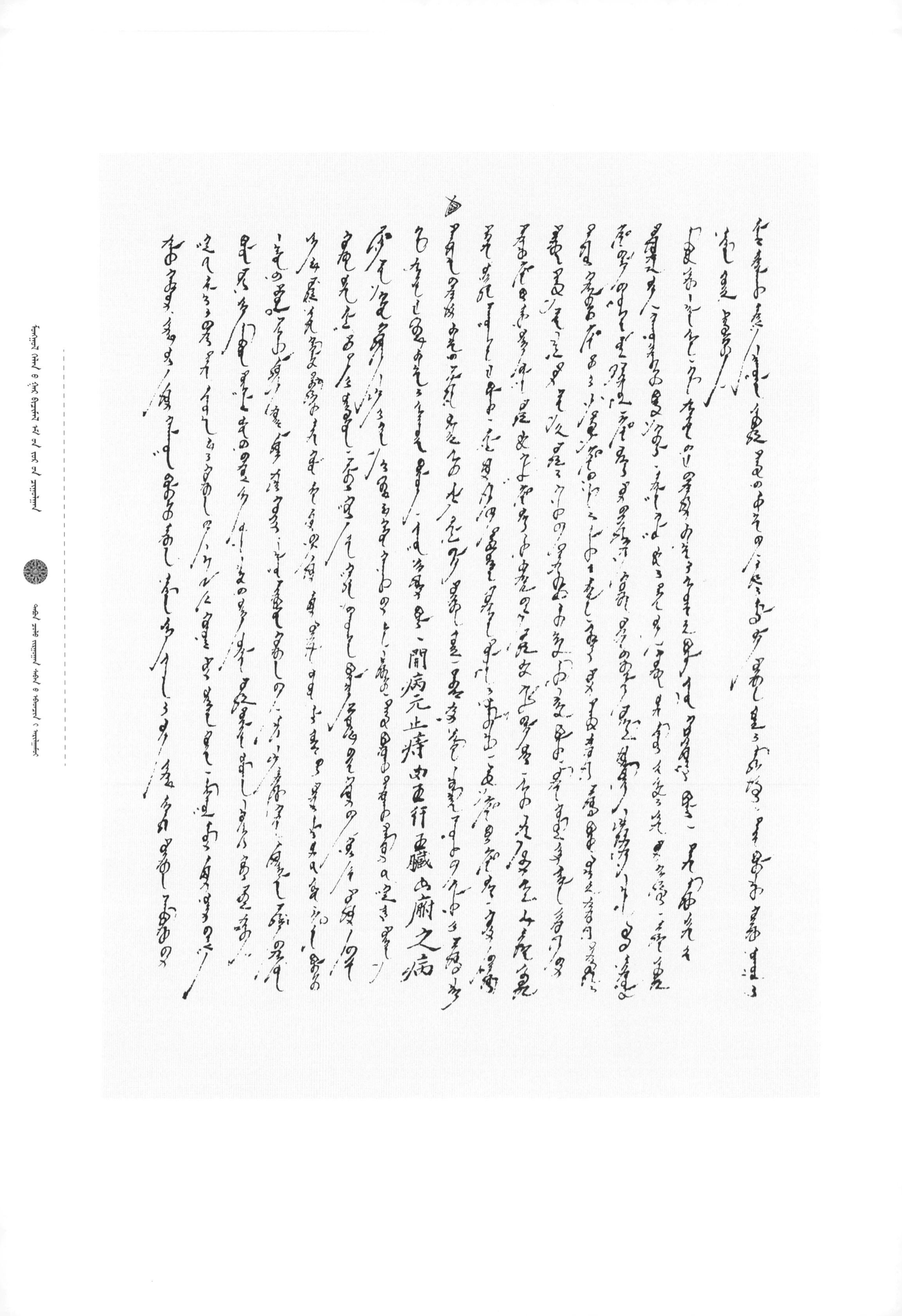

開病元止痔由五行五臟由腑之病

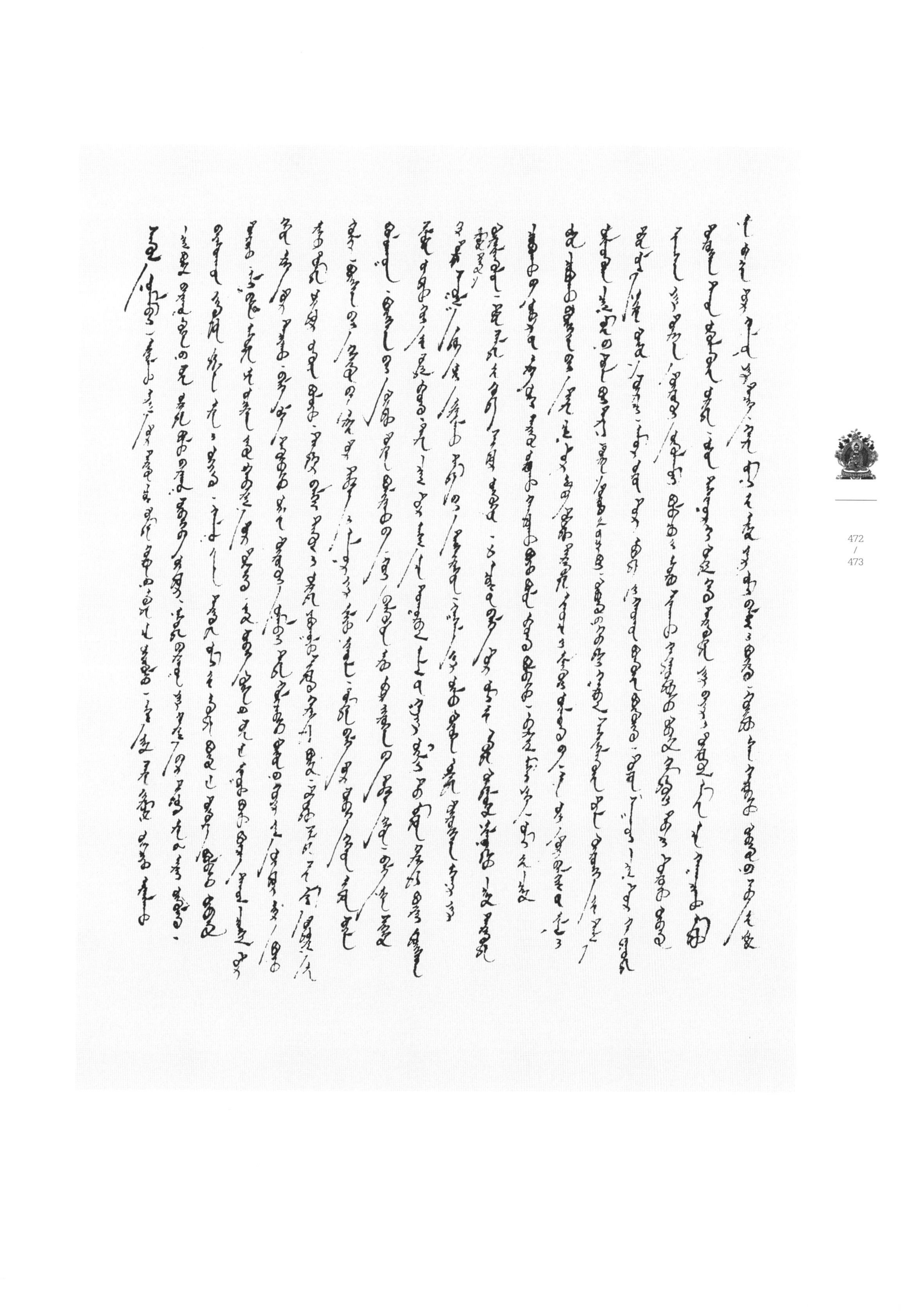

[illegible]

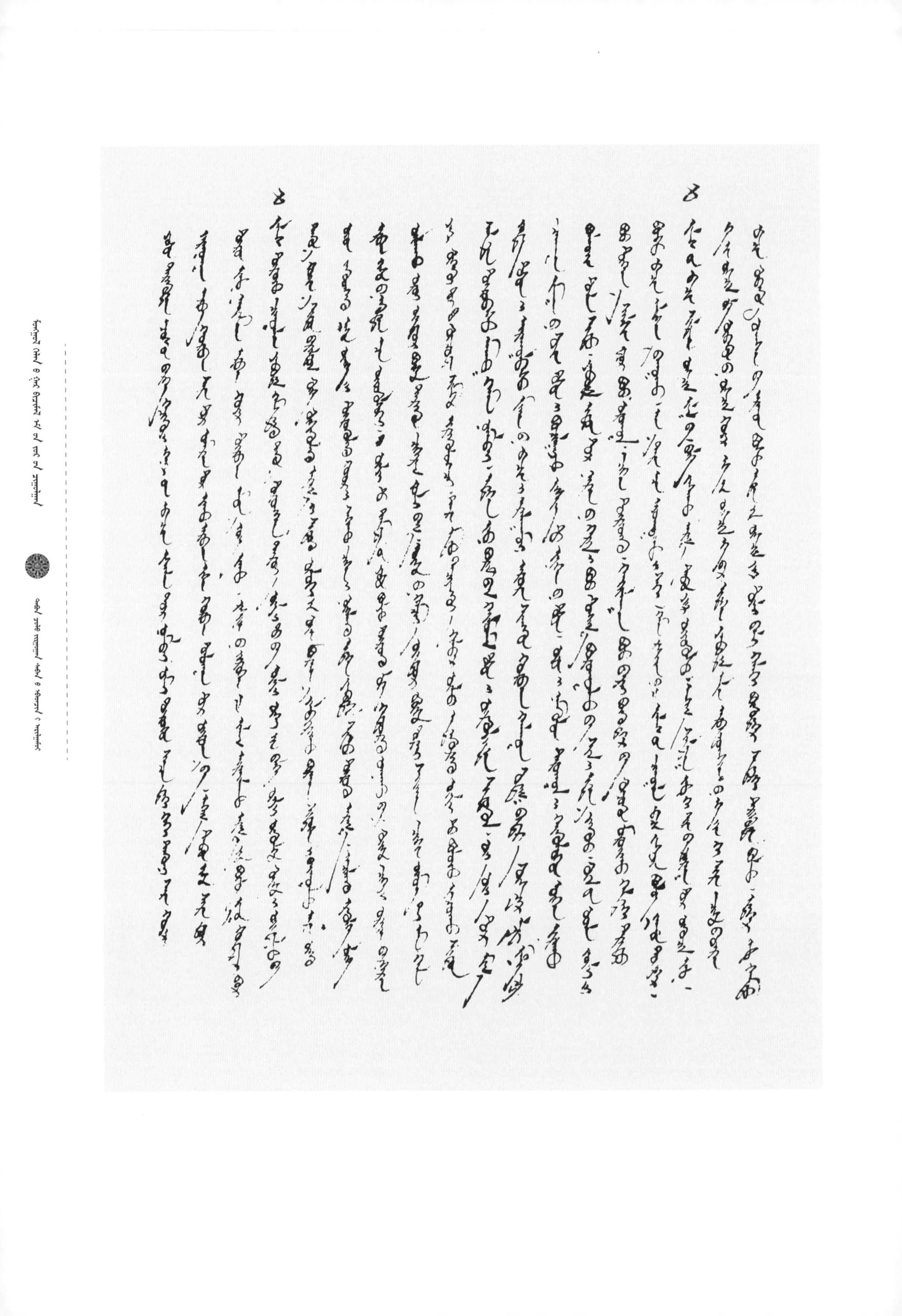

[illegible]

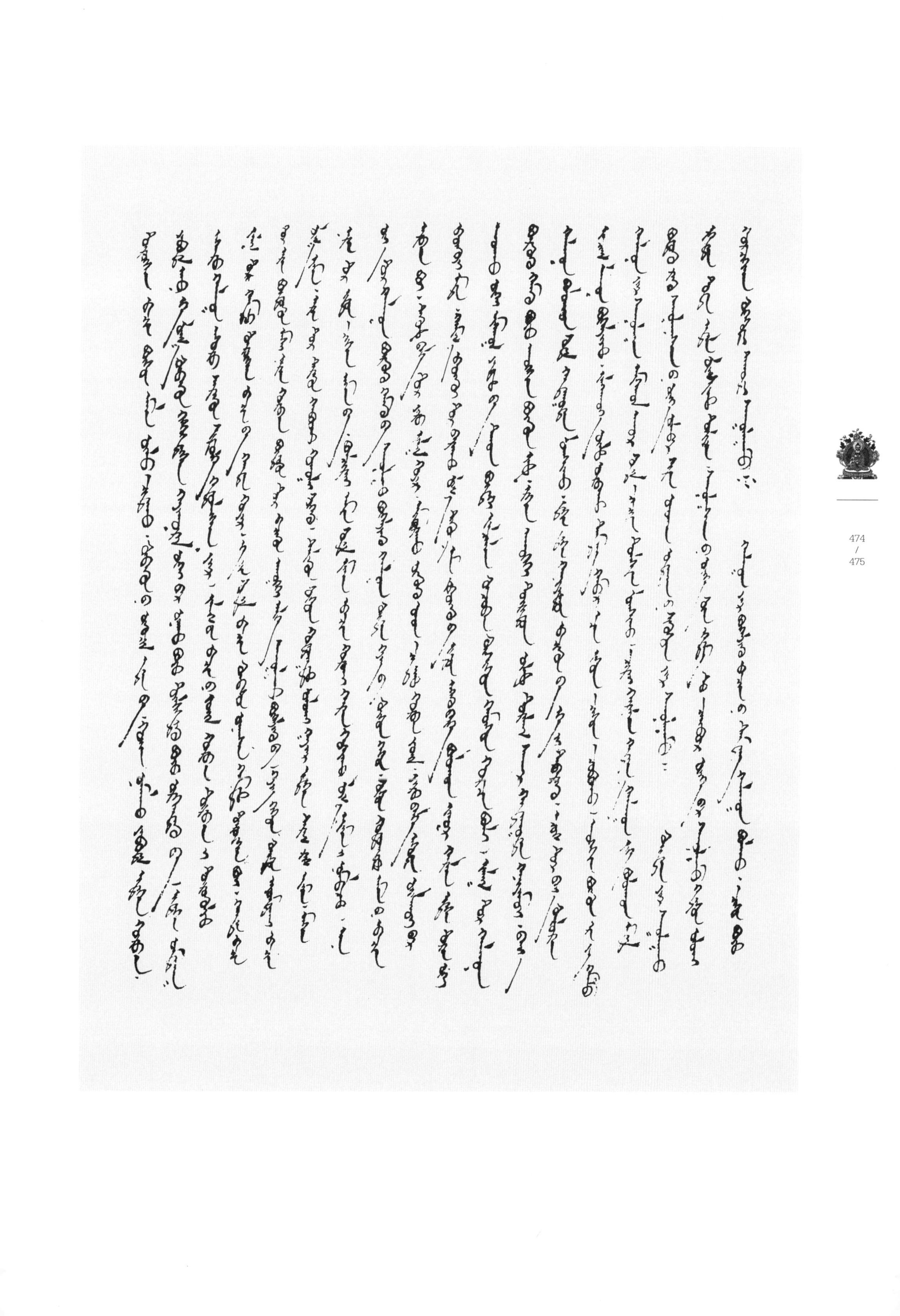

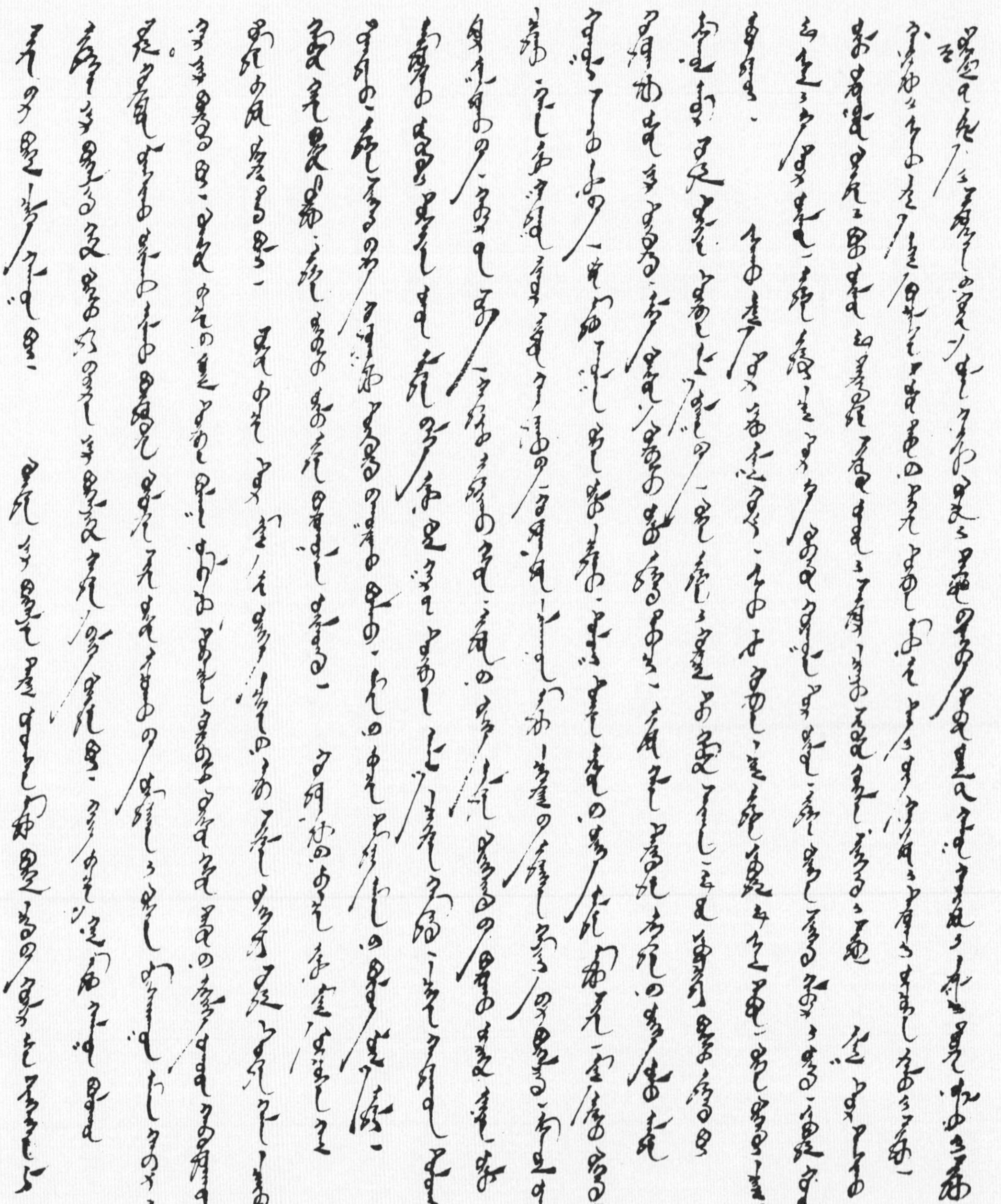

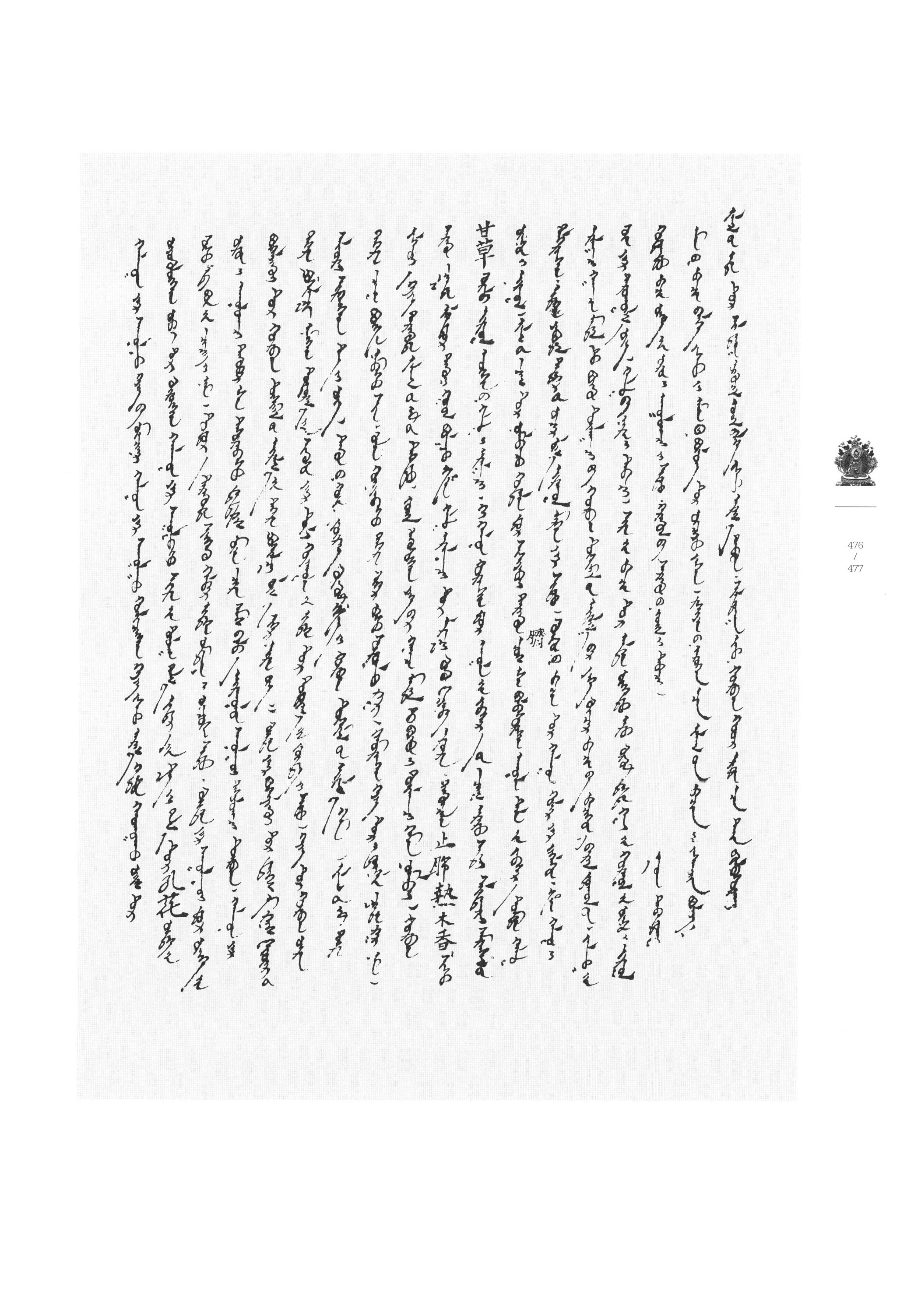

[illegible]

甘草 [illegible] 臍 [illegible]

[illegible] 上肺熱 [illegible] 木香 [illegible]

[illegible] 孔花 [illegible]

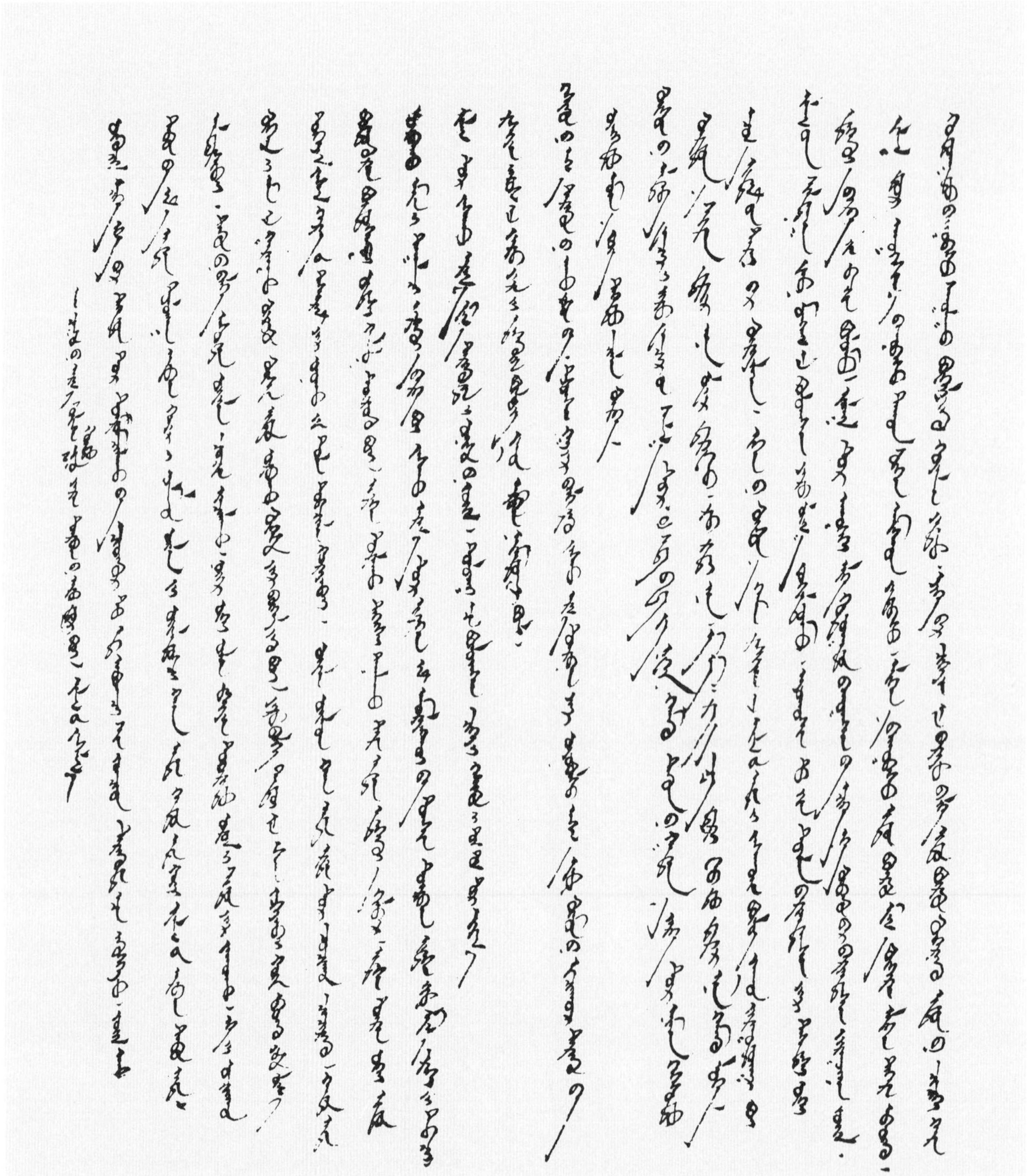

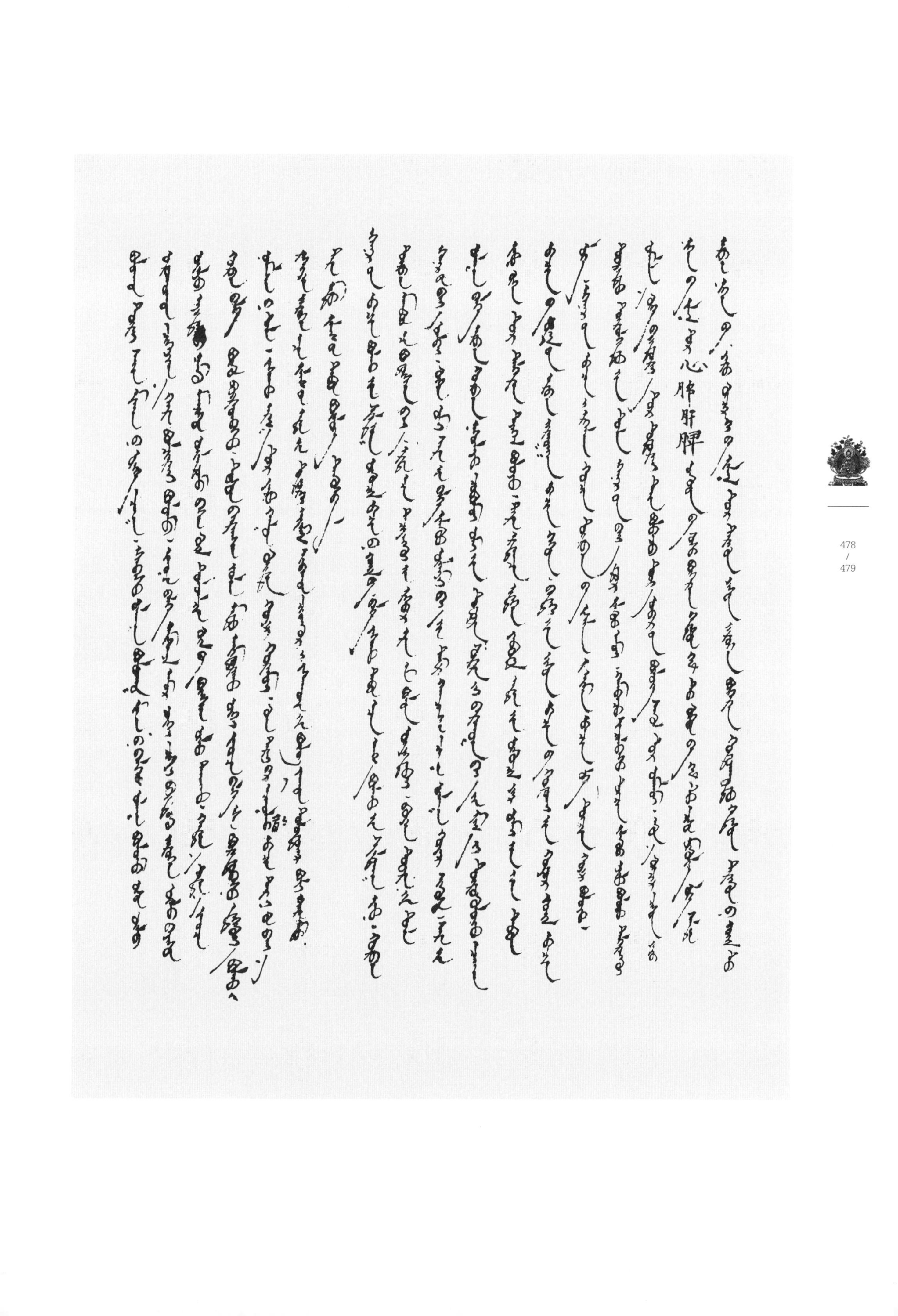

心肺肝脾

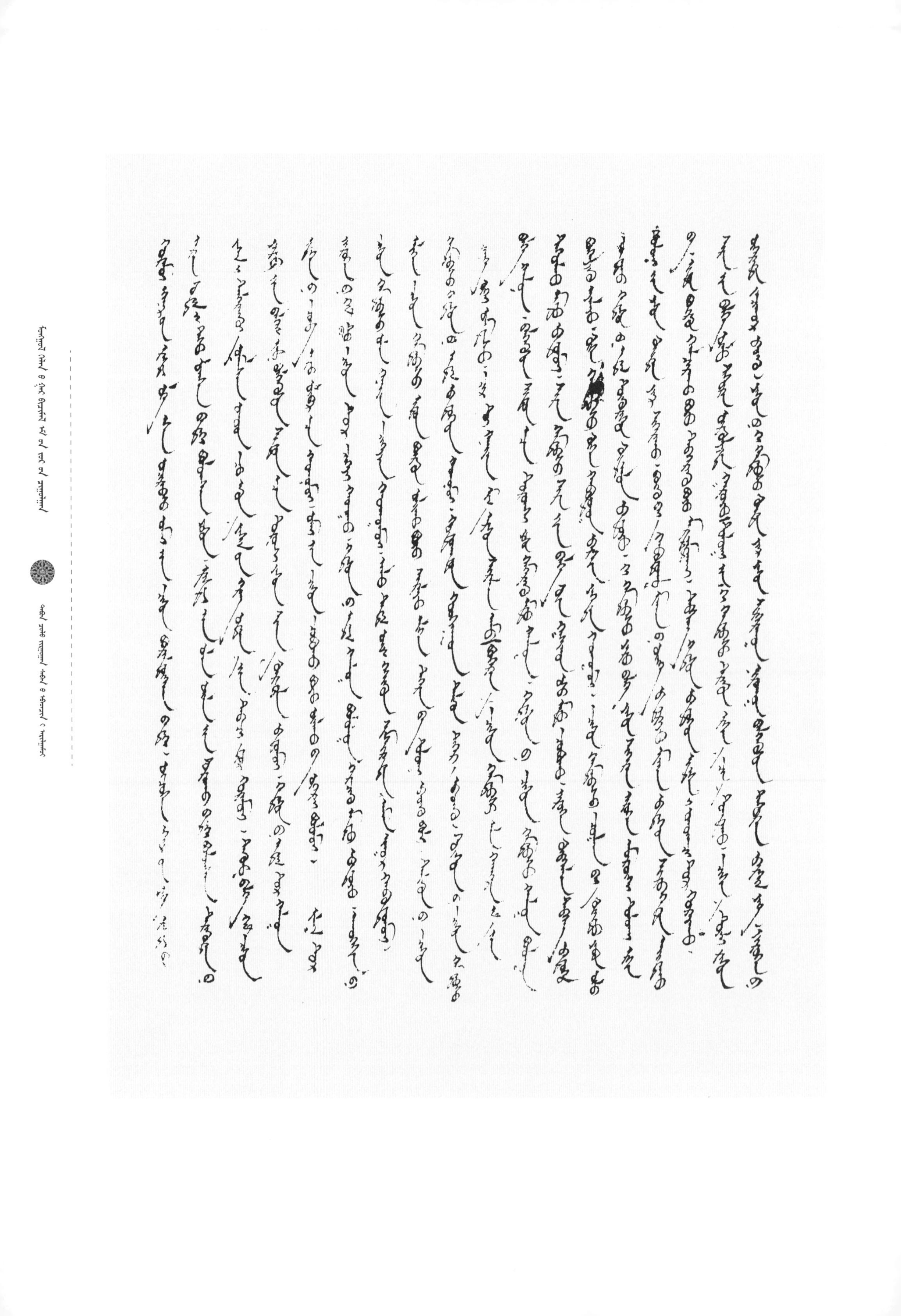

[illegible]

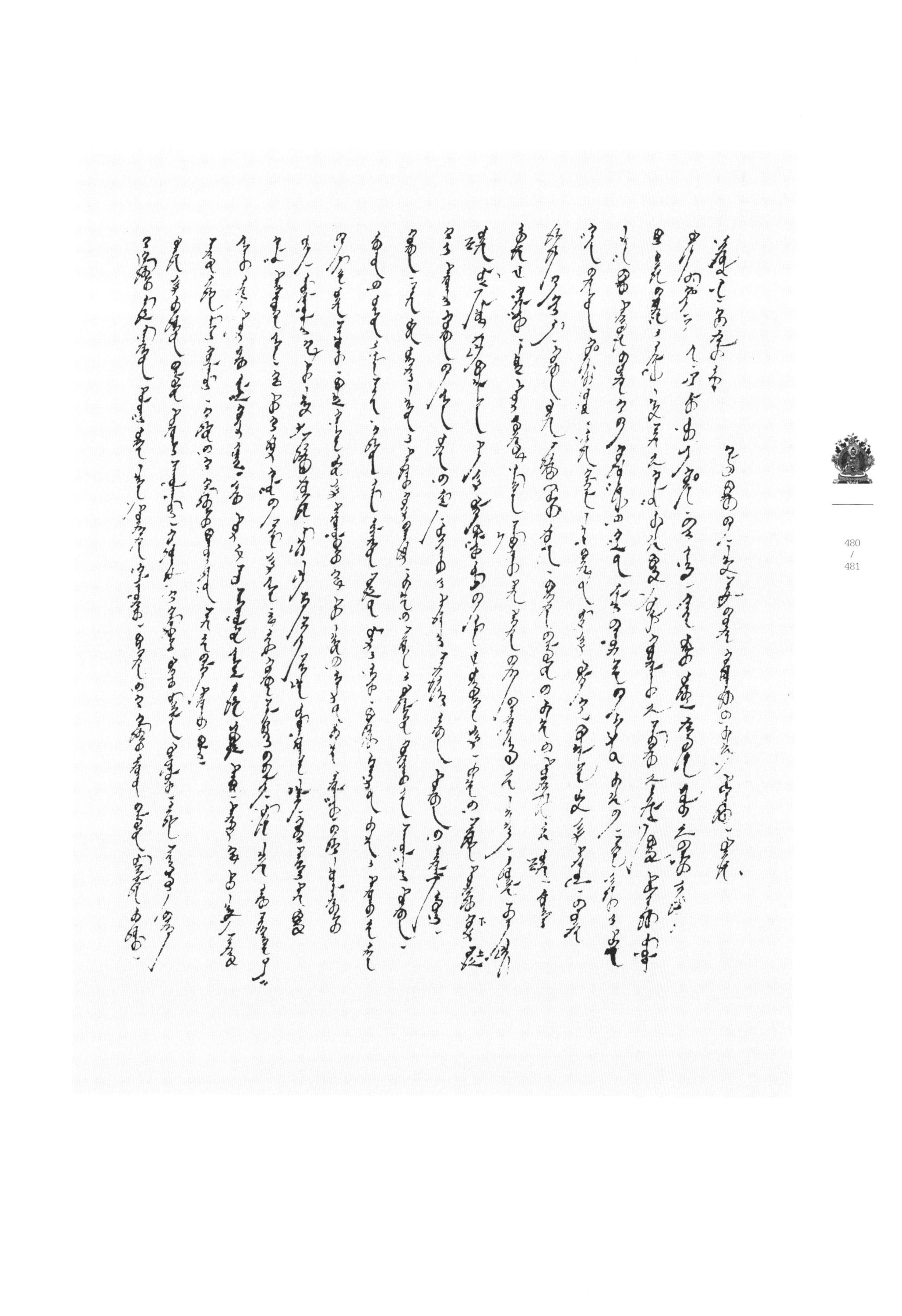

[illegible]

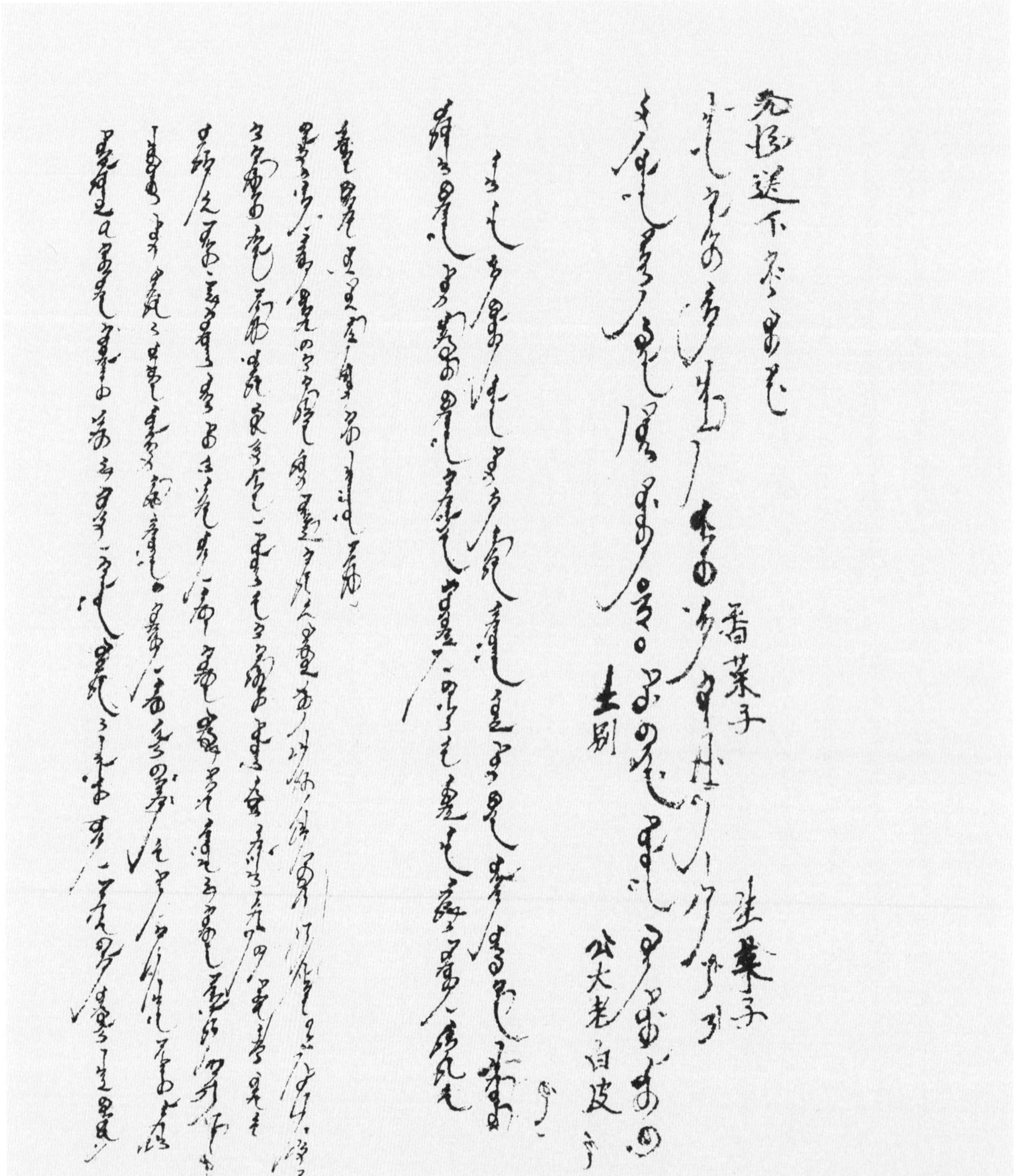
香菜子
公大老白皮

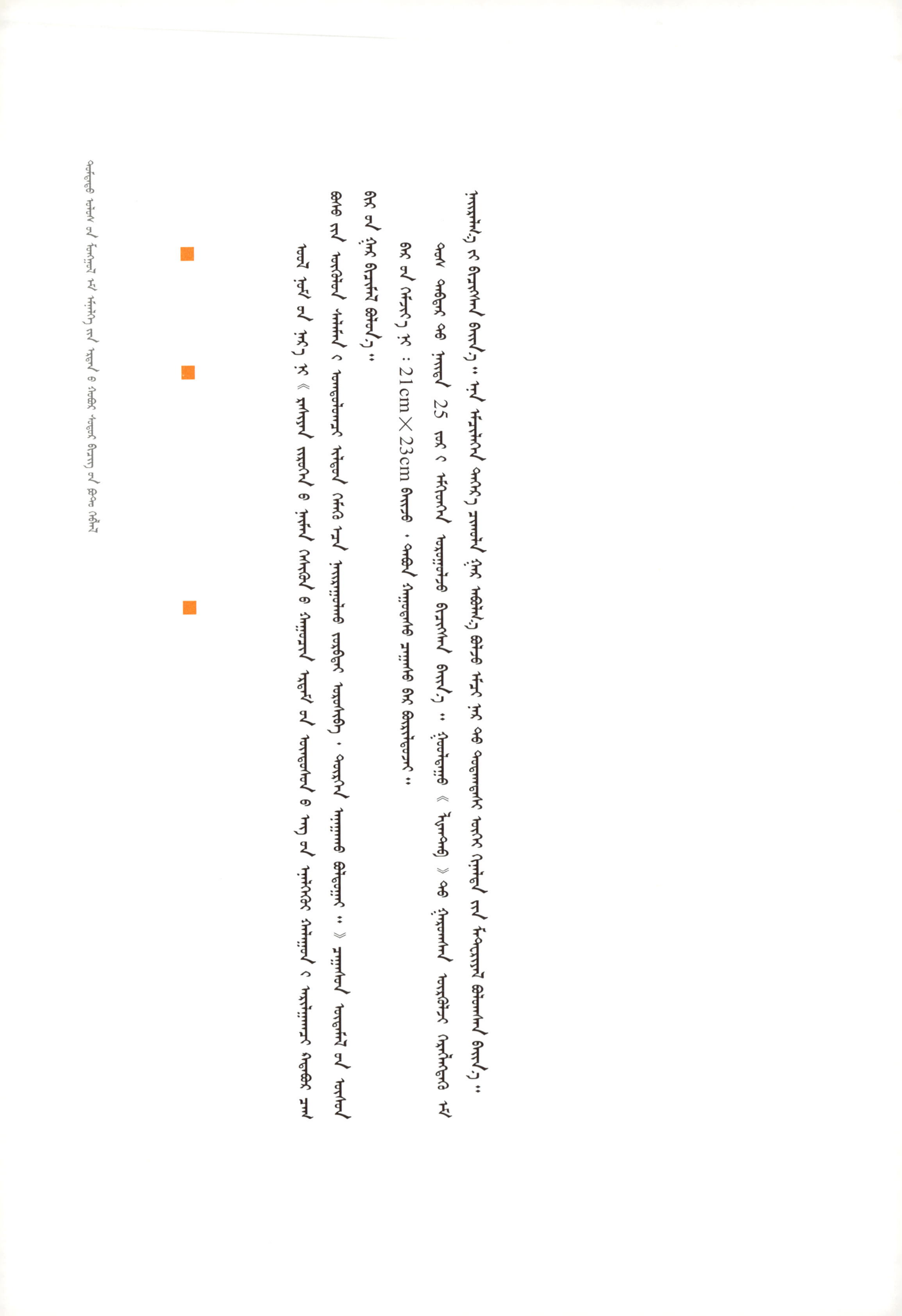

ᠪᠣᠳᠣ ᠶᠢᠨ ᠬᠡᠮᠵᠢᠶ᠎ᠡ ᠨᠢ : 21cm×23cm ᠪᠣᠯᠤᠭᠰᠠᠨ᠂ ᠮᠣᠩᠭᠣᠯ ᠦᠰᠦᠭᠡᠷ ᠪᠢᠴᠢᠭᠳᠡᠭᠰᠡᠨ ᠪᠣᠯᠪᠠᠴᠤ ᠨᠢᠭᠡ ᠪᠣᠯᠳᠠᠭ᠃

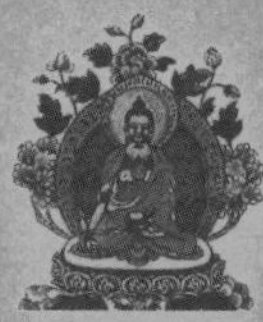

Prescriptions of Lhan Thabs

兰塔布之药方

《ᠯᠠᠨᠲᠠᠪ》 ᠤᠨ [illegible]

11

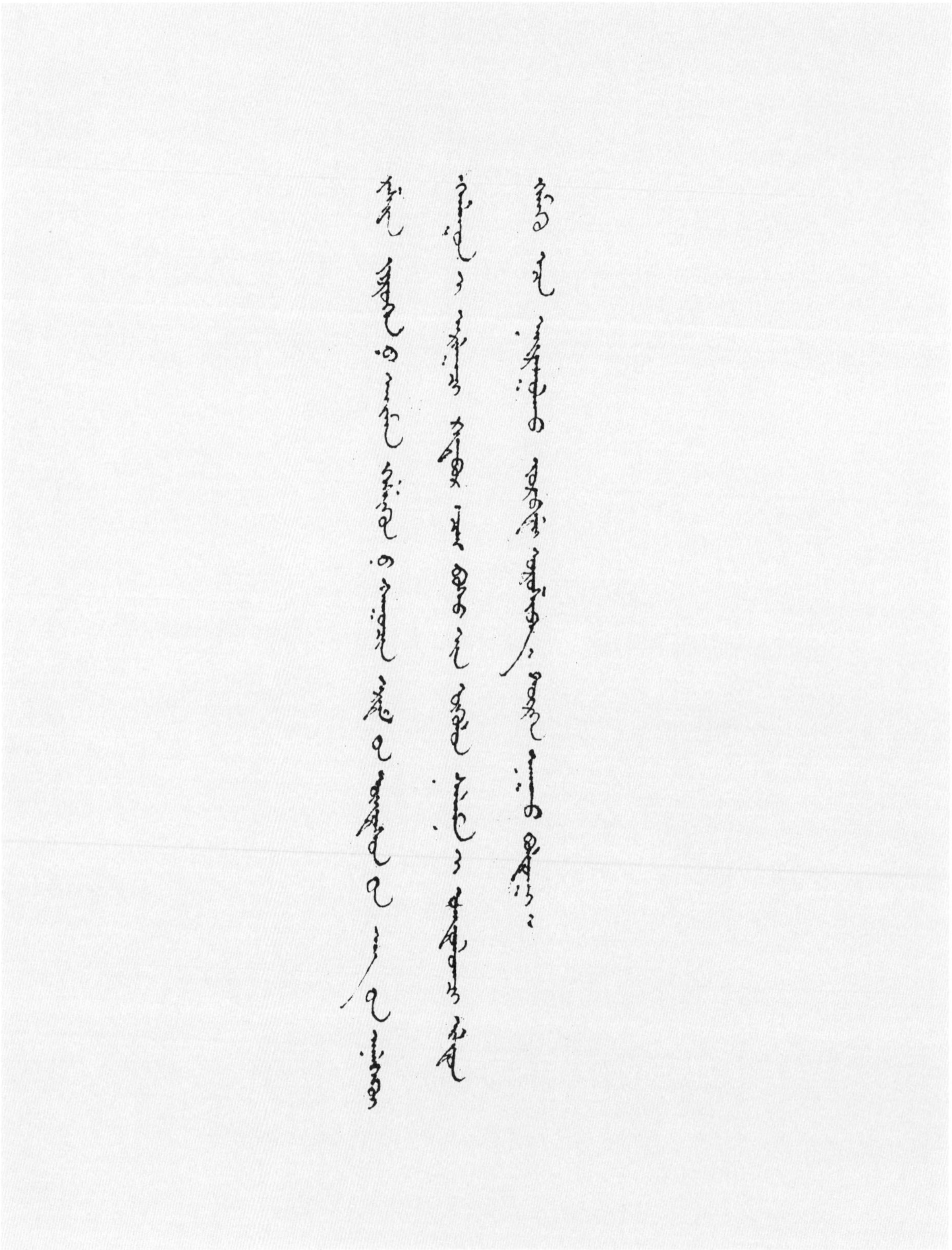

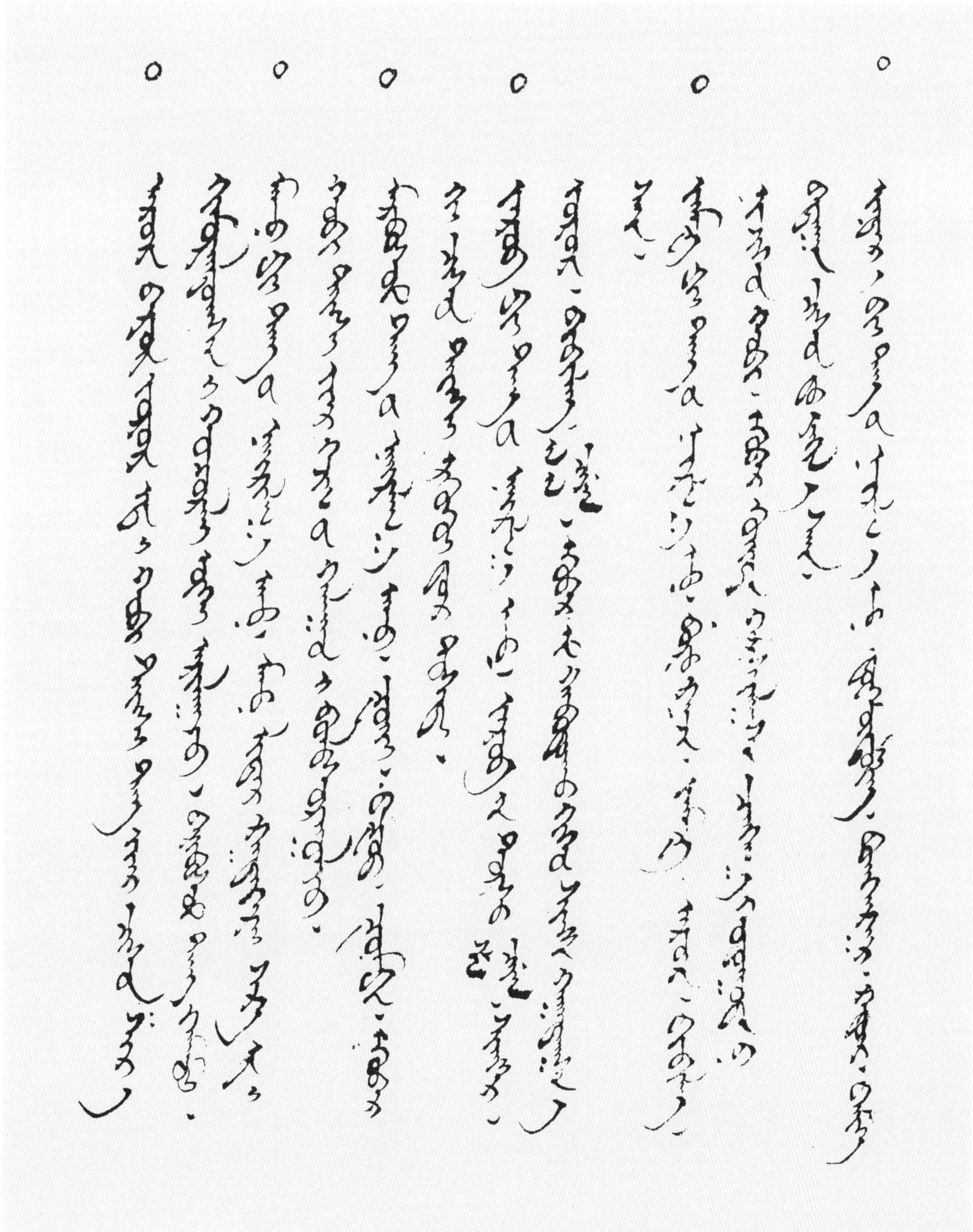

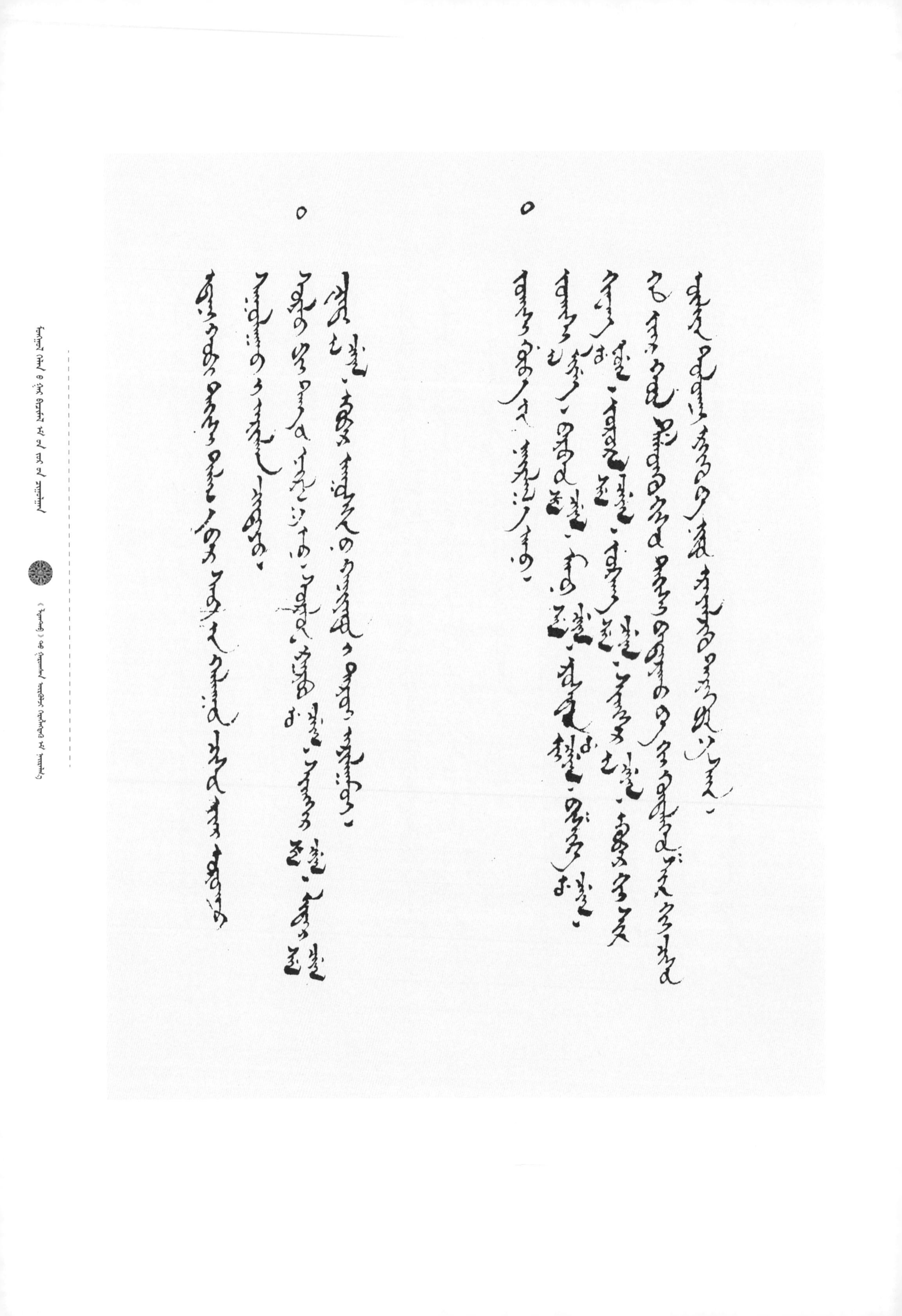

[illegible]

[illegible]

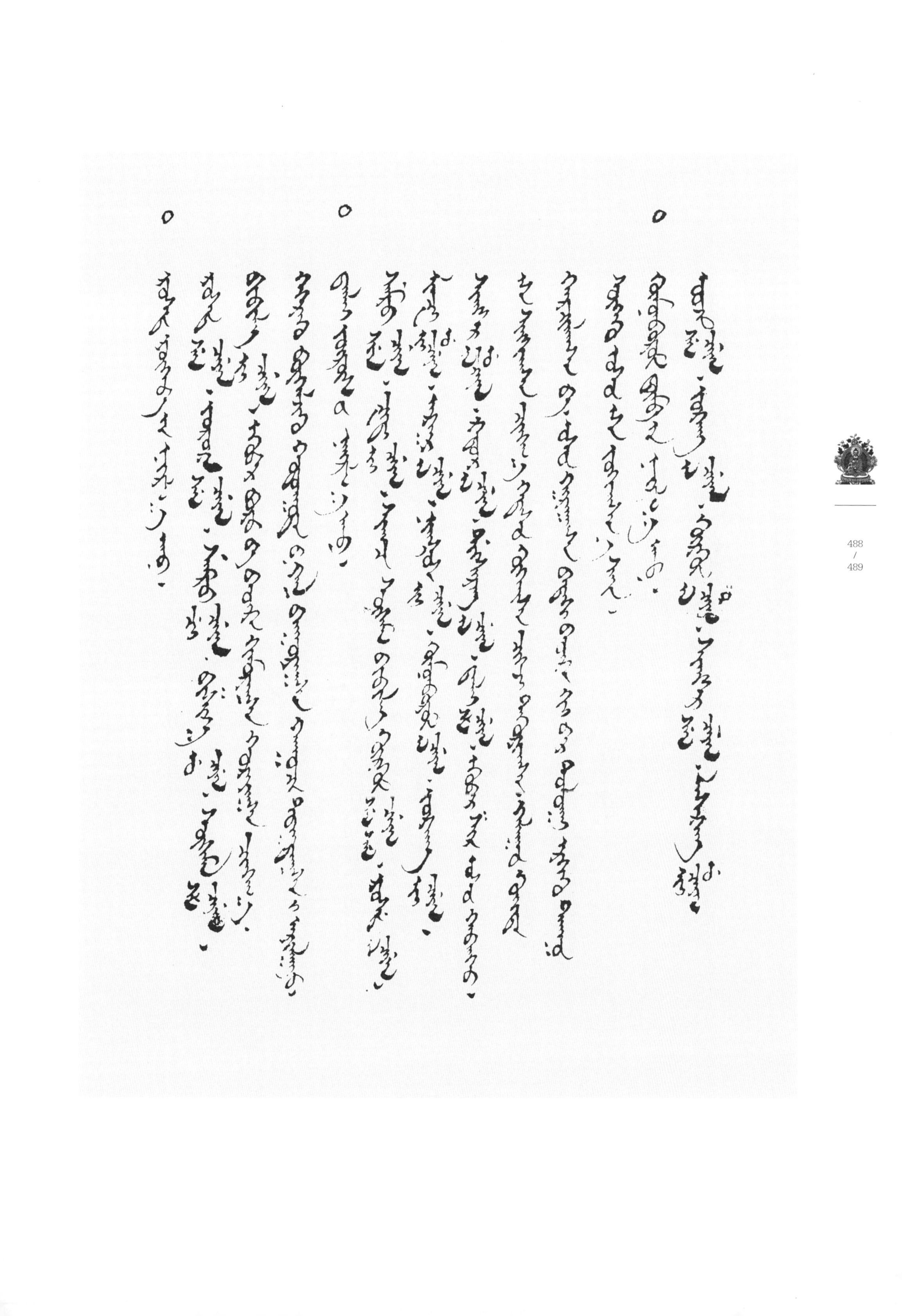

[illegible]

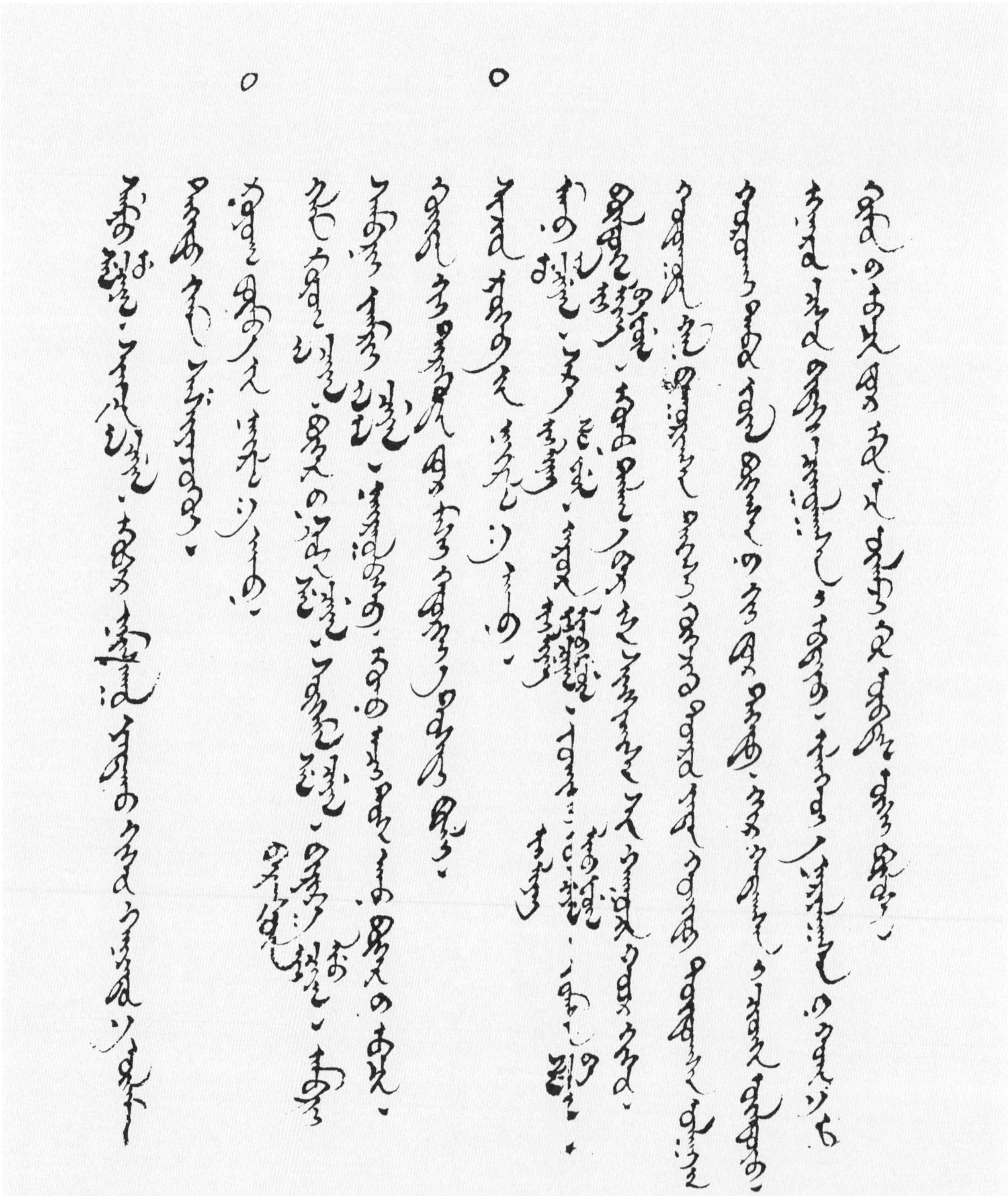

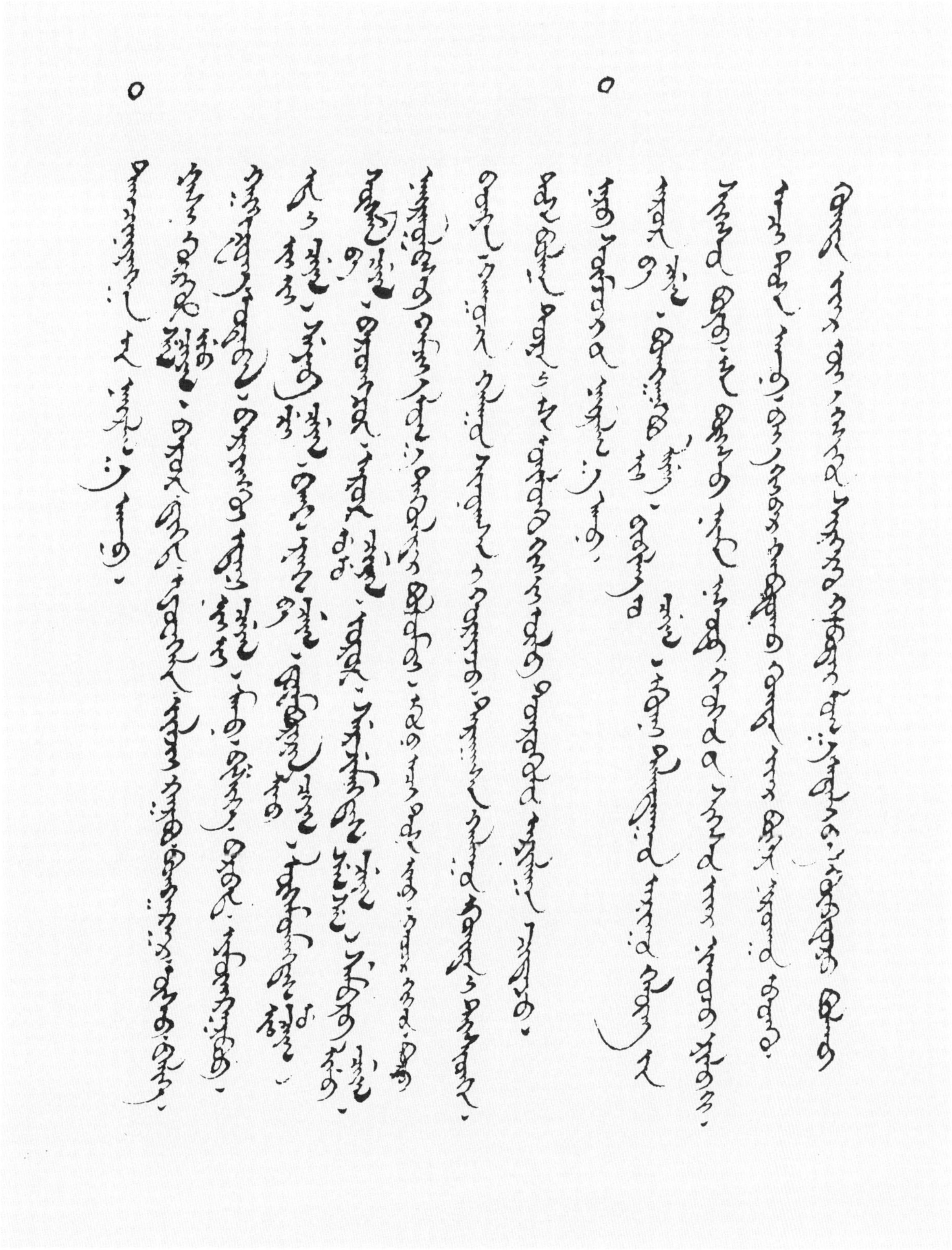

[illegible]

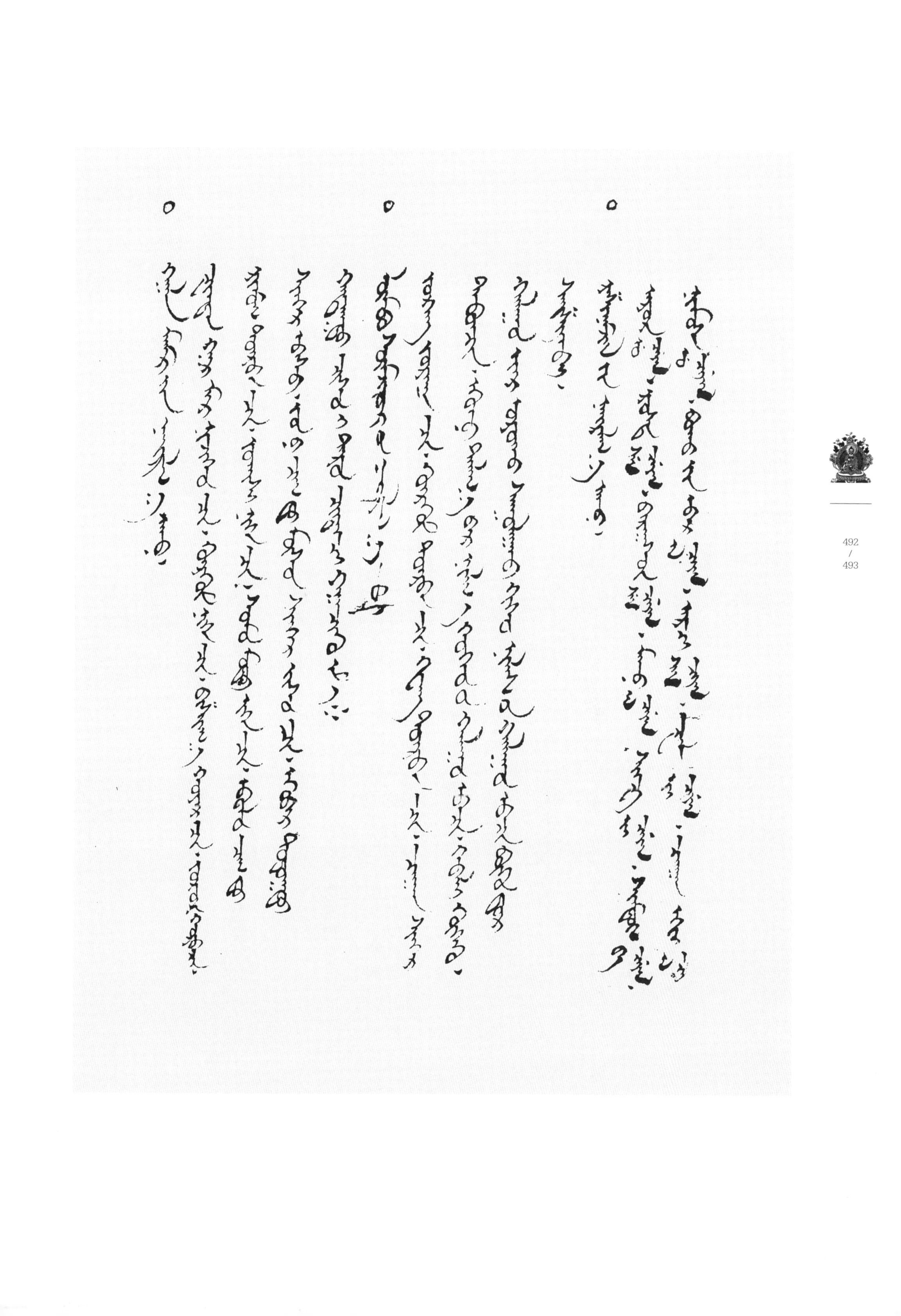

[illegible]

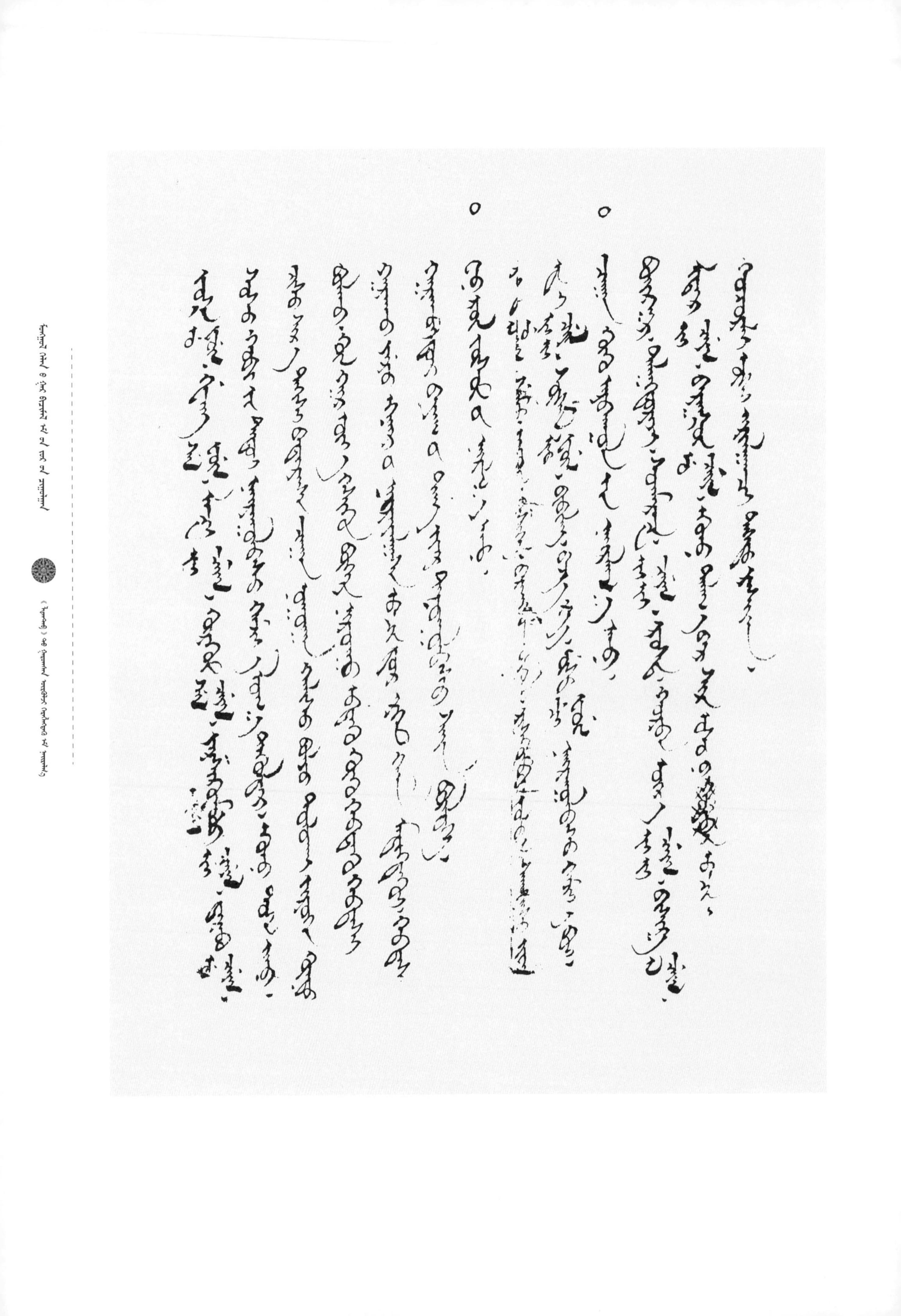

[illegible]
[illegible]
[illegible]
[illegible]
[illegible]
[illegible]
[illegible]
[illegible]
○ [illegible]
[illegible]
[illegible]
○ [illegible]
[illegible]
[illegible]
[illegible]

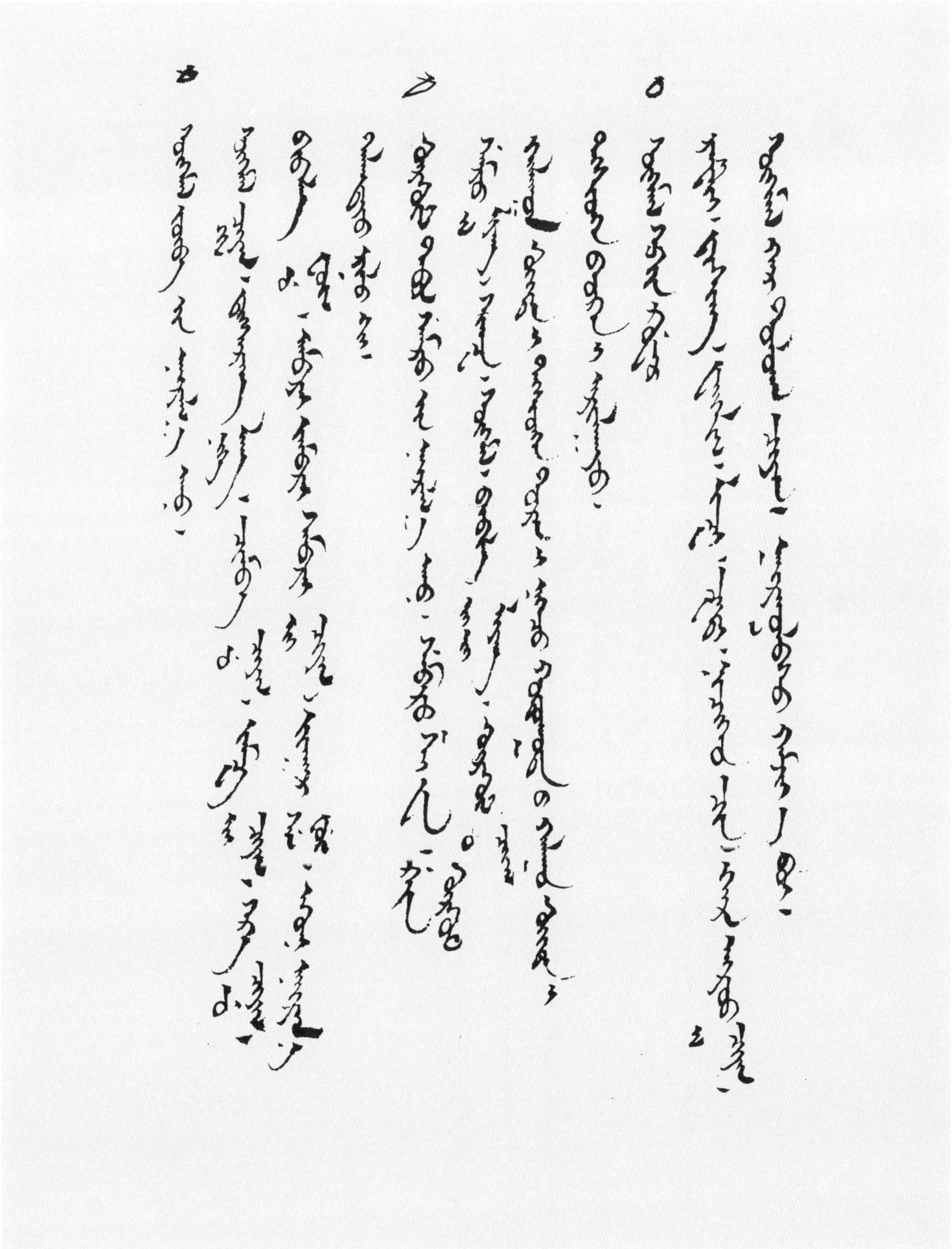

ᠬᠠᠷᠠᠨ ᠪᠢᠴᠢᠭ ᠦᠨ ᠬᠠᠪᠲᠠᠰᠤ ᠬᠠᠪᠲᠠᠰᠤᠨ ᠤ ᠨᠢᠭᠤᠷ ᠪᠢᠴᠢᠭᠰᠡᠨ ᠳᠡᠪᠲᠡᠷ ᠪᠣᠯᠤᠨ᠎ᠠ :: ᠲᠣᠪᠴᠢᠶᠠᠯᠠᠭᠰᠠᠨ ᠣᠨ ᠴᠠᠭ ᠢ ᠲᠣᠳᠣᠷᠬᠠᠢ ᠦᠭᠡᠢ :: ᠲᠣᠭᠠᠴᠠᠭᠠᠨ ᠤ ᠨᠢᠭᠤᠷ ᠬᠠᠭᠤᠳᠠᠰᠤ ᠶᠢᠨ ᠨᠢ ᠲᠣᠪᠴᠢᠶᠠᠯᠠᠯᠲᠠ《ᠲᠡᠩᠭᠡᠷ ᠪᠣᠷᠬᠠᠨ ᠤ ᠲᠣᠭᠠᠨ ᠤ ᠨᠢ ᠡᠳ ᠦᠨ ᠳᠡᠪᠲᠡᠷ》ᠭᠡᠵᠦ ᠲᠡᠮᠳᠡᠭᠯᠡᠭᠰᠡᠨ ᠪᠣᠯᠤᠨ᠎ᠠ ::

ᠪᠢᠴᠢᠭ ᠦᠨ ᠬᠡᠮᠵᠢᠶ᠎ᠡ ᠨᠢ : 22cm × 24.5cm ᠪᠣᠯᠤᠨ ᠂ ᠮᠥᠷ 38 ᠨᠢᠭᠤᠷ ᠲᠠᠢ ::

ᠨᠢᠭᠤᠷ ᠪᠦᠷᠢ ᠳᠦ ᠮᠥᠷ 33 ᠦᠰᠦᠭ ᠦᠨ ᠲᠣᠭ᠎ᠠ ᠲᠠᠢ (ᠨᠠᠢ) ᠢ ᠪᠢᠴᠢᠭᠰᠡᠨ ᠲᠡᠮᠳᠡᠭᠯᠡᠭᠰᠡᠨ ᠪᠣᠯᠤᠨ᠎ᠠ :: ᠨᠢᠭᠤᠷ ᠪᠦᠷᠢ ᠳᠦ ᠲᠣᠭᠠᠨ ᠤ ᠨᠢ ᠡᠳ ᠢ ᠪᠢᠴᠢᠭᠰᠡᠨ ᠲᠣᠪᠴᠢᠶᠠᠨ ᠪᠣᠯᠤᠨ᠎ᠠ :: ᠬᠠᠮᠲᠤ ᠲᠠᠢ ᠲᠣᠪᠴᠢᠶᠠᠯᠠᠭᠰᠠᠨ ᠤ ᠪᠡᠷ ᠭᠠᠭᠴᠠ ᠪᠡᠷ ᠢ ᠬᠡᠪᠯᠡᠵᠦ ᠂ ᠲᠣᠭᠠᠴᠠᠭᠰᠠᠨ ᠤ ᠲᠣᠭ᠎ᠠ ᠪᠠᠨ ᠤ ᠲᠡᠮᠳᠡᠭᠯᠡᠭᠰᠡᠨ ᠳᠦ ᠳᠠᠭᠠᠯᠳᠤᠭᠤᠯᠤᠭᠰᠠᠨ ᠨᠢᠭᠤᠷᠯᠠᠭᠰᠠᠨ ᠨᠢᠭᠤᠷᠯᠠᠭᠤᠯ ᠪᠣᠯᠤᠨ᠎ᠠ :: ᠲᠣᠭ᠎ᠠ ᠢ ᠢᠯᠡᠷᠭᠡᠢᠯᠡᠭᠰᠡᠨ ᠪᠠᠷᠢᠮᠲᠠ ᠪᠠᠢᠳᠠᠯ ᠢ

ᠰᠢᠯᠢᠭᠳᠡᠮᠡᠯ ᠪᠣᠯᠤᠨ᠎ᠠ ::

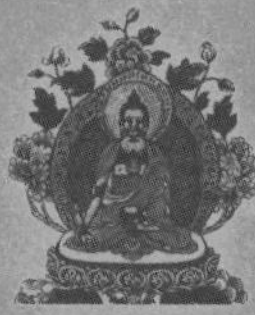

The Manual of Yaowang Miraculous Prescriptions

药王灵丹药方手册

12

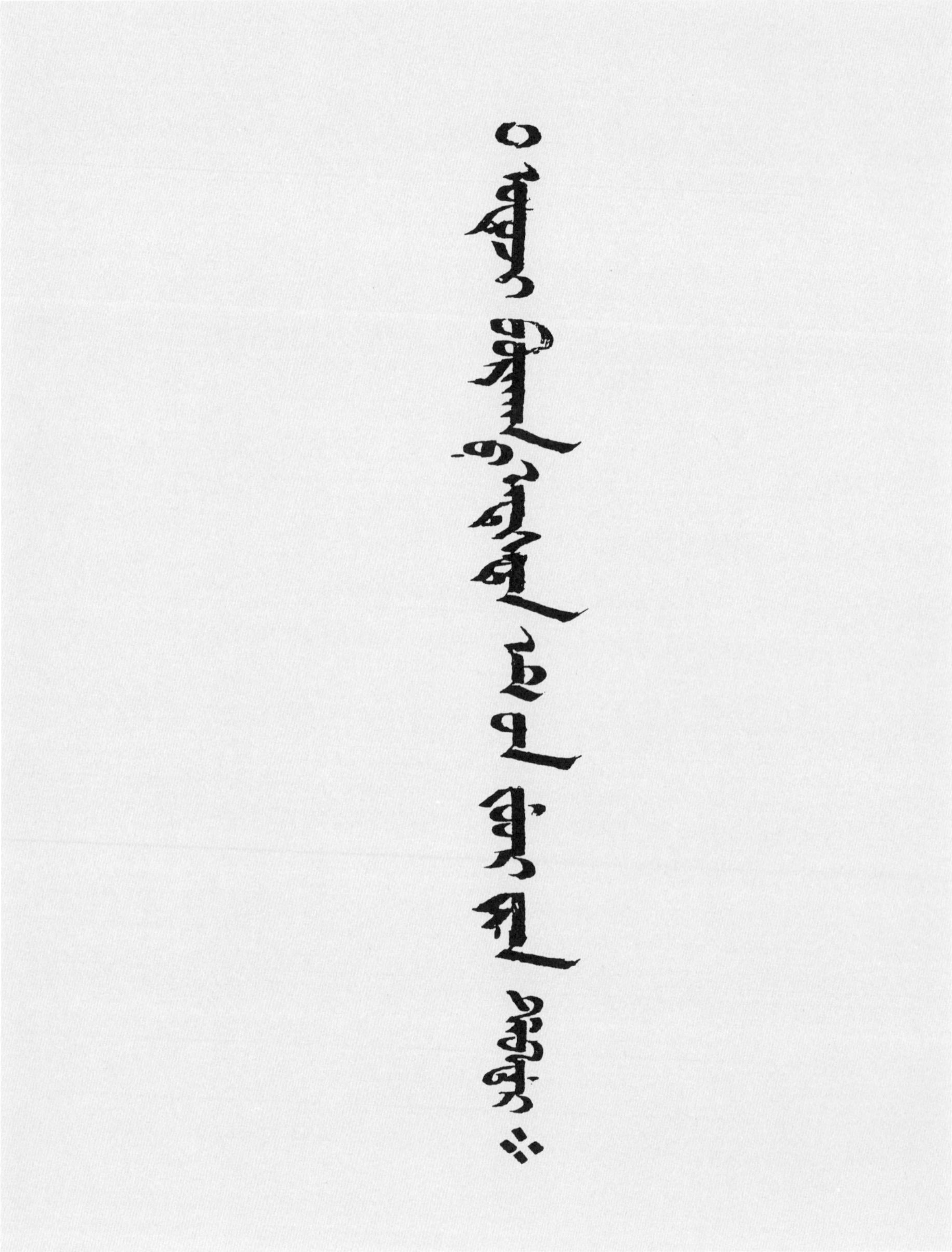

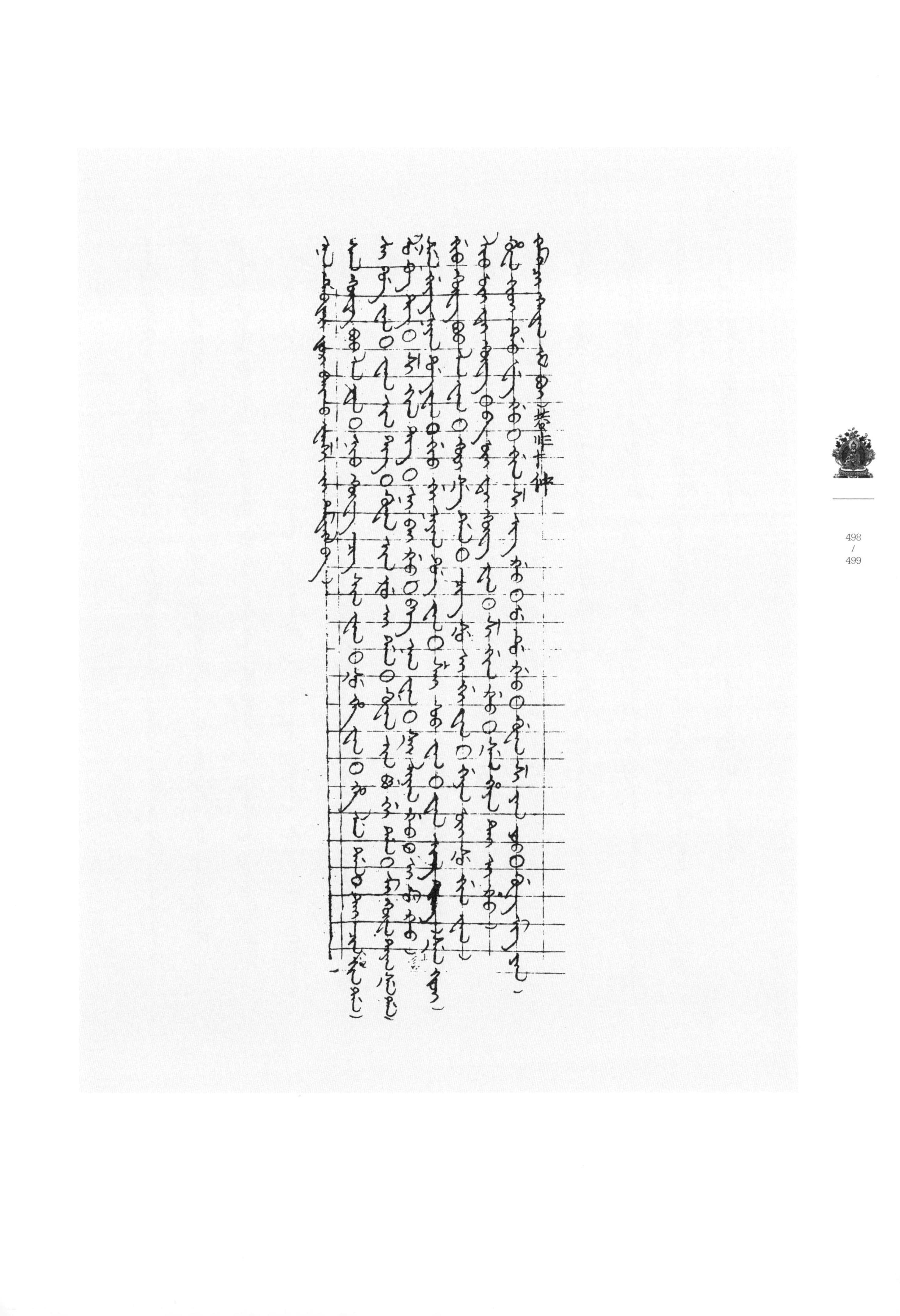

卷卌十一

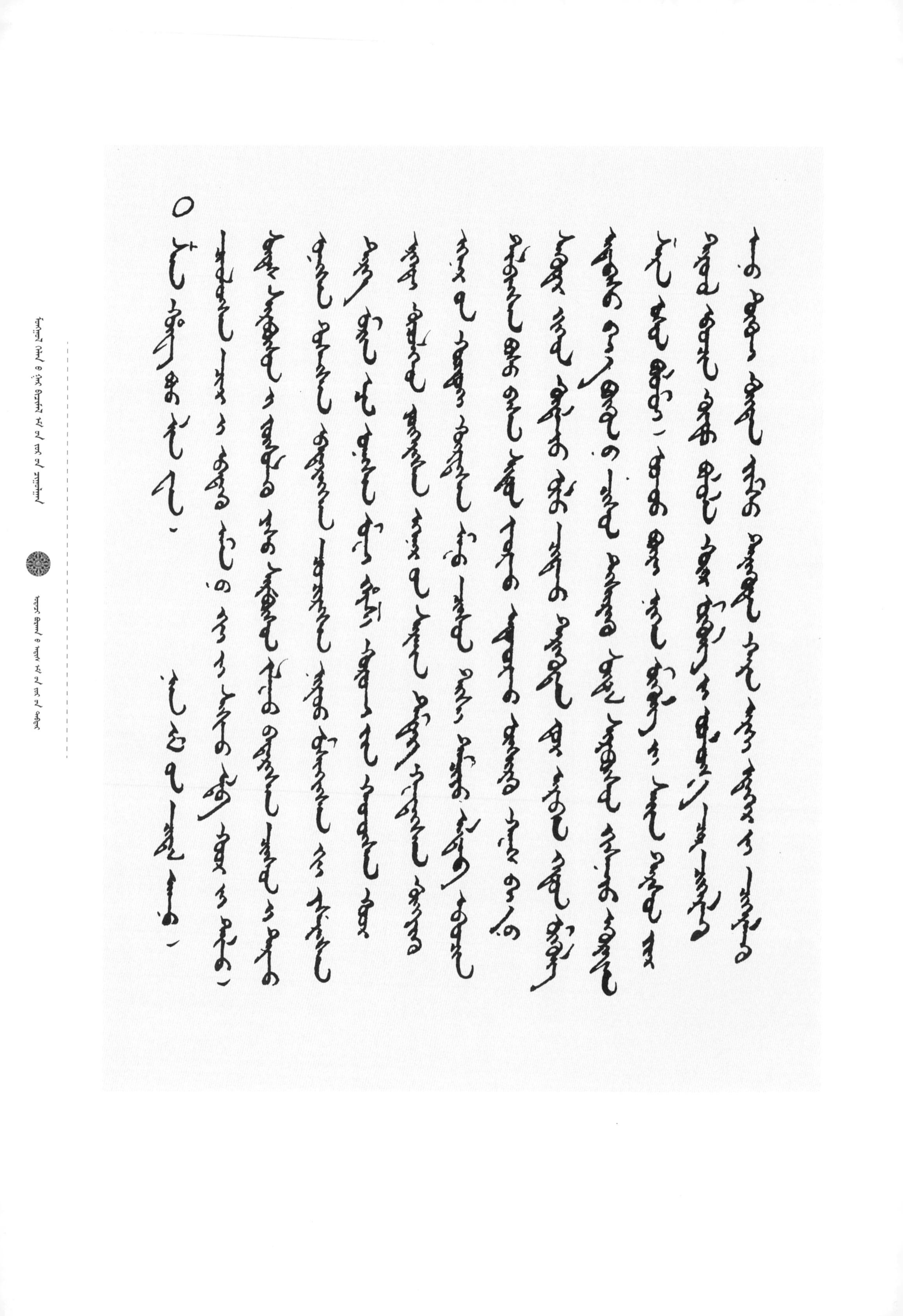

[illegible]

[illegible]

[illegible]

[illegible]

[illegible]

[illegible]

[illegible]

[illegible]

[illegible]

[illegible]

[illegible]

[illegible]

[illegible]

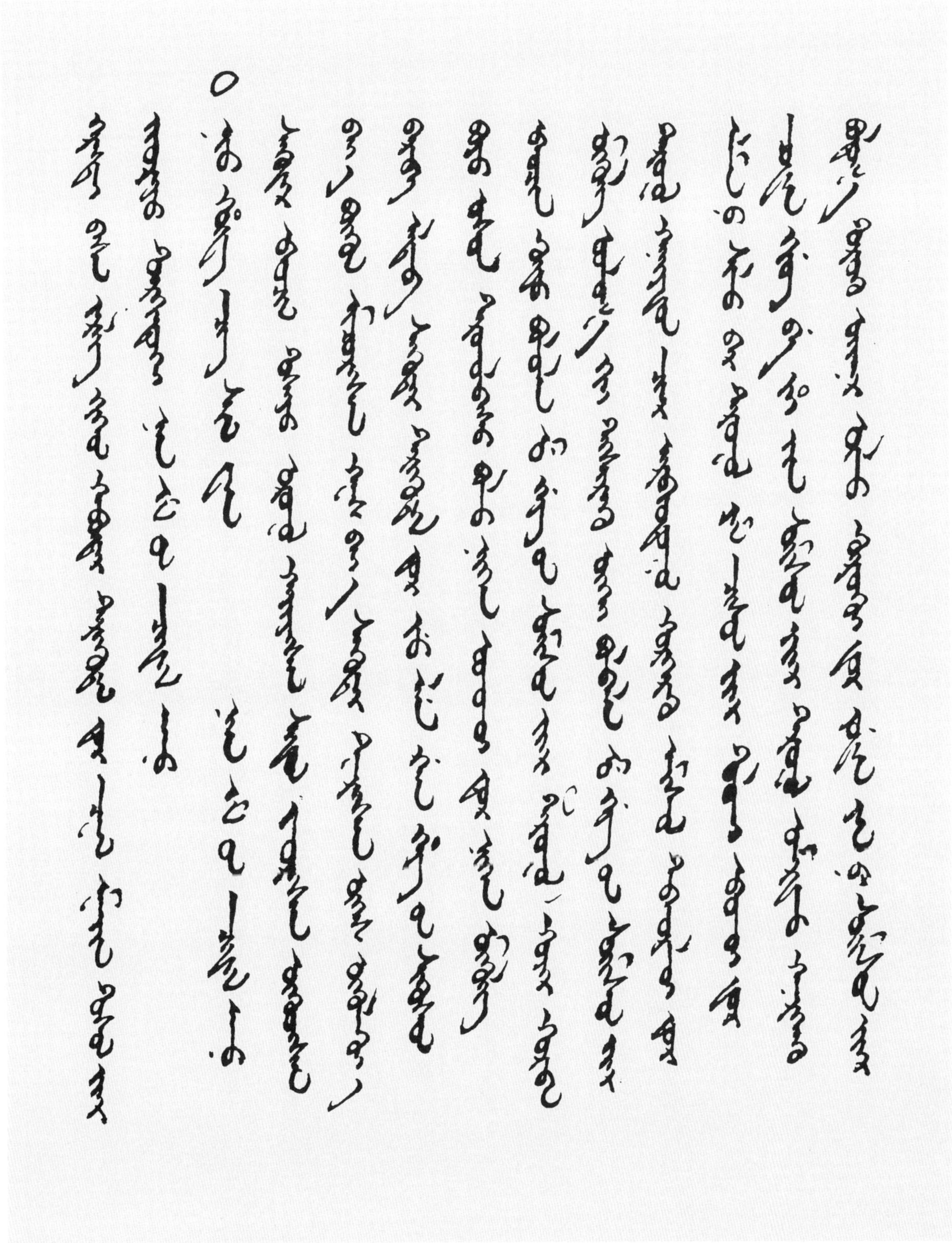

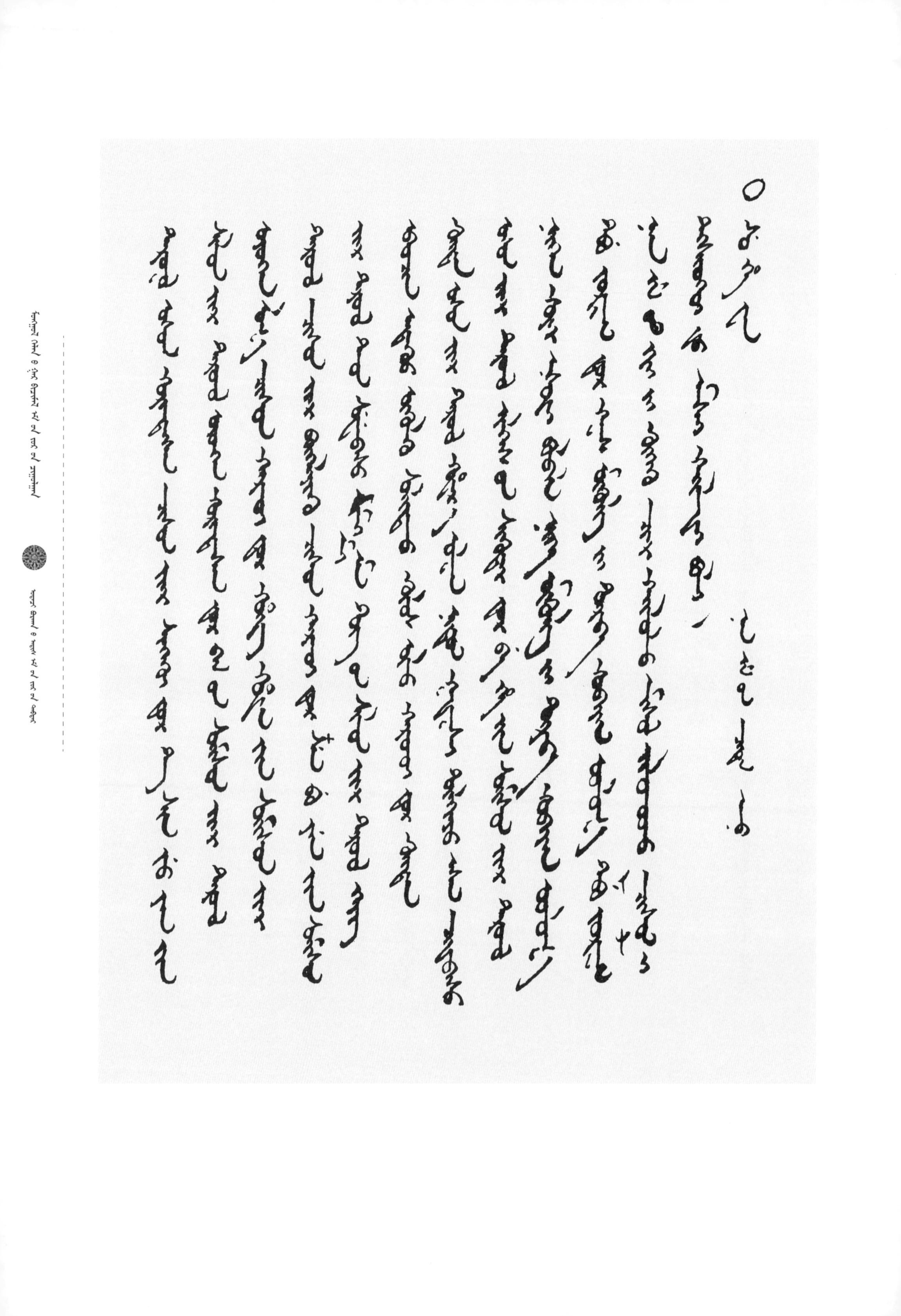

[illegible]

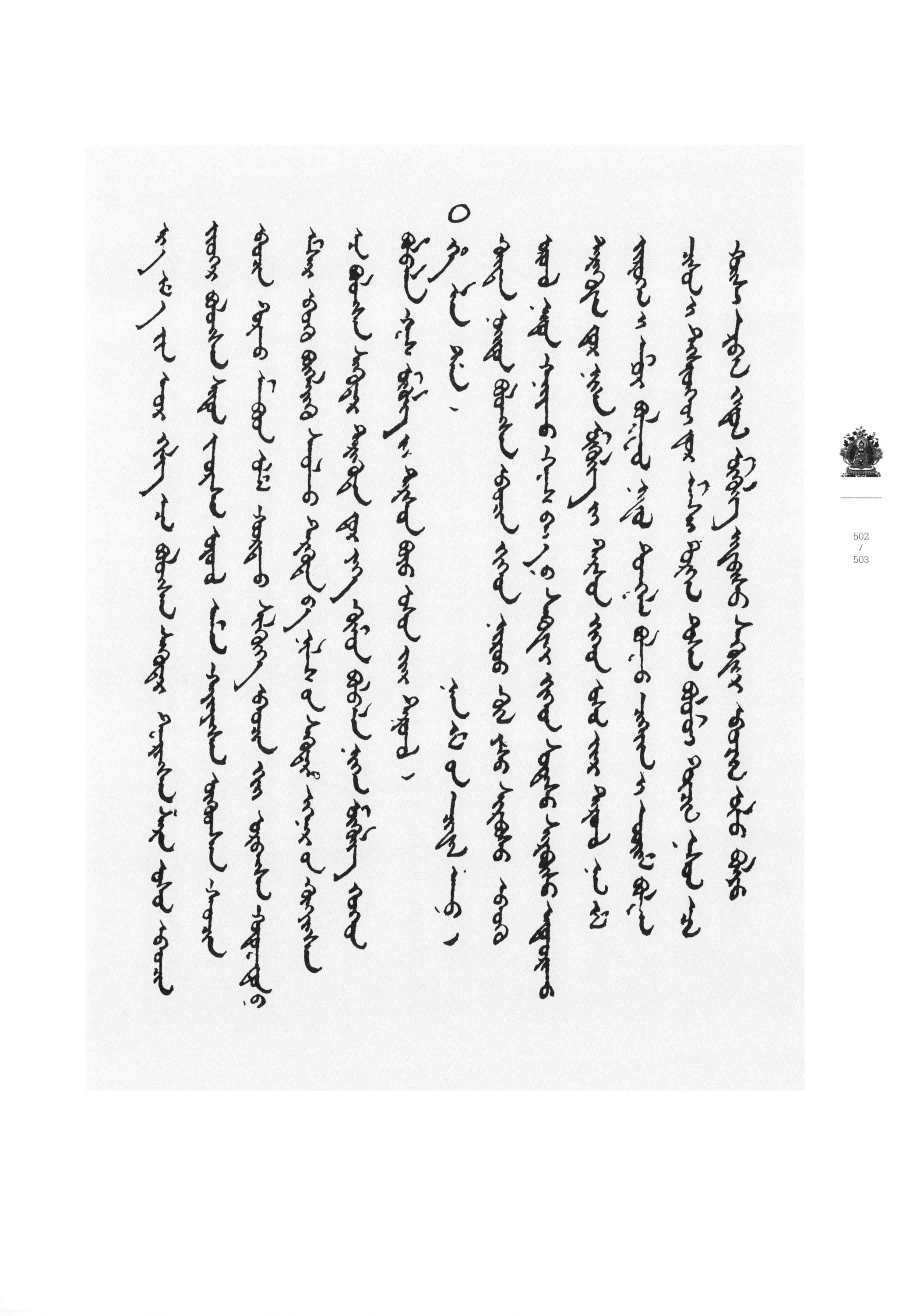

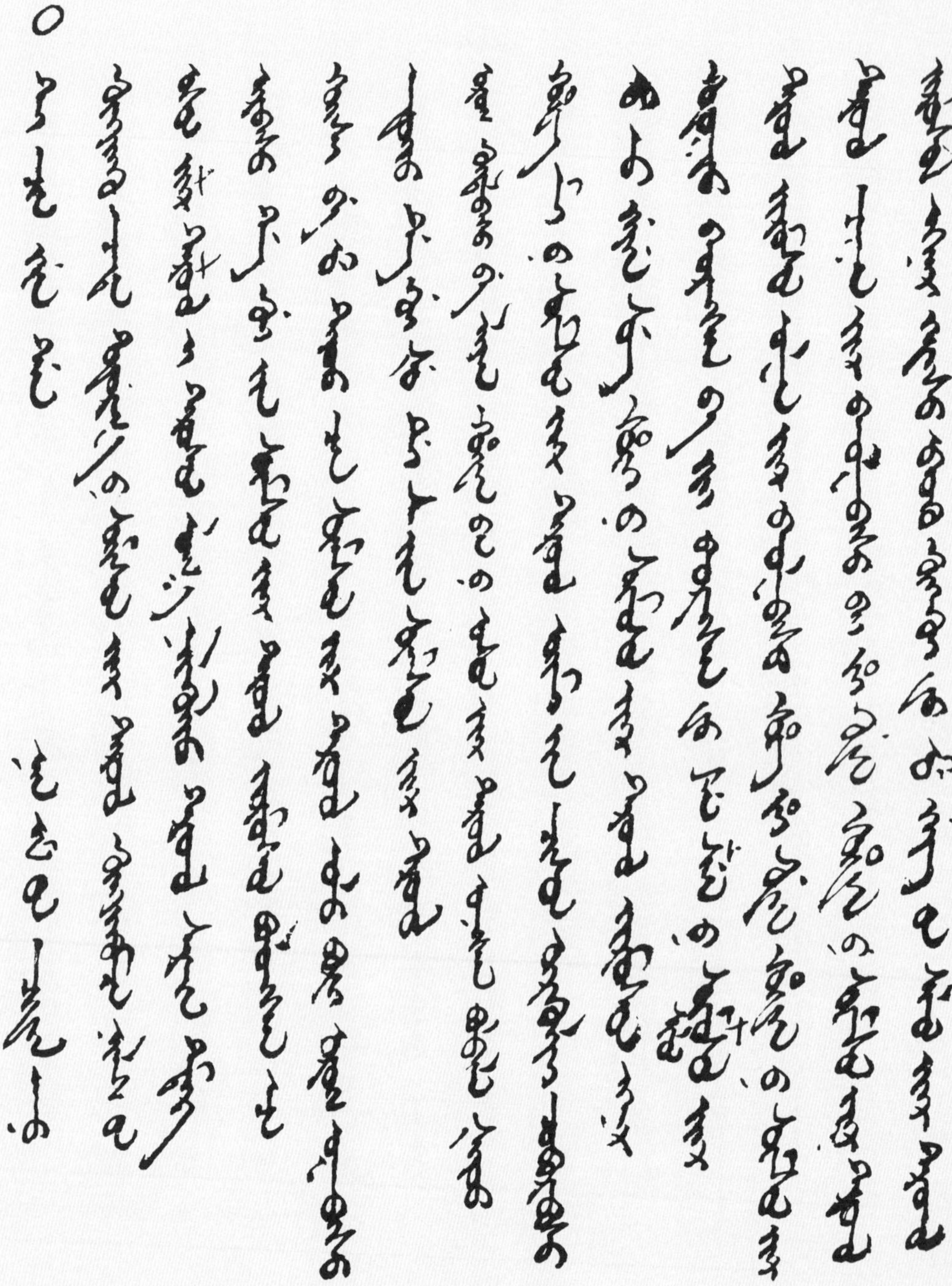

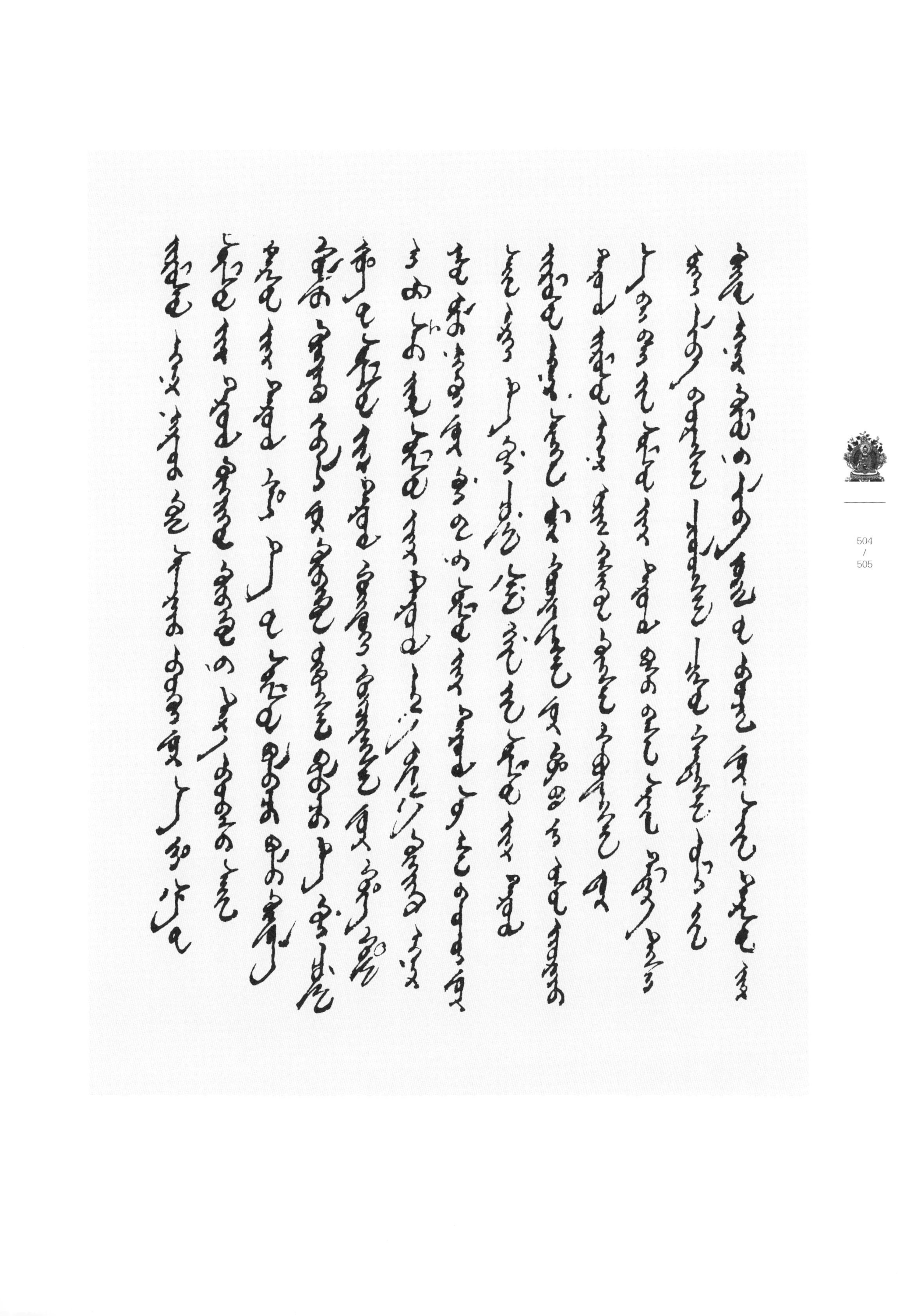

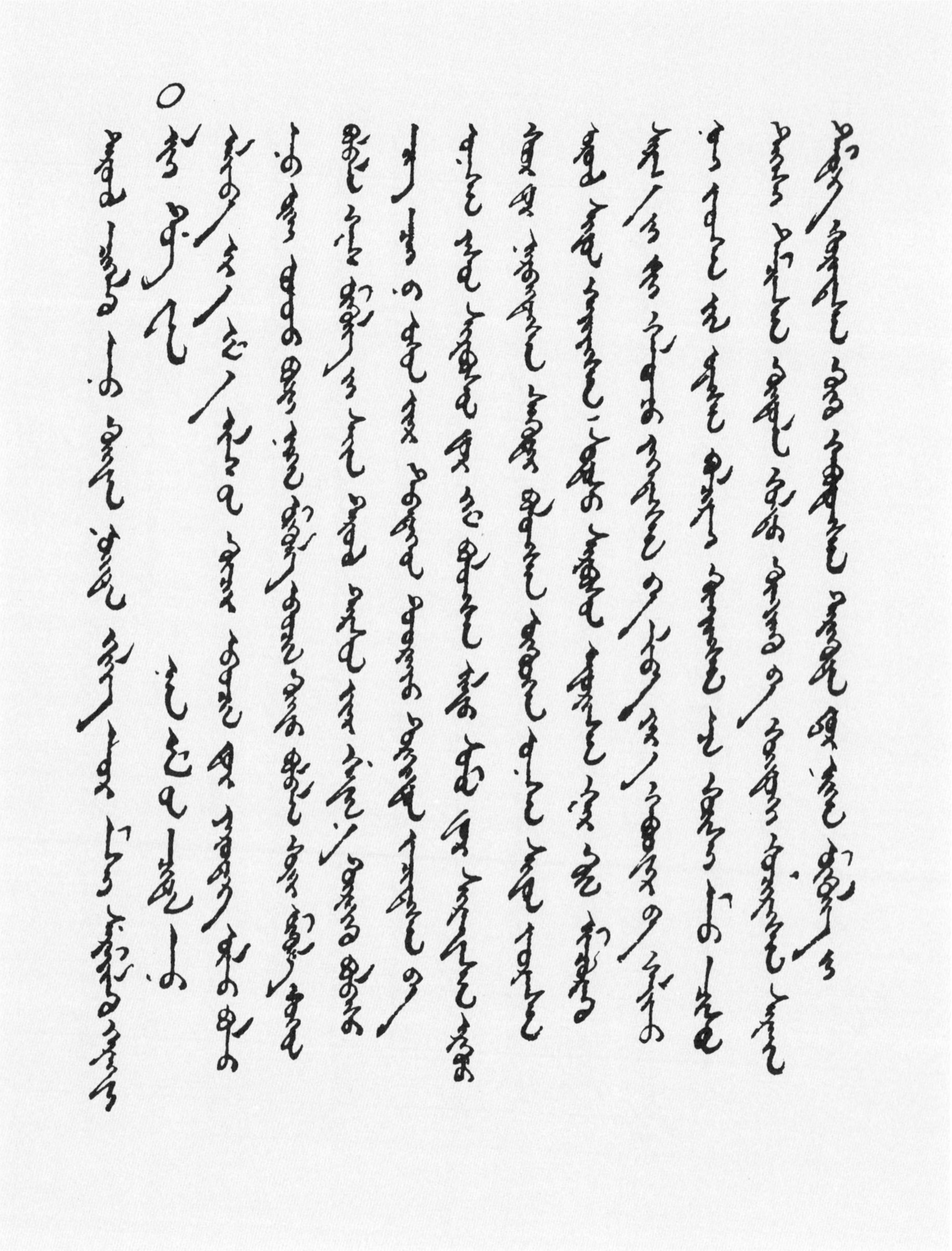

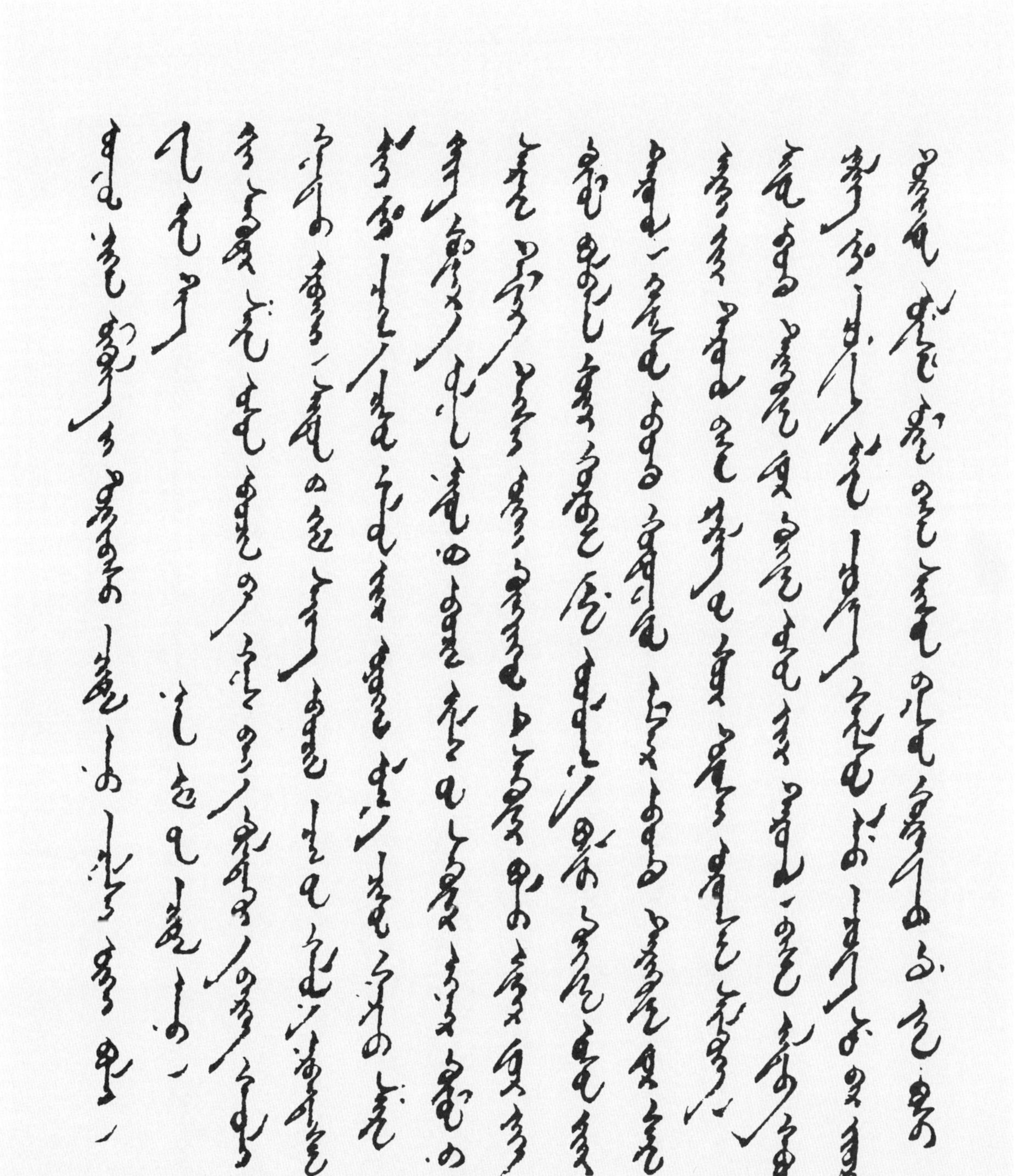

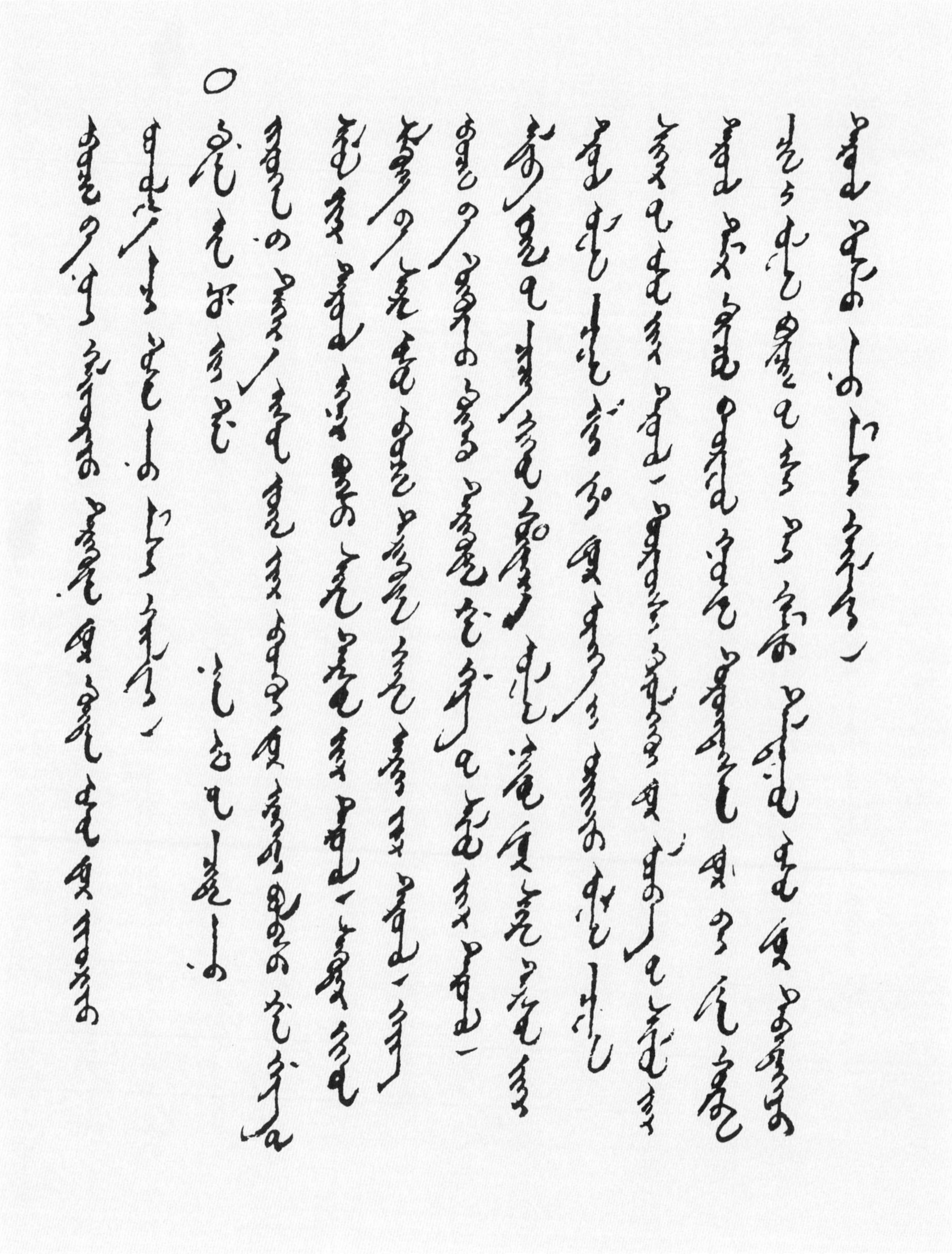

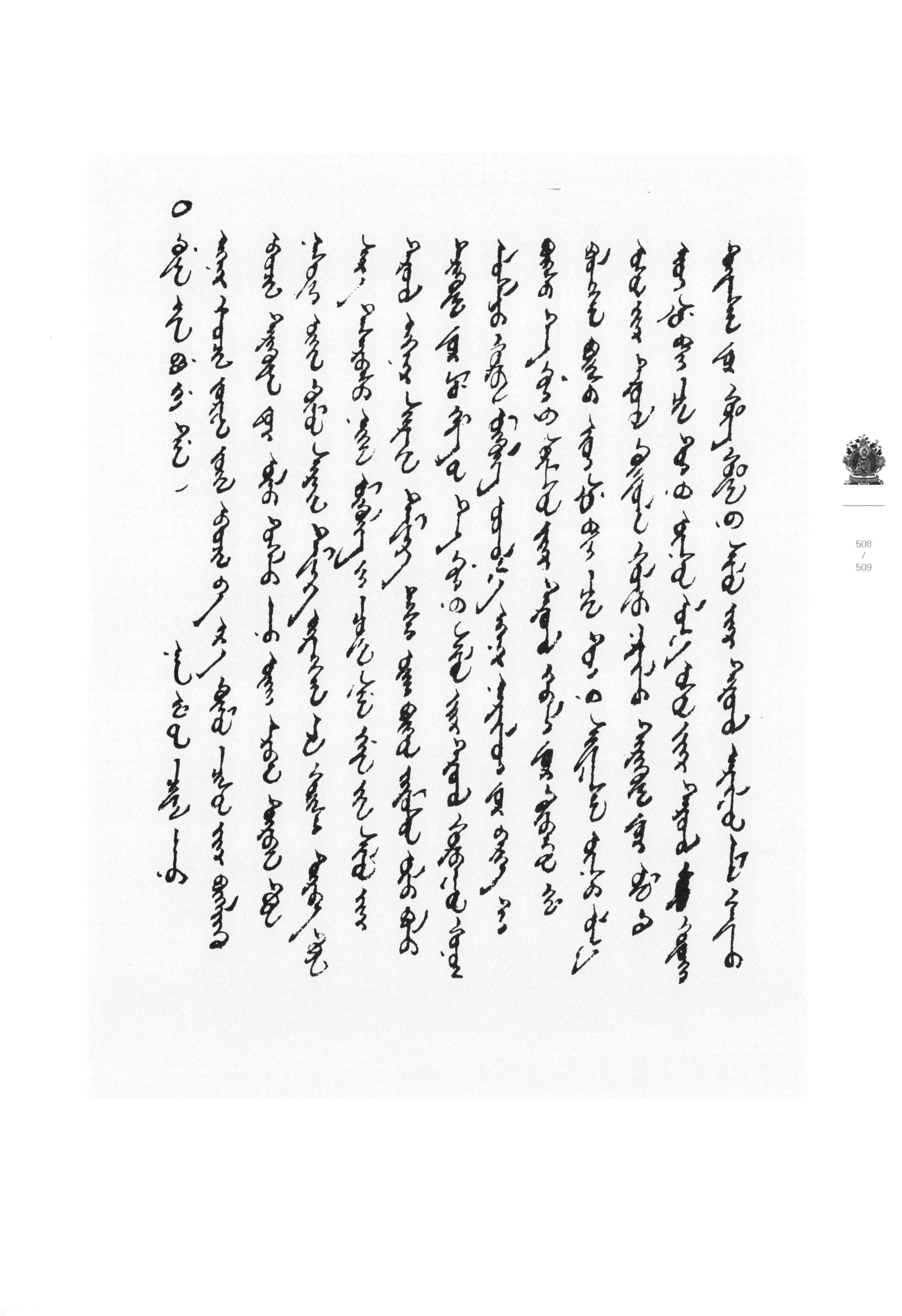

[illegible]

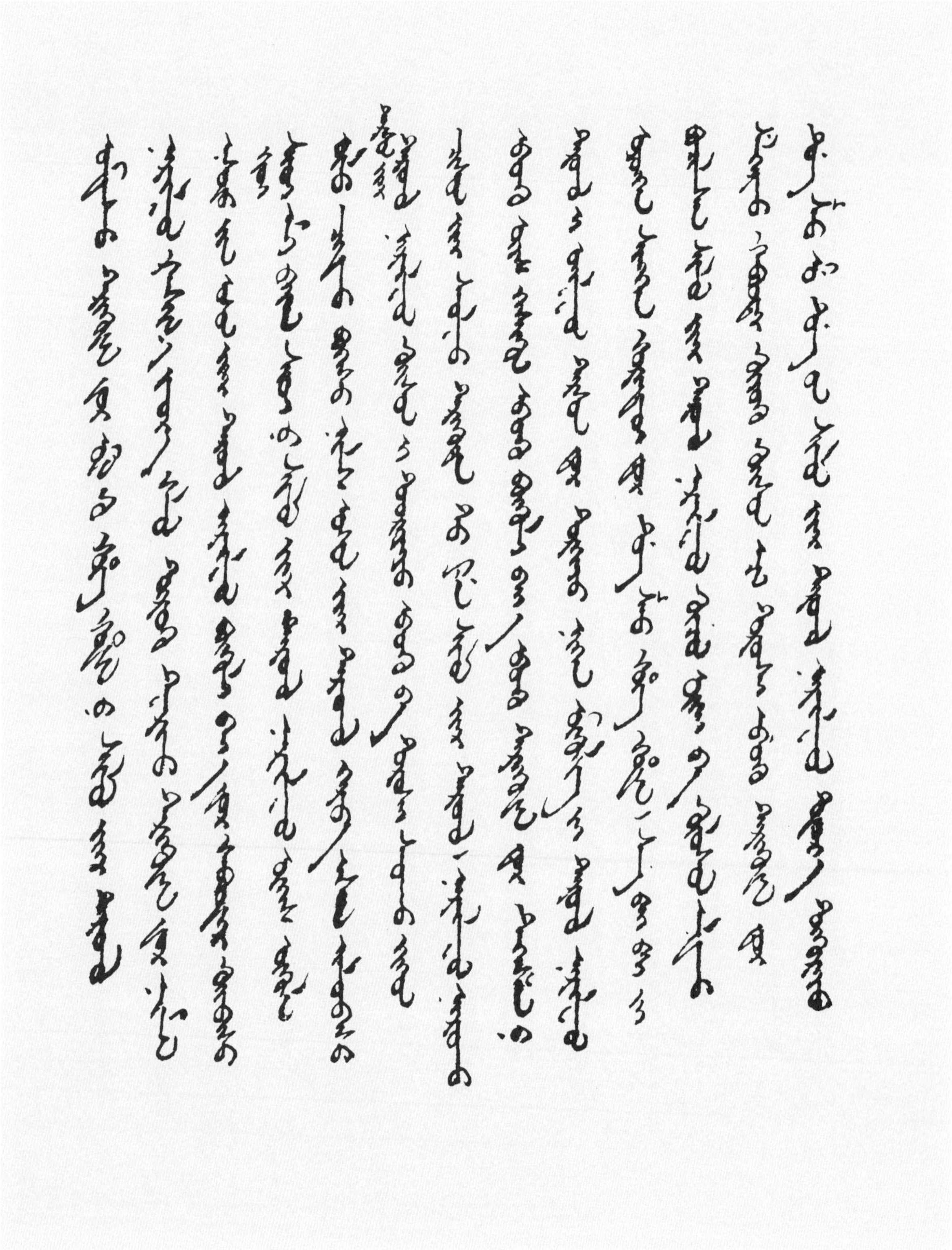

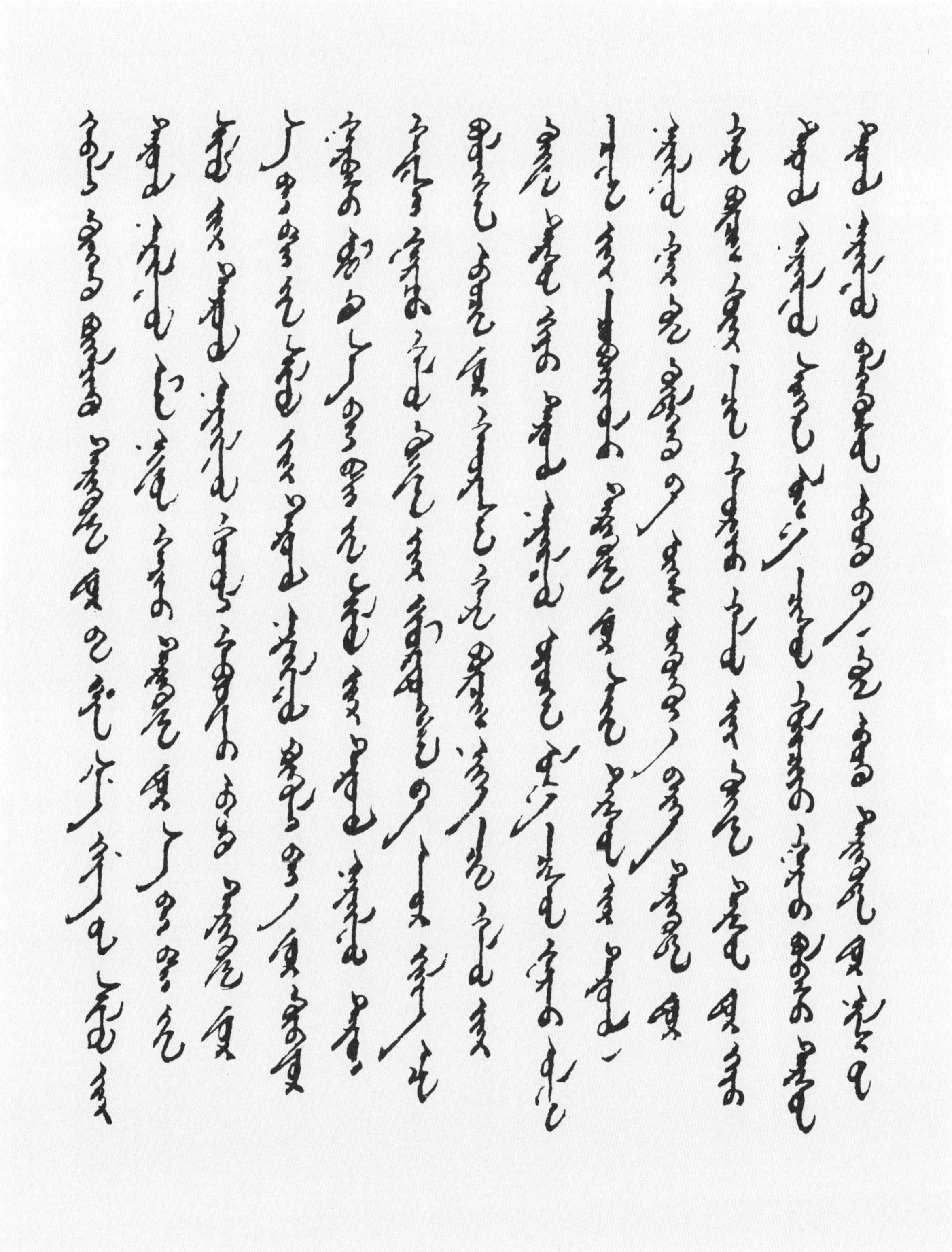

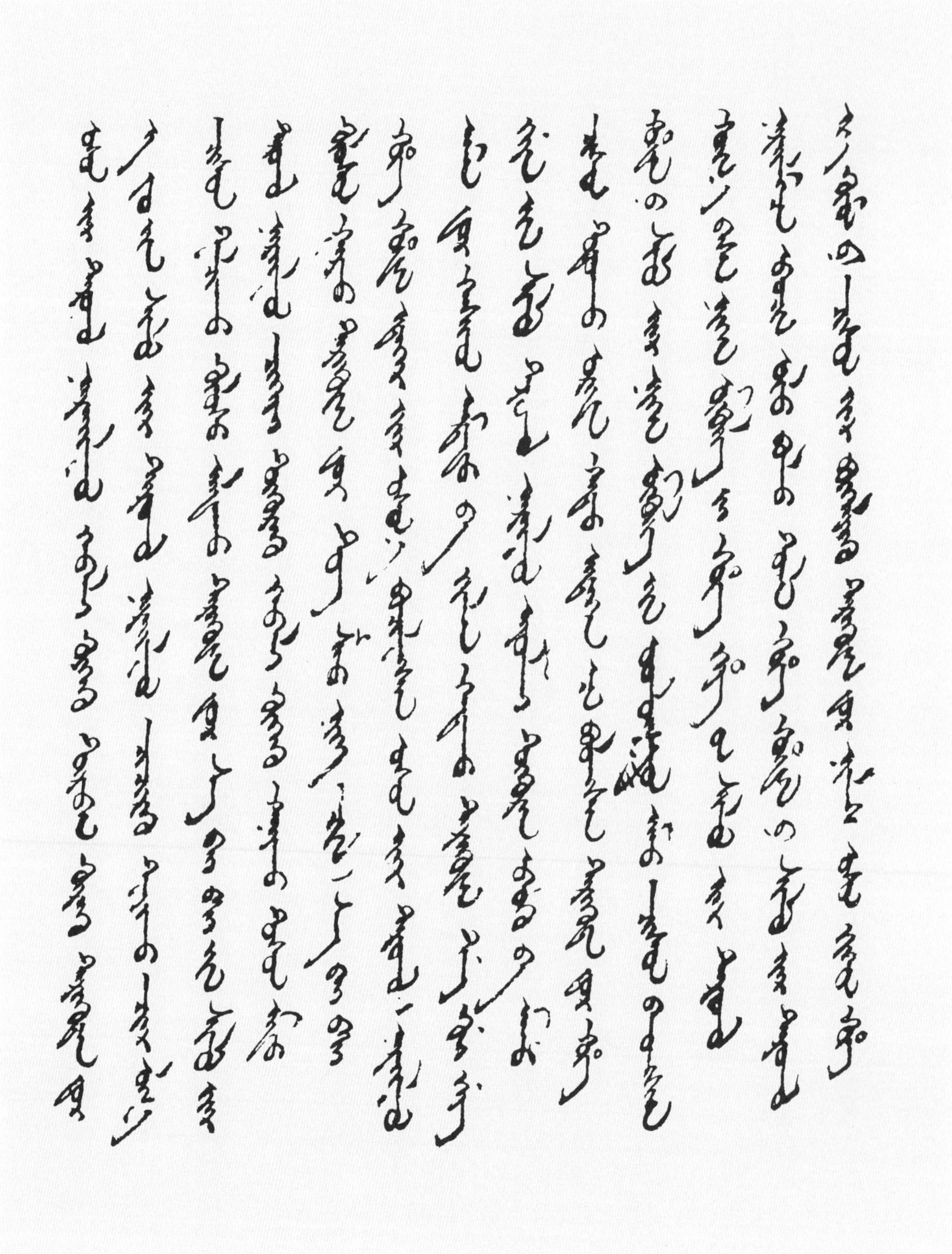

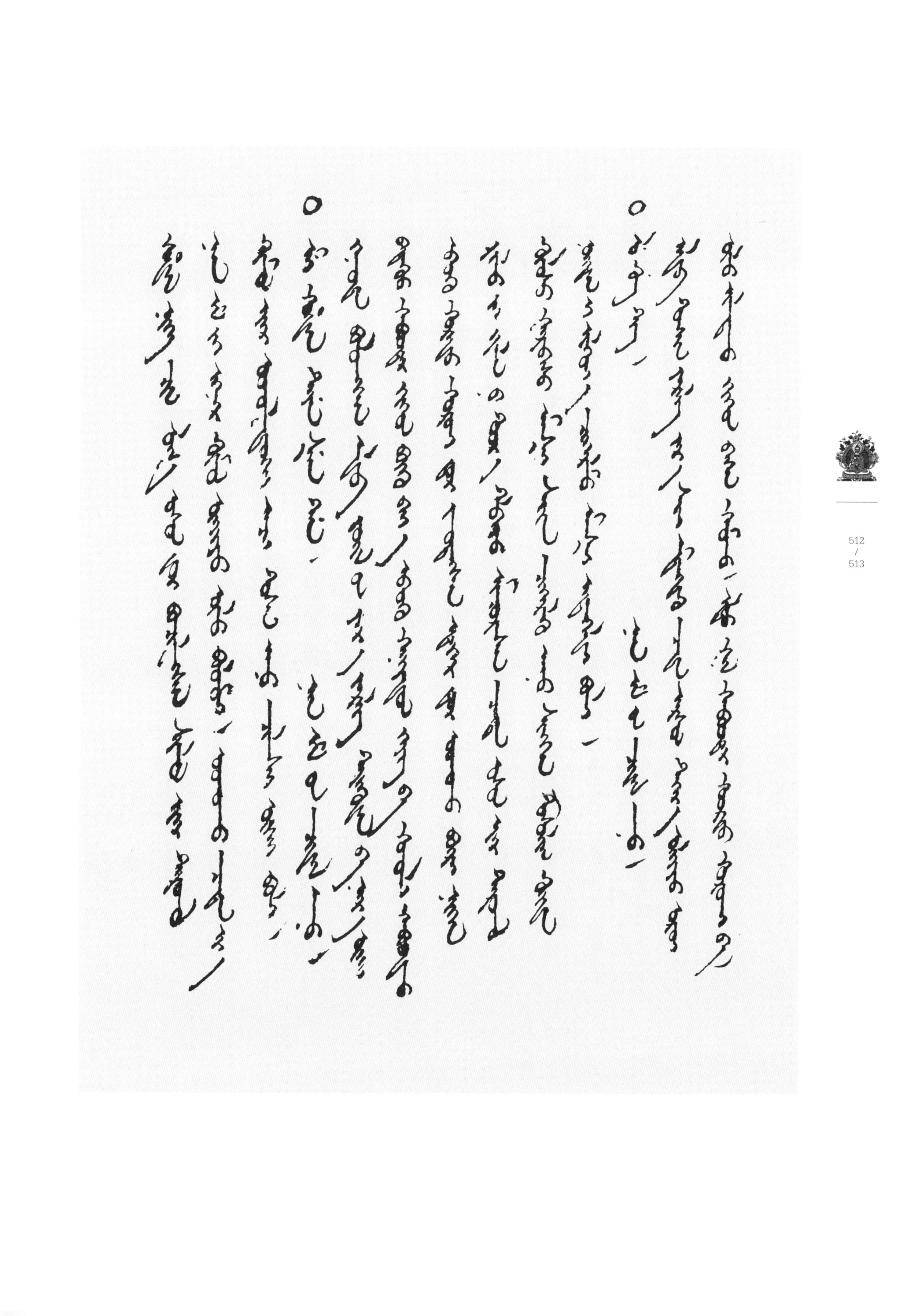

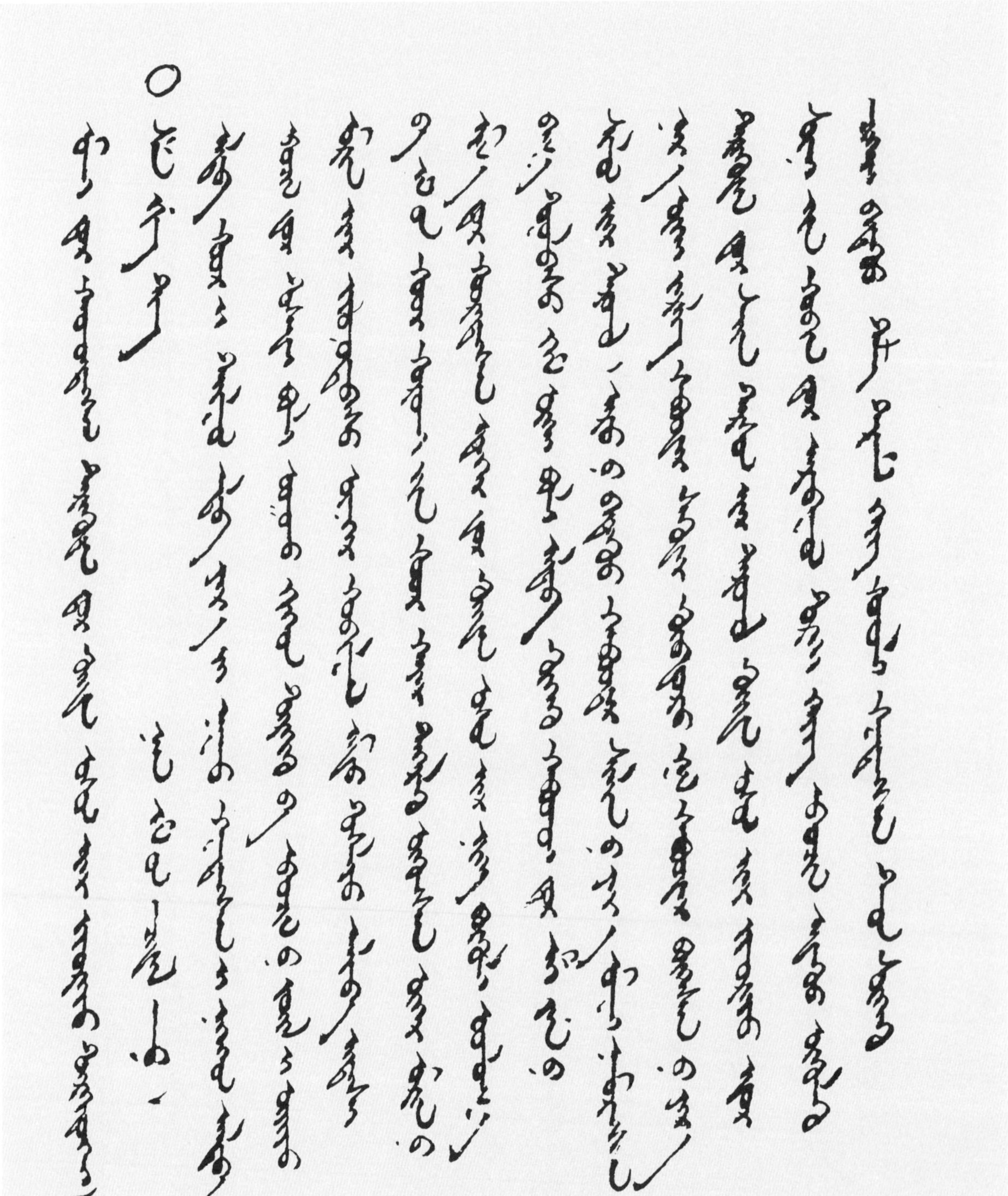

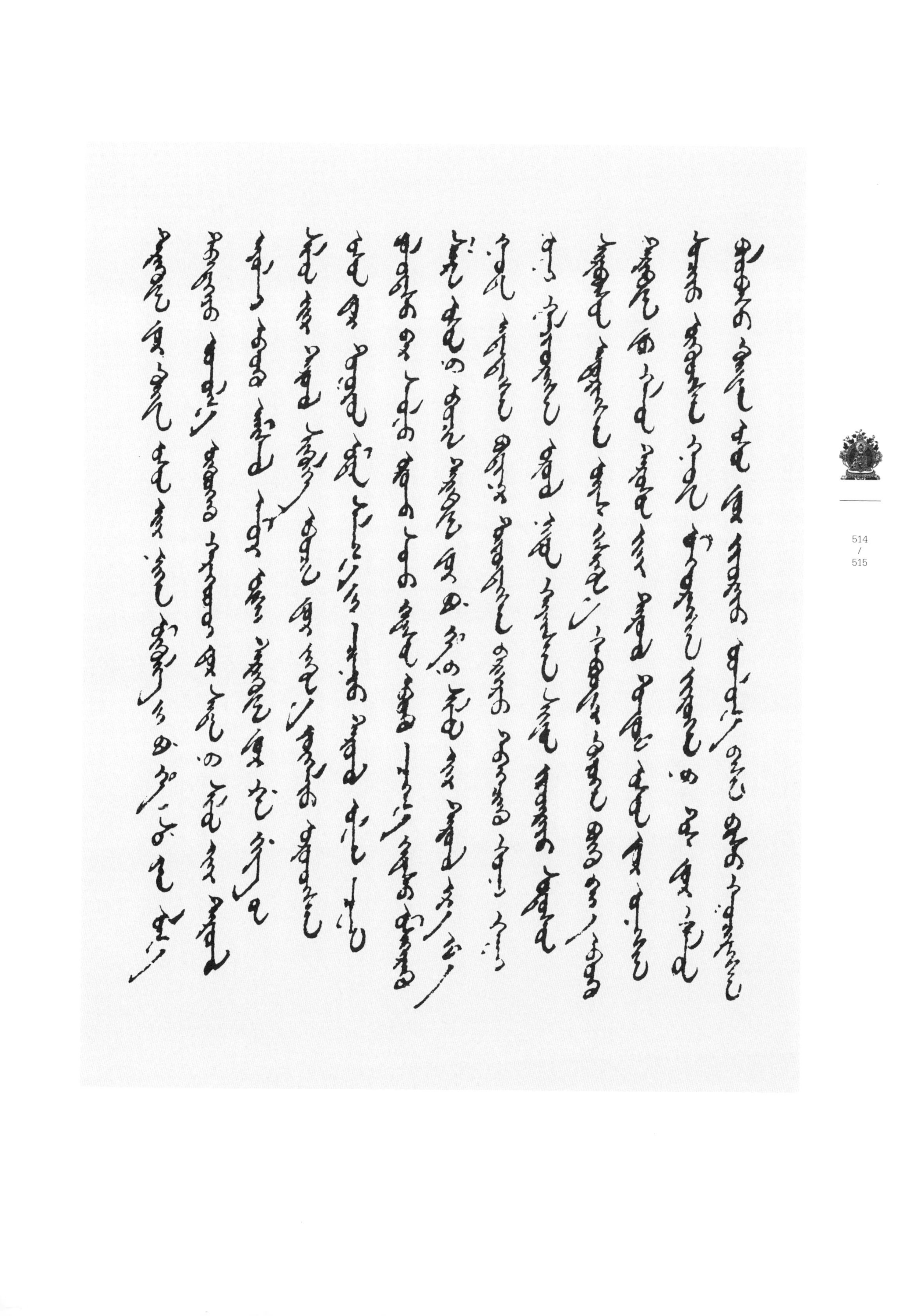

[illegible]

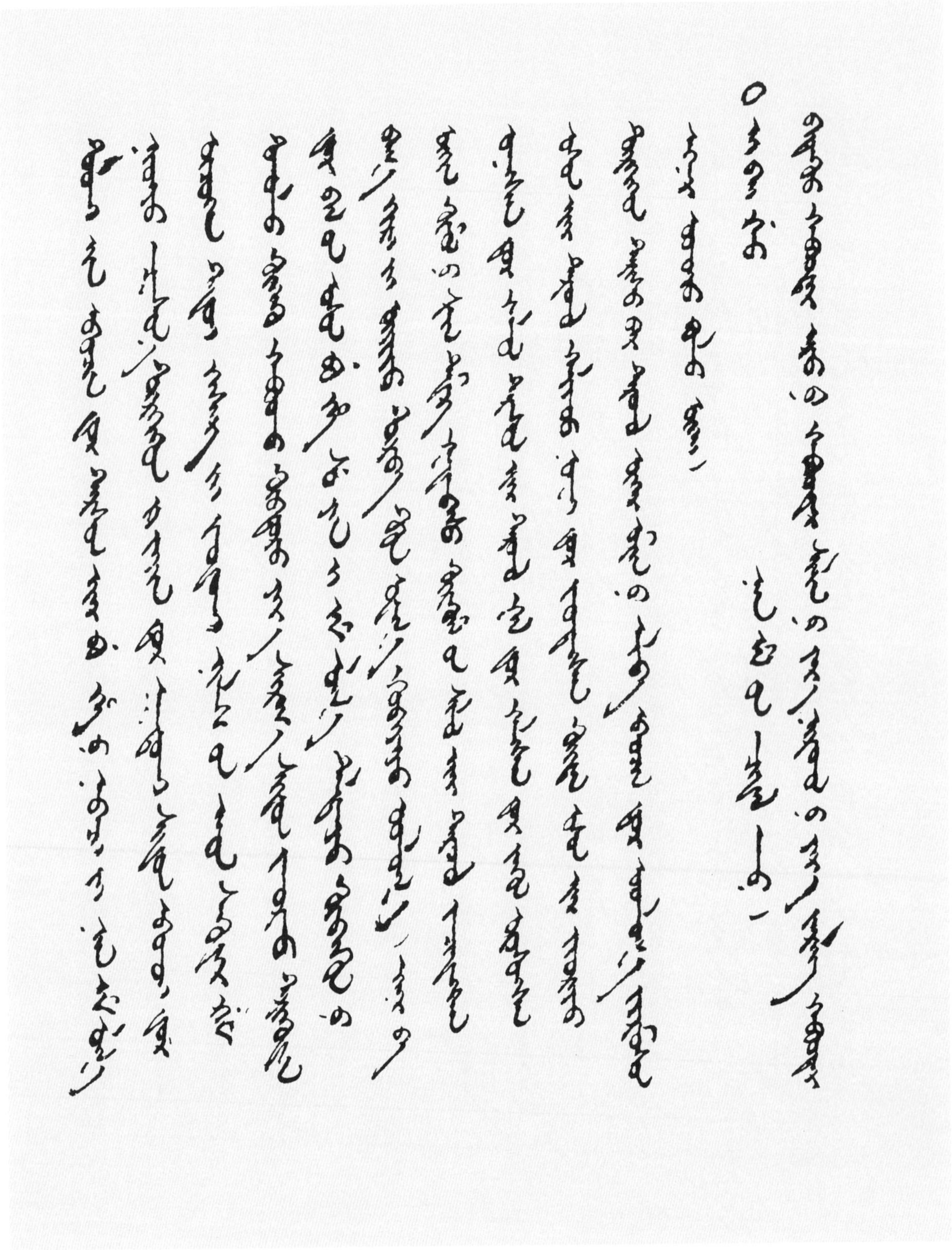

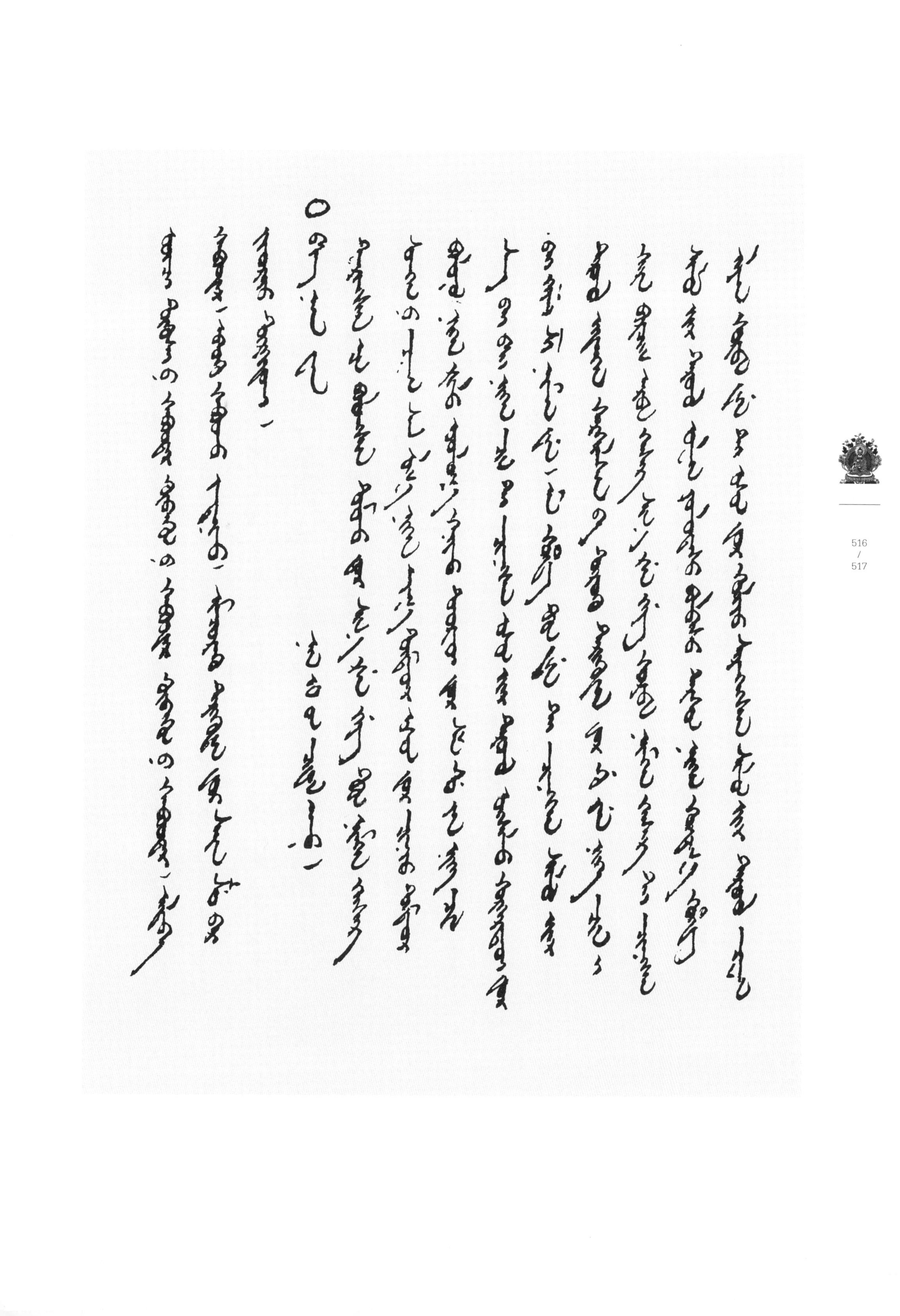

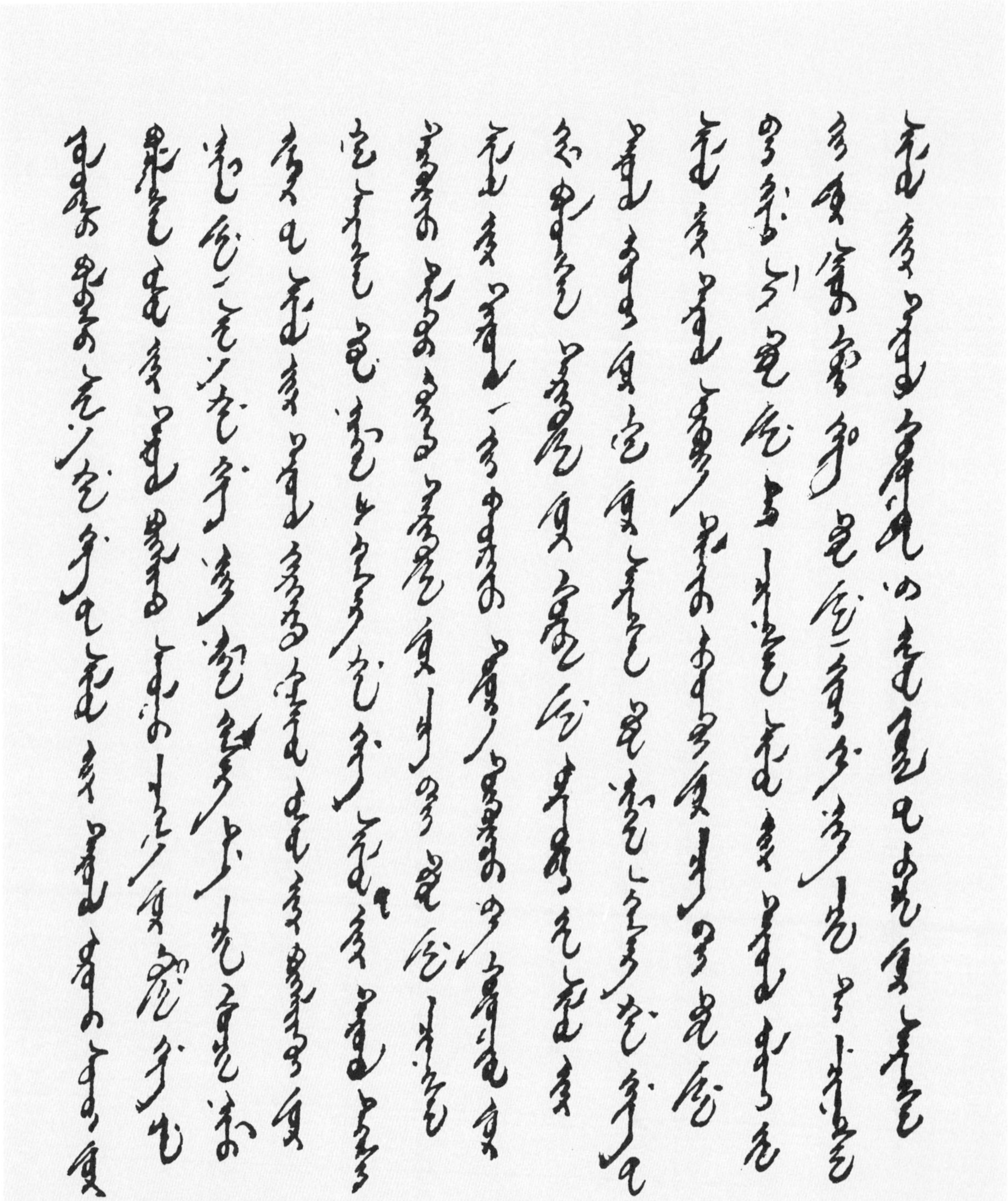

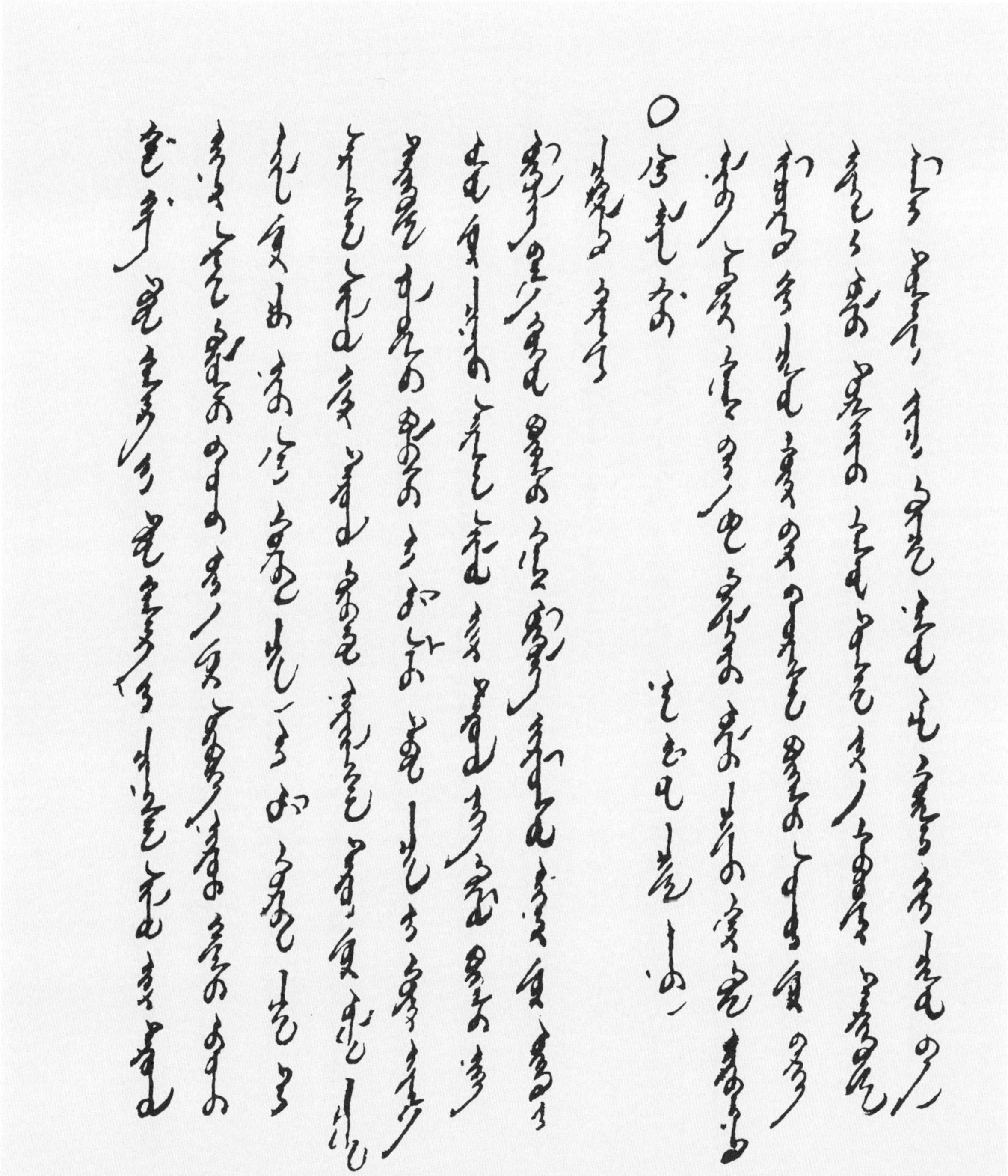

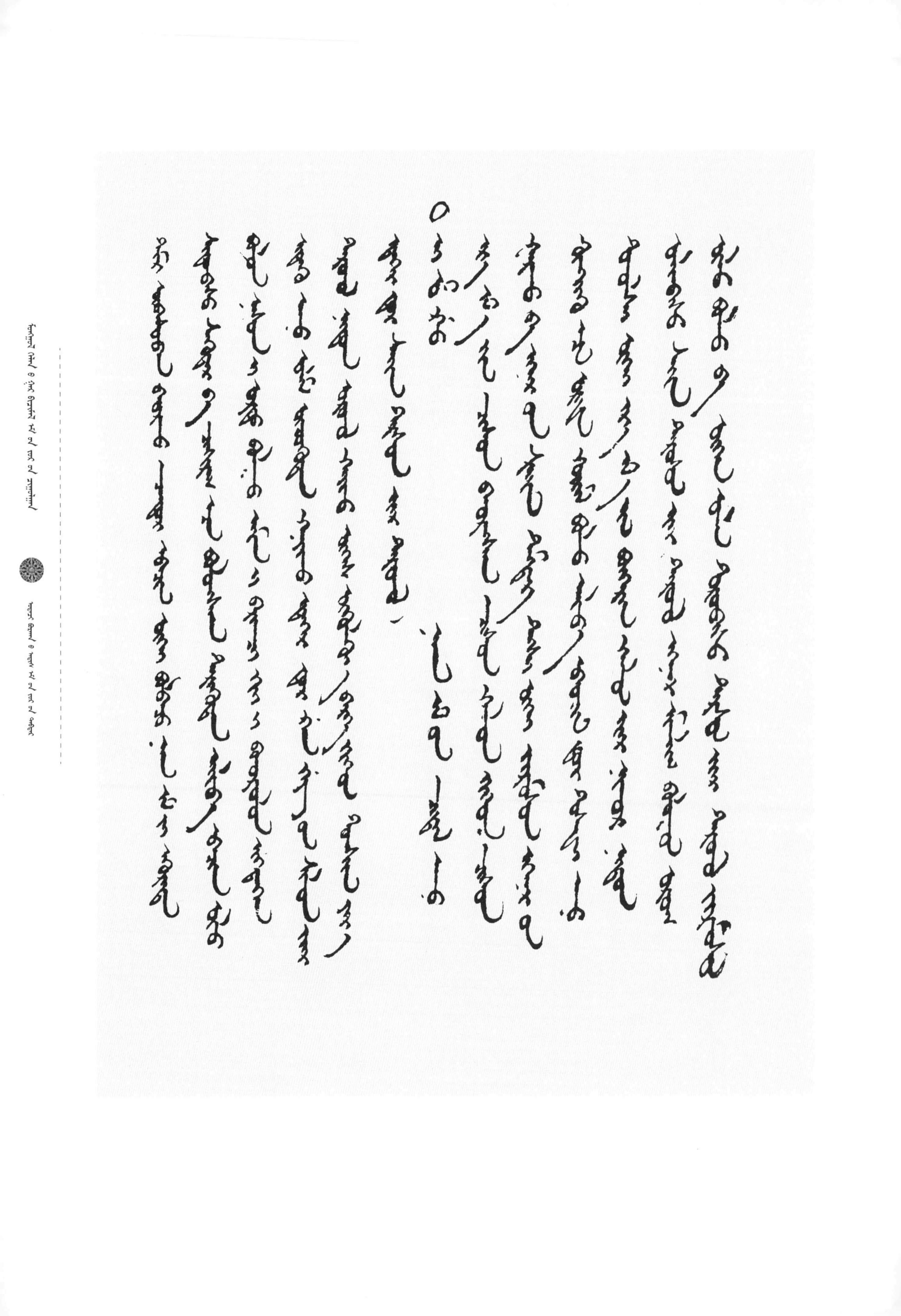

[illegible]

[illegible]

[illegible]

[illegible]

[illegible]

[illegible]

[illegible]

[illegible]

[illegible]

[illegible]

[illegible]

[illegible]

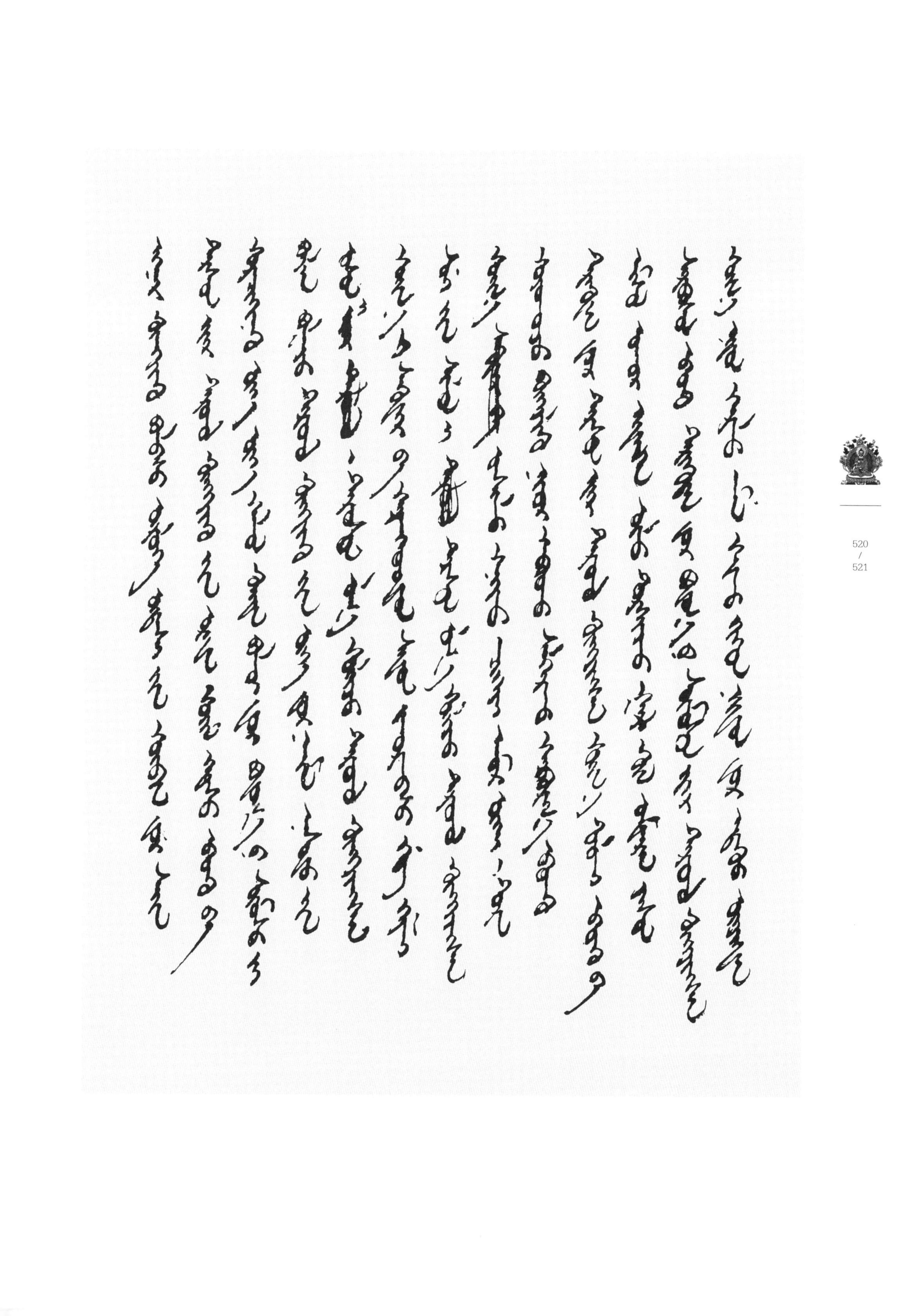

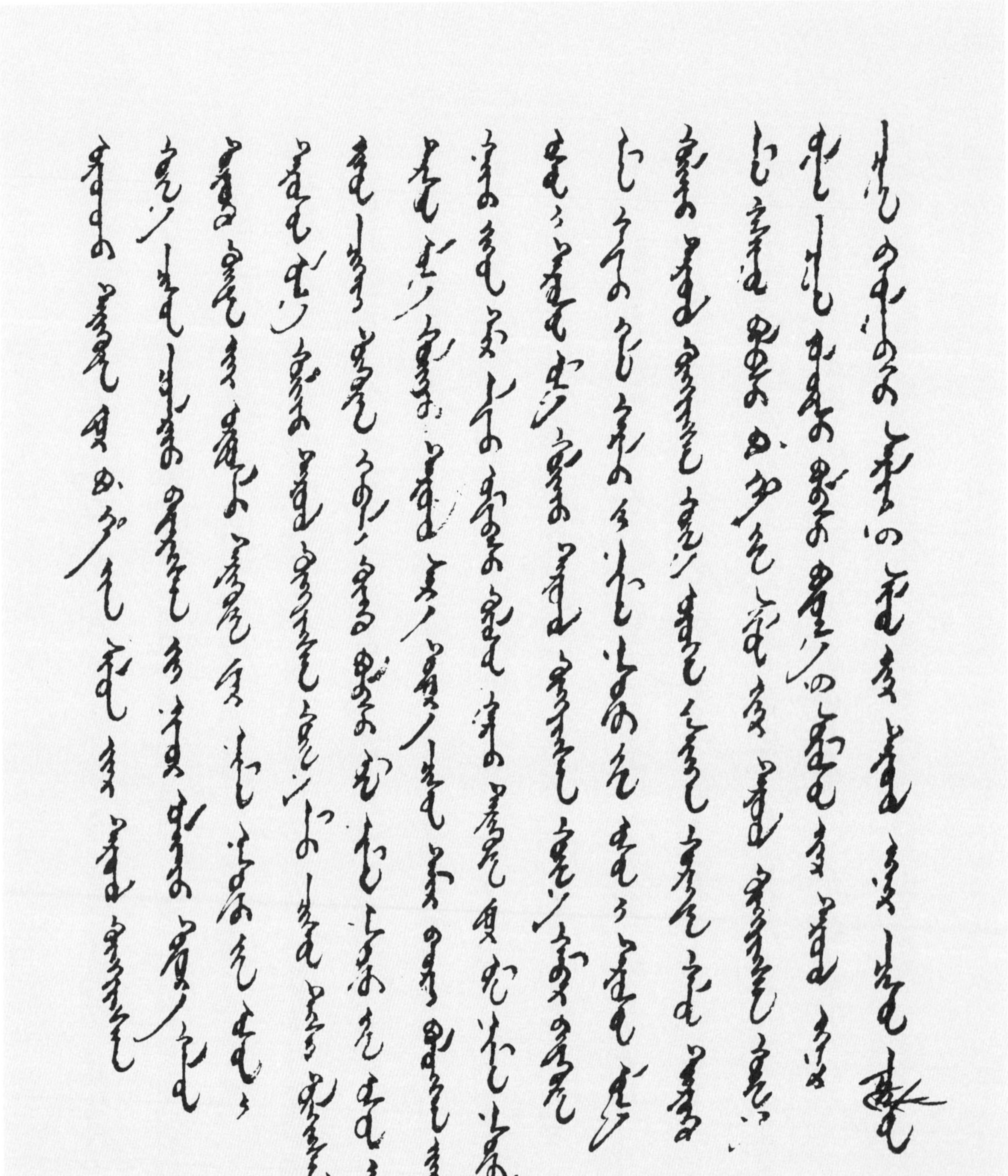

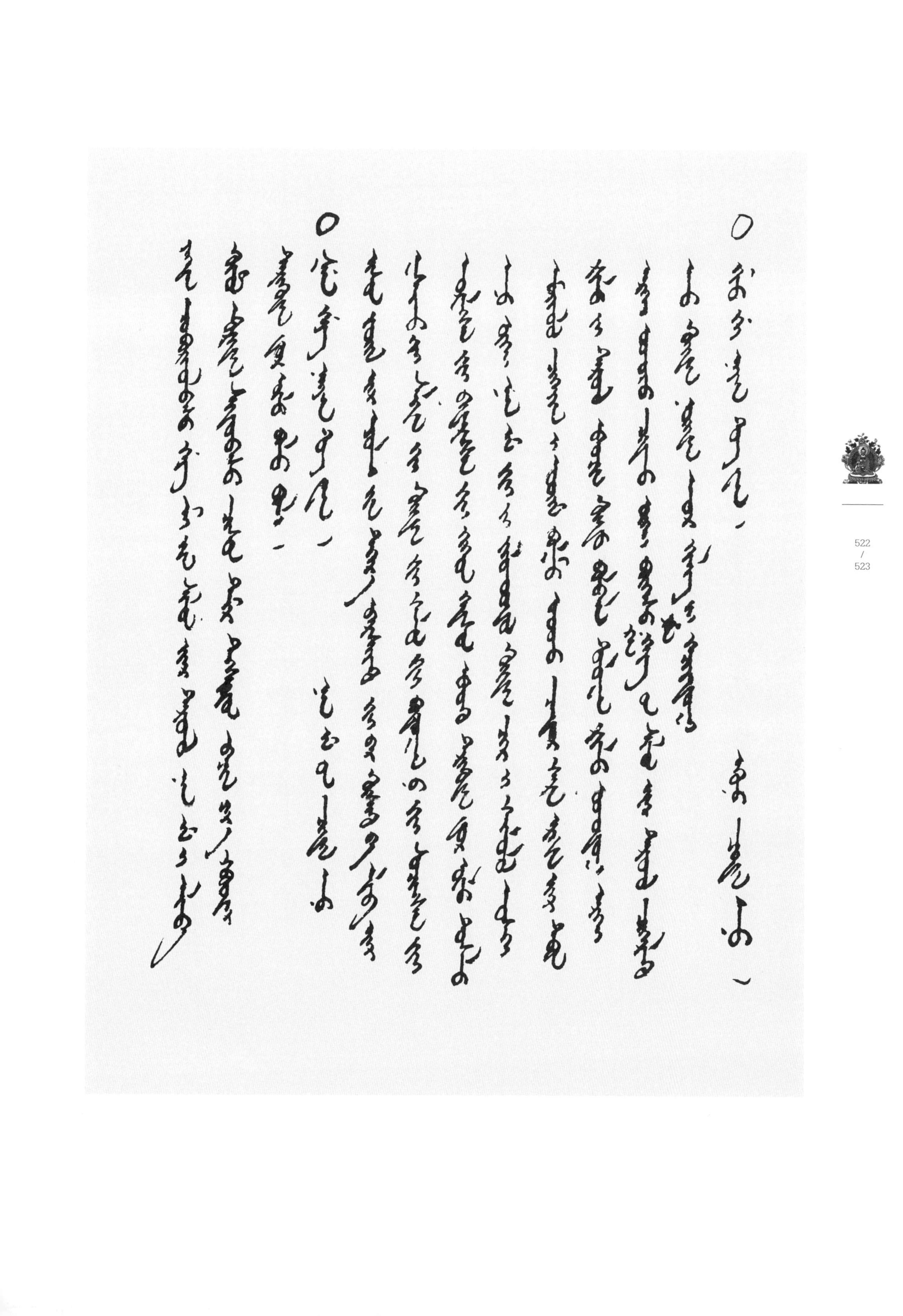

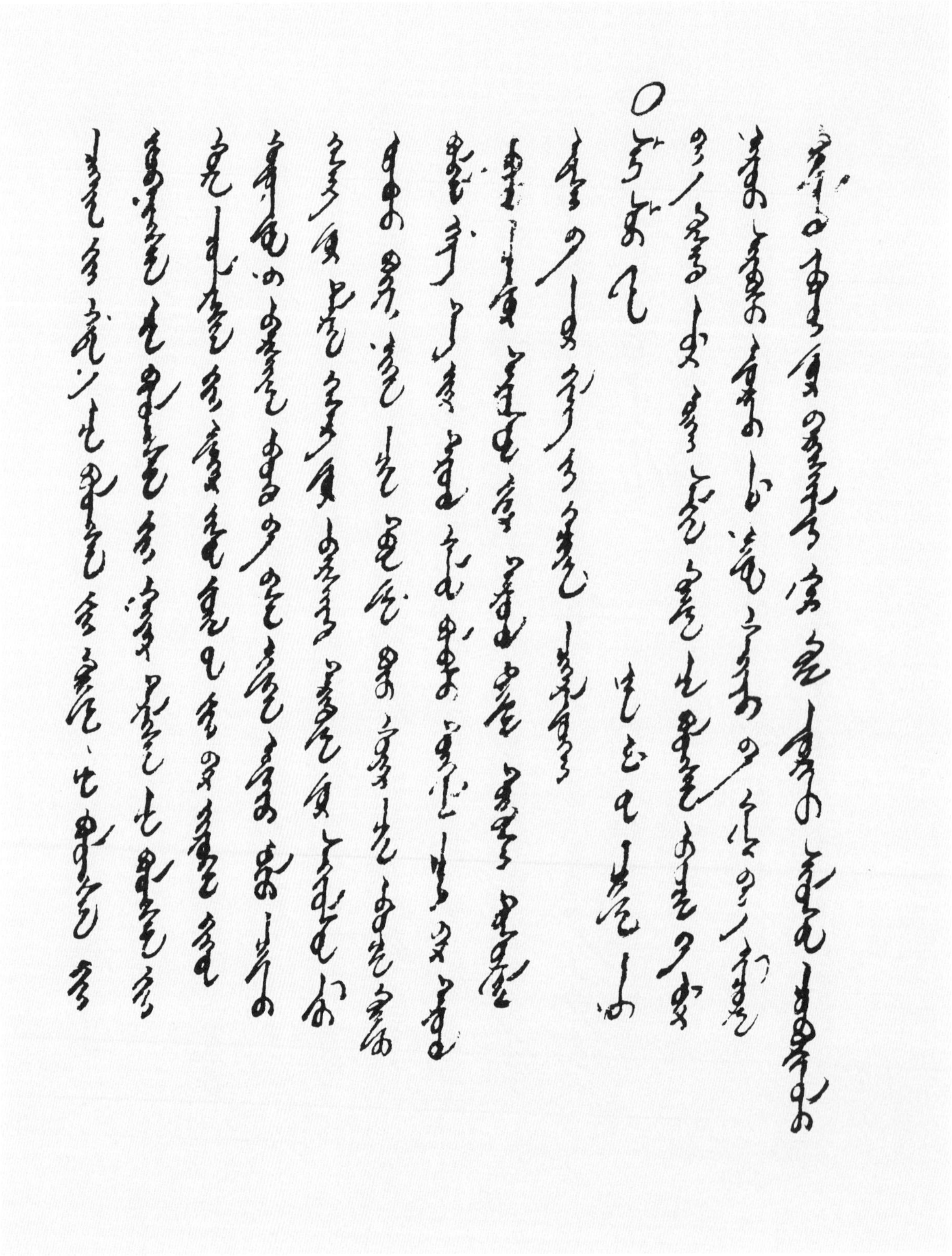

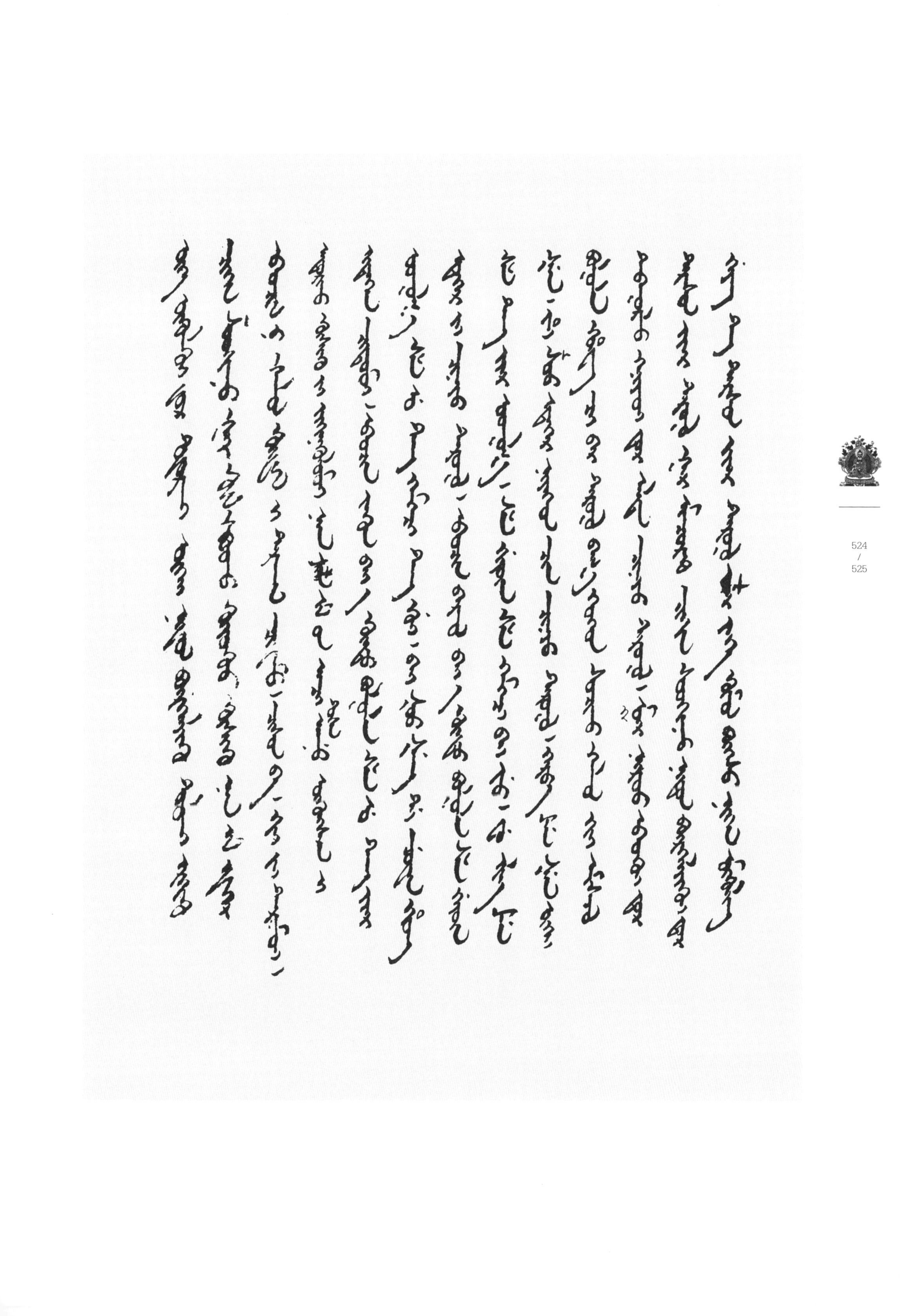

[illegible]

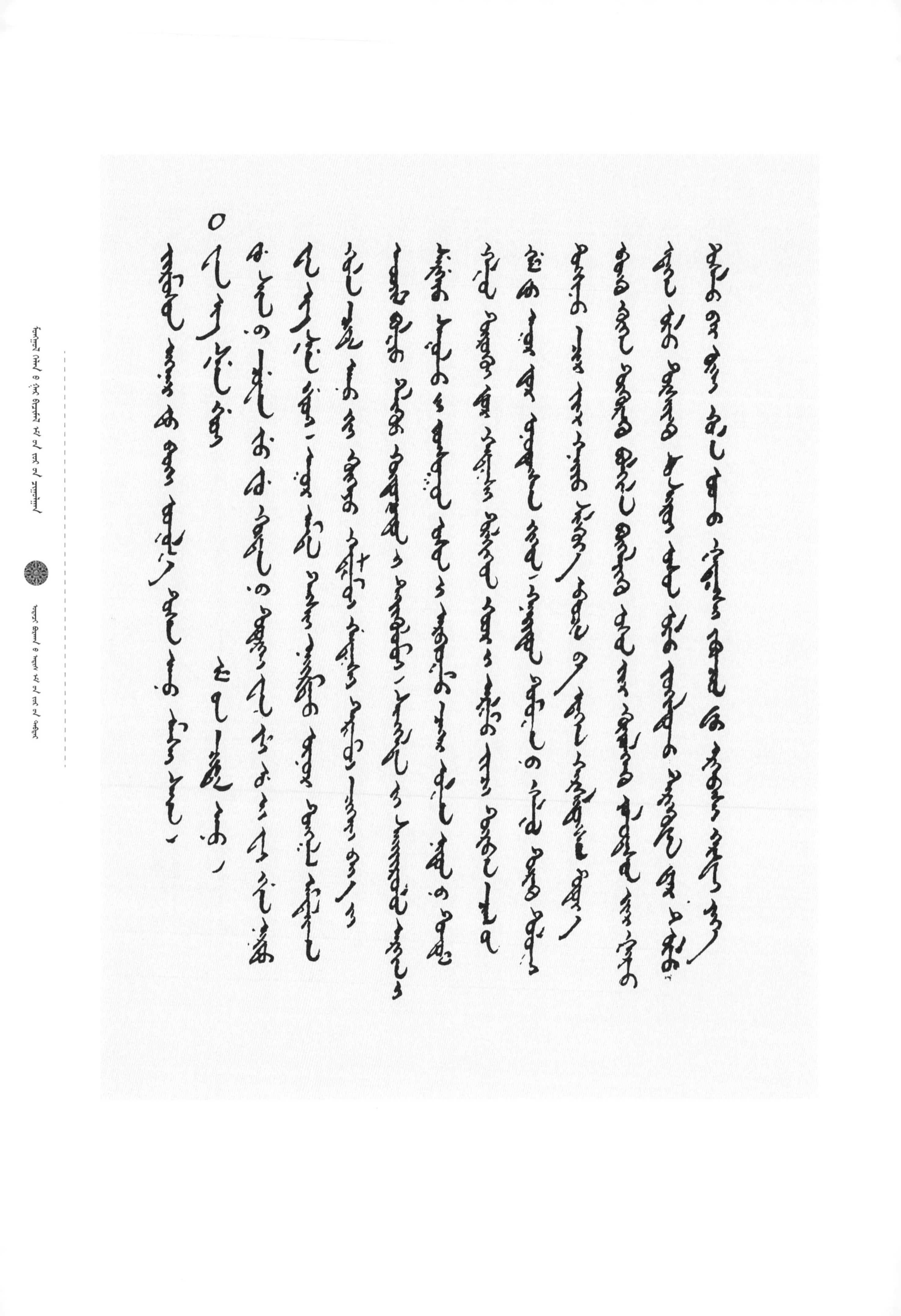

[illegible]

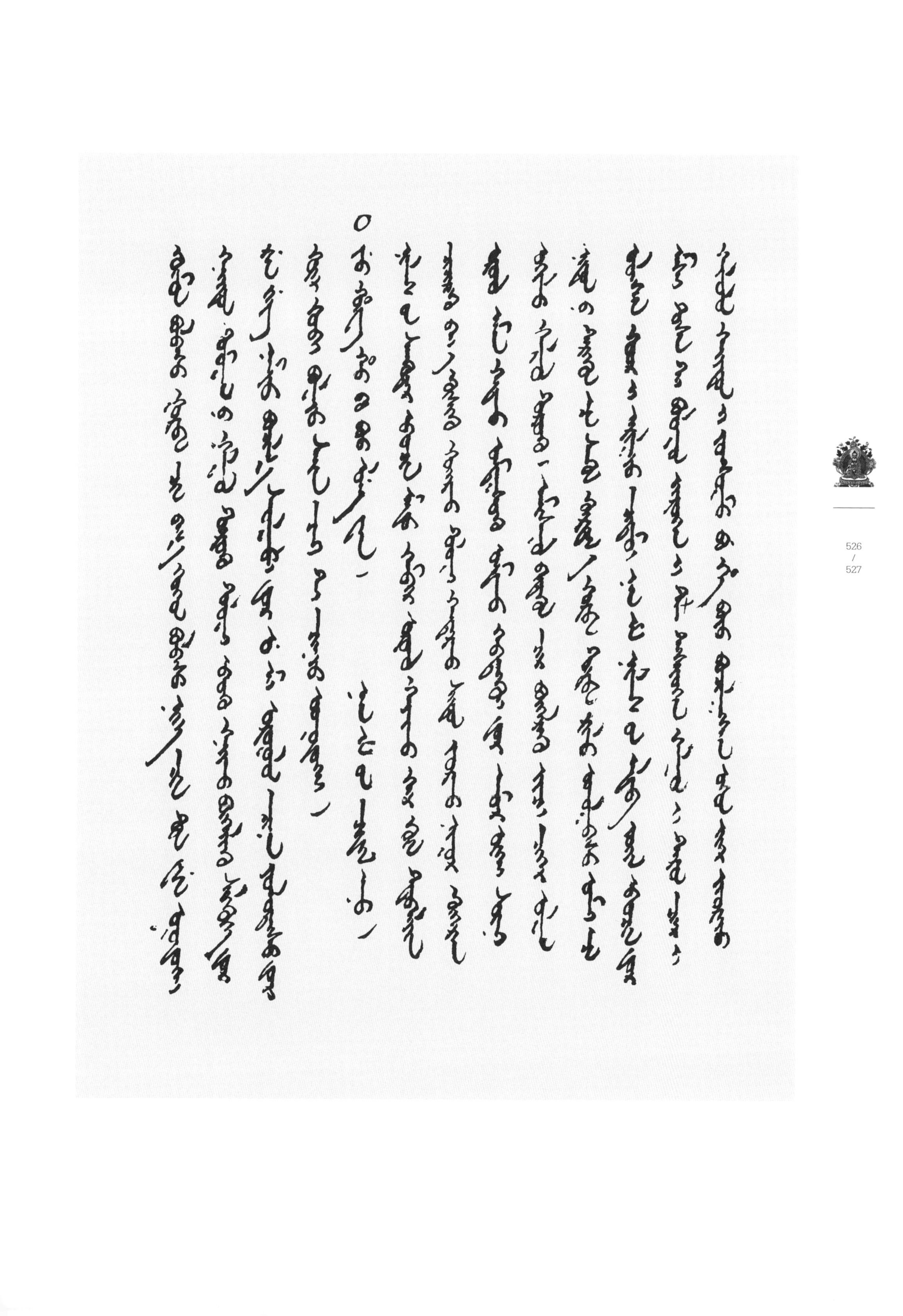

[illegible]

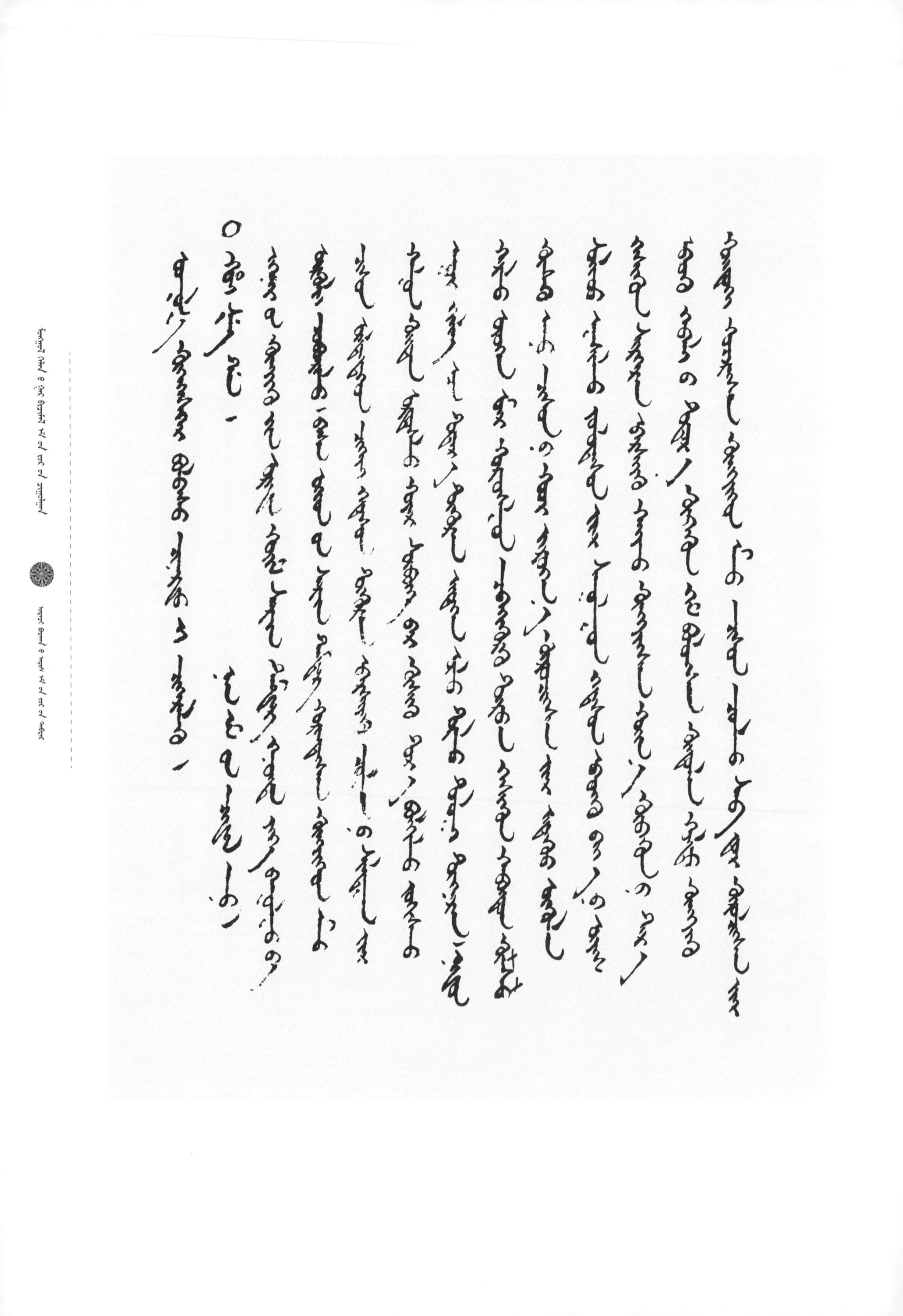

[illegible]

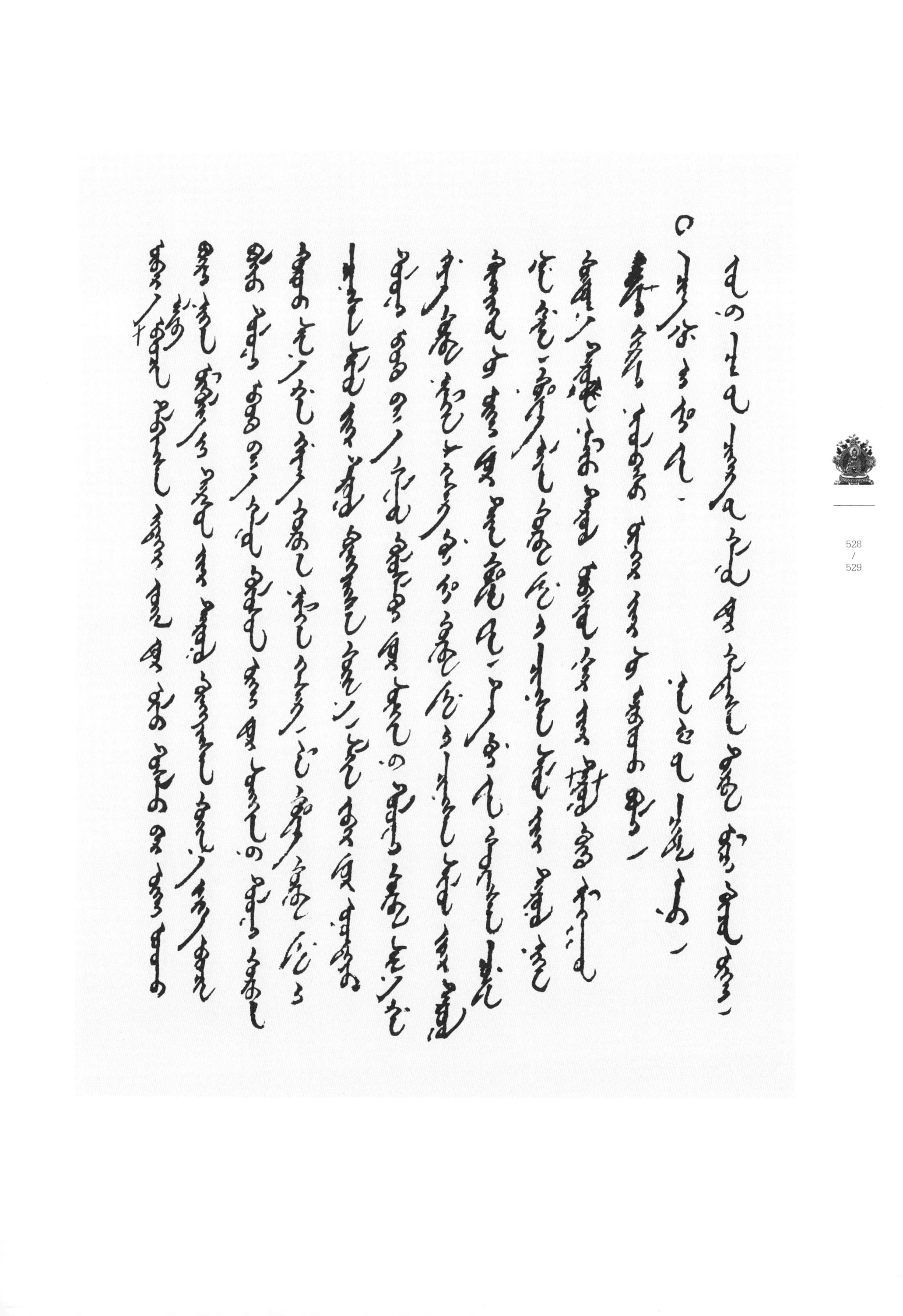

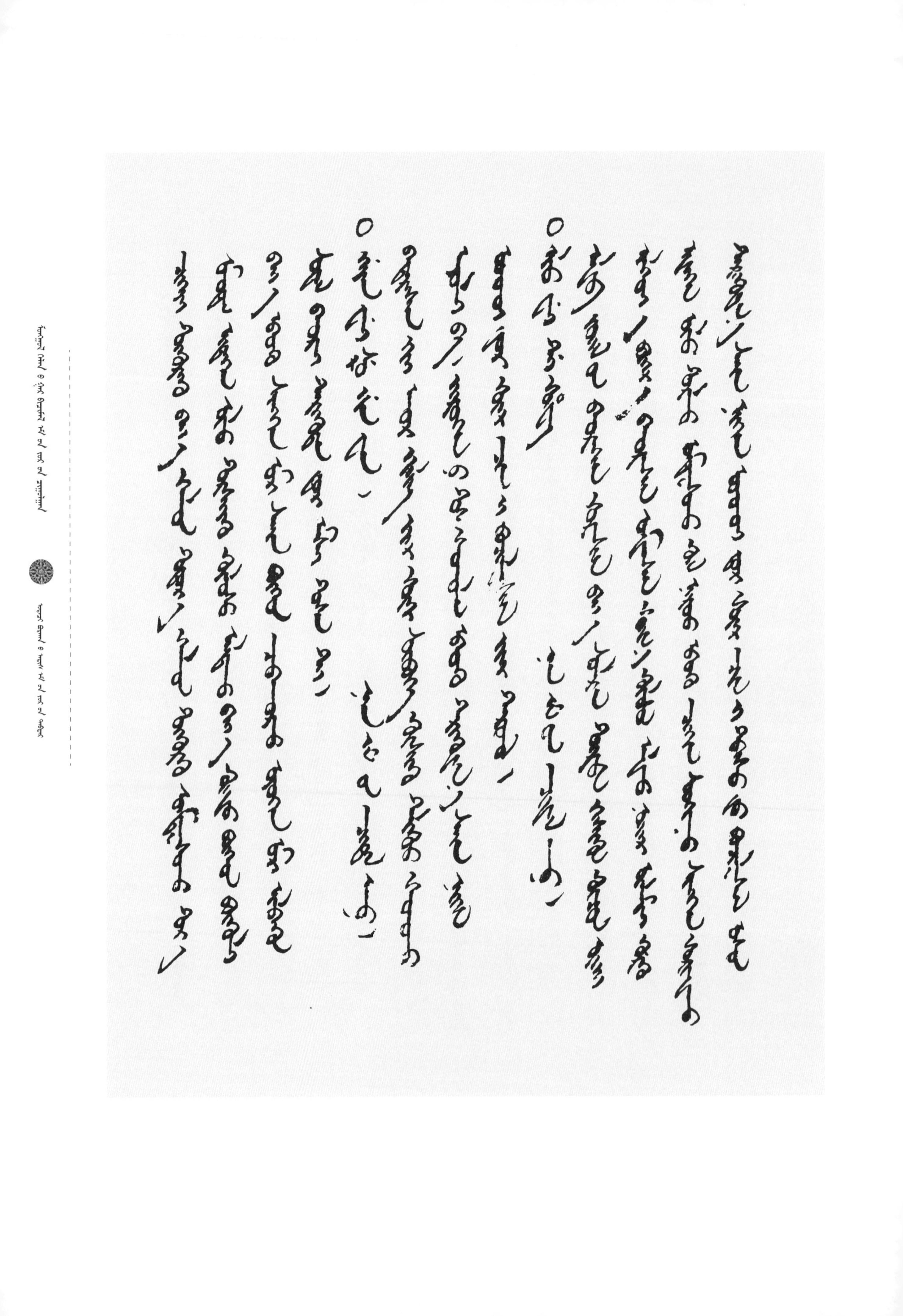

[illegible]

[illegible]

[illegible]

[illegible]

○ [illegible]

[illegible]

[illegible]

[illegible]

○ [illegible]

[illegible]

[illegible]

[illegible]

[illegible]

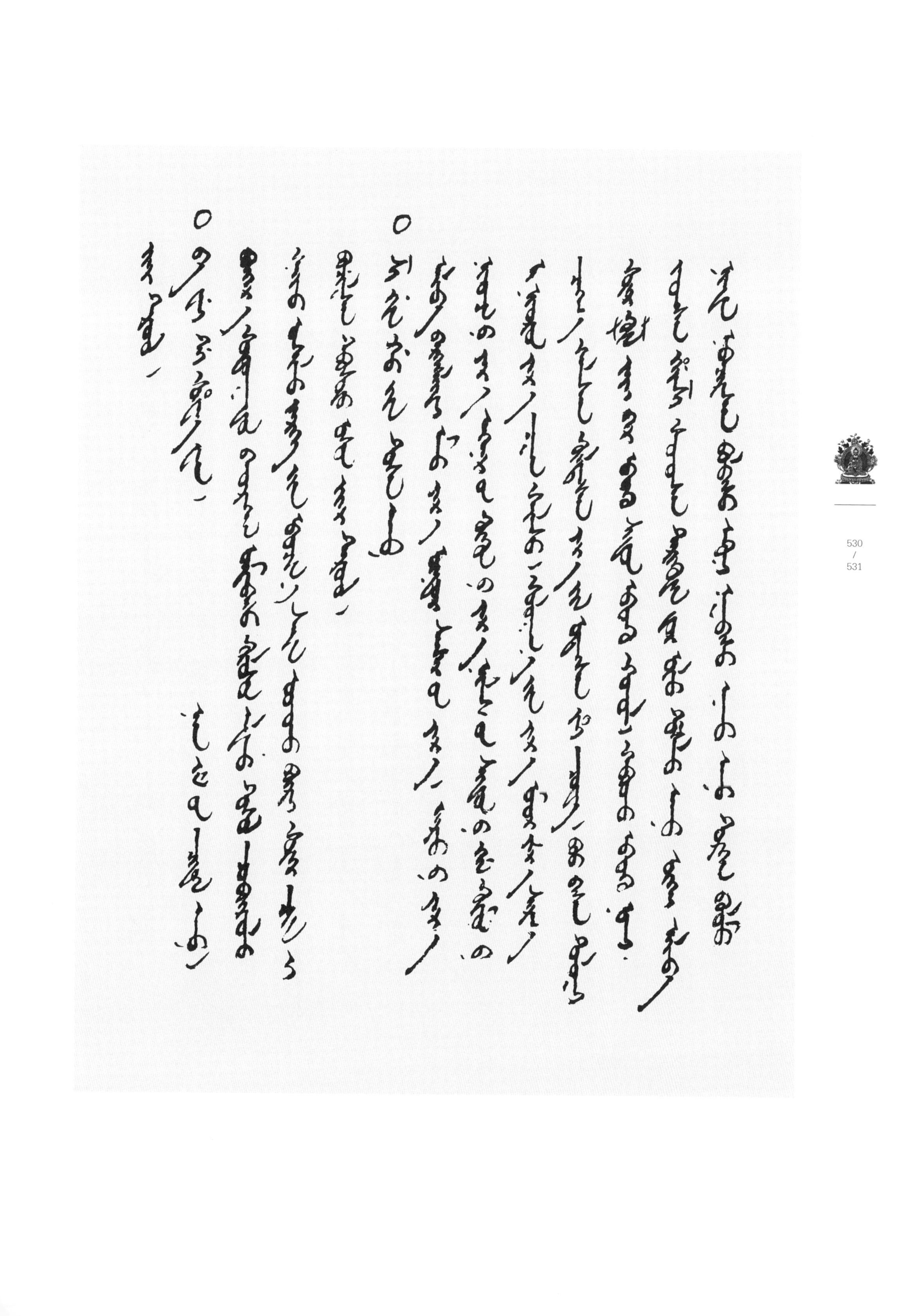

[illegible]

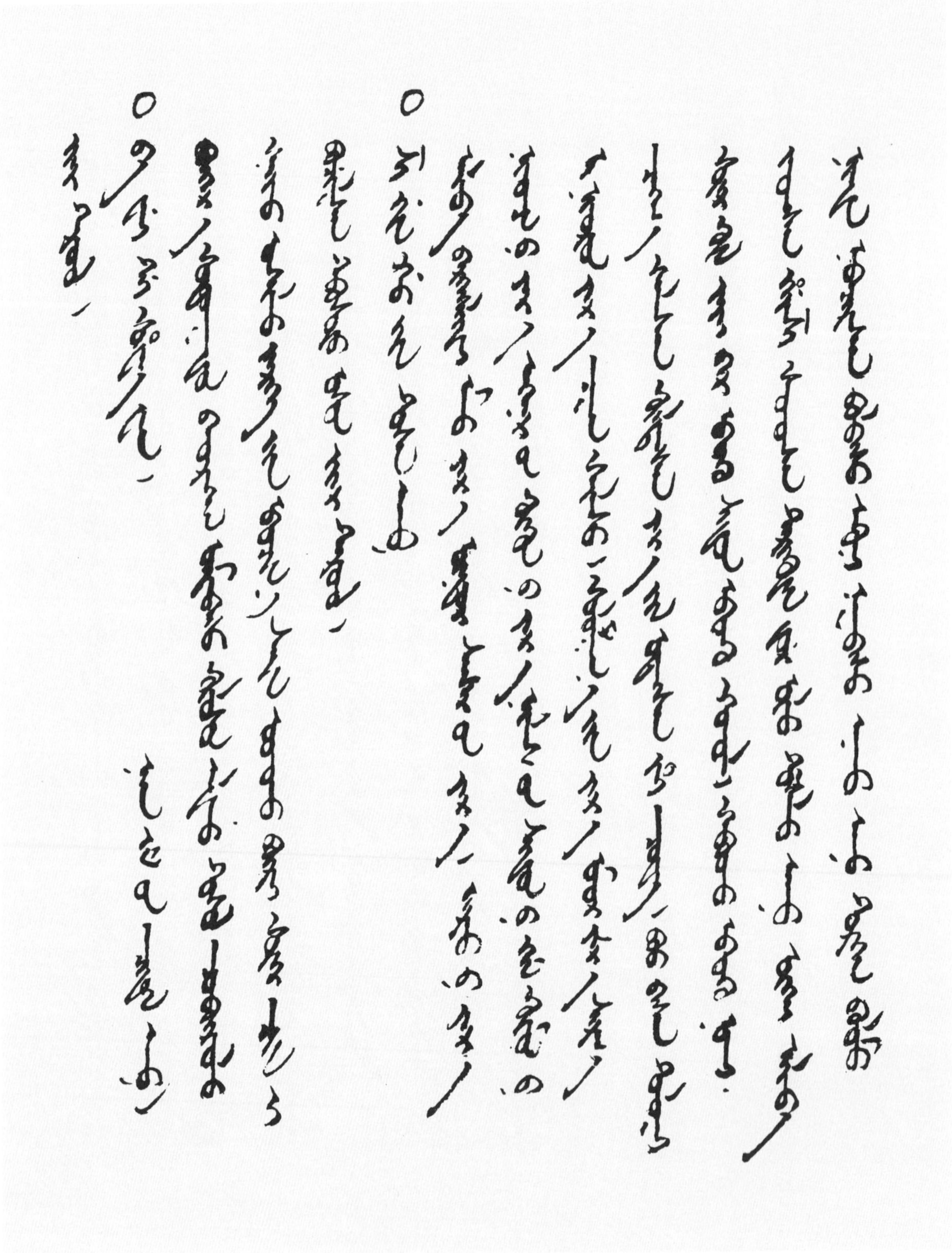

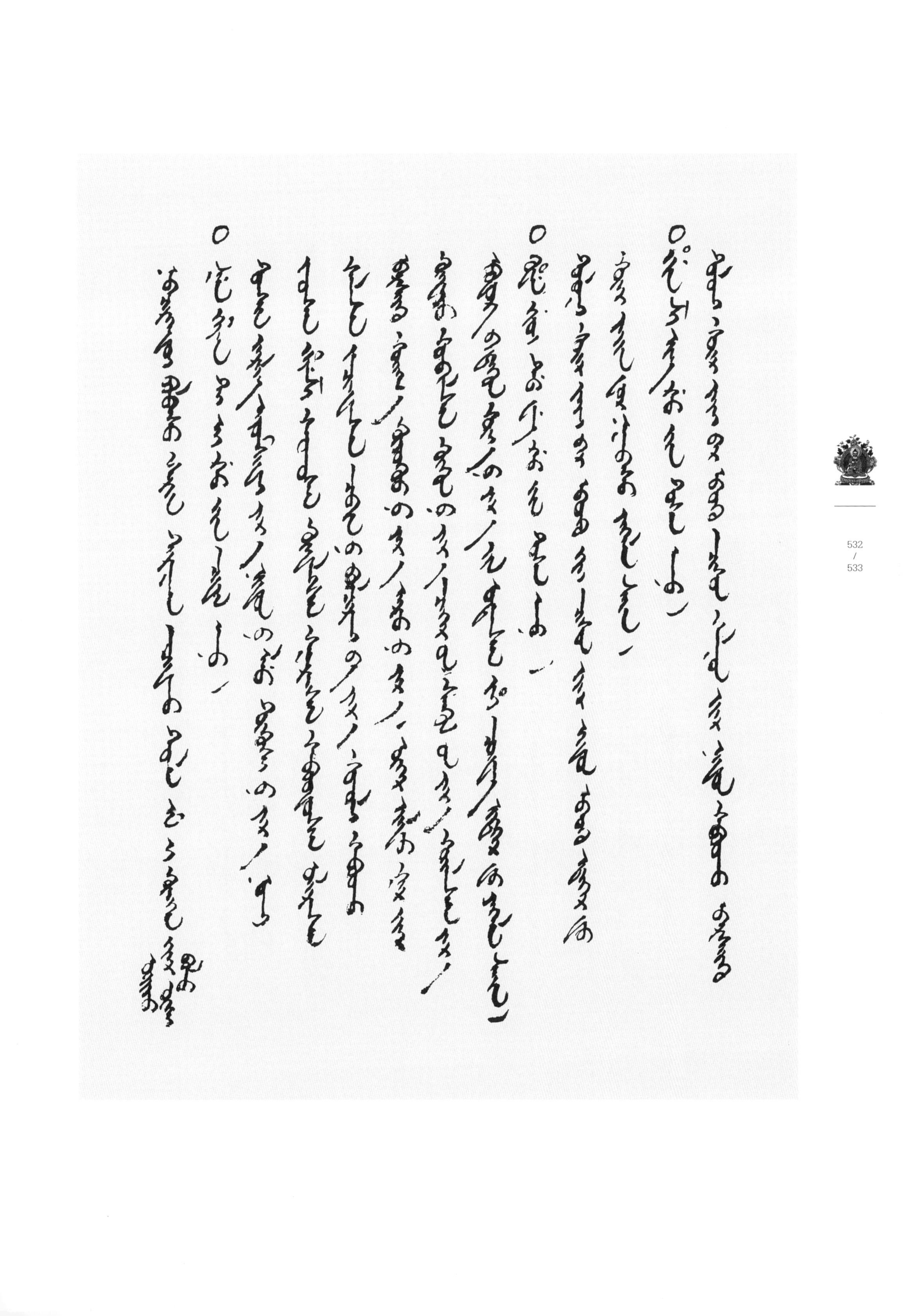

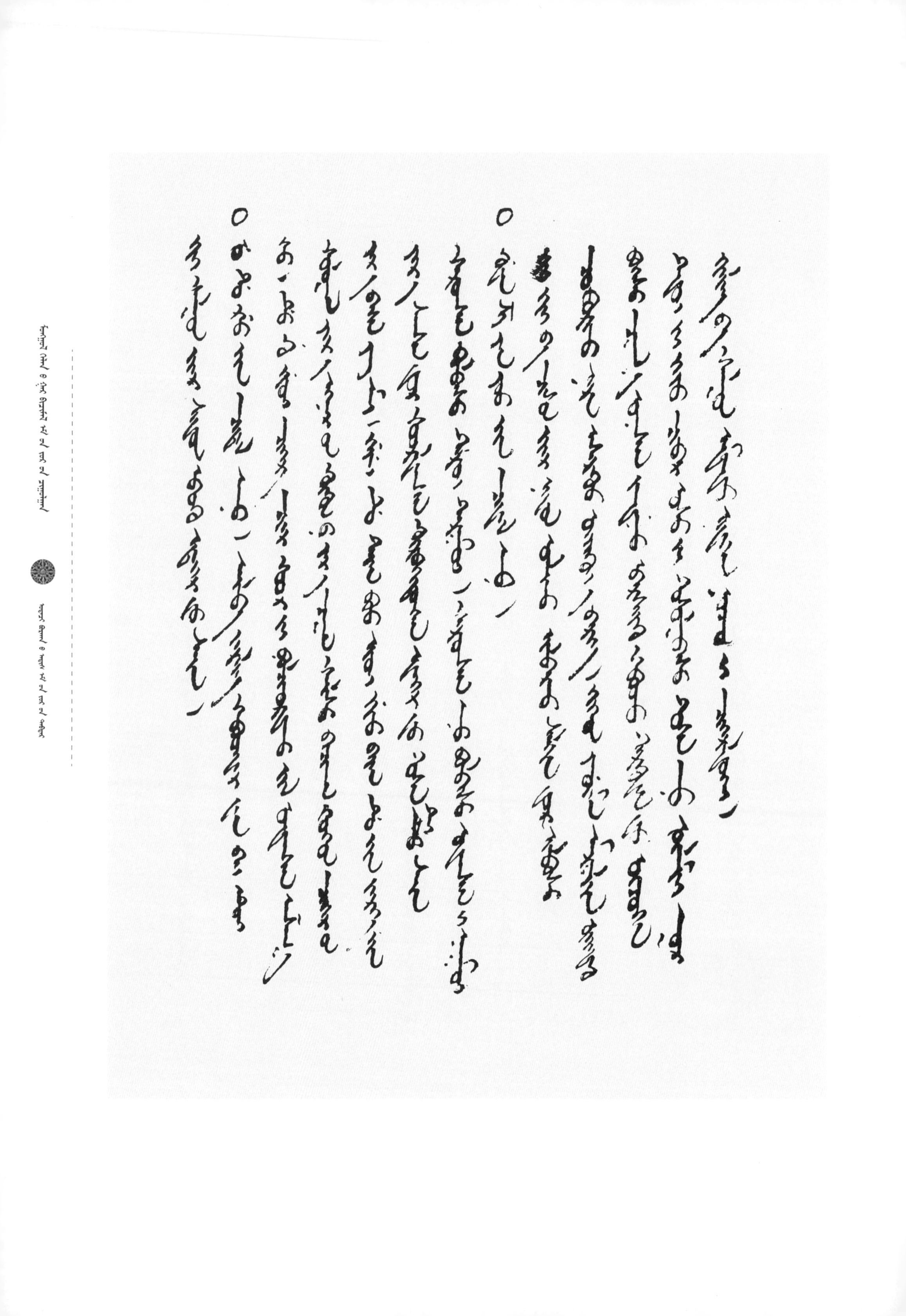

[illegible]
[illegible]
[illegible]
[illegible]
[illegible]

○ [illegible]
[illegible]
[illegible]
[illegible]
[illegible]
[illegible]

○ [illegible]
[illegible]

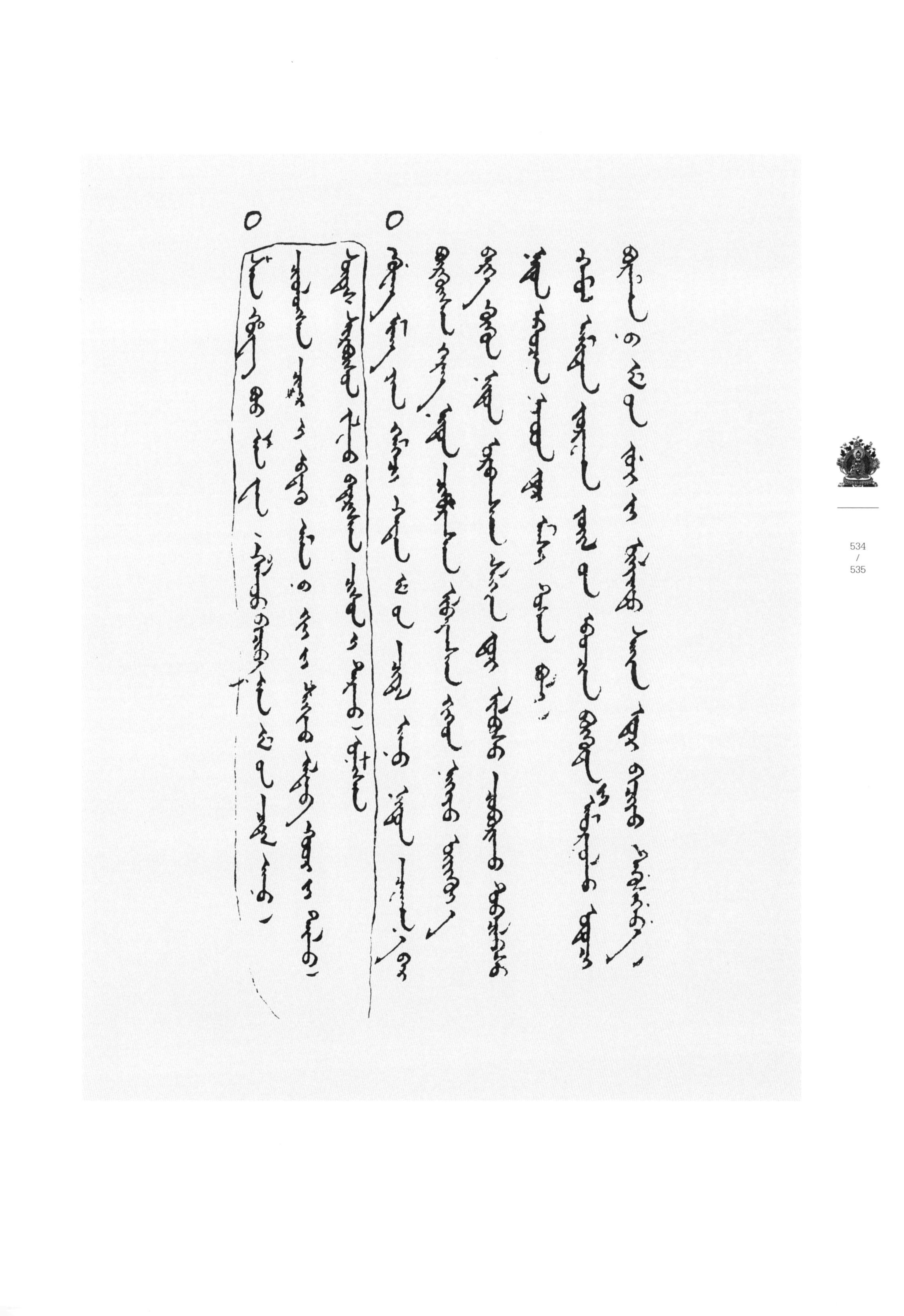

ᠣᠷᠣᠰᠢᠵᠤ ᠵᠠᠭᠤᠨ ᠨᠢᠭᠡ ᠰᠤᠳᠤᠯᠤᠭᠰᠠᠨ ᠠᠴᠠ ᠲᠣᠭᠲᠠᠭᠠᠭᠰᠠᠨ ᠬᠡᠮᠵᠢᠶᠡᠨ ᠦ ᠬᠡᠮᠵᠢᠶ᠎ᠡ ᠲᠡᠭᠦᠨ ᠠᠴᠠ ::
ᠨᠢᠭᠡ ᠤ ᠪᠢᠴᠢᠭᠯᠡᠭᠰᠡᠨ ᠬᠠᠮᠤᠭ ᠰᠤᠳᠤᠷ ᠤᠨ ᠳᠡᠪᠲᠡᠷ ᠤ ᠰᠤᠪᠤᠳ ᠰᠤᠷᠭᠠᠯ ᠤᠨ ᠳᠠᠭᠤᠤ ᠨᠣᠮᠤᠨ ᠤ ᠪᠢᠴᠢᠭ ᠪᠣᠯᠤᠨ᠎ᠠ :: ᠲᠤᠰ ᠪᠡ ᠰᠤᠳᠤᠷ ᠤᠨ ᠬᠡᠮᠵᠢᠶ᠎ᠡ ᠨᠢ ᠲᠠᠷᠠᠬᠤ ᠭᠠᠷ ᠤᠨ ᠲᠤᠰ ᠲᠡᠭᠦᠨ
ᠪᠢᠴᠢᠭᠯᠡᠭᠰᠡᠨ ᠪᠢᠴᠢᠭ ᠮᠠᠲᠠᠷ ᠪᠣᠯᠤᠨ᠎ᠠ :: ᠨᠢᠭᠡ ᠪᠡ ᠲᠤᠰ ᠳᠠᠭᠤ ᠨᠢ ᠰᠤᠪᠤᠳ ᠪᠡᠷ ᠲᠤᠰᠬᠠᠯ ᠢ ᠲᠠᠯᠠ ᠰᠤᠳᠤᠯᠤᠭᠰᠠᠨ ᠲᠣᠭᠲᠠᠭᠠᠭᠰᠠᠨ ᠣᠷᠣᠰᠢᠵᠤ ᠲᠠᠯᠠ ᠬᠠᠮᠤᠭᠯᠠᠭᠰᠠᠨ ᠪᠤᠯᠤᠭᠰᠠᠨ ᠢ ᠲᠠᠶᠢᠯᠪᠤᠷᠢ ᠪᠣᠯᠤᠨ᠎ᠠ ::
ᠡᠨᠡ ᠪᠢᠴᠢᠭ ᠰᠤᠷᠠᠭᠠᠯᠳᠠ ᠨᠢᠭᠡ ᠰᠤᠳᠤᠷ ᠤᠨ ᠳᠡᠪᠲᠡᠷ ᠦᠨ ᠰᠢᠨᠵᠢᠯᠡᠯ ᠲᠤᠬᠠᠢ ᠪᠡᠷ ᠲᠤᠰ ᠤ ᠪᠢᠴᠢᠭᠯᠡᠭᠰᠡᠨ ᠮᠠᠨ ᠪᠣᠯᠤᠨ ᠲᠠᠢᠯᠪᠤ ᠰᠤᠳᠤᠷ ᠤᠨ ᠨᠢ ᠬᠡᠮᠵᠢᠶ᠎ᠡ ᠢ
ᠪᠢᠴᠢ ᠨᠢ ᠥᠨᠳᠥᠷ ᠢ : 22cm × 23.5cm ᠪᠣᠯᠤᠨ᠎ᠠ᠂ ᠨᠡᠢᠲᠡ 21 ᠨᠢᠭᠤᠷ ᠲᠠᠢ ::
ᠡᠨᠡ ᠪᠢᠴᠢᠭ ᠮᠠᠲᠠᠷ ᠲᠠᠷᠠᠭᠰᠠᠨ ᠪᠢᠴᠢ ᠨᠢ ᠰᠢᠨ᠎ᠡ ᠪᠠᠢᠳᠠᠯ ᠪᠢᠴᠢᠭ ᠮᠠᠲᠠᠷ ᠪᠣᠯᠤᠨ᠎ᠠ :: ᠲᠤᠰᠬᠠᠢ ᠨᠢ ᠰᠤᠷᠤᠭ ᠢ ᠪᠢᠴᠢᠭ ᠨᠢ ᠰᠢᠨᠵᠢᠯᠡ ᠪᠡᠷ ᠪᠠᠢᠭᠤᠯ ᠰᠤᠳᠤᠯᠤᠭᠰᠠᠨ ᠲᠤᠰ ᠲᠤᠰᠬᠠᠢ ᠲᠠᠢ ᠪᠣᠯᠤᠨ᠎ᠠ ::

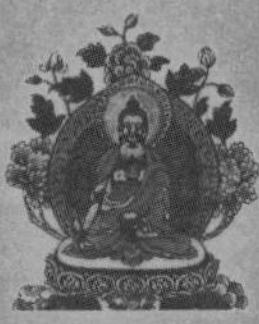

Collected Works of Prescriptions

杂方集

13

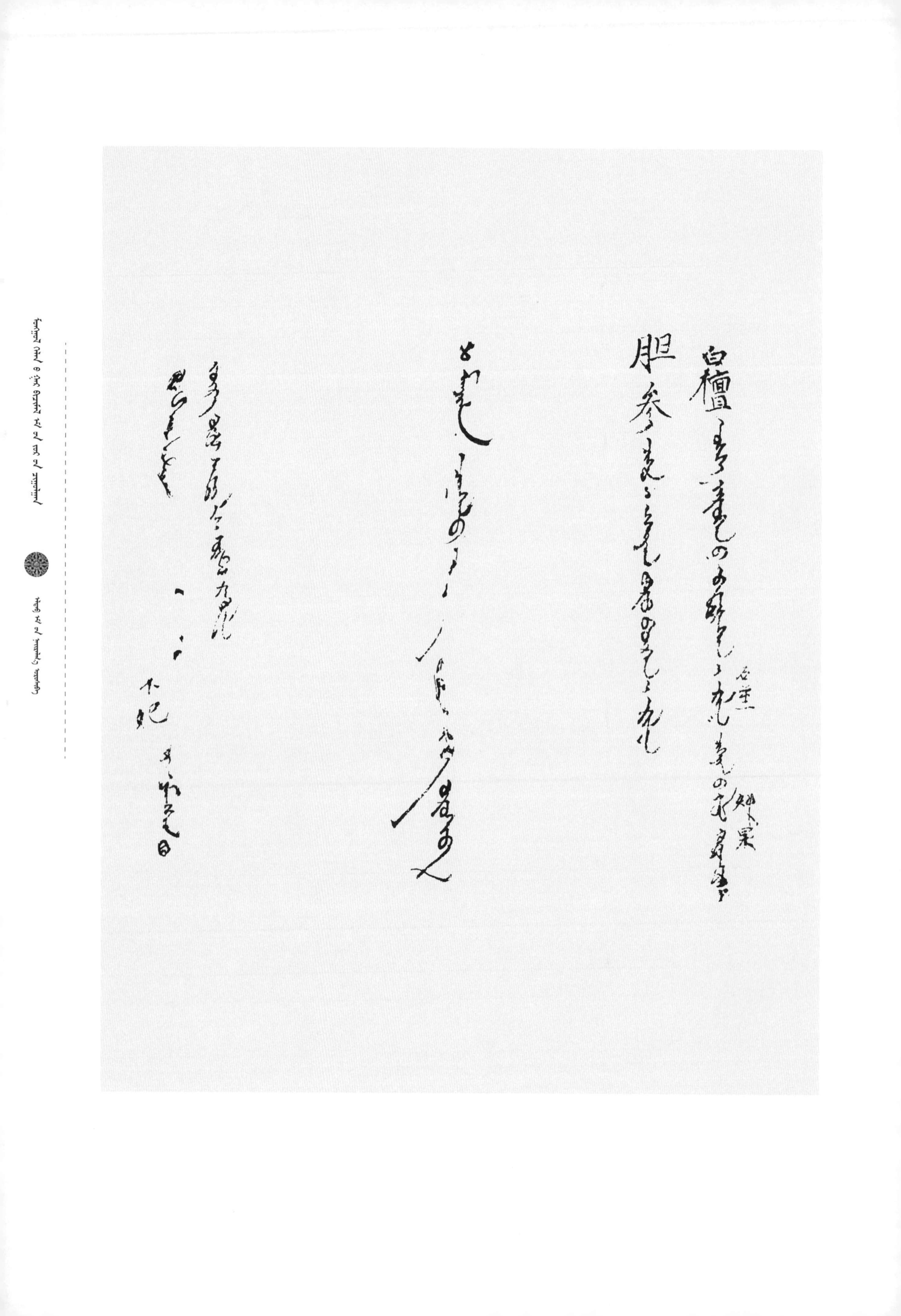

白檀 [illegible]

胆参 [illegible]

[illegible]

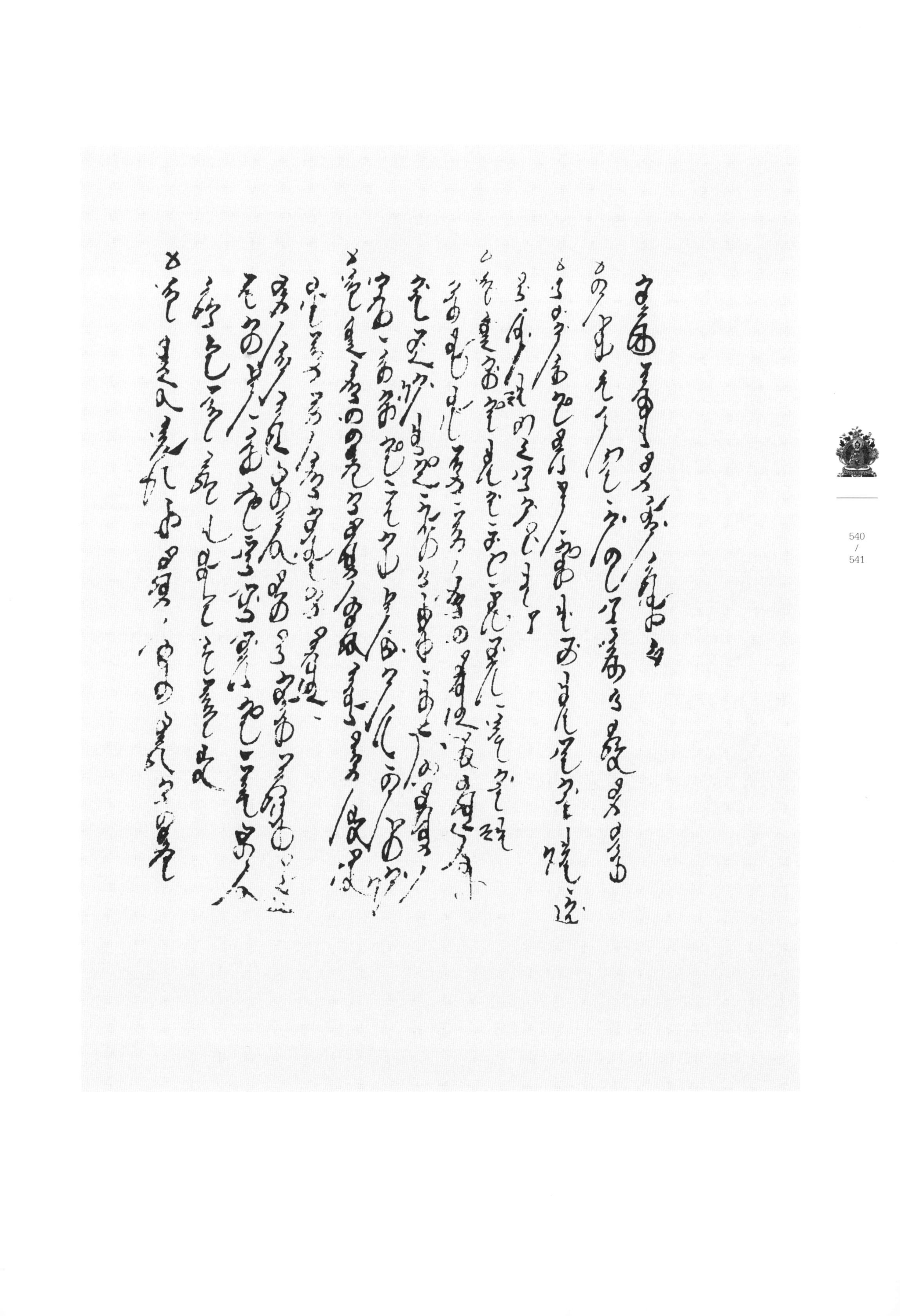

[illegible]

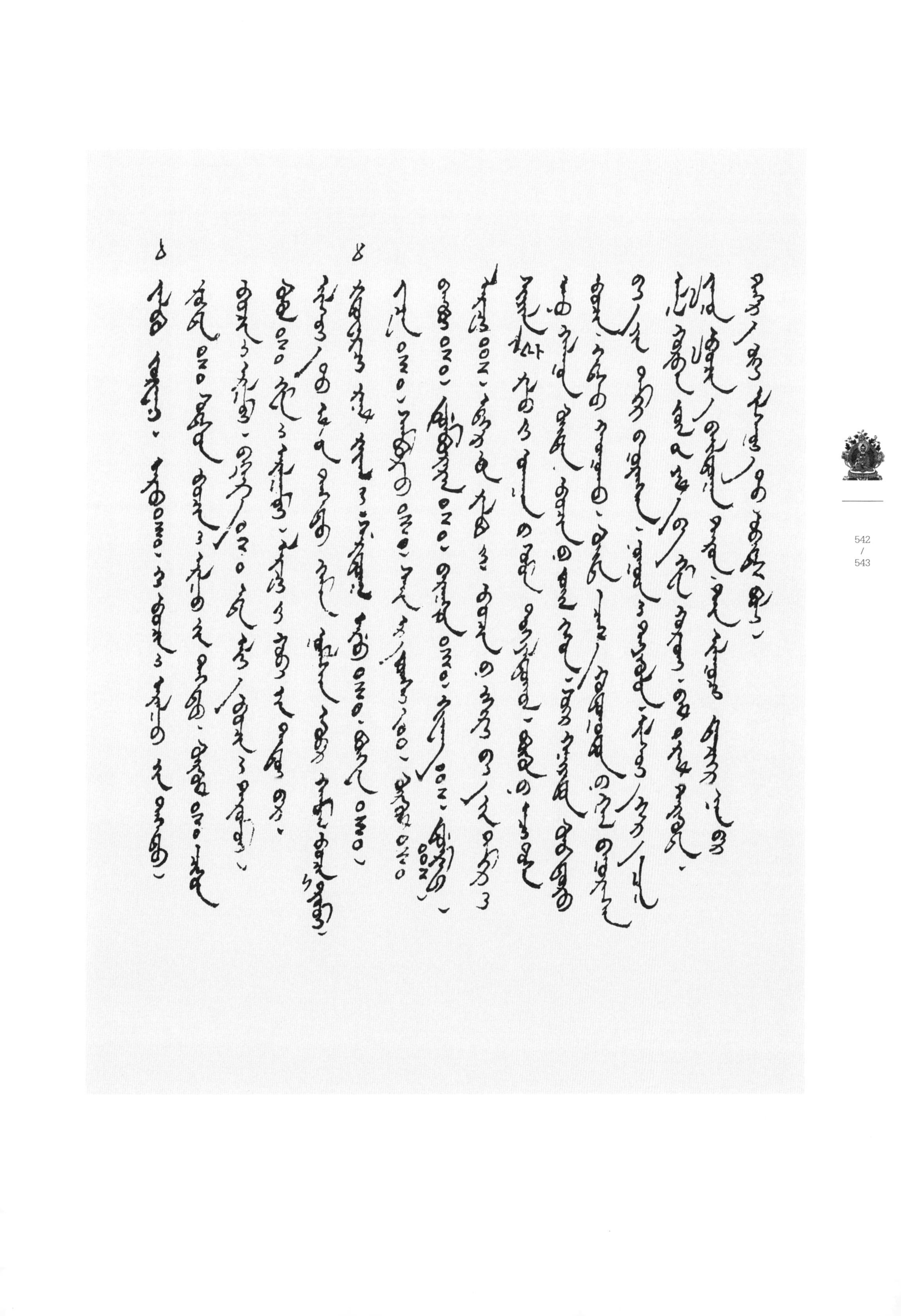

[illegible]

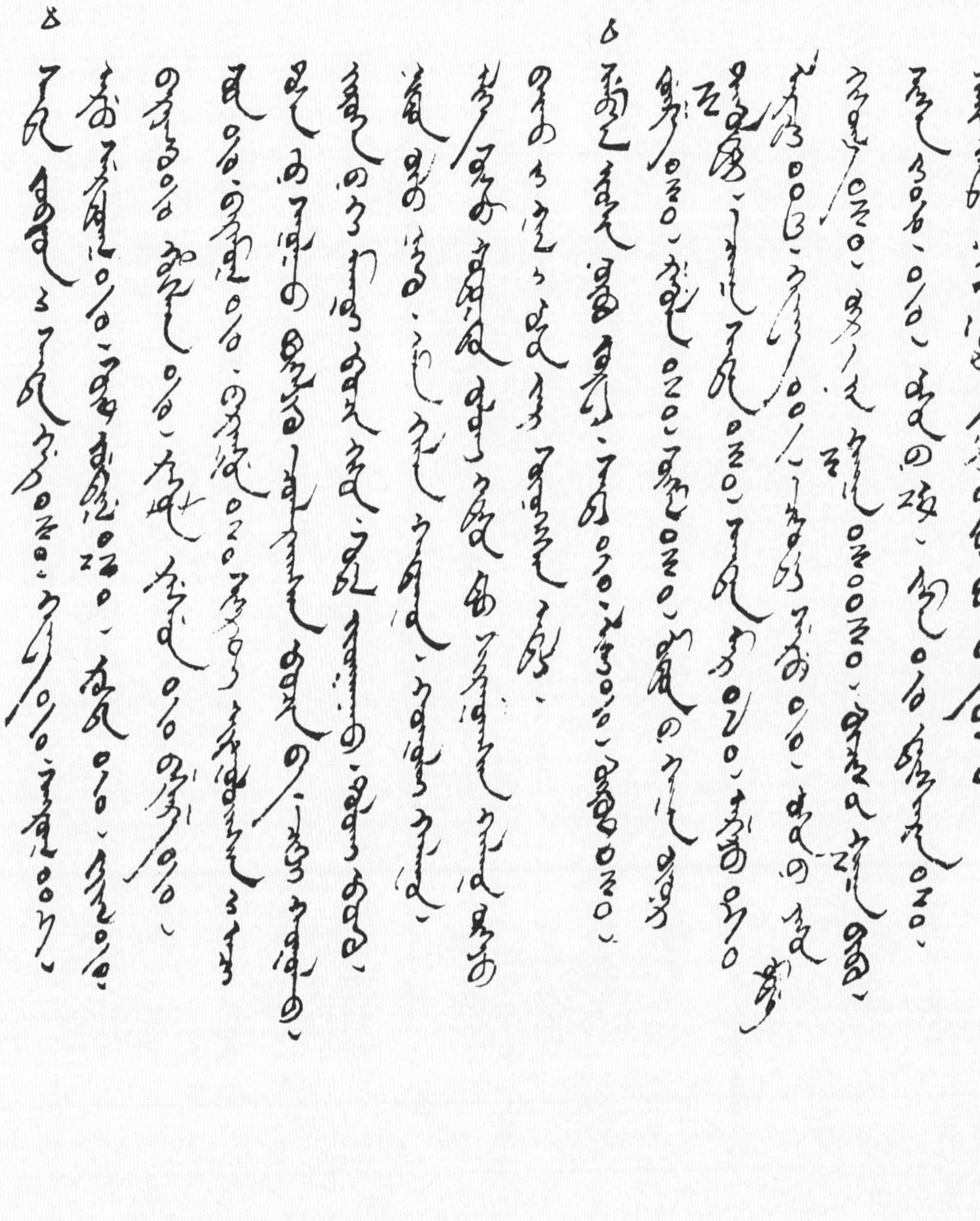

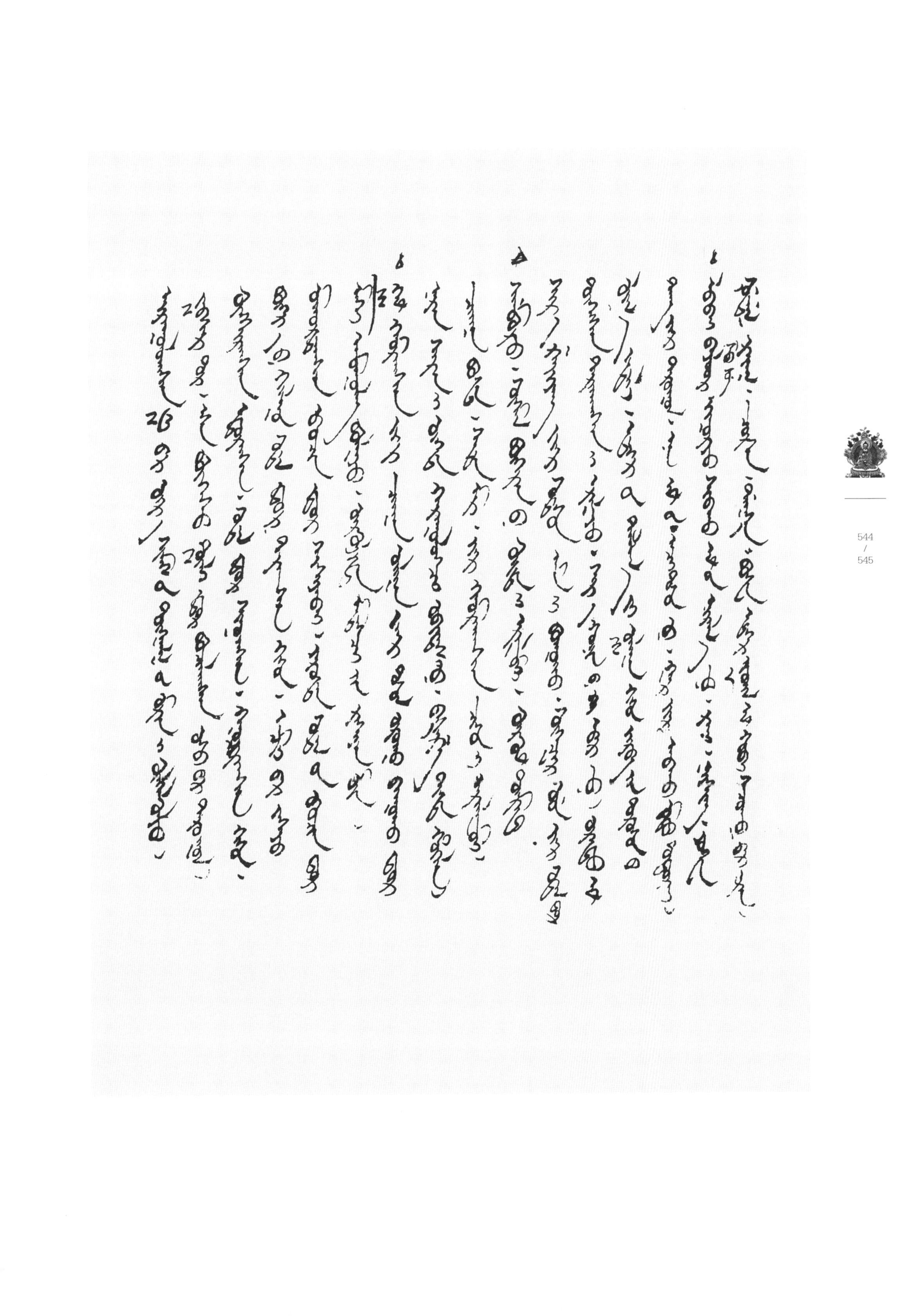

[illegible]

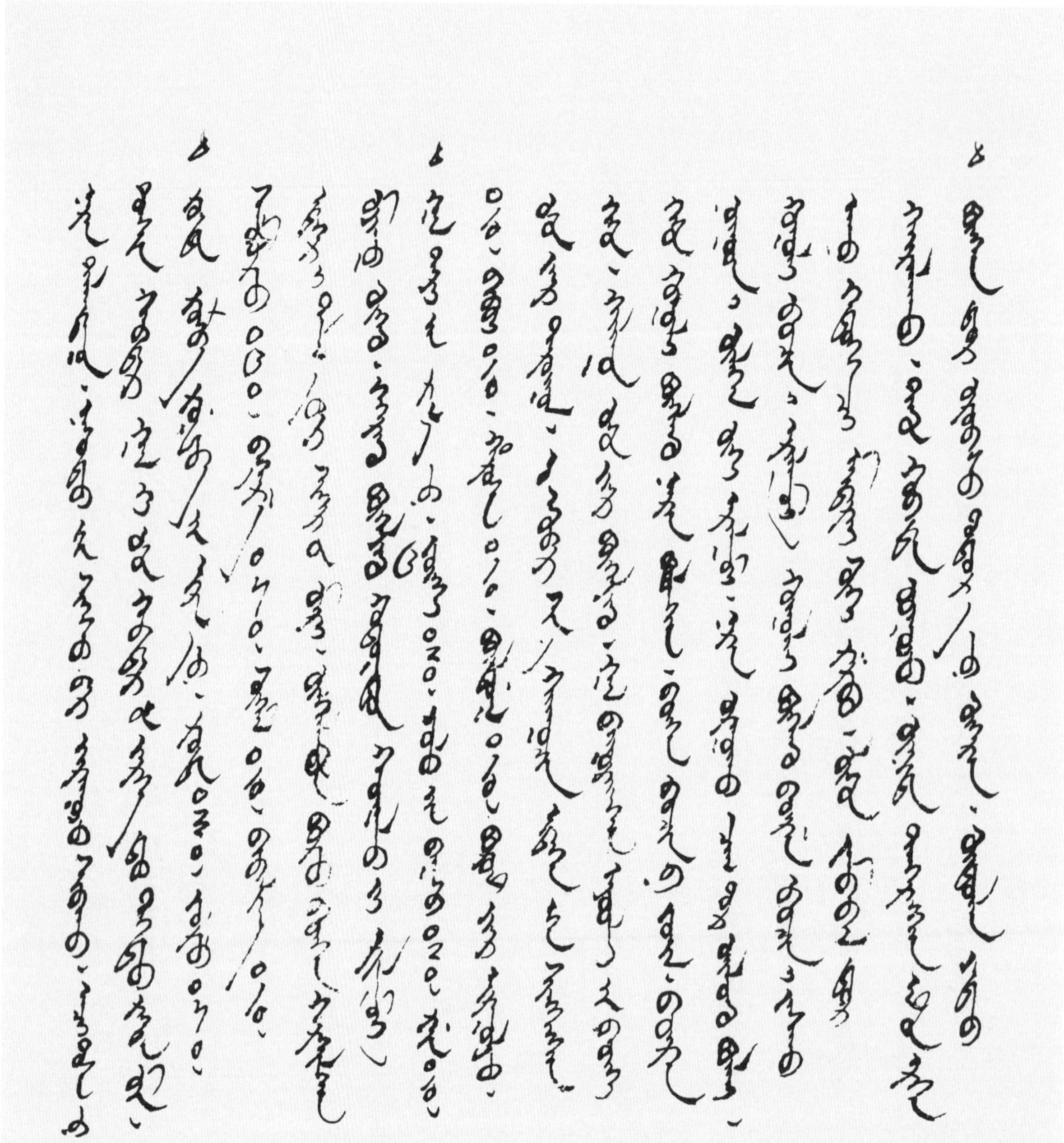

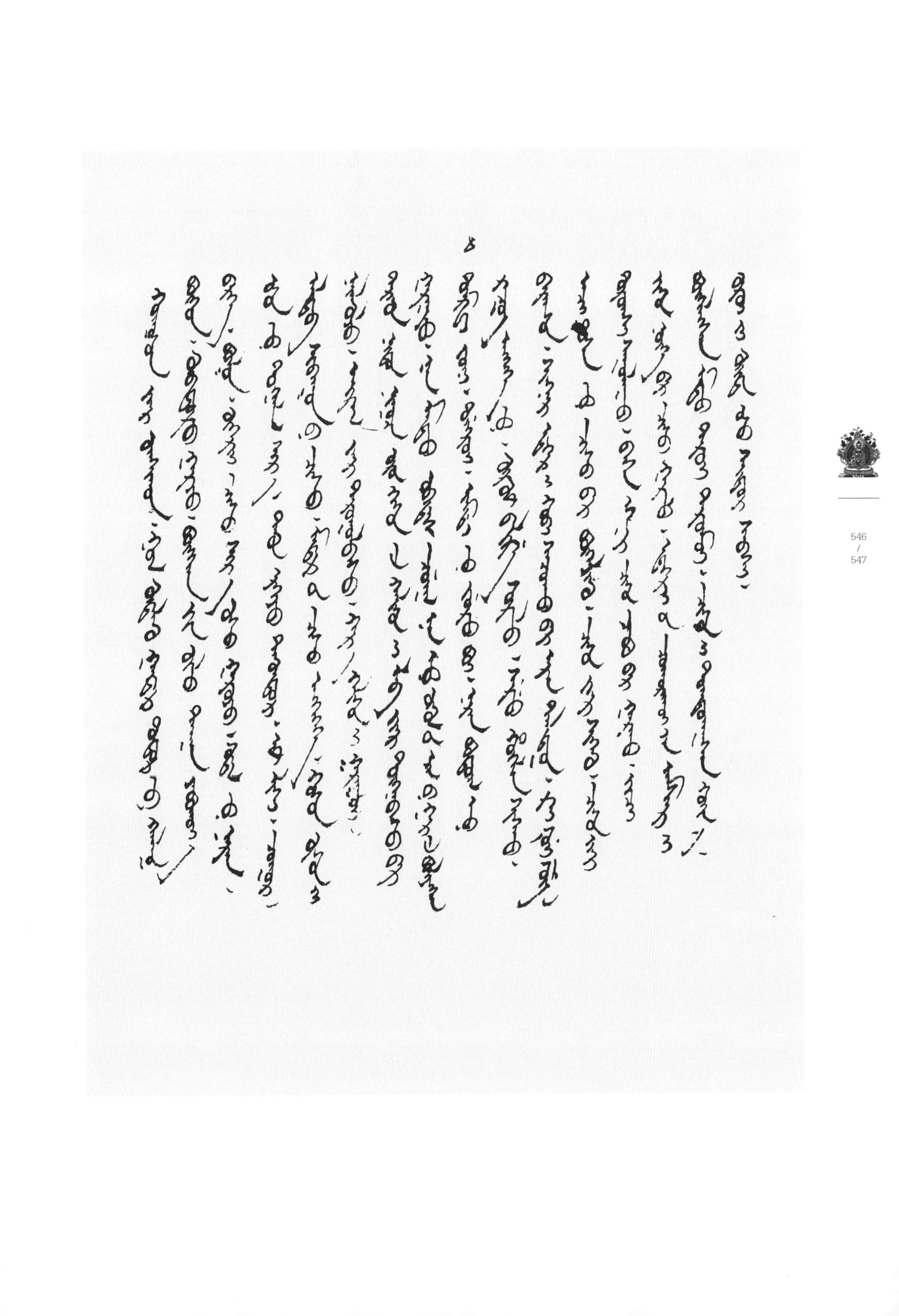

[illegible]

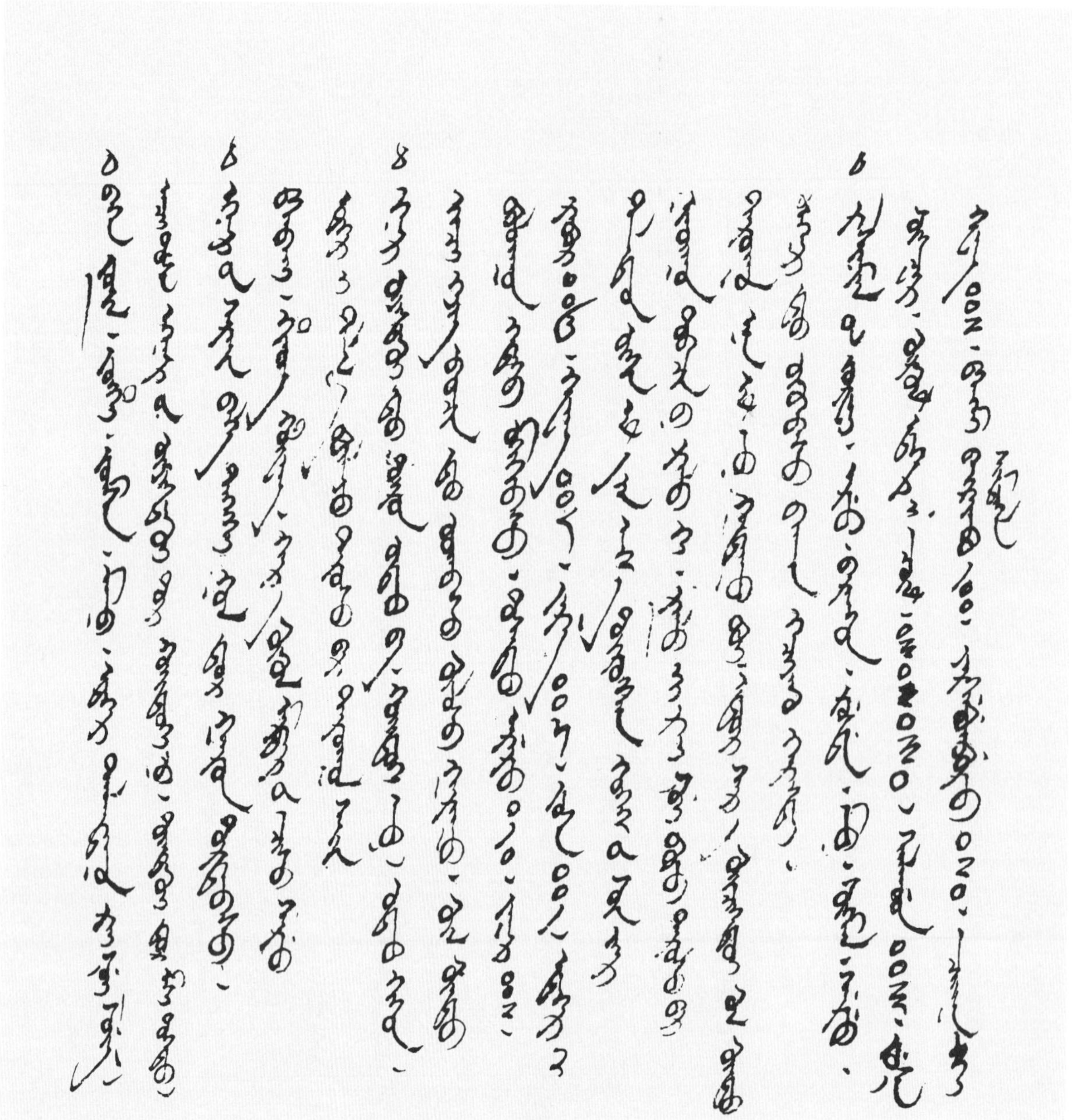

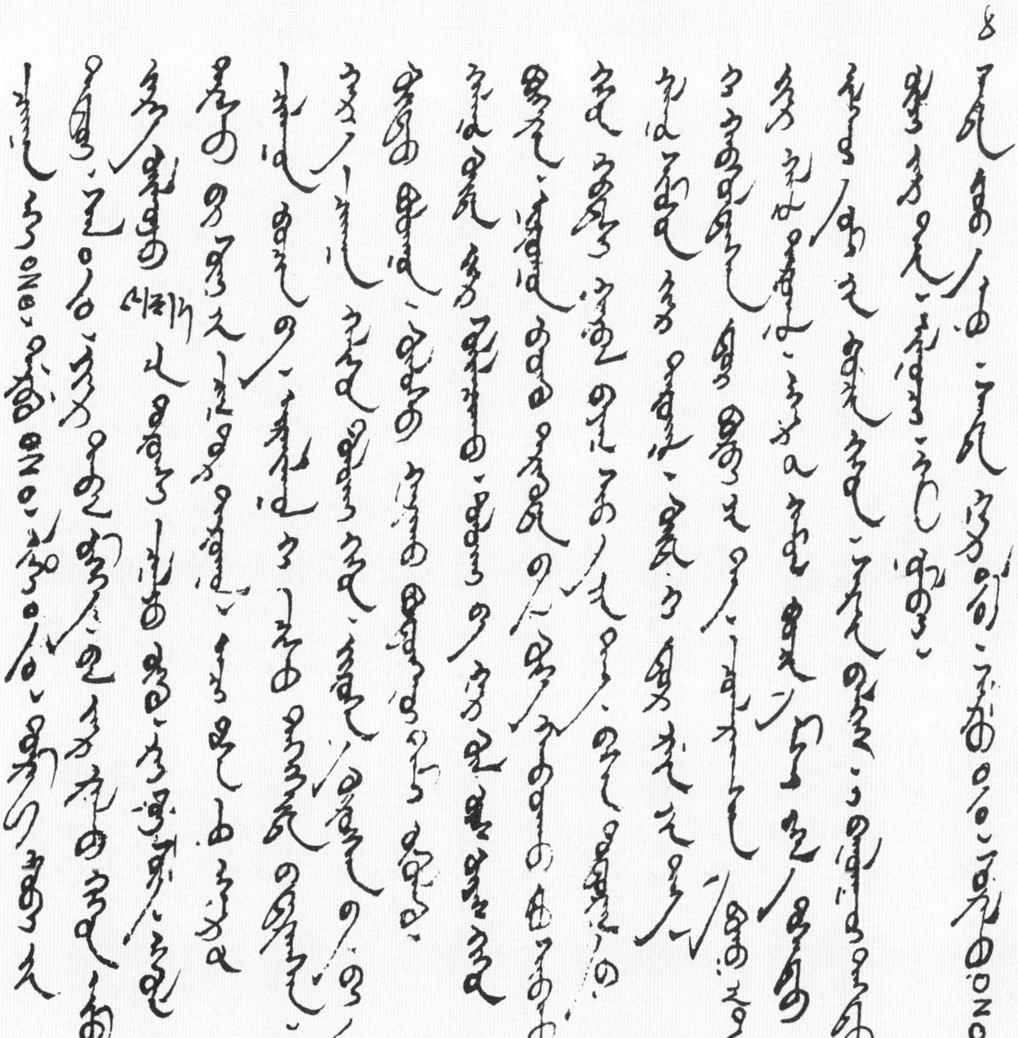

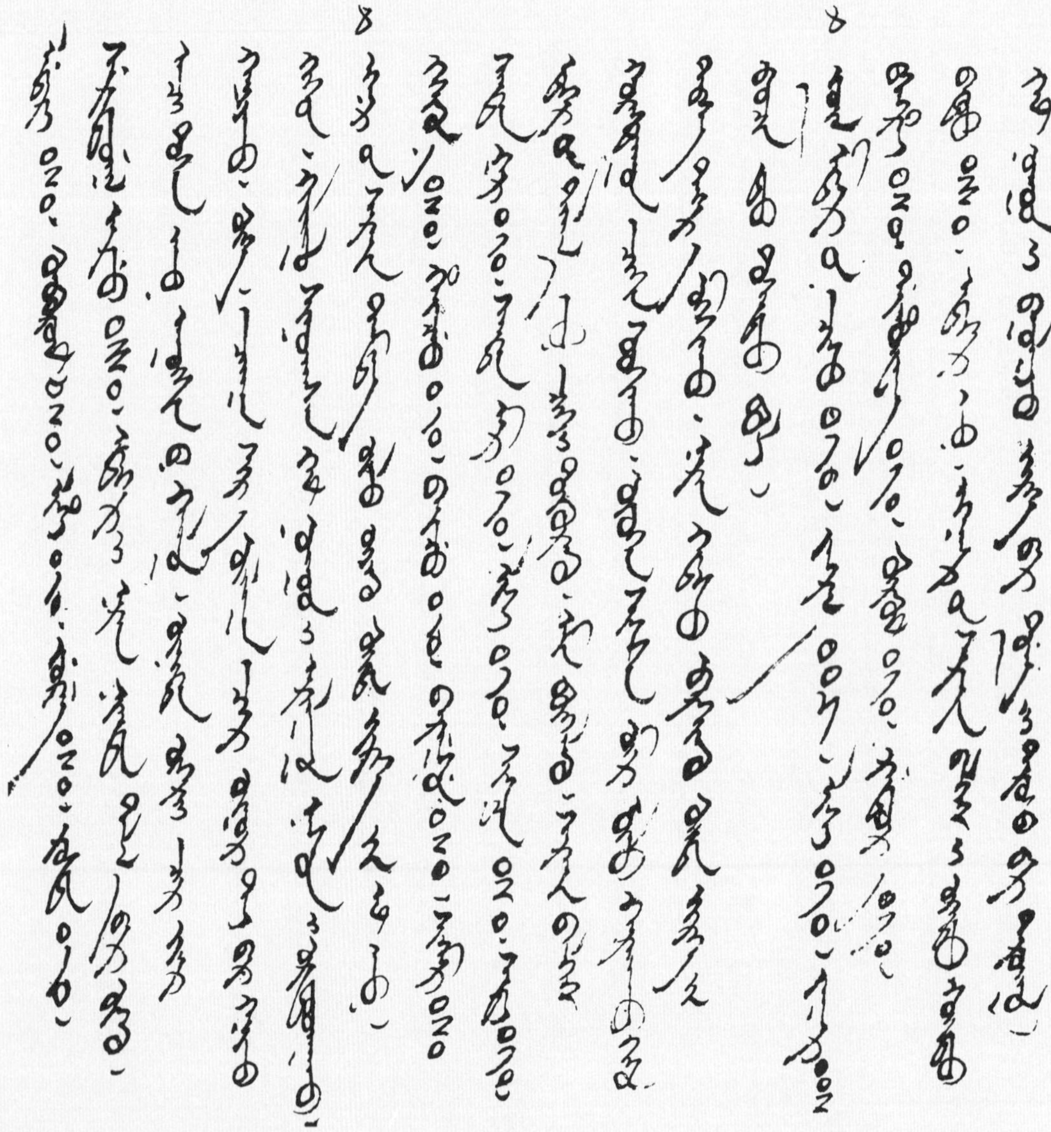

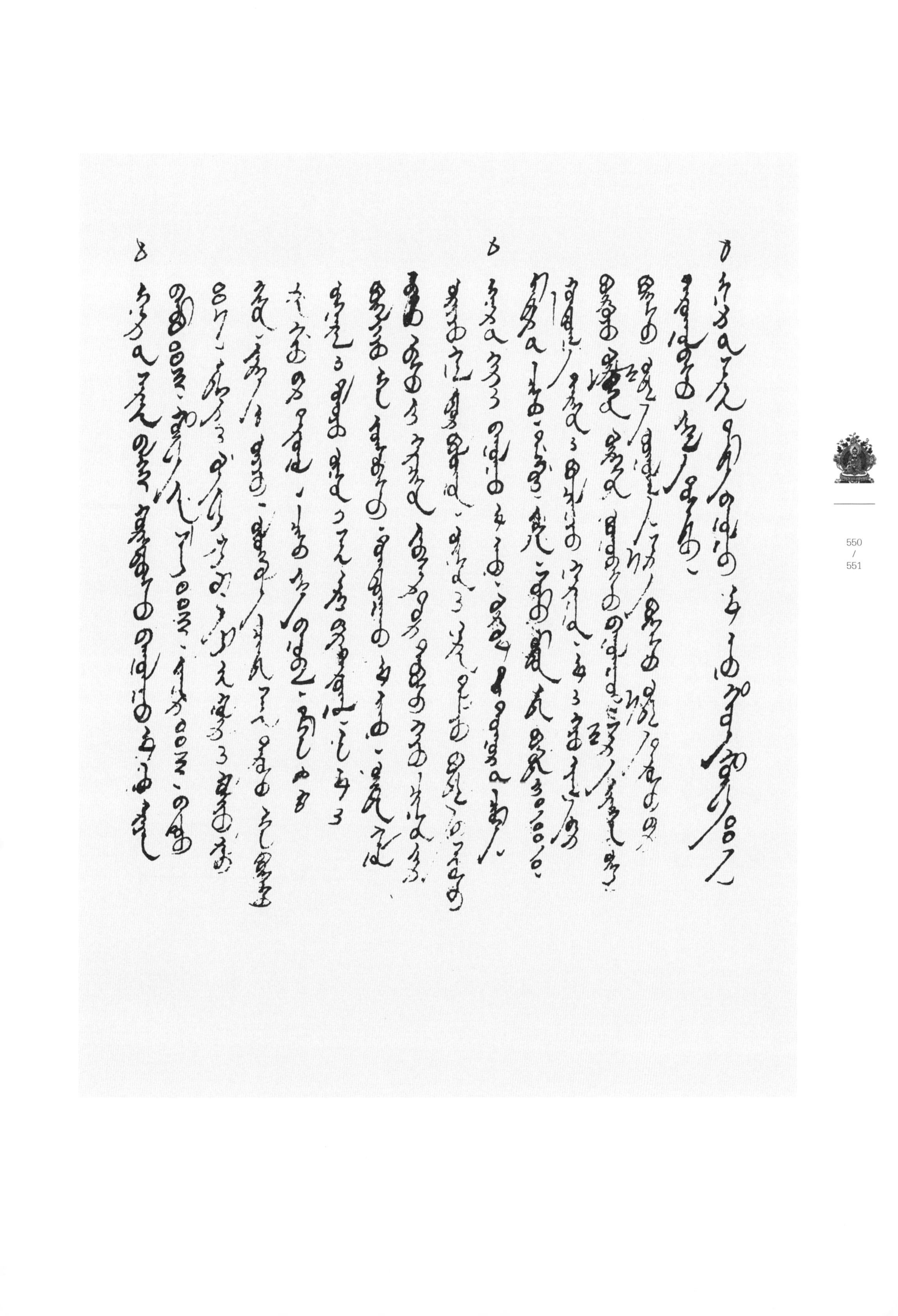

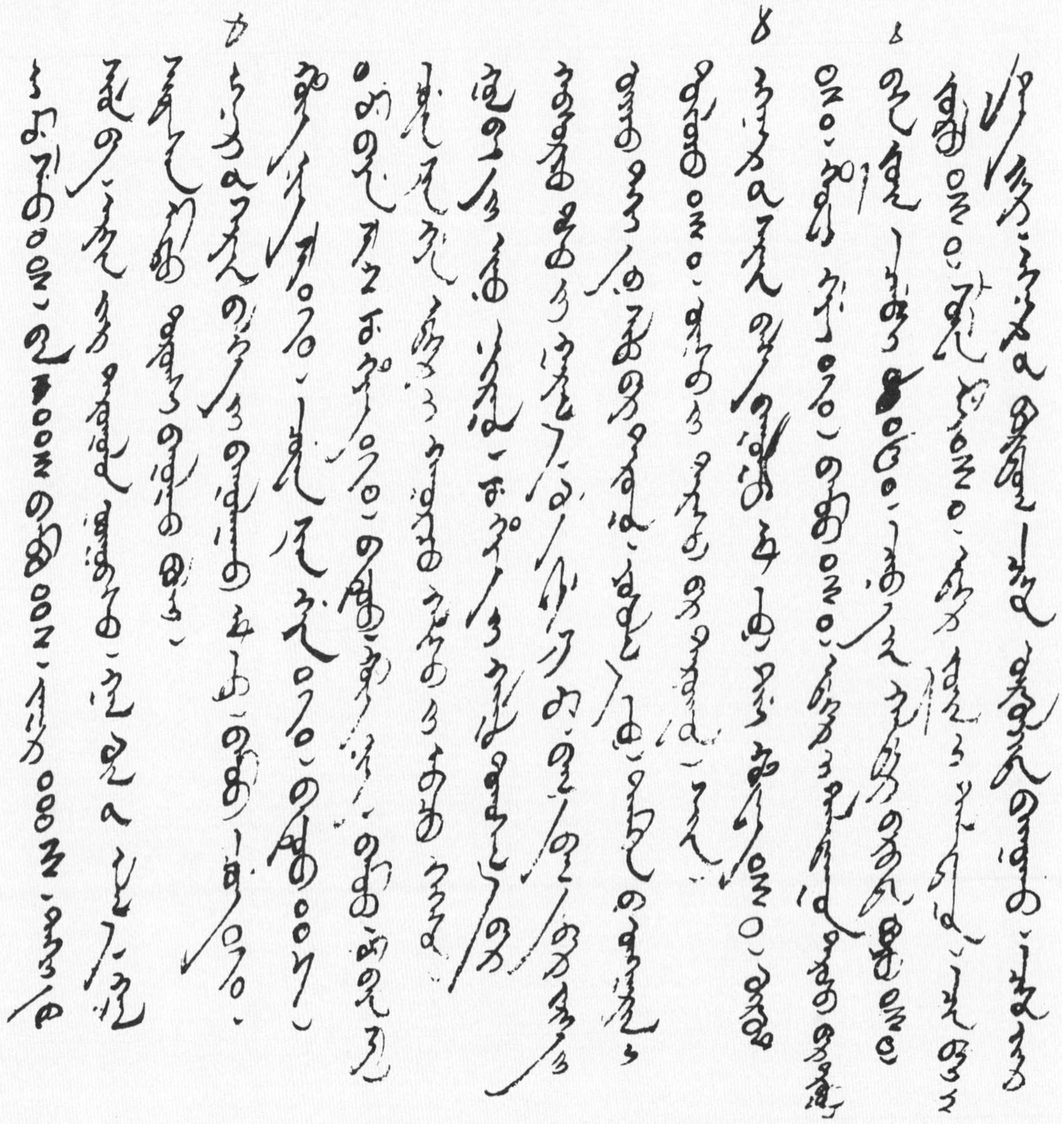

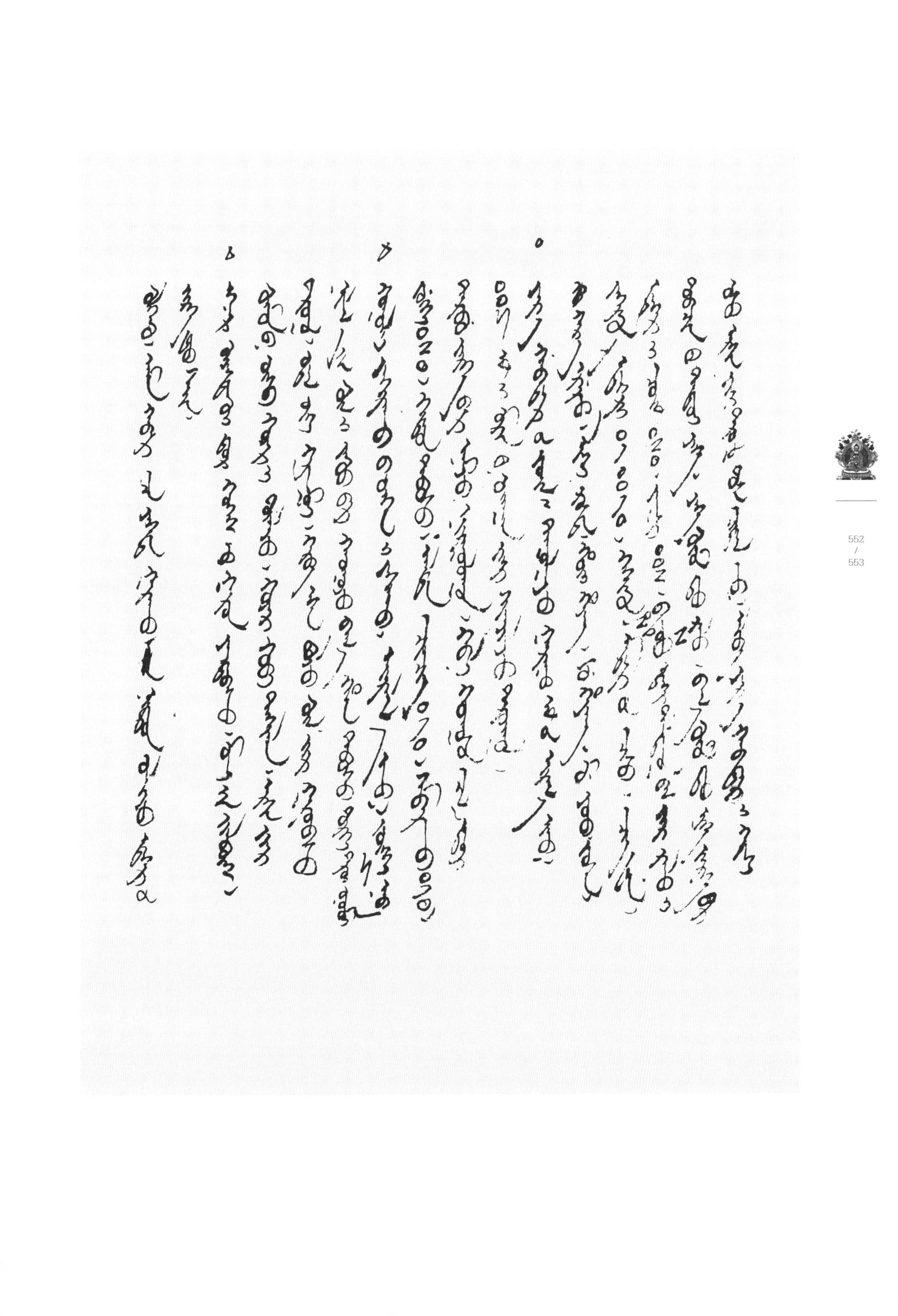

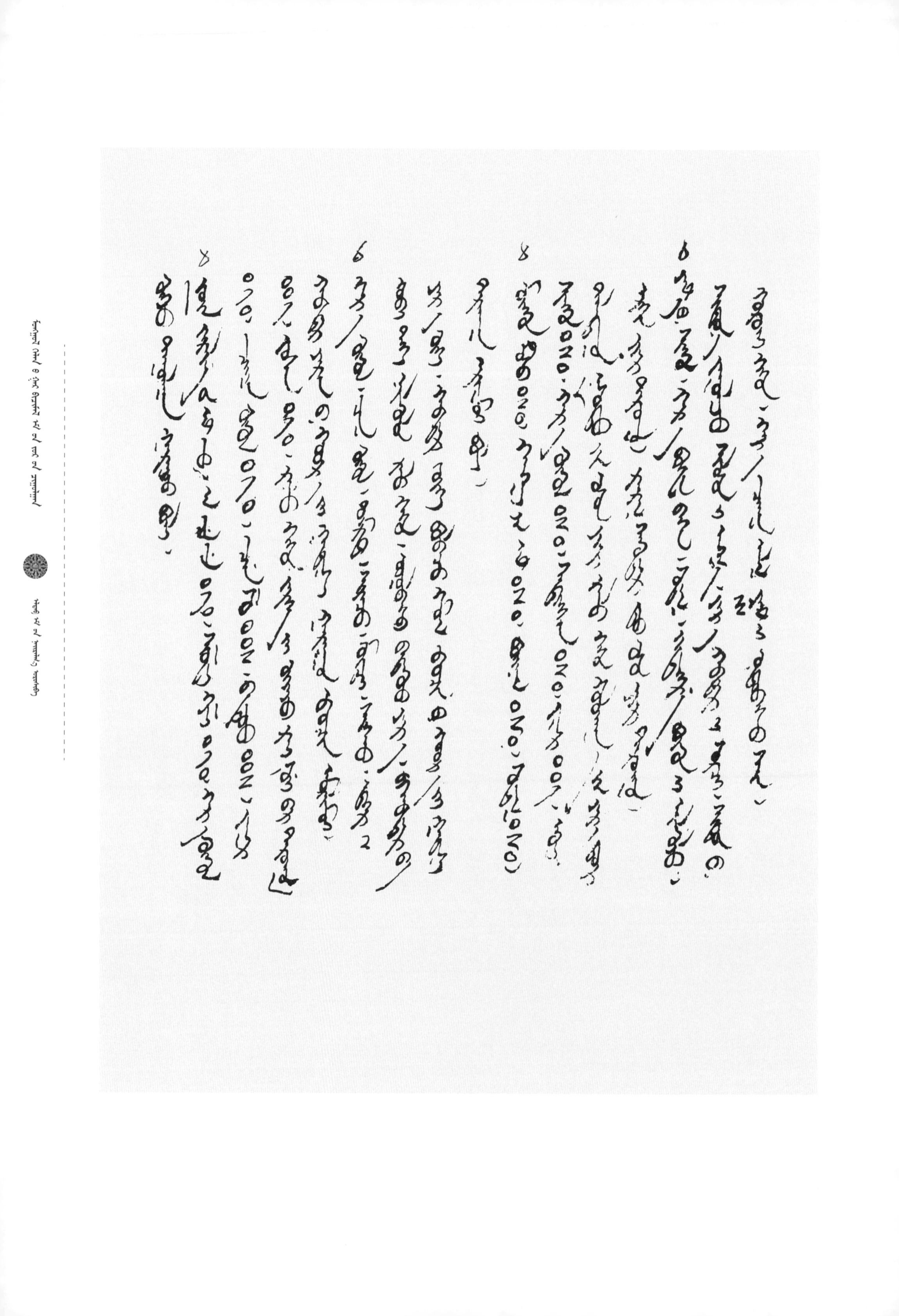

[illegible]

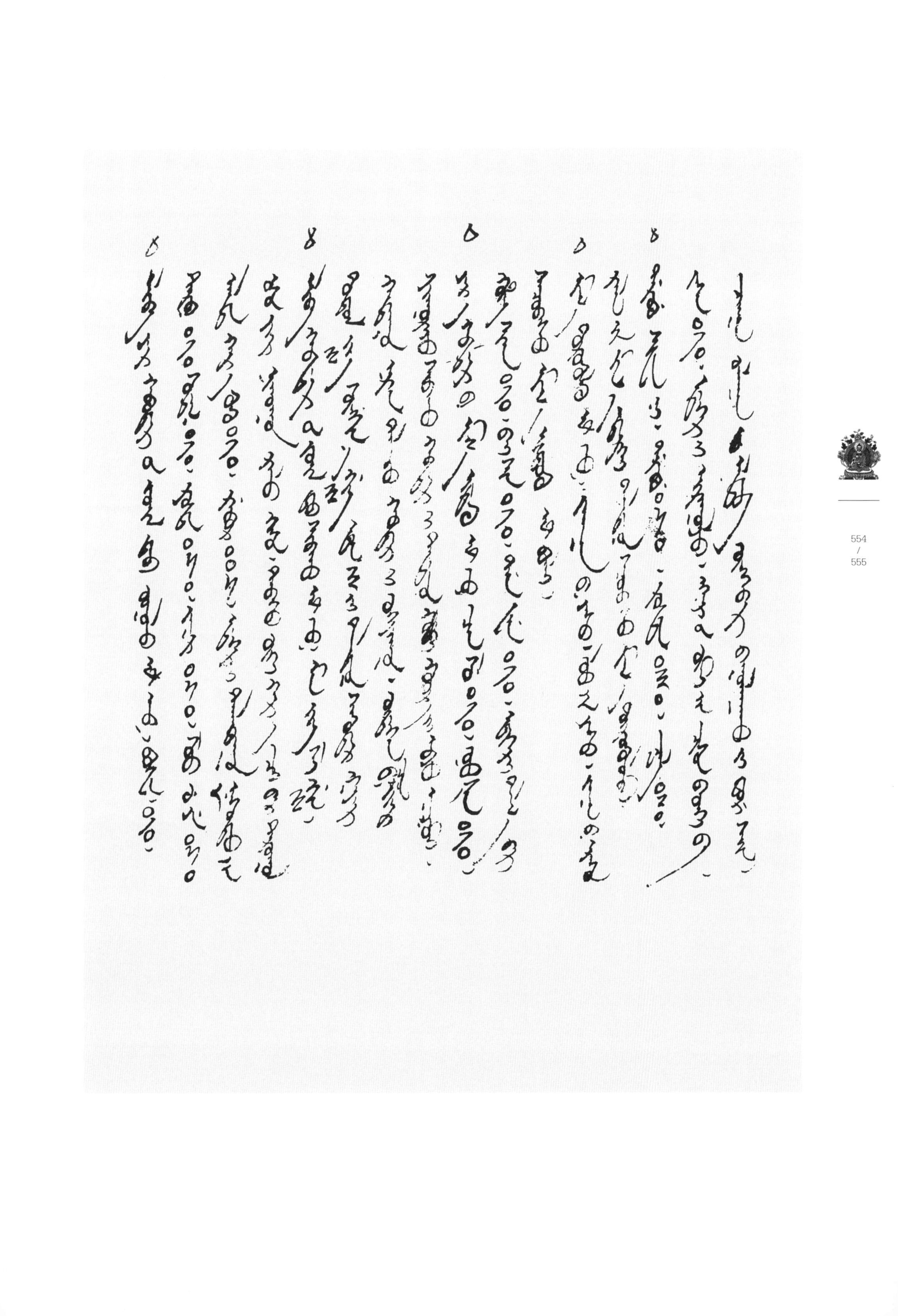

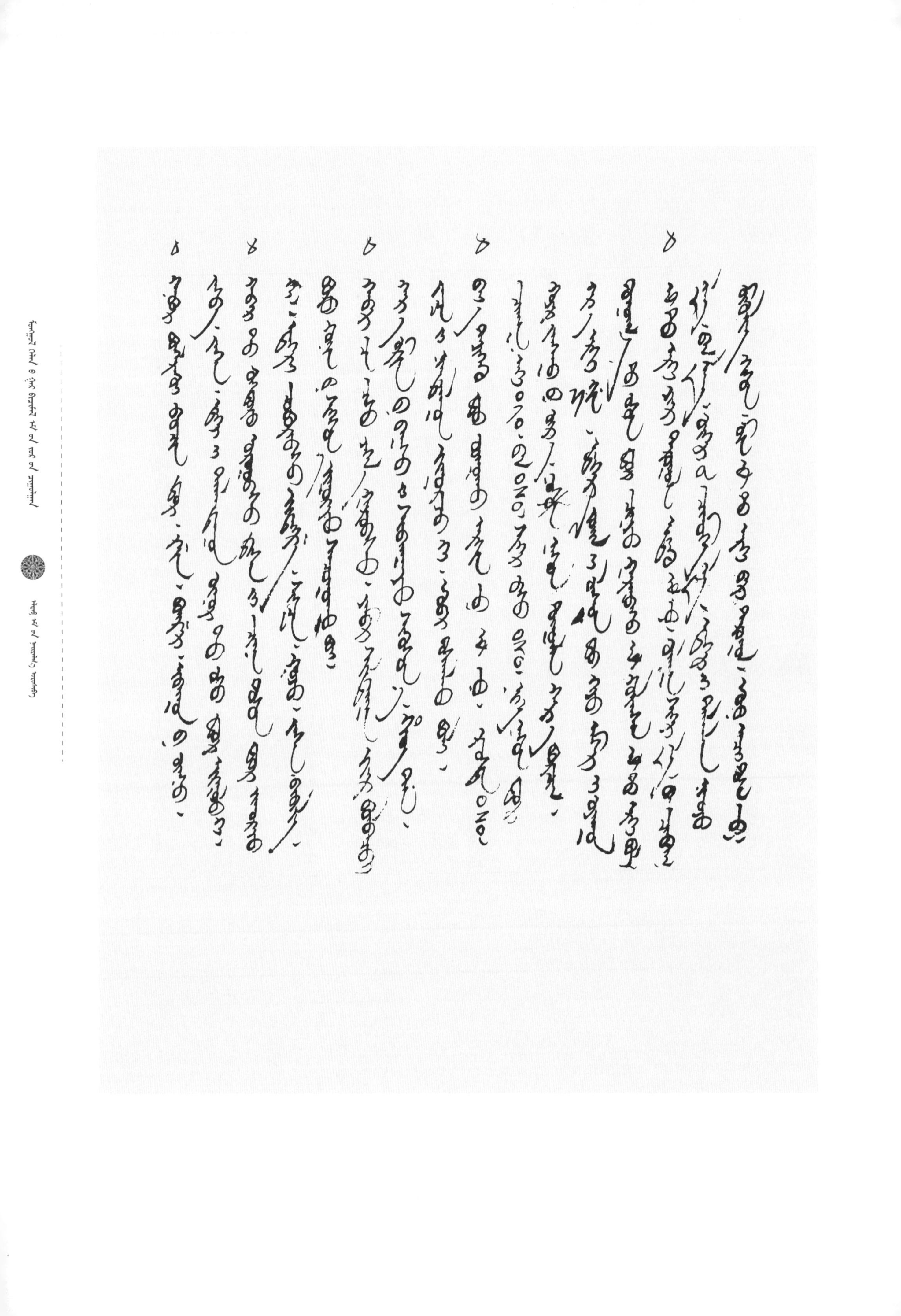

[illegible]

[illegible]

[illegible]

[illegible]

[illegible]

[illegible]

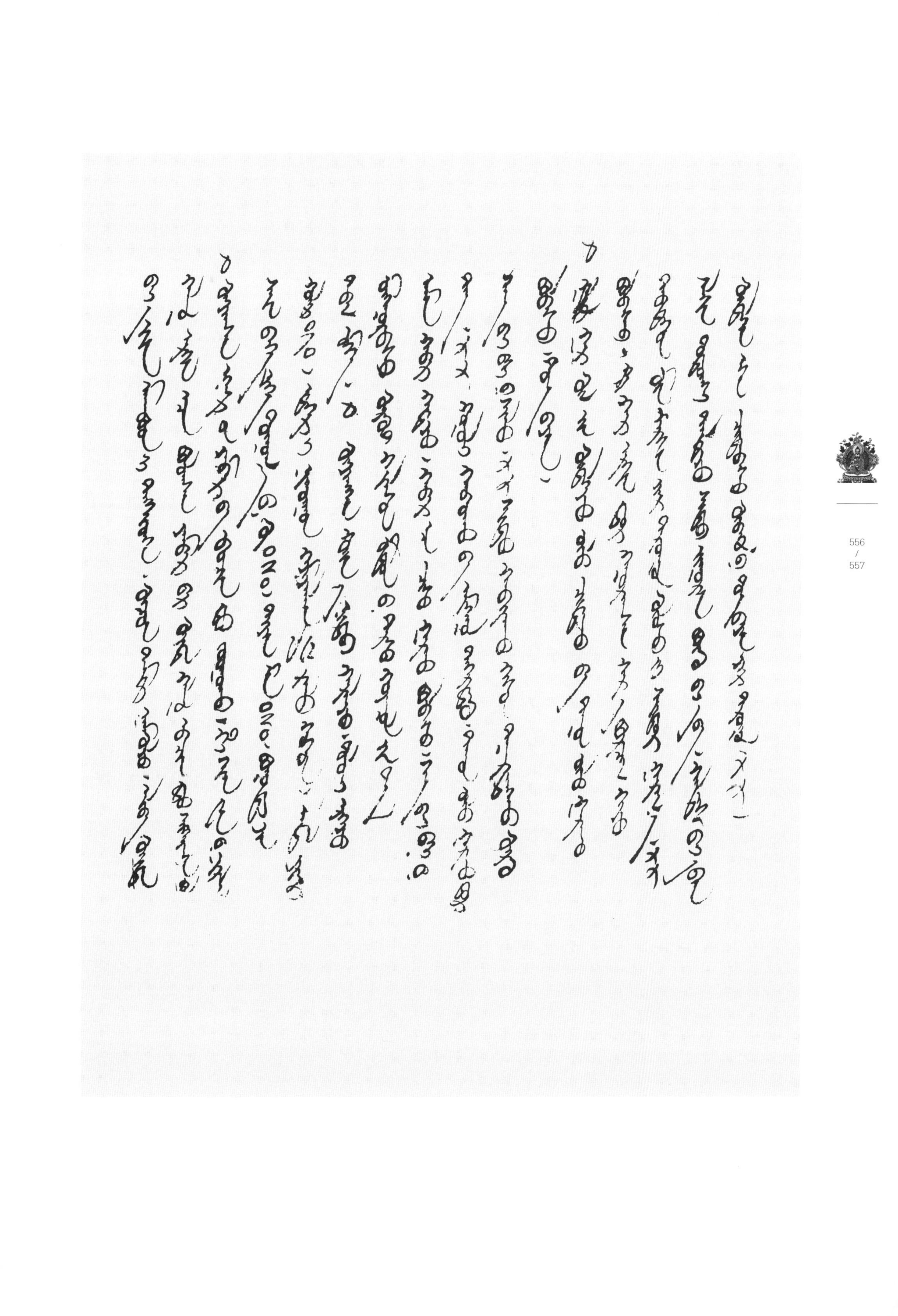

[illegible]

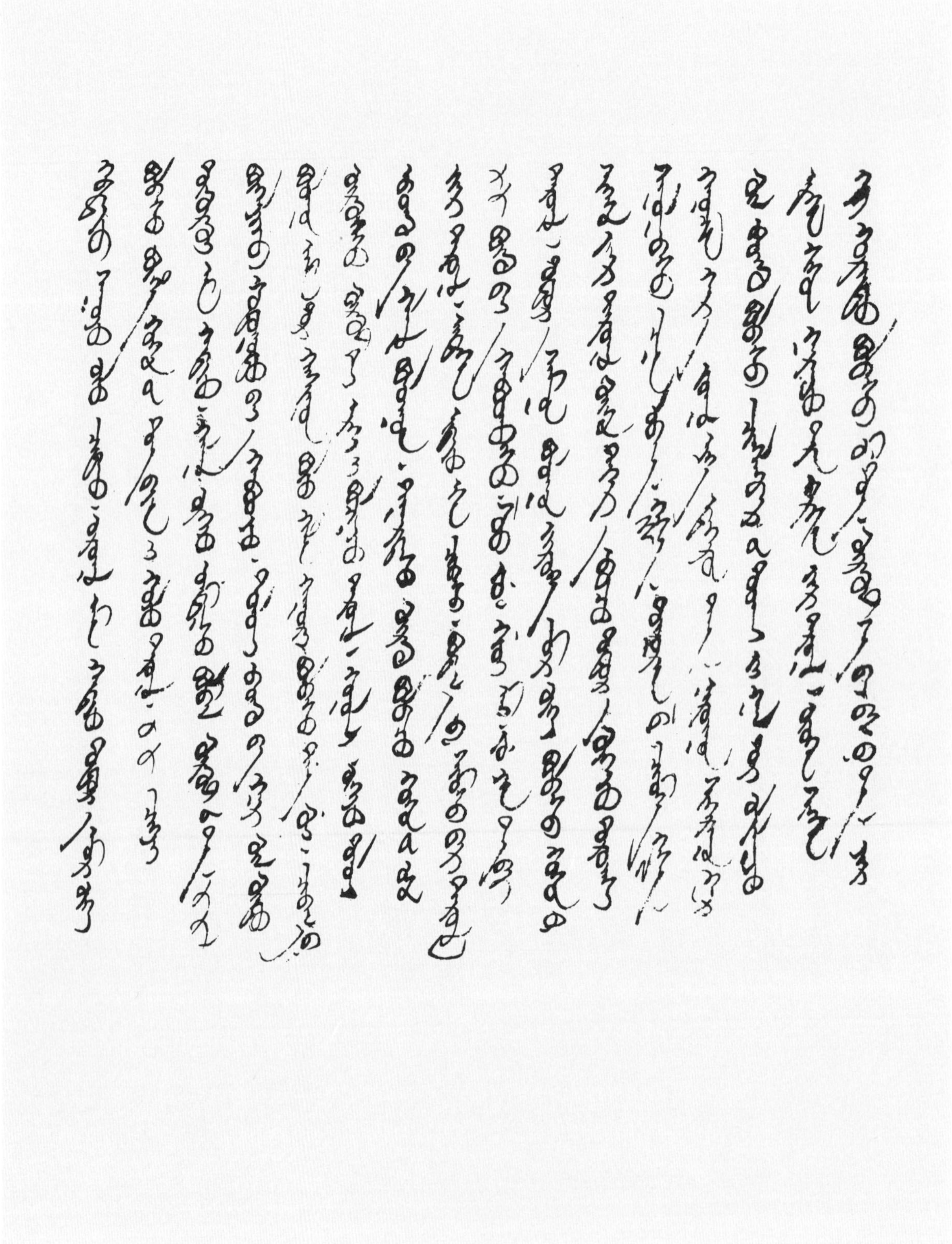

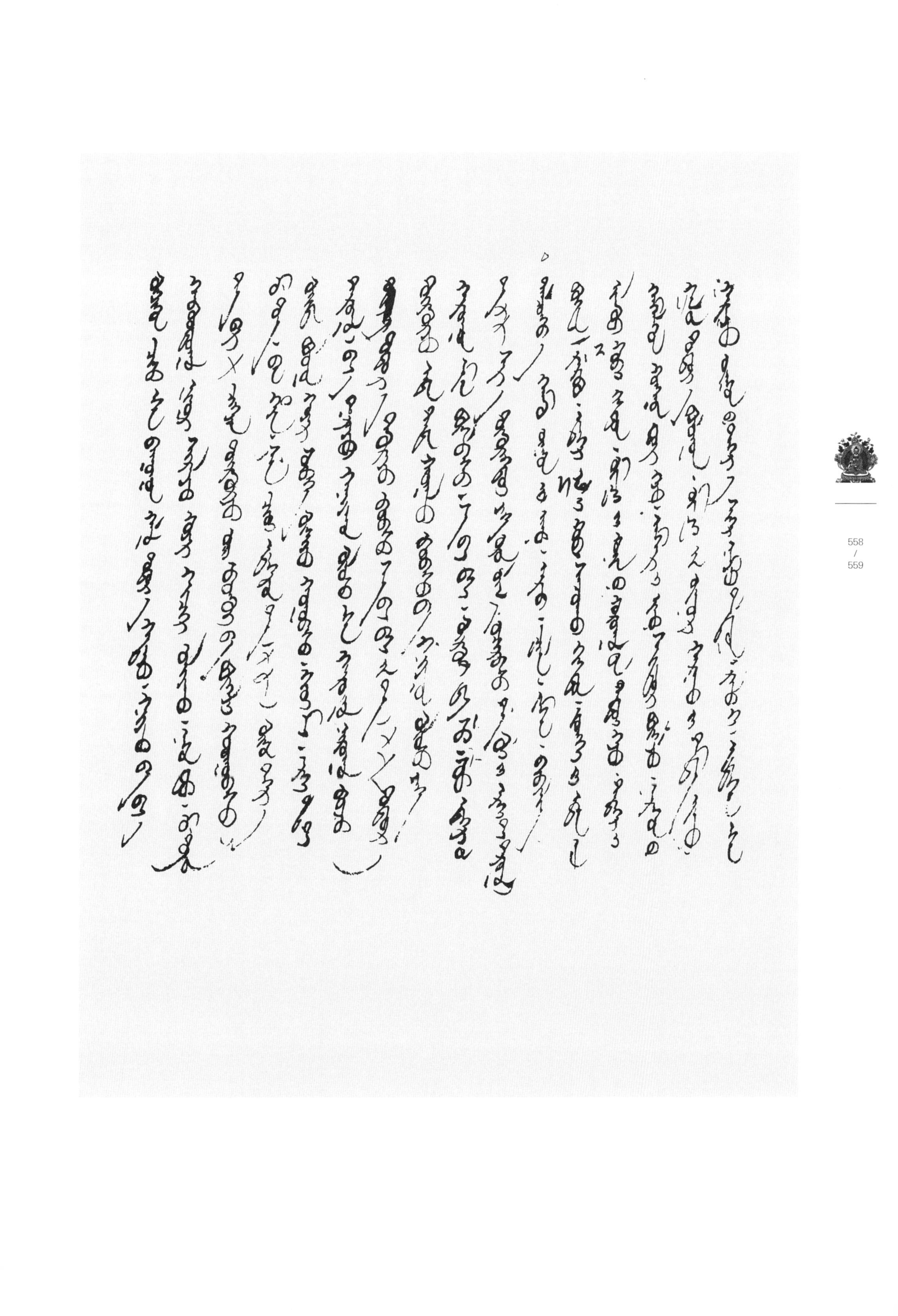

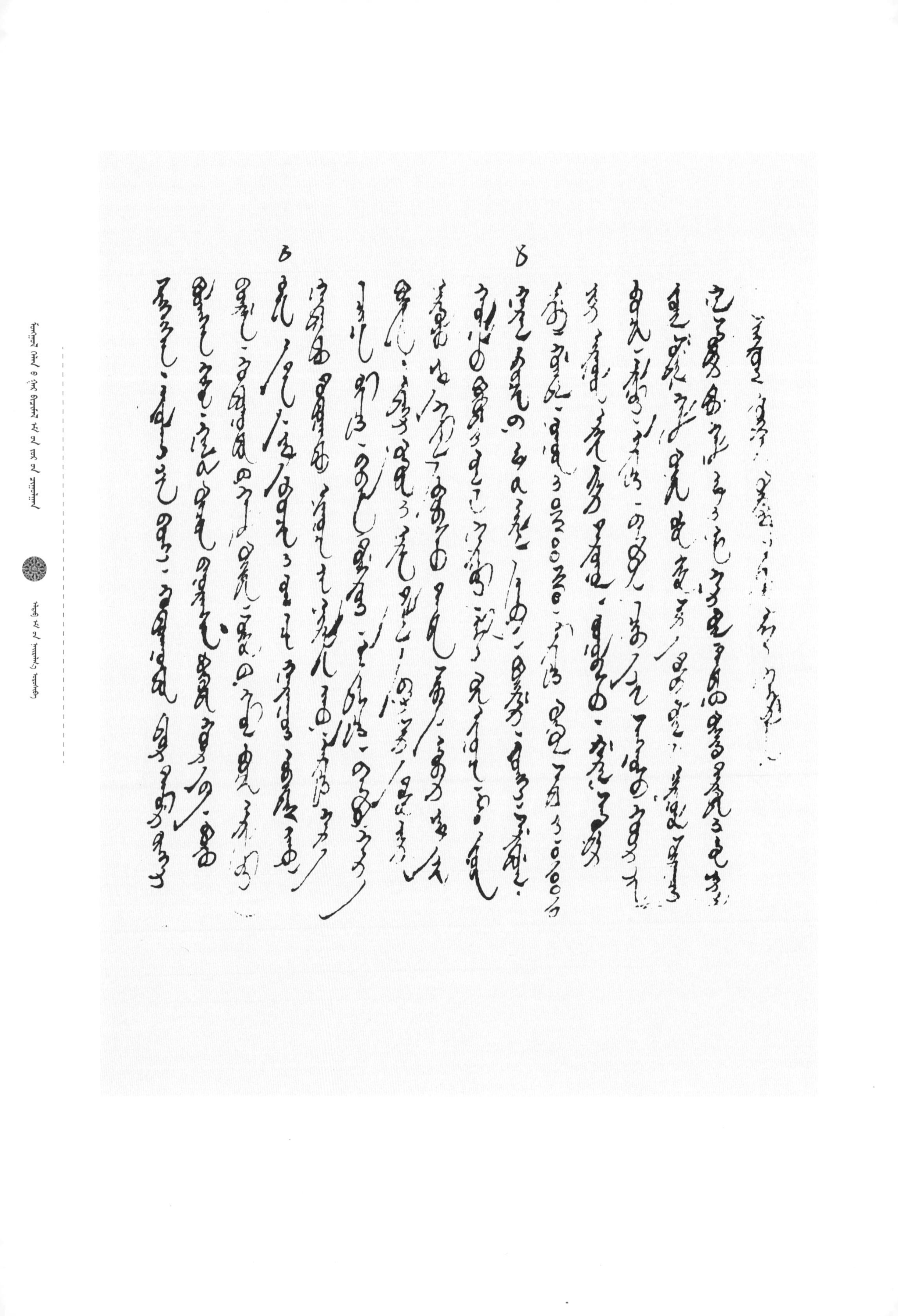

[illegible]

[illegible]

[illegible]

[illegible]

[illegible]

[illegible]

[illegible]

[illegible]

[illegible]

[illegible]

[illegible]

[illegible]

[illegible]

[illegible]

[illegible]

《ᠮᠣᠩᠭᠣᠯ ᠤᠨ ᠤᠯᠠᠮᠵᠢᠯᠠᠯᠲᠤ ᠰᠣᠶᠣᠯ ᠤᠨ ᠴᠢᠨᠠᠷ ᠤᠨ ᠨᠣᠮ ᠪᠢᠴᠢᠭ ᠤᠨ ᠴᠤᠪᠤᠷᠠᠯ 》

ᠮᠣᠩᠭᠣᠯ ᠬᠡᠯᠡ ᠶᠢᠨ ᠦᠭᠡᠰ ᠦᠨ ᠰᠤᠳᠤᠯᠭ᠎ᠠ ᠶᠢᠨ ᠲᠣᠯᠢ ᠶᠢᠨ ᠬᠡᠷᠡᠭᠯᠡᠭᠡ

ᠬᠠᠮᠲᠤ ᠮᠣᠩᠭᠣᠯ ᠤᠨ ᠦᠨᠳᠦᠰᠦᠲᠡᠨ ᠦ ᠬᠡᠯᠡ ᠪᠢᠴᠢᠭ ᠤᠨ ᠬᠦᠷᠢᠶᠡᠯᠡᠩ ᠨᠡᠶᠢᠲᠡᠯᠡᠪᠡ
ᠬᠦᠮᠦᠨ ᠰᠤᠷᠭᠠᠯ ᠤᠨ ᠬᠡᠪᠯᠡᠯ ᠦᠨ ᠬᠣᠷᠢᠶ᠎ᠠ ᠶᠢᠨ ᠬᠡᠪᠯᠡᠯ ᠦᠨ ᠦᠢᠯᠡᠳᠪᠦᠷᠢ

*

ᠦᠪᠦᠷ ᠮᠣᠩᠭᠣᠯ ᠤᠨ ᠰᠤᠷᠭᠠᠨ ᠬᠦᠮᠦᠵᠢᠯ ᠦᠨ ᠬᠡᠪᠯᠡᠯ ᠦᠨ ᠬᠣᠷᠢᠶ᠎ᠠ ᠬᠡᠪᠯᠡᠪᠡ
ᠦᠪᠦᠷ ᠮᠣᠩᠭᠣᠯ ᠤᠨ ᠰᠢᠨ᠎ᠡ ᠬᠤᠸᠠ ᠪᠢᠴᠢᠭ ᠤᠨ ᠳᠡᠯᠭᠡᠭᠦᠷ ᠲᠠᠷᠬᠠᠭᠠᠪᠠ
2018 ᠣᠨ ᠤ 7 ᠰᠠᠷ᠎ᠠ ᠳᠤ ᠨᠢᠭᠡᠳᠦᠭᠡᠷ ᠤᠳᠠᠭ᠎ᠠ ᠳᠠᠷᠤᠮᠠᠯᠠᠪᠠ
2018 ᠣᠨ ᠤ 7 ᠰᠠᠷ᠎ᠠ ᠳᠤ ᠨᠢᠭᠡᠳᠦᠭᠡᠷ ᠬᠡᠪᠯᠡᠯ
ᠦᠨ᠎ᠡ : 480.00 ᠶᠤᠸᠠᠨ